The authors dedicate this book to the memory of Christopher Dyer Saudek, whose vision and passion for the care of patients with diabetes made this guide a reality.

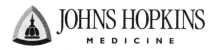

JOHNS HOPKINS

DIABETES GUIDE

Treatment and Management of Diabetes

2012 EDITION

Edited by
Christopher D. Saudek, MD
Rita Rastogi Kalyani, MD, MHS
Frederick L. Brancati, MD, MHS

Foreword by
Ronald J. Daniels
President, The Johns Hopkins University

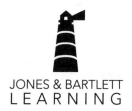

JONES & BARTLETT
LEARNING

World Headquarters

Jones & Bartlett Learning	Jones & Bartlett Learning Canada	Jones & Bartlett
40 Tall Pine Drive	6339 Ormindale Way	Learning International
Sudbury, MA 01776	Mississauga, Ontario L5V 1J2	Barb House, Barb Mews
978-443-5000	Canada	London W6 7PA
info@jblearning.com		United Kingdom
www.jblearning.com		

Jones & Bartlett Learning books and products are available through most bookstores and online booksellers. To contact Jones & Bartlett Learning directly, call 800-832-0034, fax 978-443-8000, or visit our website, www.jblearning.com.

Substantial discounts on bulk quantities of Jones & Bartlett Learning publications are available to corporations, professional associations, and other qualified organizations. For details and specific discount information, contact the special sales department at Jones & Bartlett Learning via the above contact information or send an email to specialsales@jblearning.com.

The authors, editors, and publisher have made every effort to provide accurate information. However, they are not responsible for errors, omissions, or for any outcomes related to the use of the contents of this book and take no responsibility for the use of the products and procedures described. Treatments and side effects described in this book may not be applicable to all people; likewise, some people may require a dose or experience a side effect that is not described herein. Drugs and medical devices are discussed that may have limited availability controlled by the Food and Drug Administration (FDA) for use only in a research study or clinical trial. Research, clinical practice, and government regulations often change the accepted standard in this field. When consideration is being given to use of any drug in the clinical setting, the healthcare provider or reader is responsible for determining FDA status of the drug, reading the package insert, and reviewing prescribing information for the most up-to-date recommendations on dose, precautions, and contraindications, and determining the appropriate usage for the product. This is especially important in the case of drugs that are new or seldom used.

Production Credits

Senior Acquisitions Editor: Nancy Anastasi Duffy
Special Projects Editor: Kathy Richardson
Associate Production Editor: Laura Almozara
Marketing Manager: Rebecca Rockel
Manufacturing and Inventory Control
    Supervisor: Amy Bacus

Composition: diacriTech, Chennai, India
Cover Design: Scott Moden
Cover Image of Insulin Molecule:
    © Kenneth Eward/Photo
    Researchers, Inc.
Printing and Binding: Cenveo
Cover Printing: Cenveo

Library of Congress Cataloging Information

ISBN 978-1-4496-1337-2

Application for CIP data submitted.

6048

Printed in the United States of America
15 14 13 12 11   10 9 8 7 6 5 4 3 2 1

Table of Contents

Section 4: Medications 387

Section 5: Clinical Tests 549

Index 601

List of Contributors

Editors

Christopher D. Saudek, MD (in memoriam)
Professor of Medicine
Division of Endocrinology and Metabolism
The Johns Hopkins University School of Medicine
Baltimore, MD

Rita Rastogi Kalyani, MD, MHS
Assistant Professor of Medicine
Division of Endocrinology and Metabolism
The Johns Hopkins University School of Medicine
Baltimore, MD

Frederick L. Brancati, MD, MHS
Professor of Medicine and Epidemiology
Director, Division of General Internal Medicine
Director, Diabetes Prevention & Control Core, Baltimore DRTC
The Johns Hopkins University School of Medicine
Baltimore, MD

Authors

Bassam G. Abu Jawdeh, MD
Postdoctoral Fellow
Division of Nephrology
The Johns Hopkins University School of Medicine
Baltimore, MD

Nada Alachkar, MD
Assistant Professor
Division of Nephrology
The Johns Hopkins University School of Medicine
Baltimore, MD

Reza Alavi, MD, MHS, MBA
Postdoctoral Fellow
Division of General Internal Medicine
The Johns Hopkins University School of Medicine
Baltimore, MD

Martinson K. Arnan, MD, MPA
Resident
Division of Neurology
The Johns Hopkins University School of Medicine
Baltimore, MD

Douglas W. Ball, MD
Associate Professor of Medicine and Oncology
Division of Endocrinology and Metabolism
The Johns Hopkins University School of Medicine
Baltimore, MD

Nancyellen Brennan, CRNP, CDE
Senior Diabetes Nurse Practitioner
The Johns Hopkins Comprehensive Diabetes Center
Division of Endocrinology and Metabolism
The Johns Hopkins University School of Medicine
Baltimore, MD

Todd T. Brown, MD, PhD
Assistant Professor of Medicine
Division of Endocrinology and Metabolism
The Johns Hopkins University School of Medicine
Baltimore, MD

Kathleen Burks, MSN, CRNP
Nurse Practitioner
Division of Neurology
The Johns Hopkins University School of Medicine
Baltimore, MD

Shivam Champaneri, MD
Postdoctoral Fellow
Division of Endocrinology and Metabolism
The Johns Hopkins University School of Medicine
Baltimore, MD

Gregory O. Clark, MD
Assistant Professor
Division of Endocrinology and Metabolism
University of Texas Southwestern Medical Center
Dallas, TX

Jeanne M. Clark, MD, MPH
Associate Professor of Medicine and Epidemiology
Division of General Internal Medicine
The Johns Hopkins University School of Medicine
Baltimore, MD

David W. Cooke, MD
Associate Professor of Pediatrics
Division of Pediatric Endocrinology
The Johns Hopkins University School of Medicine
Baltimore, MD

Rachel Derr, MD, PhD
Adult Endocrinologist
Center for Medicine, Endocrinology and Diabetes
Atlanta, GA

Joanne Dintzis, CRNP, CDE
Senior Diabetes Nurse Practitioner
The Johns Hopkins Inpatient Diabetes Management Service
Division of Endocrinology and Metabolism
The Johns Hopkins University School of Medicine
Baltimore, MD

Ari Eckman, MD
Adult Endocrinologist
Chief, Division of Diabetes, Endocrinology & Metabolism
Trinitas Regional Medical Center
Elizabeth, NJ

Ana Emiliano, MD
Adult Endocrinologist
Sinai Hospital of Baltimore
Baltimore, MD

Rebecca Gottesman, MD, PhD
Assistant Professor of Neurology
Cerebrovascular Division
The Johns Hopkins University School of Medicine
Baltimore, MD

Sheldon H. Gottlieb, MD
Associate Professor of Medicine
Division of Cardiology
The Johns Hopkins University School of Medicine
Baltimore, MD

Sherita Hill Golden, MD, MHS
Associate Professor of Medicine and Epidemiology
Director, Inpatient Diabetes Management Service
Division of Endocrinology and Metabolism
The Johns Hopkins University School of Medicine
Baltimore, MD

Nadeen Hosein, MD, MS
Adult Endocrinologist
San Diego, CA

Mary Huizinga, MD, MPH
Assistant Professor (Part-time)
Division of General Internal Medicine
The Johns Hopkins University School of Medicine
Associate, McKinsey & Company
Washington, DC

Sachin D. Kalyani, MD
Ophthalmologist
Rutzen Eye Specialists & Laser Center
Severna Park, MD

Mariana Lazo, MD, ScM, PhD
Postdoctoral Fellow
Clinical Epidemiology
The Johns Hopkins
    University Bloomberg
    School of Public Health
Baltimore, MD

Emily Loghmani, MS, RD, LDN, CDE
Senior Nutritionist
The Johns Hopkins
    Comprehensive Diabetes
    Center
Division of Endocrinology
    and Metabolism
The Johns Hopkins
    University School of
    Medicine
Baltimore, MD

Simeon Margolis, MD, PhD
Professor Emeritus of
    Medicine
Division of Endocrinology
    and Metabolism
The Johns Hopkins
    University School of
    Medicine
Baltimore, MD

Nisa M. Maruthur, MD, MHS
Assistant Professor
Division of General
    Internal Medicine
The Johns Hopkins
    University School of
    Medicine
Baltimore, MD

Nestoras Mathioudakis, MD
Postdoctoral Fellow
Division of Endocrinology
    and Metabolism
The Johns Hopkins
    University School of
    Medicine
Baltimore, MD

Ali Mohamadi, MD
Pediatric Endocrinologist
Chevy Chase, MD

Kendall F. Moseley, MD
Postdoctoral Fellow
Division of Endocrinology
    and Metabolism
The Johns Hopkins
    University School of
    Medicine
Baltimore, MD

Donna I. Myers, MD
Assistant Professor of
    Medicine
Division of Nephrology
The Johns Hopkins
    University School of
    Medicine
Baltimore, MD

Wanda K. Nicholson, MD, MPH, MBA
Associate Professor
    of Obstetrics and
    Gynecology
University of North
    Carolina School
    of Medicine at
    Chapel Hill
Chapel Hill, NC

Octavia Pickett-Blakely, MD, MHS
Instructor of Medicine
Division of Gastroenterology
University of Pennsylvania
Philadelphia, PA

Brian Pinto, PharmD, MBA
Clinical Pharmacist
Division of Clinical
    Pharmacology
Assistant Director,
    Medication Policy and
    Clinical Informatics
The Johns Hopkins
    Hospital
Baltimore, MD

Michael Polydefkis, MD, MHS
Associate Professor of
    Neurology
Director, Johns Hopkins
    Cutaneous Nerve
    Laboratory
Director, Bayview EMG
    Laboratory
The Johns Hopkins
    University School of
    Medicine
Baltimore, MD

Naresh Punjabi, MD, PhD
Professor of Medicine and
    Epidemiology
Division of Pulmonary and
    Critical Care Medicine
The Johns Hopkins
    University School of
    Medicine
Baltimore, MD

Amin Sabet, MD
Instructor in Medicine
Division of Endocrinology,
  Diabetes & Metabolism
Beth Israel Deaconess
  Medical Center, Harvard
  Medical School
Boston, MA

Lipika Samal, MD, MPH
Instructor of Medicine
Division of General
  Internal Medicine and
  Primary Care
Brigham and Women's
  Hospital, Harvard
  Medical School
Boston, MA

Lee J. Sanders, DPM
Clinical Professor
  (Adjunct)
Department of Podiatric
  Medicine
Temple University School
  of Podiatric Medicine
Consultant, Veterans
  Affairs Medical Center
  Podiatry Service
Lebanon, PA

**Vanessa Walker Harris,
MD**
Postdoctoral Fellow
Division of Endocrinology
  and Metabolism
The Johns Hopkins
  University School of
  Medicine
Baltimore, MD

**Donna Westervelt, CRNP,
MS, CDE**
Diabetes Nurse Practitioner
Johns Hopkins Bayview
  Diabetic Neuropathy
  Center
The Johns Hopkins
  University School of
  Medicine
Baltimore, MD

Melissa Yates, MD
Assistant Professor
  of Gynecology and
  Obstetrics
Division of Reproductive
  Endocrinology
The Johns Hopkins
  University School of
  Medicine
Baltimore, MD

Hsin-Chieh Yeh, PhD
Assistant Professor
  of Medicine and
  Epidemiology
Division of General
  Internal Medicine
The Johns Hopkins
  University School of
  Medicine
Baltimore, MD

Foreword

More than a century ago, when Sir William Osler published his landmark medical textbook *The Principles and Practice of Medicine*, little was known about diabetes. There were limited treatment options, which included encouraging patients to maintain personal hygiene and "lead an even, quiet life if possible in an equable climate." Opium was the chief medicinal treatment suggested as "diabetic patients seem to have a special tolerance for this drug."

As someone who was diagnosed relatively late in life with type 1 diabetes, I have been the very direct beneficiary of the tremendous advances we have seen since the publication of Osler's text.

In fact, the clinical field has witnessed a proliferation of complex and sometimes revolutionary developments in the past several years alone. While patients continue the constant and often exhausting work of managing nutrition, glucose monitoring, physical activity, and medications, medical professionals have to keep up with an evolving knowledge base.

This is the reason for this guide.

The information provided here represents concise, practical, evidence-based knowledge from more than 40 Johns Hopkins-affiliated experts, all leaders in their fields.

From its early years, as evidenced by Osler's *Principles*, Johns Hopkins has sought to share its clinical and basic science knowledge with the world. Perhaps no one better embodies that commitment than Dr. Christopher Saudek, the late editor-in-chief of this book.

Whether founding the Johns Hopkins Comprehensive Diabetes Center, launching a phenomenally successful nationwide awareness campaign as president of the American Diabetes Association, initiating innovative diabetes management programs in the developing world, or quietly reminding his own patients of the tenets of self-care, he was a passionate and purposeful educator.

I am surely biased by the fact that he was my physician. When Chris passed away in 2010, Johns Hopkins lost one of its best—a gifted and dedicated clinician and scientist, an engaging teacher, but most of all, a compassionate and caring human being.

This guide adds to his passionate commitment to improve the lives of people with diabetes, and the care afforded to them. I am thankful for his work, and that of Dr. Rita Kalyani, Dr. Frederick Brancati, and their many collaborators on this text.

Ronald J. Daniels
President, The Johns Hopkins University

Preface

You have in your hands something unique. It is not a textbook of diabetes, although it includes most of what you could find at greater length in a textbook. It is not just a summary of guidelines, although all the relevant guidelines are included. It is not a set of review articles evaluating levels of evidence, although the content does distinguish evidence-based information from expert comments. Finally, what you have is not influenced by device or pharmaceutical sponsorship.

This *Diabetes Guide* is, rather, a thorough, independent, concise summary of clinically relevant information designed specifically to provide easy access for the busy healthcare professional.

The management of diabetes is vastly more complicated now than it was even a few years ago. Diagnostic criteria have changed, novel glucose monitoring options have emerged, oral agents have proliferated, and new insulins have come into common use, as have new dietary recommendations, and even insulin pumps. This *Diabetes Guide* was written in a comprehensive fashion in order to cover these advances. There are more than 140 different sections, each formatted for easy access, to help you with the basics as well as the fine points of advanced diabetes care.

You may turn to this book with a relatively straightforward question: What is the dose of the new incretin mimetic, exenatide, and what are the potential side effects? You may want to review current guidelines on diabetes management, learn more about a particular complication of diabetes, or clarify the interpretation of a laboratory result. Whatever the question, we have written the *Diabetes Guide* with the expectation that you can find the answer within minutes, without having to wade through pages of text and equivocations.

The sections are grouped according to the following categories: Overview, Management, Complications and Comorbidities, Medications, and Clinical Tests. You will see immediately that the entire book is written using bullets rather than full sentences. But our bullets are not a substitute for thoroughness, accuracy, or rigor; they simply reduce your reading time so you can quickly move along. References are provided if you want to pursue the primary data. In addition, an overview section on key studies in diabetes care succinctly summarizes the findings from over 50 historical studies that are often quoted as the basis for current recommendations. And one of the more popular features of the guide is the Expert Opinion section, in which the authors provide insight into how they actually manage diabetes in the "real world." Needless to say, each section has been extensively reviewed and edited.

The authors are clinicians who see patients regularly. They are either currently or were previously on the full-time staff at Johns Hopkins, specializing in the areas they write about. They represent a diversity of disciplines and include physicians, pharmacists, podiatrists, nurses, dieticians, and educators.

This *Diabetes Guide* is based on the concept of the *Johns Hopkins ABX Guide: Diagnosis and Treatment of Infectious Diseases* by Dr. John Bartlett. The initial version of the *Diabetes Guide* was developed, funded, and provided online for the healthcare professionals of Trinidad and Tobago, with Trinidad and Tobago-specific sections and authors. We gratefully recognize the support of the government of Trinidad and Tobago in this effort.

Acknowledgments

We would like to thank the Johns Hopkins Division of Endocrinology and Metabolism and the division's director, Paul Ladenson, for his encouragement and guidance of this project. Thanks also to Myron Weisfeldt, Chair of the Department of Medicine, for his support of this guide. The entire POC-IT Center team—Nicole Sokol, Danielle Meinsler, Steve Libowitz, and Paul Auwaerter—are to be especially recognized for the numerous hours put in behind the scenes. Thanks also to Jones & Bartlett Learning publishers, especially Laura Almozara, Daniel Stone, and Nancy Duffy, for their efficient organization and much appreciated effort in producing this book.

Thanks in particular to our authors whose enthusiasm for diabetes and wide-ranging expertise led to the unique guide in front of you. We also could not be more grateful for President Ron Daniels' candid foreword.

On a more personal note, we would like to thank Susan Saudek and children, Mark, Debbie, Tina, and Tony, and the many family members who brought such joy to the life of C.D.S.

R.R.K. would like to thank her family including her parents, Ashok and Kanchan, and brother, Kapil, for their unconditional support; and, especially, her husband, Sachin, and children, Shaan and Sonia, for the life and inspiration they bring to each day.

F.L.B. would like to thank both his families—the one at home and the one at Hopkins.

And lastly, we would like to thank our patients for being our greatest teachers and the reason for this book.

The Editors

SECTION 1
OVERVIEW

INTRODUCTION TO DIABETES

Christopher D. Saudek, MD, and Rita Rastogi Kalyani, MD, MHS

OVERVIEW OF DIABETES

- Diabetes mellitus is a common, chronic disease defined by hyperglycemia (high blood glucose), with multiple other metabolic abnormalities (i.e., acidosis) often present.
- The pathophysiology of diabetes is characterized by relative or absolute insulin insufficiency, due to either decreased insulin sensitivity and/or insulin secretory insufficiency.
- Insulin is the key hormone regulating uptake of glucose from the blood into most cells (primarily muscle and fat cells, not central nervous system cells). Insulin is released into the blood by beta cells found in pancreatic Islets of Langerhans, in response to rising levels of blood glucose, typically after eating. Insulin also controls conversion of glucose to glycogen for storage in liver and muscle cells. Higher insulin levels increase anabolic processes such as cell growth, protein synthesis, and fat storage. Lower insulin levels result in catabolism and, in particular, can trigger ketosis or breakdown of fat.
- Diabetes mellitus ("sugar diabetes") is unrelated to diabetes insipidus except that they can both cause polyuria.
- About 23.6 million people, or 7.8%, of the US population had diagnosed diabetes in 2007 (CDC), over 40% of those >20 years old had either diabetes or prediabetes (Cowie). Approximately 40% of total diabetes is undiagnosed.
- The number of people with diabetes in the US will almost double to 44.1 million in the next 25 years (Huang).
- Diabetes is the 7th-leading cause of death in the US, responsible for about one-third of expenditures in Medicare, and the leading cause of blindness among working age adults (due to diabetic retinopathy and macular edema), nontraumatic amputations, end-stage renal disease and dialysis, and peripheral neuropathy.
- Diagnosis and classification: type 2 diabetes (insulin resistance and relative insulin secretory defect) constitutes 90%–95% of cases; type 1 diabetes (absolute insulin deficiency) constitutes 5%–10% of cases; and other types (i.e., unusual genetic forms) constitute 1%–5% of cases. Gestational diabetes is diabetes that is first diagnosed during pregnancy.
- Type 2 diabetes is highly associated with increased adiposity, particularly central (abdominal), and positive family history.
- Type 1 diabetes is highly associated with specific genetic markers and is more prevalent in people of northern European ancestry.

COMPLICATIONS AND COMORBIDITIES OF DIABETES

- Acute complications: a direct, immediate consequence of hyperglycemia and other metabolic abnormalities, which resolve upon correction of these abnormalities. Examples: excessive thirst (polydipsia), frequent urination (polyuria), blurry vision, fatigue, ketoacidosis.
- Polyuria and polydipsia usually occur when blood glucose increases above urinary filtering threshold of 180 mg/dl. Blurry vision occurs due to osmolar shifts from hyperglycemia within the lens.

- Chronic complications: occur over years or decades of diabetes, and are difficult or impossible to reverse. Examples include microvascular complications (i.e., small vessel disease) such as retinopathy, neuropathy, and nephropathy or macrovascular complications (i.e., large vessel disease) such as coronary heart disease, peripheral vascular disease, or stroke.
- Pathophysiology for both microvascular and macrovascular complications are similar; both occur due to oxidative damage from long-term, uncontrolled hyperglycemia, resulting in plaque formation, narrowing of small- and large-sized blood vessels and ischemic damage to end organ tissues.
- Cardiovascular disease can be fatal. The risk of cardiovascular disease is increased 2–4 times by diabetes.
- Other common complications include poor wound healing, increased susceptibility to infections, erectile dysfunction, and gastroparesis.
- Many comorbidities associated with diabetes may influence management including HIV, cystic fibrosis, polycystic ovarian syndrome (PCOS), postpancreatectomy diabetes, and Cushing's syndrome. Sleep apnea and depression are also common.
- Diabetes during pregnancy may be associated with neonatal and maternal complications if not optimally managed.

MANAGEMENT OF DIABETES AND ASSOCIATED COMPLICATIONS

- Prevention of diabetes, or the progression from prediabetes to diabetes, particularly by healthy lifestyle and obesity management, would be the ideal.
- Once the diagnosis of diabetes is established, treatment includes a medical nutrition plan, physical activity and exercise, pharmacologic therapy as indicated with oral agents (sulfonylureas and secretagogues, alpha-glucosidase inhibitors, thiazolidinediones, metformin, DPP-IV inhibitors), noninsulin injectables (incretin mimetics) or insulin (basal insulins and bolus insulins), regular monitoring by the healthcare professional, and, most importantly, education of the patient about living with diabetes.
- In 2004–2006, 57% of people with diabetes took oral medications only, 16% insulin only, 13% combined insulin and oral agents, and 14% no medication (CDC).
- Bariatric surgery may be offered to individuals with severe obesity and lead to improvement of diabetes.
- Medications used to treat complications and comorbidities of diabetes may exacerbate hyperglycemia including antipsychotics, thiazide diuretics, beta-blockers, niacin, and several antibiotics.
- External insulin pump therapy is often successful for treatment in type 1 diabetes where appropriate.
- Chronic microvascular complications of diabetes can be delayed or prevented by optimal glycemic control (i.e., A1c <7%) as demonstrated in several key studies including the Diabetes Complications and Control Trial (DCCT) in type 1 diabetes and the UK Prospective Diabetes Study (UKPDS) in type 2 diabetes.
- To reduce retinopathy, neuropathy, and nephropathy, blood glucose control is most important.
- To reduce cardiovascular disease, address tobacco abuse, obesity, hypertension (goal <130/80 mmHg), and dyslipidemia (i.e., LDL <100 mg/dl). Glycemic control is also important as demonstrated in recent studies (DCCT/EDIC, UKPDS long-term follow-up).

OVERVIEW

- Both elevated blood glucose and other cardiovascular risk factors should be treated to reduce cardiovascular disease.
- A1c targets may be higher in children and the elderly.
- Management of acute complications such as ketoacidosis, severe hyperglycemia, diabetic foot, or myocardial infarction should include regular follow-up to establish good outpatient care.
- Optimally, a team is available to address the needs of the patient, including a nurse educator, nutritionist, primary care physician, podiatry, ophthalmology, and other specialties as indicated.
- An informed, involved patient is the essential center of every successful diabetes care plan.

CLINICAL TESTING IN DIABETES

- Longitudinal monitoring includes self-monitoring of blood glucose by the patient, and preventive screening by the healthcare professional of blood pressure, hemoglobin A1c, serum lipids, urine microalbumin, retinal examinations, and foot examinations.
- Routine vaccinations of influenza and pneumonia should be given.
- Other laboratory tests should be considered for evaluation of important diabetes comorbidities including sex hormones for assessment of hypogonadism, vitamin D and bone mineral density for assessment of bone disease, liver function tests for nonalcoholic fatty liver disease, and testing for anemia.
- Autoantibodies may be useful to help distinguish type 1 diabetes from type 2 diabetes.
- Continuous glucose monitoring systems may be of benefit in patients with difficult-to-control diabetes and lead to improvement of glycemic control.

EXPERT OPINION

- Diabetes is manageable. Its complications are not inevitable with optimal glycemic control and cardiovascular risk factor management, and can be treated if they occur.
- Diabetes nevertheless is a serious disease, which can and does cause devastating complications and premature death, particularly if not well treated.
- Diabetes is a major and growing burden to society, due primarily to its long-term complications, but also because of its longitudinal care and the growing population of elderly individuals.
- Societal issues surrounding diabetes, including employment discrimination and driving with diabetes, remain important to address.

REFERENCES

Cowie CC, Rust KF, Ford ES, et al. Full accounting of diabetes and pre-diabetes in the U.S. population in 1988–1994 and 2005–2006. *Diabetes Care,* 2009; Vol. 32: pp. 287–94.

    Comments: A recent publication from NIDDK reporting an alarming 40% of people age >20 years in the US with either diabetes or prediabetes.

Huang ES, Basu A, O'Grady M, et al. Projecting the future diabetes population size and related costs for the U.S. *Diabetes Care,* 2009; Vol. 32: pp. 2225–9.

    Comments: Modeled projection of rates of diabetes in the US over the next 25 years.

American Diabetes Association. *http://www.diabetes.org/.*

    Comments: The American Diabetes Association is a reliable source of diabetes information, and has multi-faceted programs for people with diabetes.

Centers for Disease Control and Prevention. Diabetes Data and Trends. *http://apps.nccd.cdc.gov/DDTSTRS/default.aspx*.

> **Comments:** Centers for Disease Control and Prevention (CDC) is an excellent source of reliable data on diabetes in the US.

International Diabetes Federation. Diabetes Facts and Figures. *http://www.idf.org/Facts_and_Figures*.

> **Comments:** International Diabetes Federation (IDF) is an excellent source of reliable data on diabetes worldwide, as well as educational programs.

Juvenile Diabetes Research Foundation International. *http://www.jdrf.org/*.

> **Comments:** The Juvenile Diabetes Research Foundation is an important funder of diabetes research, as well as source of reliable diabetes information.

National Diabetes Education Program. *http://www.ndep.nih.gov/*.

> **Comments:** The National Diabetes Education Program has useful, multicultural education information and resources.

National Diabetes Information Clearinghouse (NDIC). *http://diabetes.niddk.nih.gov/*.

> **Comments:** The National Institute of Diabetes, Digestive, and Kidney Diseases has reliable diabetes information.

DIAGNOSIS AND CLASSIFICATION OF DIABETES

Christopher D. Saudek, MD

CLASSIFICATION

- Diabetes is classified as type 1 (formerly called juvenile-onset or insulin-dependent diabetes mellitus), type 2 (formerly called adult-onset or noninsulin dependent diabetes mellitus), gestational, or other specific types.
- **Type 1 diabetes:** complete or almost complete insulin deficiency, usually caused by autoimmunity. Clinical features: younger onset (usually but not always before 30 years old), normal body weight, usually no family history of diabetes, insulin treatment required immediately or within about a year, positive GAD, IA2 and/or islet cell antibodies (see Autoantibodies in Type 1 Diabetes, p. 582), susceptibility to ketoacidosis (see p. 38), and unstable blood glucoses.
- **Type 1b or idiopathic diabetes:** an unusual form of phenotypic type 1 diabetes with almost complete insulin deficiency, a strong hereditary component, and no evidence of autoimmunity. Reported mainly in Africa and Asia.
- **Latent autoimmune diabetes of adulthood (LADA):** a form of type 1 diabetes with adult onset, slowly progressive, eventual insulin requirement but may respond to oral agents initially, usually no ketoacidosis on presentation, positive GAD, IA2 and/or islet cell antibodies (see LADA, p. 142).
- **Type 2 diabetes:** insulin resistance with preserved endogenous insulin secretion but inadequate to overcome the resistance. About 90% of all diabetes, more in Asians and Africans. Clinical features: older onset (often >35 years old, though recently occurring more often in youth), overweight or obese, strong family history of diabetes, response to oral agents usually for some years, and relatively stable blood glucose levels.
- At presentation, in the setting of acute illness, or as type 2 patients become increasingly insulin deficient, ketoacidosis may occur ("**ketosis-prone type 2 diabetes**") (Umpierrez).
- **Gestational diabetes mellitus (GDM):** diagnosed first during pregnancy. Usually a precursor to type 2 diabetes, but may be first onset of type 1 diabetes.

- **Other specific subtypes of diabetes:** those with a more well-defined cause. Examples: postpancreatectomy, Cushing's syndrome, HIV-associated diabetes, cystic fibrosis-related diabetes, certain drugs such as glucocorticoids, genetic syndromes such as maturity onset diabetes of the young (MODY), and infections such as coxsackievirus B (see American Diabetes Association Guidelines on Diagnosis and Classification for detailed list of specific subtypes).

DIAGNOSIS

- Criteria for the diagnosis of diabetes for nonpregnant adults in stable state (not acutely ill): (1) Fasting plasma glucose (FPG) ≥126 mg/dl (7 mmol/l); (2) random plasma glucose ≥200 mg/dl (11.1 mmol/l) with symptoms of hyperglycemia; (3) plasma glucose >200 mg/dl (11.1 mmol/l) 2 hours after 75-gram oral glucose tolerance test (OGTT); or (4) newly recommended criterion: hemoglobin A1c ≥6.5% (ADA Standards of Medical Care in Diabetes).
- For FPG and OGTT, patients ingest no calories for at least 8 hours prior to testing and should have adequate carbohydrate intake for several days prior to the test.
- Diagnosis of diabetes should ideally be confirmed on a different day.
- Diagnosis of "prediabetes" or "categories of increased risk for diabetes" includes impaired fasting glucose (IFG) defined as FPG 100–125 mg/dl, and impaired glucose tolerance (IGT) defined as plasma glucose 140–199 mg/dl 2 hours after OGTT. Both are not necessarily present in the same patient. Newly recommended criterion: hemoglobin A1c 5.7–6.4%.
- Screening for diabetes should be performed in adults ≥45 years of age or all adults with BMI ≥25 kg/m² and additional risk factors for diabetes.
- Criteria for GDM described elsewhere (see p. 121).

EXPERT OPINION

- Specific glucose criteria should be used to confirm the diagnosis of diabetes or prediabetes.
- The classification of diabetes is usually obvious, but not always.
- Each of the clinical characteristics of type 1 or type 2 diabetes has exceptions. For instance, some people with type 2 are normal body weight and have ketoacidosis; some with type 1 are overweight.
- When in doubt, GAD, IA2 and/or islet cell antibodies can be assayed. If positive, they generally confirm the diagnosis of type 1; if negative, however, type 1 cannot be ruled out.
- Many people with type 2 diabetes do eventually need insulin therapy but not all, so insulin independence is not part of the definition of type 2 diabetes.
- It is worth diagnosing the specific type of diabetes to appropriately direct treatment; for instance, type 1 diabetes always requires insulin, almost always multiple doses.
- We do not find routine measurement of insulin level or C-peptide to be clinically useful, as normal insulin secretion may be seen in type 2 diabetes or in type 1 diabetes during a "honeymoon period."
- Use of the terms "type 1.5" or "type 3" diabetes is not preferred. Some cases cannot be definitively diagnosed, but these other terms have no specific meaning.
- In the clinical setting, use of FPG (or the newly recommended hemoglobin A1c) are likely more convenient than a full OGTT.

REFERENCES

American Diabetes Association. Standards of medical care in diabetes—2011. *Diabetes Care,* 2011; Vol. 34 Suppl 1: pp. S11–61.

Comments: The annually updated standards of medical care, which include diagnosis and classification.

American Diabetes Association. Diagnosis and classification of diabetes mellitus. *Diabetes Care,* 2010; Vol. 33 Suppl 1: pp. S62–9.

Comments: The annually updated diagnosis and classification of diabetes including a complete etiological classification of diabetes with subtypes.

International Expert Committee International Expert Committee report on the role of the A1C assay in the diagnosis of diabetes. *Diabetes Care,* 2009; Vol. 32: pp. 1327–34.

Comments: An ADA committee that recently recommended use of A1c for diagnosis; not officially endorsed by ADA.

Saudek CD, Herman WH, Sacks DB, et al. A new look at screening and diagnosing diabetes mellitus. *J Clin Endocrinol Metab,* 2008; Vol. 93: pp. 2447–53.

Comments: Publication by a panel that reviews the literature and presents arguments in favor of use of A1c for diagnosis.

Genuth S, Alberti KG, Bennett P, et al. Follow-up report on the diagnosis of diabetes mellitus. *Diabetes Care,* 2003; Vol. 26: pp. 3160–7.

Comments: A follow-up expert committee report that lowered the criterion for IFG to 100 mg/dl.

Report of the Expert Committee on the Diagnosis and Classification of Diabetes Mellitus. *Diabetes Care,* 1997; Vol. 20: pp. 1183–97.

Comments: This committee report established diagnostic criteria for the modern era, changing the FPG criterion to 126 mg/dl, and establishing the names type 1 and type 2, and impaired fasting glucose (IFG).

Umpierrez GE, Casals MM, Gebhart SP, et al. Diabetic ketoacidosis in obese African-Americans. *Diabetes,* 1995; Vol. 44: pp. 790–5.

Comments: A description of type 2 diabetes presenting with diabetic ketoacidosis ("ketosis-prone type 2 diabetes").

EPIDEMIOLOGY OF TYPE 1 DIABETES

Rita Rastogi Kalyani, MD, MHS

INCIDENCE AND PREVALENCE OF TYPE 1 DIABETES MELLITUS (T1DM) IN THE US

- In the SEARCH for Diabetes in Youth Study, incidence of T1DM highest among youth aged 10–14 years (25.9 per 100,000 person years) in 2002–2003 (SEARCH for Diabetes in Youth Study Group).
- Incidence rate similar by gender (incidence rate ratio ~1).
- Overall, highest incidence rates of T1DM observed in non-Hispanic white youth across all age groups (15.1–32.9 per 100,000 person years).
- Prevalence of T1DM ~0.15% in US (2001).
- Prevalence of T1DM was lower for youth aged 0–9 years (0.78 cases per 1000 youth) compared to those 10–19 years (2.28 cases per 1000 youth)
- Across all ages, non-Hispanic whites had the highest prevalence of T1DM (1.03 and 2.88 cases per 1000 youth in younger and older youth, respectively).
- Among youth <10 years at diagnosis, T1DM most common (>85%) regardless of race/ethnicity. Among youth >10 years at diagnosis, T1DM most common in non-Hispanic white adolescents (85.1%) compared to minority youth including Hispanic (53.9%), African American (42.2%), Asian/Pacific Islander (30.3%), and American Indian (13.8%), for whom type 2 diabetes is relatively more common.

MANAGEMENT AND OUTCOMES OF T1DM IN US YOUTH

- In Wisconsin Diabetes Registry cohort with T1DM, all incident cases (≤30 years of age) documented between 1987–1992 were actively followed for up to 20 years (Palta).
- Glucose checking and glycemic control deteriorated considerably during adolescence.
- After 14–20 years diabetes duration (mean age 30 years), only 22% of individuals had A1c <7%.
- 96% were on insulin pump or 3 or more daily insulin injections.
- 22% were obese (BMI ≥30 kg/m²) and 36% were overweight (BMI 25–29 kg/m²).
- 76% reported checking glucose at least 3 times a day.
- Hypoglycemia common, occurring ≥2–4 times/week in 26%–32% of individuals.
- Retinopathy onset much delayed and severity decreased over the last 2 decades.
- Annual incidence of T1DM increased two-fold over 10 years in Wisconsin, mostly in younger and heavier children (Evertsen).

GLOBAL INCIDENCE AND PREVALENCE OF T1DM

- The age-adjusted incidence of T1DM ranged between 0.1 per 100,000/year in China and Venezuela to 40.9 per 100,000/year in Finland (DIAMOND project group).
- Annual increase in incidence worldwide was 2.8% per year (95% CI 2.4%–3.2%) between 1990–1999.
- All continents showed statistically significant increases during this time (4.0% in Asia, 3.2% in Europe, 5.3% in North America), except Central America and the West Indies where incidence decreased 3.6%.
- In most populations, girls and boys are equally affected.
- Increases in incidence from 1990–1999 highest in the youngest age group.
- Environmental risk factors early in life cited as possibly contributing to the increasing incidence: enteroviral infections in pregnant women, older maternal age (39–42 years), preeclampsia, cesarean section delivery, increased birth weight, early introduction of cow's milk proteins, and an increased rate of postnatal growth (weight and height). Vitamin D supplementation may be protective. Viruses may initiate autoimmunity toward the beta cell, while other exposures may overload beta cell and accelerate diabetes development (Soltesz).
- In general, incidence increases with age, peaking at puberty. After puberty, incidence rate significantly drops in young women, but remains relatively high in males up to age 29–35 years. In Finland, the overall boy-to-girl ratio of incidence was 1.1; at the age of 13 years, it was 1.7 (1.4–2.0) (Harjutsalo).
- Assuming present trends in Europe continue, based on 20 population-based EURODIAB registers, scientists predict doubling of new cases of type 1 diabetes in European children <5 years between 2005 and 2020, and 70% rise in prevalent cases younger than 15 years (Patterson).

REFERENCES

American Diabetes Association. Standards of medical care in diabetes—2011. *Diabetes Care*, 2011; Vol. 34 Suppl 1: pp. S11–61.
  Comments: Outlines standards of medical care for diabetes including A1c goals by age group for T1DM.

Evertsen J, Alemzadeh R, Wang X. Increasing incidence of pediatric type 1 diabetes mellitus in Southeastern Wisconsin: relationship with body weight at diagnosis. *PLoS ONE*, 2009; Vol. 4: p. e6873.
  Comments: Describes increasing incidence of type 1 diabetes between 1995 and 2004 in Wisconsin youth.

Palta M, LeCaire T. Managing type 1 diabetes: trends and outcomes over 20 years in the Wisconsin Diabetes Registry cohort. *WMJ*, 2009; Vol. 108: pp. 231–5.

Comments: Describes diabetes management and acute and chronic complications from diabetes among youth with type 1 diabetes followed for up to 20 years in Wisconsin Diabetes Registry cohort.

Patterson CC, Dahlquist GG, Gyürüs E, et al. Incidence trends for childhood type 1 diabetes in Europe during 1989–2003 and predicted new cases 2005–20: a multicentre prospective registration study. *Lancet*, 2009; Vol. 373: pp. 2027–33.

Comments: Population-based study of 20 EURODIAB registers in 17 countries that registered children diagnosed with diabetes before their 15th birthday between 1989–2003. Describes trends in incidence during this time and predicted new cases in 2005–2020.

Harjutsalo V, Sjöberg L, Tuomilehto J. Time trends in the incidence of type 1 diabetes in Finnish children: a cohort study. *Lancet*, 2008; Vol. 371: pp. 1777–82.

Comments: Children with newly diagnosed type 1 diabetes in Finland who were listed on public registers in 1980–2005 were included in a cohort study and followed for trends in diabetes incidence.

Soltesz G, Patterson CC, Dahlquist G, et al. Worldwide childhood type 1 diabetes incidence—what can we learn from epidemiology? *Pediatr Diabetes*, 2007; Vol. 8 Suppl 6: pp. 6–14.

Comments: Describes global epidemiology of type 1 diabetes, and trends in incidence and risk factors in early life.

Writing Group for the SEARCH for Diabetes in Youth Study Group, Dabelea D, Bell RA, et al. Incidence of diabetes in youth in the United States. *JAMA*, 2007; Vol. 297: pp. 2716–24.

Comments: Estimates incidence rates for youth <20 years of age in the US for years 2002–2003 by age, gender, race/ethnicity, and type of diabetes.

SEARCH for Diabetes in Youth Study Group, Liese AD, D'Agostino RB, et al. The burden of diabetes mellitus among US youth: prevalence estimates from the SEARCH for Diabetes in Youth Study. *Pediatrics*, 2006; Vol. 118: pp. 1510–8.

Comments: Estimates national prevalence of diabetes in youth <20 years of age in 2001 in the United States according to age, gender, race/ethnicity, diabetes type.

DIAMOND Project Group. Incidence and trends of childhood type 1 diabetes worldwide 1990–1999. *Diabet Med*, 2006; Vol. 23: pp. 857–66.

Comments: The incidence of type 1 diabetes was analyzed in children aged <14 years from 114 populations in 112 centers in 57 countries. A total of 43,013 cases were diagnosed in the 84 million children. Average annual increase in incidence 2.8%.

EPIDEMIOLOGY OF TYPE 2 DIABETES

Rita Rastogi Kalyani, MD, MHS

PREVALENCE OF TYPE 2 DIABETES IN THE US

- Crude prevalence of diagnosed diabetes in adults ≥20 years rose from 5.1% (1988–1994) to 7.7% (2005–2006) (Cowie).
- In 2005–2006, crude prevalence of all diabetes in adults ≥20 years was 12.9%, of which 40% was undiagnosed (fasting plasma glucose ≥7 mmol/l and/or 2-hour glucose ≥11.1 mmol/l).
- In adults ≥20 years, crude prevalence of impaired fasting glucose was 25.7% and impaired glucose tolerance 13.8%; 30% had either.

- One-third of elderly had diabetes; three-quarters had diabetes or prediabetes.
- Compared with non-Hispanic whites, age- and sex-standardized prevalence of diagnosed diabetes was twice as high in non-Hispanic blacks and Mexican Americans.

ECONOMIC BURDEN OF DIABETES IN THE US

- People with diagnosed diabetes incur average medical expenditures approximately 2.3 times higher than what expenditures would be in the absence of diabetes.
- In the US, approximately 1 in 5 healthcare dollars is spent caring for someone with diagnosed diabetes, while 1 in 10 healthcare dollars is attributed directly to diabetes.
- New research suggests total cost of diabetes in 2007 was $218 billion, including $153 billion in excess medical expenditures and $65 billion in reduced national productivity.
- Medical costs attributed to diabetes include $27 billion for care to directly treat diabetes, $58 billion to treat diabetes-related chronic complications, $31 billion in general medical costs.
- Largest components of medical expenditures attributable to diabetes: hospital inpatient care (50% of total cost); diabetes medication and supplies (12%); retail prescriptions to treat complications (11%); physician office visits (9%).
- Average cost per case: $2,864 for undiagnosed diabetes, $9,975 for diagnosed diabetes ($9677 for type 2 and $14,856 for type 1), and $443 for prediabetes (medical costs only).
- For each American, regardless of diabetes status, this burden represents a cost of approximately $700 annually.
- Indirect costs include absenteeism from work, reduced work productivity, unemployment from disease-related comorbidity, lost productive capacity due to early mortality.
- For the Medicare-eligible population, the diabetes population will rise from 8.2 million in 2009 to 14.6 million in 2034; associated spending is estimated to rise from $45 billion to $171 billion.
- Information here from the American Diabetes Association; Dall TM, Zhang Y, Chen YJ, et al.; and Basu A, O'Grady M, et al.

GLOBAL PREVALENCE OF TYPE 2 DIABETES

- World prevalence of diabetes among adults (20–79 years) was 6.4% or 285 million adults in 2010 (Shaw).
- By 2030, prevalence of diabetes will increase to 7.7% or 439 million adults.
- Anticipated 69% increase in diabetes in developing countries and 20% increase in developed countries between 2010 and 2030.
- Top 10 countries for diabetes prevalence in 2010: Nauru (31%), United Arab Emirates (19%), Saudi Arabia (17%), Mauritius (16%), Bahrain (15%), Reunion (15%), Kuwait (15%), Oman (13%), Tonga (13%), Malaysia (12%).
- Top 10 countries for number of people aged 20–79 years with diabetes in 2010 (millions): India (50.8), China (43.2), United States (26.8), Russian Federation (9.6), Brazil (7.6), Germany (7.5), Pakistan (7.1), Japan (7.1), Indonesia (7.0), Mexico (6.8).
- In 2030, projected that top countries for numbers of people with diabetes will remain India (87 million), China (62.6 million), and United States (36 million).

GLOBAL ECONOMIC BURDEN OF DIABETES

- 12% of global healthcare expenditures ($1330 USD/person) anticipated to be spent on diabetes in 2010 (Zhang).

- Global healthcare expenditure on diabetes expected to total $376 billion USD in 2010, and $490 billion USD in 2030.
- Top 10 countries with highest national *total* healthcare expenditures (USD) estimated for 2010: United States ($197 billion), Germany ($28 billion), Japan ($22 billion), France ($17 billion), Canada ($11 billion), Italy ($11 billion), United Kingdom ($8 billion), Spain ($7 billion), China ($5 billion), Mexico ($5 billion).
- Top 10 countries with highest national healthcare expenditures (USD) *per person with diabetes* for 2010: United States ($7383), Luxembourg ($7268), Iceland ($7001), Norway ($6933), Switzerland ($5995), Monaco ($5866), Ireland ($5035), Austria ($4007), Canada ($3914), Slovenia ($1626).
- Top 10 countries with highest *percentage* of national health expenditure on diabetes: Nauru (41%), Saudi Arabia (21%), Mauritius (20%), Tuvalu (19%), Bahrain (19%), Tonga (18%), Oman (18%), Qatar (18%), Seychelles (18%), Malaysia (16%).
- In 2030, projected that United States will continue to spend the most on diabetes, with $264 billion USD or 54% of world total.

GLOBAL MORBIDITY AND MORTALITY ATTRIBUTABLE TO DIABETES

- Total number of excess deaths attributable to diabetes worldwide was 3.96 million in age group 20–79 years (6.8% of global all ages mortality) for year 2010, calculated using computerized WHO disease model (Roglic).
- Top 10 leading causes of burden of disease (by disability-adjusted life years) for high-income countries for 2001: (1) ischemic heart disease, (2) cerebrovascular disease, (3) unipolar depressive disorders, (4) dementia, (5) lung cancer, (6) hearing loss, (7) COPD, (8) diabetes, (9) alcohol use, (10) osteoarthritis (Lopez).
- In low- and middle-income countries, communicable diseases (i.e., HIV/AIDS, respiratory infections, diarrheal diseases, malaria, tuberculosis) and perinatal conditions associated with relatively greater burden of disease in 2001.
- Diabetes accounted for the following percentage of deaths in adults: Africa (6%), North America (15.7%).
- Beyond age 49 years, diabetes constituted a higher proportion of deaths in females than males in all regions, reaching 25% in some regions and age groups.
- As diabetes prevalence increases, overall morbidity and mortality from diabetes will likely also increase, especially in low- and middle-income countries.

REFERENCES

Roglic G, Unwin N. Mortality attributable to diabetes: estimates for the year 2010. *Diabetes Res Clin Pract*, 2010; Vol. 87: pp. 15–9.

Comments: Estimates of underlying mortality and relative risk of dying for people with diabetes compared to those without diabetes using a computerized disease model.

Shaw JE, Sicree RA, Zimmet PZ. Global estimates of the prevalence of diabetes for 2010 and 2030. *Diabetes Res Clin Pract*, 2010; Vol. 87: pp. 4–14.

Comments: Based on studies from 91 countries, estimated prevalence of diabetes for 216 countries for 2010 and 2030.

Zhang P, Zhang X, Brown J, et al. Global healthcare expenditure on diabetes for 2010 and 2030. *Diabetes Res Clin Pract*, 2010; Vol. 87: pp. 293–301.

Comments: Country-by-country expenditures for 193 countries estimated based on diabetes prevalence, population estimates, and healthcare expenditures for years 2010 and 2030.

Cowie CC, Rust KF, Byrd-Holt DD, et al. Prevalence of diabetes and high risk for diabetes using A1c criteria in the U.S. population in 1988–2006. *Diabetes Care*, 2010; Vol. 33: pp. 562–8.

    Comments: Using data from National Health and Nutrition Examination Survey 1988–2006, provides estimates for prevalence of diabetes and high risk for diabetes using HbA1c. The authors conclude that HbA1c alone detects much lower prevalence of diabetes than glucose criteria.

Dall TM, Zhang Y, Chen YJ, et al. The economic burden of diabetes. *Health Aff (Millwood)*, 2010; pp. 297–303.

    Comments: Provides more updated estimates of spending on diabetes in 2007 for US.

Cowie CC, Rust KF, Ford ES, et al. Full accounting of diabetes and pre-diabetes in the U.S. population in 1988–1994 and 2005–2006. *Diabetes Care*, 2009; Vol. 32: pp. 287–94.

    Comments: Using data from National Health and Nutrition Examination Survey in 1988–2004 and 2005–2006, provides estimates for prevalence of diabetes and prediabetes in the US using glucose criteria.

Huang ES, Basu A, O'Grady M, et al. Projecting the future diabetes population size and related costs for the U.S. *Diabetes Care*, 2009; Vol. 32: pp. 2225–9.

    Comments: Using a novel population-level model, projected that the number of people with diagnosed and undiagnosed diabetes will increase from 23.7 million (2009) to 44.1 million (2034), and annual diabetes-related spending is expected to increase from $113 billion to $336 billion in US. For the Medicare-eligible population, associated spending is estimated to rise from $45 billion to $171 billion.

American Diabetes Association. Economic costs of diabetes in the U.S. in 2007. *Diabetes Care*, 2008; Vol. 31: pp. 596–615.

    Comments: Using a prevalence-based approach, estimates healthcare costs attributable to diabetes in the US.

Lopez AD, Mathers CD, Ezzati M, et al. Global and regional burden of disease and risk factors, 2001: systematic analysis of population health data. *Lancet*, 2006; Vol. 367: pp. 1747–57.

    Comments: The global burden of disease and risk factors for 2001 was calculated for 136 diseases, including diabetes, using mortality, incidence, prevalence, and disability-adjusted life years.

KEY STUDIES IN DIABETES CARE: PREVENTION AND GLYCEMIC CONTROL

Christopher D. Saudek, MD, and Rita Rastogi Kalyani, MD, MHS

PURPOSE

- To provide easy access to many of what the editors consider the most important original studies in diabetes research.
- To quickly see the original data upon which we practice evidence-based medicine in diabetes.

PREVENTION OF DIABETES

- **Type 2 Diabetes (The Da Qing IGT and Diabetes Study, 1997):** in Da Qing, China, 557 people with IGT were randomized to dietary treatment, exercise, both, or control. The 6-year conversion to diabetes was 67.7% in the control group; diet reduced the conversion to 44%, exercise to 41%, and both to 46%. Concluded an overall reduction of conversion to diabetes of 31% by diet and/or exercise after adjustment for differences in baseline BMI and fasting glucose (Pan). Long-term follow-up showed sustained benefits of lifestyle intervention with 40% reduction in relative risk of diabetes at 20 years (Li).
- **Type 2 Diabetes (Diabetes Prevention Program, 2002):** DPP randomly assigned 3234 adults (mean age 51 years, BMI 34 kg/m²) with impaired glucose tolerance (IGT)

and elevated fasting plasma glucose >95 mg/dl to intensive lifestyle counseling (ILS), metformin 850 mg twice daily or placebo. Over a mean follow-up of 2.8 years, the DPP demonstrated the incidence of diabetes was reduced by 58% from ILS, and 31% from metformin (Knowler).

- **Type 2 Diabetes (Finnish Diabetes Prevention Study, 2002):** randomized 552 people with IGT to lifestyle counseling or control. After 3.2 years, conversion to diabetes occurred in 23% of controls and 11% of people in the lifestyle group. The reduction was identical to that of the Diabetes Prevention Program (Tuomilento).

- **Type 2 Diabetes (Troglitazone In the Prevention Of Diabetes, 2002):** TRIPOD randomly treated 133 women with previous gestational diabetes using troglitazone or placebo. After 30 months, 12.1% of controls had diabetes, compared to 5.4% on troglitazone. While troglitazone was subsequently removed from the market due to liver toxicity, the study was continued unblinded using pioglitazone, with persistent demonstration of less diabetes and preserved beta-cell function (Buchanan).

- **Type 2 Diabetes (Diabetes REduction Assessment with ramipril and rosiglitazone Medication trial, 2008):** the DREAM trial randomized 5269 patients with impaired glucose tolerance or impaired fasting glucose without known cardiovascular disease or renal insufficiency to ramipril versus placebo and rosiglitazone versus placebo. Rosiglitazone increased heart failure (hazard ratio 7.04, 95% CI 1.60–31.0) and significantly reduced the renal outcome by 20% ($p = 0.01$); prevention of diabetes was independently associated with prevention of the renal outcomes ($p < 0.001$) (Dagenais).

- **Type 1 Diabetes (Diabetes Prevention Trial-Type 1 Study Group, 2002):** the DPT-1 studied, in addition to oral insulin, low-dose parenterally administered ultralente insulin to prevent development of type 1 diabetes in very high-risk people. As with the oral insulin, insulin injections given before diabetes manifested had no effect in delaying or preventing the onset of type 1 diabetes mellitus (T1DM) (DPT-1 Study Group).

- **Type 1 Diabetes (Herold et al., 2002):** in 2005, this small study demonstrated a proof of principle, that immune-modulation could slow insulin loss in type 1 diabetes. 24 subjects were treated with a nonactivated humanized monoclonal antibody against CD3-hOKT3gamma1(Ala-Ala) or placebo, within 6 weeks of diagnosis of T1DM. 9 of the 12 who received the antibody improved their insulin response, versus 2 of the 12 who received placebo. Fever, rash, and myalgias were noted. The study ushered in multiple attempts at immune-modulation to improve insulin response in recently diagnosed T1DM.

- **Type 1 Diabetes (Keymeulen et al., 2005):** in a phase 2 placebo-controlled trial of humanized aglycosylated antibody against CD3 (ChAglyCD3), 80 patients with type 1 diabetes were assigned to receive the CD3 antibody or placebo for 6 consecutive days. Residual beta-cell function was better maintained for up to 18 months in the CD3 antibody group, with an increasing insulin dose needed in the placebo but not antibody group. In patients with residual beta-cell function at or above the 50th percentile initially, the mean insulin dose was 0.22 IU/kg/day with the CD3 antibody versus 0.61 IU/kg/day with placebo ($p < 0.001$).

BENEFITS OF LONG-TERM GLYCEMIC CONTROL

- **Hemoglobin as an index of glycemic control (Koenig et al., 1976):** early report on the use of hemoglobin A1c (versus hemoglobin A1a + 1b) as an index of blood glucose control. Five subjects who were in poor glycemic control were intensively managed for

3 months, and a corresponding fall in hemoglobin A1c was demonstrated. Hemoglobin A1c reflected average glycemia over the previous weeks to months and was proposed as a useful way to monitor the degree of glucose control.

- **Type 1 Diabetes (Diabetes Control and Complications Trial, 1993):** DCCT was the definitive, NIH-sponsored study of whether glycemic control affects complications. 1441 people with type 1 diabetes with no retinopathy at baseline (primary intervention group) or mild retinopathy (secondary prevention group), randomized into "intensive" or "conventional" glycemic control. Over a mean follow-up of 6.5 years, the intensive treatment group achieved an average hemoglobin A1C of 7.2% compared with 9.1% in the conventional treatment group. The progression of DR was reduced by 76% in the primary intervention group, and 54% in the secondary-intervention group. In both cohorts combined, intensive control reduced urinary microalbumin excretion by 39%, albuminuria by 54%, and clinical neuropathy by 60%. However, hypoglycemia was 2–3 times higher with intensive control. Many earlier and subsequent publications have come from DCCT (DCCT).

- **Type 1 Diabetes, long-term follow-up (Epidemiology of Diabetes Interventions and Complications Research Group, 2000):** EDIC was the first report describing the long-term follow-up of the DCCT 4 years after the trial ended and found that although hemoglobin A1c equalized in the people treated with intensive or conventional control, the difference in progression of retinopathy and nephropathy persisted, favoring those who had been intensively treated (DCCT/EDIC).

- **Type 2 Diabetes (Kumamoto Trial, 1995):** randomized 110 patients with type 2 diabetes to multiple insulin injection (MIT) or conventional insulin injection therapy for 6 years. In the primary prevention cohort, the MIT group had developed significantly less retinopathy (7.7% vs 32%) and nephropathy (7.7% vs 28.0%) compared to conventional group. In the secondary prevention cohort, the MIT group had significantly less progression of retinopathy (19.2% vs 44.0%) and nephropathy (11.5% vs 32.0%) compared to conventional group. Based on this study, the glycemic threshold at which to prevent onset and progression of diabetic microangiopathy was found to be HbA1c <6.5%, fasting blood glucose <110 mg/dl, and 2-hour postprandial blood glucose <180 mg/dl (Ohkubo).

- **Type 2 Diabetes (UK Prospective Diabetes Study Group 33, 1998):** UKPDS 33 evaluated the effect of glycemic control with either sulfonylureas or insulin on risk of developing complications in 3867 patients with newly diagnosed type 2 diabetes. Over 10 years, hemoglobin A1c averaged 7.0% in the intensive control group versus 7.9% in the conventional control group. Intensive control reduced any diabetes-related endpoint by 12% (p = 0.029); reduced diabetes-related death by 10% (p = 0.34); and reduced microvascular endpoints by 25% (p = 0.0099). Reduction in risk was of borderline significance for myocardial infarction (p = 0.052). No significant difference between sulfonylureas or insulin, and more hypoglycemia in intensive group (p < 0.0001). Concluded that intensive blood glucose control with either sulfonylureas or insulin substantially reduced risk of microvascular complications but not macrovascular disease in type 2 diabetes (UKPDS 33).

- **Type 2 Diabetes, long-term follow-up (UKPDS, 2008):** long-term follow-up of 3277 patients who had resumed usual clinical care after undergoing a period of intensive or conventional glycemic control during UKPDS, evaluated 6–10 years later. A1c between groups equalized after the first year, but the sulfonylurea-insulin group had a continued

9% risk reduction of all diabetes endpoints (p = 0.04), and 24% risk reduction of microvascular disease (p = 0.01). There was also a 15% reduced risk of myocardial infarction (p = 0.01), and 13% decreased risk of death from any cause (p = 0.001). Similar or greater risk reduction was seen for the group intensively treated with metformin. This follow-up indicates continued benefit of even transient, early intensive therapy for a wide range of endpoints in type 2 diabetes (Holman).

- **Type 2 Diabetes, multifactorial intervention (Steno-2, 2003):** this trial tested the effect of multifactorial intervention on development of cardiovascular disease in type 2 diabetes, as distinct from testing only the effect of glucose control. 160 patients with persistent microalbuminuria were assigned to either conventional treatment or more intense interventions using a combination of behavioral modification and pharmacologic therapy. After 7.8 years follow-up, there was a significant reduction in cardiovascular disease as well as microvascular complications by about 50% (Gaede).

- **Type 2 Diabetes, multifactorial intervention long-term follow-up (Steno-2, 2008):** similar to the long-term follow-up of DCCT (EDIC) and of UKPDS, this result demonstrated a prolonged benefit in type 2 diabetes of multiple risk factor control, including a reduced rate of all-cause death and cardiovascular disease (Gaede).

- **Limits of intensive control (Action to Control Cardiovascular Risk in Diabetes Study Group, 2008):** the ACCORD study randomized 10,251 people with diabetes, all at high risk for cardiovascular disease, to very intense glycemic targets (A1c <6.0% vs target 7%–7.9%). Study was stopped early because there were more deaths in the intensive group (253 vs 207, p = 0.04). However, there were fewer nonfatal CV events in the intensive group, which also had far more side effects of the medications. The cause of the excess deaths is still debated, and several similar studies (ADVANCE, VA Diabetes Trial) did not confirm ACCORD findings. A reasonable conclusion is that the pharmacologic treatment designed to lower A1c to under 6% is not indicated, particularly in older people predisposed to heart disease (ACCORD).

- **Limits of intensive control (Action in Diabetes and Vascular Disease Preterax and Diamicron Modified Release Controlled Evaluation, 2008):** ADVANCE randomized 11,140 patients with type 2 diabetes to standard glucose control (A1c 7.3%) versus intensive glucose control (A1c 6.5%) using gliclazide (modified release) and other drugs as needed. After 5 years, intensive control associated with significantly reduced major macrovascular and microvascular events combined by 10% compared to the standard control group. This was primarily due to decreased incidence of nephropathy, reduced by 21%; no significant effect on retinopathy. No significant differences in mortality reported. Severe hypoglycemia, however, was more common in the intensive control group compared to standard control group (2.7% vs 1.5%, hazard ratio 1.86, 95% CI 1.42–2.40) (ADVANCE).

- **Limits of intensive control (Veteran Affairs Diabetes Trial, 2009):** VADT randomized 1791 military veterans with type 2 diabetes to intensive (A1c 6.9%) versus standard (8.4%) glucose control. After a median follow-up of 5.6 years, 12% decreased risk of first major cardiovascular event. No difference in mortality between groups or in rates of microvascular complications with exception of albuminuria. However, hypoglycemia occurred in 24.1% of the intensive-therapy group compared to 17.6% of the standard-therapy group (Duckworth).

OVERVIEW

BENEFITS OF INPATIENT GLYCEMIC CONTROL

- **Intensive care (van den Berghe et al., 2001):** Van den Berghe changed concepts of inpatient care with this study of 1548 patients in a single-center ICU setting on mechanical ventilation, randomly assigned to receive intensive insulin therapy (maintenance of blood glucose at a level between 80 and 110 mg/dl) or conventional treatment (insulin only for glucose >215 mg/dl, and target 180–200 mg/dl on admission). Only 13% previously had diabetes and 5% were on insulin. After 1 year, intensive insulin therapy reduced mortality from 8.0% with conventional treatment to 4.6% (p < 0.04). The benefit was primarily due to mortality benefits on patients who were in the ICU for >5 days. Other morbidities were also decreased by intensive insulin therapy including bloodstream infections (46% reduction), acute renal failure requiring dialysis or hemofiltration (41% reduction), number of red blood cell transfusion (50% reduction), and critical illness polyneuropathy (44% reduction). Subsequent studies by Van den Berghe extended the findings to other inpatient acute care settings.

- **Intensive care (Normoglycemia in Intensive Care Evaluation-Survival Using Glucose Alogorithm Regulation, 2009):** the NICE-SUGAR study, a large multicenter trial, randomized 6104 patients admitted to the ICU who were expected to stay >3 days to either intensive glycemic control (target 81–108 mg/dl) versus conventional (<180 mg/dl). Conventional control was associated with less mortality (24.9% mortality vs 27.5% in intensive control group, p < 0.02). Severe hypoglycemia was also more common in the intensive-control group versus conventional-control group (6.8% vs 0.5%; p < 0.001). This study challenged the notion that intensive insulin control in the ICU is beneficial (Finfer).

- **Intensive care (Clinical Review, 2009):** Van den Berge, who started the trend toward tight glycemic control in ICUs prior to the NICE-SUGAR study, reviews the literature, in a valid attempt to reconcile the discrepant results described previously. She suggests that no single glucose target can be set based on the current evidence but that maintaining glucose levels as close to normal as possible in the ICU setting, without evoking unacceptable fluctuations, hypoglycemia, or hypokalemia, is reasonable (van den Berghe).

EXPERT OPINION

- The series of studies cited previously, and more could be added, are consistent in their conclusion: the conversion from prediabetes (early glucose intolerance) to type 2 diabetes can be reduced. Lifestyle changes are the most effective intervention, and a series of oral agents, particularly metformin, are also effective.

- The prevention of type 1 diabetes has proven far more difficult. The window of opportunity is generally considered to be the time between demonstration of positive islet markers for the active autoimmune process (e.g., IA2) and established type 1 diabetes. Studies are underway, with considerable promise, designed to manipulate the immune process that is damaging beta cells.

- The earlier studies, first in type 1 diabetes then in type 2 diabetes, were definitive in showing that better glycemic control reduces retinopathy and nephropathy, particularly. Inevitably, subsequent, recent studies addressed "how low should you go?" by pushing the glucose down even to the ACCORD target of HbA1c <6%. These studies, cited previously, were far more equivocal as the rate of hypoglycemia and

potential risk of increased mortality overtook the benefit of glycemic control at a HbA1c level of <6%.
- The original single-center studies by Van den Berge et al. spurred a move toward very aggressive glycemic control of inpatients. The subsequent multicenter NICE SUGAR study, however, found that risks of severe hypoglycemia outweighed benefits. This has led many, including our hospital, to moderate the goal of inpatient glycemia.

REFERENCES

Duckworth W, Abraira C, Moritz T, et al. Glucose control and vascular complications in veterans with type 2 diabetes. *NEJM*, 2009; Vol. 360: pp. 129–39.
  Comments: A summary of the results of the VADT study.

Knowler WC, Fowler SE, Hamman RF, et al. 10-year follow-up of diabetes incidence and weight loss in the Diabetes Prevention Program Outcomes Study. *Lancet*, 2009; Vol. 374: pp. 1677–86.
  Comments: A summary of the results of the DPPOS follow-up study.

NICE-SUGAR Study Investigators, Finfer S, Chittock DR, et al. Intensive versus conventional glucose control in critically ill patients. *NEJM*, 2009; Vol. 360: pp. 1283–97.
  Comments: A summary of the results of the NICE-SUGAR study.

Van den Berghe G, Schetz M, Vlasselaers D, et al. Clinical review: Intensive insulin therapy in critically ill patients: NICE-SUGAR or Leuven blood glucose target? *J Clin Endocrinol Metab*, 2009; Vol. 94: pp. 3163–70.
  Comments: Clinical review comparing NICE-SUGAR and the Leuven study.

DREAM Trial Investigators, Dagenais GR, Gerstein HC, et al. Effects of ramipril and rosiglitazone on cardiovascular and renal outcomes in people with impaired glucose tolerance or impaired fasting glucose: results of the Diabetes REduction Assessment with ramipril and rosiglitazone Medication (DREAM) trial. *Diabetes Care*, 2008; Vol. 31: pp. 1007–14.
  Comments: A summary of the results of the DREAM Trial Study.

Li G, Zhang P, Wang J, et al. The long-term effect of lifestyle interventions to prevent diabetes in the China Da Qing Diabetes Prevention Study: a 20-year follow-up study. *Lancet*, 2008; Vol. 371: pp. 1783–9.
  Comments: A summary of the results of the Da Qing follow-up study.

Holman RR, Paul SK, Bethel MA, et al. 10-year follow-up of intensive glucose control in type 2 diabetes. *NEJM*, 2008; Vol. 359: pp. 1577–89.
  Comments: A summary of the results of the UKPDS follow-up study.

Action to Control Cardiovascular Risk in Diabetes Study Group, Gerstein HC, Miller ME, et al. Effects of intensive glucose lowering in type 2 diabetes. *NEJM*, 2008; Vol. 358: pp. 2545–59.
  Comments: A summary of the results of the ACCORD study.

Gaede P, Lund-Andersen H, Parving HH, et al. Effect of a multifactorial intervention on mortality in type 2 diabetes. *NEJM*, 2008; Vol. 358: pp. 580–91.
  Comments: A summary of the results of the Multifactorial Intervention Long-term Follow-up (Steno-2) study.

ADVANCE Collaborative Group, Patel A, MacMahon S, et al. Intensive blood glucose control and vascular outcomes in patients with type 2 diabetes. *NEJM*, 2008; Vol. 358: pp. 2560–72.
  Comments: A summary of the results of the ADVANCE study.

Lindström J, Ilanne-Parikka P, Peltonen M, et al. Sustained reduction in the incidence of type 2 diabetes by lifestyle intervention: follow-up of the Finnish Diabetes Prevention Study. *Lancet*, 2006; Vol. 368: pp. 1673–9.
  Comments: A summary of the results of the Finnish Diabetes Prevention follow-up study.

Keymeulen B, Vandemeulebroucke E, Ziegler AG, et al. Insulin needs after CD3-antibody therapy in new-onset type 1 diabetes. *NEJM*, 2005; Vol. 352: pp. 2598–608.
  Comments: A hallmark study describing use of CD3-antibody for type 1 diabetes prevention.

Gaede P, Vedel P, Larsen N, et al. Multifactorial intervention and cardiovascular disease in patients with type 2 diabetes. *NEJM*, 2003; Vol. 348: pp. 383–93.
Comments: A summary of the results of the Multifactorial Intervention (Steno-2) study.

Knowler WC, Barrett-Connor E, Fowler SE, et al. Reduction in the incidence of type 2 diabetes with lifestyle intervention or metformin. *NEJM*, 2002: Vol. 346; pp. 393–403.
Comments: A summary of the results of the Diabetes Prevention Program (DPP).

Buchanan TA, Xiang AH, Peters RK, et al. Preservation of pancreatic beta-cell function and prevention of type 2 diabetes by pharmacological treatment of insulin resistance in high-risk hispanic women. *Diabetes*, 2002; Vol. 51: pp. 2796–803.
Comments: A summary of the results of the TRIPOD Study.

Diabetes Prevention Trial—Type 1 Diabetes Study Group. Effects of insulin in relatives of patients with type 1 diabetes mellitus. *NEJM*, 2002; Vol. 346; pp. 1685–91.
Comments: A summary of the results of the DPT Study.

Herold KC, Hagopian W, Auger JA, et al. Anti-CD3 monoclonal antibody in new-onset type 1 diabetes mellitus. *NEJM*, 2002; Vol. 346: pp. 1692–8.
Comments: A hallmark study describing use of anti-CD3 antibody for type 1 diabetes prevention.

Tuomilehto J, Lindstr, Eriksson JG, et al. Prevention of type 2 diabetes mellitus by changes in lifestyle among subjects with impaired glucose tolerance. *NEJM*, 2001; Vol. 344: pp. 1343–50.
Comments: A summary of the results of the Finnish Diabetes Prevention Study.

van den Berghe G, Wouters P, Weekers F, et al. Intensive insulin therapy in the critically ill patients. *NEJM*, 2001; Vol. 345: pp. 1359–67.
Comments: A summary of the results of the Leuven study.

The Diabetes Control and Complications Trial/Epidemiology of Diabetes Interventions and Complications Research Group. Retinopathy and nephropathy in patients with type 1 diabetes four years after a trial of intensive therapy. *NEJM*, 2000; Vol. 342: pp. 381–9.
Comments: A summary of the results of the EDIC Study.

UK Prospective Diabetes Study (UKPDS) Group. Intensive blood-glucose control with sulphonylureas or insulin compared with conventional treatment and risk of complications in patients with type 2 diabetes (UKPDS 33). *Lancet*, 1998; Vol. 352: pp. 837–53.
Comments: A summary of the results of UK Prospective Diabetes Study Group 33.

Pan XR, Li GW, Hu YH, et al. Effects of diet and exercise in preventing NIDDM in people with impaired glucose tolerance. The Da Qing IGT and Diabetes Study. *Diabetes Care*, 1997; Vol. 20: pp. 537–44.
Comments: A summary of the results of the Da Qing IGT and Diabetes Study.

Ohkubo Y, Kishikawa H, Araki E, et al. Intensive insulin therapy prevents the progression of diabetic microvascular complications in Japanese patients with non-insulin-dependent diabetes mellitus: a randomized prospective 6-year study. *Diabetes Res Clin Pract*, 1995; Vol. 28: pp. 103–17.
Comments: A summary of the results of the Kumamoto Trial study.

The Diabetes Control and Complications Trial Research Group. The effect of intensive treatment of diabetes on the development and progression of long-term complications in insulin-dependent diabetes mellitus. *NEJM*, 1993; Vol. 329: pp. 977–86.
Comments: A summary of the results of the Diabetes Control and Complications Trial Research Group (DCCT) Study.

Koenig RJ, Peterson CM, Jones RL, et al. Correlation of glucose regulation and hemoglobin A1c in diabetes mellitus. *NEJM*, 1976; Vol. 295: pp. 417–20.
Comments: One of the earliest studies describing use of hemoglobin A1c as an index of glycemic control.

KEY STUDIES IN DIABETES CARE: MANAGEMENT OF COMPLICATIONS

Christopher D. Saudek, MD, and Rita Rastogi Kalyani, MD, MHS

OVERVIEW

RETINOPATHY

- **Hemoglobin A1c predicts retinopathy (Wisconsin Study, 1988):** followed 891 younger- and 987 older-onset persons with diabetes over 4 years and determined retinopathy using stereoscopic fundus photographs. In younger-onset group, comparing highest versus lowest quartile of A1c, relative risk (RR) for developing: any diabetic retinopathy 1.9%, proliferative retinopathy 21.8%, progression 4.0%. Among older-onset group taking insulin, corresponding RR were 1.9%, 4.0%, 2.1%. These data, showing the positive relationship between incidence and progression of retinopathy and A1c, remained after controlling for confounders. These results were important in planning the power of the DCCT (Klein).

- **Effects of glycemic control, Type 1 Diabetes (Diabetes Control and Complications Group, 1995):** DCCT took a more detailed look at effect of intensive glycemic treatment on diabetic retinopathy in 1441 patients with type 1 diabetes. Intensive therapy reduced risk of any retinopathy by 27%. Although intensive therapy could not prevent retinopathy completely, it had a beneficial effect that began after 3 years of therapy (DCCT).

- **Effects of glycemic control, Type 1 Diabetes (Epidemiology of Diabetes Interventions and Complications Research Group, 2000):** EDIC was the first report describing the long-term follow-up of the DCCT 4 years after the trial ended and found that although hemoglobin A1c equalized in persons with type 1 diabetes treated with intensive or conventional control, the difference in progression of retinopathy (n = 1208) and nephropathy (n = 1302) persisted, favoring those who had been intensively treated (DCCT/EDIC).

- **Effects of glycemic control, Type 2 Diabetes (Kumamoto Trial, 1995):** randomized 110 patients with type 2 diabetes to multiple insulin injection (MIT) or conventional insulin injection therapy for 6 years. In the primary prevention cohort, the MIT group had developed significantly less retinopathy (7.7% vs 32%) compared to conventional group. In the secondary prevention cohort, the MIT group had significantly less progression of retinopathy (19.2% vs 44.0%) compared to conventional group. Based on this study, the glycemic threshold at which to prevent onset and progression of diabetic microangiopathy was found to be HbA1c <6.5%, fasting blood glucose <110 mg/dl, and 2-hour postprandial blood glucose <180 mg/dl (Ohkubo).

- **Effects of glycemic control, Type 2 Diabetes (UK Prospective Diabetes Study 50, 2001):** followed 1919 patients from UKPDS who had retinal photographs at diagnosis and 6 years later. 63% had no retinopathy at diagnosis but by 6 years, 22% had developed retinopathy. 37% had retinopathy at diagnosis, with 29% that progressed by 2 scale steps or more. Incidence of retinopathy associated with baseline glycemia, glycemic exposure over 6 years, higher blood pressure, and not smoking. Hyperglycemia also a risk factor for secondary progression of retinopathy (UKPDS 50).

- **Effects of blood pressure control, Type 1 Diabetes (Renin-Angiotensin System Study, 2009):** losartan and enalapril compared with placebo in 285 normotensive, normoalubminuric patients with type 1 diabetes. There was no effect of either medication on carefully assessed progression of nephropathy. There was, however, a surprising and significant reduction of progression of diabetic retinopathy from both losartan (70%) and enalopril (65%) (Mauer).

- **Effects of blood pressure control, Type 2 Diabetes (UK Prospective Diabetes Study 38, 1998):** randomized 1148 hypertensive patients with type 2 diabetes to tight control ($<150/85$ mmHg; n = 758) versus less tight control ($<180/105$ mmHg; n = 390) with median follow-up of 8.4 years and looked at various endpoints, including retinopathy, determined using retinal photography. Group assigned to tighter control had 34% reduction in retinopathy by 2 steps and 47% reduced risk of deterioration in visual acuity by 3 lines of Early Treatment Diabetic Retinopathy Study (ETDRS) chart (UKPDS 38).

- **Effects of lipid control, Type 2 Diabetes (Fenofibrate Intervention and Event Lowering in Diabetes, 2005):** the FIELD study randomized 9795 participants with type 2 diabetes to fenofibrate versus placebo. After 5 years, the primary outcome of coronary events was not significantly reduced, although it did reduce total cardiovascular events (p = 0.035). The fenofibrate group also had less retinopathy needing laser treatment (p = 0.0003) (Keech).

- **Effects of medical treatments, Type 2 Diabetes (Action to Control Cardiovascular Risk in Diabetes, 2010):** randomized 10,251 participants with type 2 diabetes who were at high risk for cardiovascular disease to receive either intensive (A1c <6) or standard treatment (A1c 7–7.9) for glycemia and also for dyslipidemia (160 mg daily of fenofibrate plus simvastatin versus placebo plus simvastatin) or for systolic blood-pressure control (<120 vs <140 mmHg). 2856 participants evaluated for the progression of diabetic retinopathy using ETDRS Severity Scale (as assessed stereoscopic fundus photographs). At 4 years, the rates of progression of diabetic retinopathy reduced significantly by 33% with intensive glycemia treatment, 40% with combination of fenofibrate and statin for intensive dyslipidemia therapy, and no significant effect with intensive blood-pressure therapy (Chew).

- **Treatment with panretinal laser photocoagulation (Diabetic Retinopathy Study, 1981):** the DRS was the first to demonstrate rigorously the beneficial effect of panretinal laser photocoagulation in reducing the risk of severe visual loss by 50% or more, providing the evidence base for treating proliferative diabetic retinopathy and the rationale for screening people with diabetes in order to make a timely diagnosis of proliferative retinopathy. However, decreases of visual acuity of one or more lines and peripheral field constriction were more frequent with the xenon technique. The findings suggest that prompt treatment is advisable if progression to severe retinopathy has occurred (DRS Research Group).

- **Treatment with focal laser photocoagulation (Early Treatment Diabetic Retinopathy Study, 1985):** the ETDRS tested whether stages of retinopathy that precede proliferative retinopathy also benefit from laser photocoagulation. 754 eyes with macular edema and mild to moderate diabetic retinopathy were randomly assigned to focal argon laser photocoagulation, and 1490 eyes were randomly assigned to deferral of laser treatment. Major findings of the ETDRS included the fact that macular edema benefits from treatment with focal (not panretinal) photocoagulation, but that the outcome of preproliferative retinopathy is not improved by laser treatment (ETDRS).

- **Treatment with vitrectomy (Diabetic Retinopathy Vitrectomy Study Report, 1988):** a randomized trial of vitrectomy versus watchful waiting in 375 eyes with proliferative diabetic retinopathy (PDR) and very poor vision. At 4 years follow-up, 44% of vitrectomized eyes had 10/20 or better vision, versus 28% in conventional group. The value of vitrectomy was proportional to the increasing severity of PDR.

NEPHROPATHY

- **Progression of nephropathy, Type 2 Diabetes (UK Prospective Diabetes Study 64, 2003):** observed 5097 participants with type 2 diabetes in UKPDS over 10 years to study natural progression of nephropathy. From diagnosis of diabetes, progression to microalbuminuria occurred at 2.0% per year, microalbuminuria to macroalbuminuria at 2.8% per year, and from macroalbuminuria to elevated plasma creatinine or renal replacement therapy at 2.3% per year. After 10 years, prevalence of microalbuminuria was 24.9%, macroalbuminuria 5.3%, and elevated creatinine or renal replacement therapy 0.8%. Death rate in those requiring renal replacement therapy was high (19.2%) (UKPDS 64).

- **Effects of glycemic control, Type 1 Diabetes (Diabetes Complications and Control Trial, 1995):** a more detailed description regarding the benefits of intensive insulin therapy on progression of diabetic nephropathy among 1441 patients with type 1 diabetes followed in the DCCT. In the primary prevention cohort, cumulative incidence of microalbumunuria was significantly reduced by 34% and albumin excretion rate was significantly reduced by 15% after the first year with intensive insulin treatment. In secondary prevention cohort, cumulative incidence of microalbumunuria significantly reduced by 43%, progression of microalbumuria significantly reduced by 56%, and clinical albumuria significantly reduced by 56% by intensive insulin treatment (DCCT).

- **Effects of glycemic control, Type 1 Diabetes (Epidemiology of Diabetes Interventions and Complications Research Group, 2000):** EDIC was the first report describing the long-term follow-up of the DCCT 4 years after the trial ended and found that although hemoglobin A1c equalized in persons with type 1 diabetes treated with intensive or conventional control, the difference in progression of nephropathy (n = 1302) persisted, favoring those who had been intensively treated (DCCT/EDIC).

- **Effects of glycemic control, Type 2 Diabetes (Kumamoto Trial, 1995):** randomized 110 patients with type 2 diabetes to multiple insulin injection (MIT) or conventional insulin injection therapy for 6 years. In the primary prevention cohort, the MIT group had developed significantly less nephropathy (7.7% vs 28.0%) compared to conventional group. In the secondary prevention cohort, the MIT group had significantly less progression of nephropathy (11.5% vs 32.0%) compared to conventional group. Based on this study, the glycemic threshold at which to prevent onset and progression of diabetic microangiopathy was found to be HbA1c <6.5%, fasting blood glucose <110 mg/dl, and 2-hour postprandial blood glucose <180 mg/dl (Ohkubo).

- **Effects of glycemic control, Type 2 Diabetes (UK Prospective Diabetes Study 33, 1998):** in UKPDS 33, more intensive blood glucose control resulted in a 24% reduced incidence of microalbuminuria, 33% reduced incidence of macroalbuminuria, and 60% reduction in plasma creatinine doubling time at 9 years (all statistically significant). Tighter blood pressure control also reduced microalbuminuria but had no effect on plasma creatinine levels at 6 years (UKPDS 33).

- **Effects of ACE inhibition, Type 1 Diabetes (The Collaborative Study Group, 1993):** randomized, controlled trial of captopril versus placebo (allowing for other blood pressure medicines) in patients with type 1 diabetes and urinary protein excretion over 500 mg/day. Captopril treatment associated with a 50% reduction in combined endpoints of death, dialysis, and transplantation, independent of differences in blood pressure. Finer measures of renal function (proteinuria, doubling of serum creatinine) were also significantly benefited by captopril. This was the first definitive demonstration of a beneficial effect of ACE-inhibition in treating hypertensive diabetes.

- **Effects of blood pressure control, Type 1 Diabetes (Renin-Angiotensin System Study, 2009):** losartan and enalapril compared with placebo in 285 normotensive, normoalbuminuric patients with type 1 diabetes. There was no effect of either medication on carefully assessed progression of nephropathy in this study (Mauer).

- **Effects of lipid control, Type 2 Diabetes (Fenofibrate Intervention and Event Lowering in Diabetes, 2005):** the FIELD study randomized 9795 participants with type 2 diabetes to fenofibrate versus placebo. After 5 years, the primary outcome of coronary events was not significantly reduced, although it did reduce total cardiovascular events (p = 0.035). The fenofibrate group also had less progression of albuminuria (p = 0.002) (Keech).

NEUROPATHY

- **Risk factors for neuropathy, Type 2 Diabetes (San Luis Valley Diabetes Study, 1997):** among 231 persons, incidence of diabetic sensory neuropathy was 6.1 per 100 person years over mean follow-up of 4.7 years. Glycemic control, current cigarette smoking, and myocardial infarction were significant independent risk factors for development of neuropathy (Sands).

- **Risk factors for neuropathy, Type 2 Diabetes (Seattle Prospective Diabetic Foot Study, 1997):** in a prospective cohort of US veterans with diabetes, 288 persons without neuropathy were followed, of whom 20% developed neuropathy over 10 years. Risk factors for incident neuropathy included age, HbA1c at baseline, height, history of foot ulcer, alcohol ingestion, current smoking, and albumin level (Adler).

- **Risk factors for neuropathy, Type 1 Diabetes (EURODIAB IDDM Complications Study, 1996):** among 3250 insulin-dependent individuals with diabetes, prevalence of neuropathy was 28% and significantly associated with age, height, duration of diabetes, HbA1c, coexistent retinopathy, smoking, HDL, cardiovascular disease, elevated diastolic blood pressure, severe ketoacidosis, increased fasting triglycerides, and microalbuminuria (Tesfaye).

- **Effects of glycemic control, Type 1 Diabetes (Diabetes Control and Complications Trial, 1993):** DCCT is the definitive, NIH-sponsored study of 1441 people with type 1 diabetes with no or mild diabetic retinopathy (DR), randomized into "intensive" or "conventional" glycemic control. Intensive control reduced clinical neuropathy by 60% in the combined primary and secondary intervention cohorts. However, hypoglycemia was 2–3 times higher with intensive control (DCCT).

- **Effects of glycemic control, Type 1 Diabetes (Epidemiology of Diabetes Interventions and Complications Research Group, 2010):** long-term follow-up of DCCT, followed 603 former intensive and 583 former conventional treatment subjects until 13–14 years after DCCT closeout, when both group had achieved similar A1c levels. Prevalence of neuropathy increased from 9% to 25% in former intensive group, and 17% to 35% in former conventional treatment group, but differences remained significant between groups. Incidence of neuropathy was lower in former intensive versus former conventional treatment group (22% vs 28%, p = 0.01) (Albers).

- **Effects of glycemic control, Type 1 Diabetes (Epidemiology of Diabetes Interventions and Complications Research Group, 2009):** long-term follow-up of DCCT, 13–14 years after DCCT closeout. Prevalence of cardiac autonomic neuropathy significantly lower in former intensive group (28.9%) versus former conventional group (35.2%, p = 0.02). Odds of cardiac autonomic neuropathy also significantly lower in former DCCT-intensive versus conventional group (odds ratio 0.69, 95% CI 0.51–0.93) (Pop-Busui).

HYPERTENSION

- **Effect of ACE inhibition on diabetic nephropathy, Type 1 Diabetes (The Collaborative Study Group, 1993):** randomized, controlled trial of captopril versus placebo (allowing for other blood pressure medicines) in patients with type 1 diabetes and urinary protein excretion over 500 mg/day. Captopril treatment associated with a 50% reduction in combined endpoints of death, dialysis, and transplantation, independent of differences in blood pressure. Finer measures of renal function (proteinuria, doubling of serum creatinine) were also significantly benefited by captopril. This was the first definitive demonstration of a beneficial effect of ACE-inhibition in treating hypertensive diabetes (Lewis).

- **Effects on nephropathy and retinopathy, Type 1 Diabetes (Renin-Angiotensin System Study, 2009):** losartan and enalopril compared with placebo in 285 normotensive, normoalbuminuric patients with type 1 diabetes. There was no effect of either medication on carefully assessed progression of nephropathy. There was, however, a surprising and significant reduction of progression of diabetic retinopathy from both losartan (70% reduction) and enalopril (65% reduction) (Mauer).

- **Effects on microvascular and macrovascular complications, Type 2 Diabetes (UK Prospective Diabetes Study 38, 1998):** UKPDS 38 was a randomized, controlled subgroup study of intensive versus conventional blood pressure control, using either ACE inhibitors or beta-blockers. Randomized 1148 hypertensive patients with type 2 diabetes to tight control (<150/85 mmHg; n = 758) versus less tight control (<180/105 mmHg; n = 390) with median follow-up of 8.4 years and looked at various endpoints including retinopathy, determined using retinal photography. Group assigned to tighter control had 34% reduction in retinopathy by 2 steps and 47% reduced risk of deterioration in visual acuity by 3 lines of ETDRS chart. Tight control versus conventional control associated with significantly reduced diabetes-related endpoints by 24%. The risk reduction was quite linear for reducing systolic blood pressure from 170–120 mmHg. Interestingly, ACE inhibitors and beta-blockers reduced cardiovascular event risk equally in a subsequent paper, discounting the notion that beta-blockers are not useful in treating hypertension in diabetes (UKPDS 38).

- **Effects on cardiovascular disease prevention, Type 2 Diabetes (The Action to Control Cardiovascular Risk in Diabetes, 2010):** In the ACCORD blood-pressure trial, a subgroup of 4733 adults were assigned in an unblinded fashion to systolic BP <120 mmHg versus <140 mmHg. The two arms had no significant differences in cardiovascular outcomes except for nonfatal stroke, which was lower in the intensive versus standard BP control arm (p = 0.03). However, the incidence of serious adverse events (i.e., hypotension, syncope) was also three times higher in the intensive arm (p<0.001). Conclusion is that, in diabetes, not necessary to adopt a goal systolic BP <120 mmHg, which may be associated with harm (Cushman).

LIPIDS

- **Effects of pravastatin on cardiovascular disease prevention (The Cholesterol And Recurrent Events Study, 1996):** CARE randomized 4159 patients to pravastatin versus placebo over 5 years. Overall, significant 24% reduction in fatal coronary event or nonfatal myocardial infarction was seen with pravastatin. Among 586 persons with diabetes, risk reduction was 25% and of borderline significance (p = 0.05) (Sacks).
- **Effects of atorvastatin on cardiovascular disease prevention (Scandinavian Survival Study [4S], 1997):** the 4S trial, in subgroup analysis of 202 people with diabetes, found that simvastatin reduced the risk of major cardiovascular events by a highly significant 55% after a median 5.4 years of follow-up. In comparison, the risk of major cardiovascular events was significantly reduced by 32% among persons without diabetes (Pyorala).
- **Effects of atorvastatin on cardiovascular disease prevention, Type 2 Diabetes (Collaborative Atorvastatin Diabetes Study, 2009):** in the CARDS study, 2838 patients with type 2 diabetes and no cardiovascular disease were treated with atorvastatin or placebo for mean 3.9 years. A 42% reduction of major cardiovascular events was found in the atorvastatin-treated group among those with and without decreased GFR (Colhoun).
- **Effects of fenofibrate on cardiovascular disease prevention, Type 2 Diabetes (Fenofibrate Intervention and Event Lowering in Diabetes, 2005):** the FIELD study randomized 9795 participants with type 2 diabetes to fenofibrate versus placebo. After 5 years, the primary outcome of coronary events was not significantly reduced, although it did reduce total cardiovascular events (p = 0.035).
- **Effects of fenofibrate on cardiovascular disease prevention, Type 2 Diabetes (The Action to Control Cardiovascular Risk in Diabetes, 2010):** in the third arm of the ACCORD study (others being glycemia and blood pressure), 5518 people with diabetes already on statin therapy were randomized to the addition of fenofibrate or placebo. Fenofibrate did not improve cardiovascular outcomes. Conclusion is that fenofibrate has no added benefit to statin therapy in diabetes overall, although certain subgroups of individuals (i.e., high triglycerides, low HDL) may obtain benefit (ACCORD).

CARDIOVASCULAR DISEASE

- **Diabetes as a cardiovascular disease equivalent (Finnish Population-Based Study, 1998):** compared the incidence of myocardial infarction (MI) over 7 years among 1373 persons without diabetes versus 1059 persons with diabetes. In persons without diabetes, MI occurred in 18.8% with previous MI versus 3.5% without previous MI. In persons with diabetes, MI occurred in 45.0% with previous MI versus 20.2% without previous MI. Persons with diabetes without previous MI had as high a risk of having a MI as persons without diabetes who had previous MI after adjustment for confounders (hazard ratio close to 1) (Haffner).
- **Fasting versus 2-hour glucose and risk of cardiovascular disease (Diabetes Epidemiology Collaborative Analysis of Diagnostic Criteria in Europe, 2003):** in one of the larger and better prospective studies, the DECODE collaboration studied 29,714 subjects for 11 years and demonstrated that both high and low fasting

glucose and high 2-hour glucose are directly associated with significantly increased cardiovascular disease risk, even at normal and mildly dysglycemic ranges and even when controlled for other known cardiovascular risk factors. This association is well proven by many subsequent analyses (DECODE Study Group).

- **Effects of glycemic control, Type 1 Diabetes (Diabetes Control and Complications Trial, 2005):** long-term follow-up of DCCT that randomly assigned 1441 patients with type 1 diabetes to intensive or conventional therapy between 1983–1993, for a mean of 6.5 years of treatment. 93% were followed until February 2005 as part of EDIC, after which time A1c became similar between groups. During mean 17 years of follow-up, intensive treatment significantly reduced risk of any cardiovascular disease event by 42% (p = 0.02), and nonfatal myocardial infarction, stroke, or death from cardiovascular disease by 57% (p = 0.02). The decline in HbA1c during DCCT was significantly associated with the majority of the beneficial cardiovascular effects conferred by intensive versus conventional treatment (Nathan).

- **Effects of glycemic control, Type 2 Diabetes (UK Prospective Diabetes Study Group Follow-up, 2008):** long-term follow-up of 3277 patients who had resumed usual clinical care after their period of intensive or conventional glycemic control during UKPDS, evaluated 6–10 years later. A1c between groups equalized after the first year, but the sulfonylurea-insulin group had a continued 9% risk reduction of all diabetes endpoints (p = 0.04), and 24% risk reduction of microvascular disease (p = 0.01). There was also a 15% reduced risk of myocardial infarction (p = 0.01), and 13% decreased risk of death from any cause (p = 0.001). Similar or greater risk reduction was seen for the group intensively treated with metformin. This follow-up indicates continued benefit of even transient, early intensive therapy for a wide range of endpoints in type 2 diabetes (Holman).

- **Effects of glycemic control, Type 1 and 2 Diabetes (Selvin et al., 2004):** this was a meta-analysis of studies testing the relationship between HbA1c and cardiovascular disease in 3 studies of type 1 diabetes (n = 1688) and 10 studies of type 2 diabetes (n = 7435). In pooled analysis, persons with type 2 diabetes had an 18% significantly higher risk of cardiovascular disease with each 1% increase in HbA1c. In type 1 diabetes, the risk of cardiovascular disease was 15% higher for each 1% increase in HbA1c, but the results were not statistically significant. In contrast, incident peripheral arterial disease was significantly higher for both type 1 and type 2 diabetes (32% and 28%, respectively) with each 1-percentage point increase in HbA1c.

- **Limits of intensive control, Type 2 Diabetes (Action to Control Cardiovascular Risk in Diabetes Study Group, 2008):** the ACCORD study randomized 10,251 people with type 2 diabetes, all at high risk for cardiovascular disease, to very intense glycemic targets (A1c <6.0% vs target 7%–7.9%). Study was stopped early because there were more deaths in the intensive group (253 vs 207, p = 0.04). However, there were fewer nonfatal cardiovascular events in the intensive group, which also had far more side effects of the medications. The cause of the excess deaths is still debated, and several similar studies (ADVANCE, VA Diabetes Trial) did not confirm ACCORD findings. A reasonable conclusion is that the pharmacologic treatment designed to lower A1c to under 6% is not indicated, particularly in older people predisposed to heart disease (ACCORD).

- **Limits of intensive control, Type 2 Diabetes (Action in Diabetes and Vascular Disease Preterax and Diamicron Modified Release Controlled Evaluation, 2008):** ADVANCE randomized 11,140 patients with type 2 diabetes to standard glucose control (A1c 7.3%) versus intensive glucose control (A1c 6.5%) using glicazide (modified release) and other drugs as needed. After 5 years, intensive control associated with significantly reduced major macrovascular and microvascular events combined by 10% compared to the standard control group. This was primarily due to decreased incidence of nephropathy (reduced by 21%), but no significant effect on retinopathy. No significant differences in mortality reported. Severe hypoglycemia, however, was more common in the intensive control group compared to standard control group (2.7% vs 1.5%, hazard ratio 1.86, 95% CI 1.42–2.40) (ADVANCE).
- **Limits of intensive control, Type 2 Diabetes (Veteran Affairs Diabetes Trial, 2009):** VADT randomized 1791 military veterans with type 2 diabetes to intensive (A1c 6.9%) versus standard (8.4%) glucose control. After a median follow-up of 5.6 years, 12% decreased risk of first major cardiovascular event. No difference in mortality between groups or in rates of microvascular complications with exception of albuminuria. However, hypoglycemia occurred in 24.1% of the intensive-therapy group compared to 17.6% of the standard-therapy group (Duckworth).

EXPERT OPINION

- The previously listed studies and others have proven beyond question that good glycemic control reduces the risk of new retinopathy and progression of established retinopathy. They also demonstrate the efficacy of laser photocoagulation when applied at the right time.
- Nephropathy is the other major microvascular complication that is proven to be reduced by good glycemic control (retinopathy being the first). Blood pressure control and blood glucose control are the main goals in avoiding the progression of microalbuminuria to "clinical" proteinuria, and subsequent ESRD.
- The benefits of glycemic control on neuropathy were largely described in the DCCT and EDIC, but several observational studies have demonstrated significant associations of hyperglycemia with development of neuropathy in both type 1 and type 2 diabetes.
- The independent effects of glycemia on cardiovascular disease have always been harder to demonstrate, presumably for several reasons: other major risk factors (i.e., lipids, blood pressure, smoking, clotting factors) are highly important in determining risk, probably more important than glycemia; the constellation of risk factors that contribute to "metabolic syndrome" (central obesity, hypertriglyceridemia, low HDL-cholesterol, hypertension, hyperglycemia) are also associated with CVD; the exact onset of hyperglycemia is difficult to know, and CVD is prevalent in the nondiabetic older population. Nevertheless, long-term follow-up of earlier studies (DCCT, UKPDS) have shown the association clearly. More recent studies, however, have failed to demonstrate a beneficial effect of too tight glycemia on CVD (i.e., ACCORD, ADVANCE, VADT).

REFERENCES

ACCORD Study Group, ACCORD Eye Study Group, Chew EY, et al. Effects of medical therapies on retinopathy progression in type 2 diabetes. *NEJM*, 2010; Vol. 363: pp. 233–44.
Comments: A summary of the results of the ACCORD study group.

ACCORD Study Group, Cushman WC, Evans GW, et al. Effects of intensive blood-pressure control in type 2 diabetes mellitus. *NEJM*, 2010; Vol. 362: pp. 1575–85.
Comments: A summary of the results of the ACCORD study on blood pressure.

ACCORD Study Group, Ginsberg HN, Elam MB, et al. Effects of combination lipid therapy in type 2 diabetes mellitus. *NEJM*, 2010; Vol. 362: pp. 1563–74.
Comments: A summary of the results of the ACCORD study on lipid therapy.

Albers JW, Herman WH, Pop-Busui R, et al. Effect of prior intensive insulin treatment during the Diabetes Control and Complications Trial (DCCT) on peripheral neuropathy in type 1 diabetes during the Epidemiology of Diabetes Interventions and Complications (EDIC) Study. *Diabetes Care*, 2010; Vol. 33: pp. 1090–6.
Comments: A summary of the results of the DCCT/EDIC research group.

Colhoun HM, Betteridge DJ, Durrington PN, et al. Effects of atorvastatin on kidney outcomes and cardiovascular disease in patients with diabetes: an analysis from the Collaborative Atorvastatin Diabetes Study (CARDS). *Am J Kidney Dis*, 2009; Vol. 54: pp. 810–9.
Comments: A summary of the results of the CARDS Study.

Duckworth W, Abraira C, Moritz T, et al. Glucose control and vascular complications in veterans with type 2 diabetes. *NEJM*, 2009; Vol. 360: pp. 129–39.
Comments: A summary of the results of the VADT study.

Mauer M, Zinman B, Gardiner R, et al. Renal and retinal effects of enalapril and losartan in type 1 diabetes. *NEJM*, 2009; Vol. 361: pp. 40–51.
Comments: A summary of the results of the Renin-Angiotensin System Study.

Pop-Busui R, Low PA, Waberski BH, et al. Effects of prior intensive insulin therapy on cardiac autonomic nervous system function in type 1 diabetes mellitus: the Diabetes Control and Complications Trial/Epidemiology of Diabetes Interventions and Complications study (DCCT/EDIC). *Circulation*, 2009; Vol. 119: pp. 2886–93.
Comments: A summary of the results of the DCCT/EDIC research group.

Action to Control Cardiovascular Risk in Diabetes Study Group, Gerstein HC, Miller ME, et al. Effects of intensive glucose lowering in type 2 diabetes. *NEJM*, 2008; Vol. 358: pp. 2545–59.
Comments: A summary of the results of the ACCORD study on glucose lowering.

ADVANCE Collaborative Group, Patel A, MacMahon S, et al. Intensive blood glucose control and vascular outcomes in patients with type 2 diabetes. *NEJM*, 2008; Vol. 358: pp. 2560–72.
Comments: A summary of the results of the ADVANCE collaborative group.

Holman RR, Paul SK, Bethel MA, et al. 10-year follow-up of intensive glucose control in type 2 diabetes. *NEJM*, 2008; Vol. 359: pp. 1577–89.
Comments: Results of the UKPDS follow-up of intensive glucose control in T2DM.

Keech A, Simes RJ, Barter P, et al. Effects of long-term fenofibrate therapy on cardiovascular events in 9795 people with type 2 diabetes mellitus (the FIELD study): randomised controlled trial. *Lancet*, 2005; Vol. 366: pp. 1849–61.
Comments: A summary of the results of the FIELD study.

Nathan DM, Cleary PA, Backlund JY, et al. Intensive diabetes treatment and cardiovascular disease in patients with type 1 diabetes. *NEJM*, 2005; Vol. 353: pp. 2643–53.
Comments: A summary of the results of the DCCT/EDIC research group.

Selvin E, Marinopoulos S, Berkenblit G, et al. Meta-analysis: glycosylated hemoglobin and cardiovascular disease in diabetes mellitus. *Ann Intern Med*, 2004; Vol. 141: pp. 421–31.
Comments: Glycosylated hemoglobin and cardiovascular disease meta-analysis.

Adler AI, Stevens RJ, Manley SE, et al. Development and progression of nephropathy in type 2 diabetes: the United Kingdom Prospective Diabetes Study (UKPDS 64). *Kidney Int*, 2003; Vol. 63: pp. 225–32.
Comments: A summary of the results of the UKPDS 64.

OVERVIEW

DECODE Study Group, European Diabetes Epidemiology Group. Is the current definition for diabetes relevant to mortality risk from all causes and cardiovascular and noncardiovascular diseases? *Diabetes Care*, 2003; Vol. 26: pp. 688–96.
Comments: A summary of the results of the DECODE study group.

Stratton IM, Kohner EM, Aldington SJ, et al. UKPDS 50: risk factors for incidence and progression of retinopathy in Type II diabetes over 6 years from diagnosis. *Diabetologia*, 2001; Vol. 44: pp. 156–63.
Comments: A summary of the results of the UKPDS 50.

The Diabetes Control and Complications Trial/Epidemiology of Diabetes Interventions and Complications Research Group. Retinopathy and nephropathy in patients with type 1 diabetes four years after a trial of intensive therapy. *NEJM*, 2000; Vol. 342: pp. 381–9.
Comments: A summary of the results of the DCCT/EDIC research group.

Haffner SM, Lehto S, Rmaa T, et al. Mortality from coronary heart disease in subjects with type 2 diabetes and in nondiabetic subjects with and without prior myocardial infarction. *NEJM*, 1998; Vol. 339: pp. 229–34.
Comments: A summary of the results of the Finnish Population-Based Study.

UK Prospective Diabetes Study (UKPDS) Group. Intensive blood-glucose control with sulphonylureas or insulin compared with conventional treatment and risk of complications in patients with type 2 diabetes (UKPDS 33). *Lancet*, 1998; Vol. 352: pp. 837–53.
Comments: A summary of the results of the UKPDS 33.

UK Prospective Diabetes Study Group. Tight blood pressure control and risk of macrovascular and microvascular complications in type 2 diabetes: UKPDS 38. *BMJ*, 1998; Vol. 317: pp. 703–13.
Comments: A summary of the results of the UKPDS 38.

UK Prospective Diabetes Study Group. Tight blood pressure control and risk of macrovascular and microvascular complications in type 2 diabetes: UKPDS 38. *BMJ*, 1998; Vol. 317; pp. 703–13.
Comments: A summary of the results of the UK Prospective Diabetes Study 38.

Adler AI, Boyko EJ, Ahroni JH, et al. Risk factors for diabetic peripheral sensory neuropathy. Results of the Seattle Prospective Diabetic Foot Study. *Diabetes Care*, 1997; Vol. 20: pp. 1162–7.
Comments: A summary of the results of the Seattle Prospective Diabetic Foot Study.

Pyorala K, Pedersen TR, Kjekshus J, et al. Cholesterol lowering with simvastatin improves prognosis of diabetic patients with coronary heart disease. A subgroup analysis of the Scandinavian Simvastatin Survival Study (4S). *Diabetes Care*, 1997; Vol. 20: pp. 614–20.
Comments: A summary of the results of the Scandinavian Survival Study (4S).

Sands ML, Shetterly SM, Franklin GM, et al. Incidence of distal symmetric (sensory) neuropathy in NIDDM. The San Luis Valley Diabetes Study. *Diabetes Care*, 1997; Vol. 20: pp. 322–9.
Comments: A summary of the results of the San Luis Valley Diabetes Study.

Sacks FM, Pfeffer MA, Moye LA, et al. The effect of pravastatin on coronary events after myocardial infarction in patients with average cholesterol levels. Cholesterol and Recurrent Events Trial investigators. *NEJM*, 1996; Vol. 335: pp. 1001–9.
Comments: A summary of the results of the CARE study.

Tesfaye S, Stevens LK, Stephenson JM, et al. Prevalence of diabetic peripheral neuropathy and its relation to glycaemic control and potential risk factors: the EURODIAB IDDM Complications Study. *Diabetologia*, 1996; Vol. 39; pp. 1377–84.
Comments: A summary of the results of the EURODIAB IDDM Complications Study.

The Diabetes Control and Complications (DCCT) Research Group. Effect of intensive therapy on the development and progression of diabetic nephropathy in the Diabetes Control and Complications Trial. *Kidney Int*, 1995; Vol. 47: pp. 1703–20.
Comments: A summary of the results of the DCCT research group.

Diabetes Control and Complications Trial Research Group (DCCT). Progression of retinopathy with intensive versus conventional treatment in the Diabetes Control and Complications Trial. *Ophthalmology*, 1995; Vol. 102: pp. 647–61.
Comments: A summary of the results of the DCCT research group.

Ohkubo Y, Kishikawa H, Araki E, et al. Intensive insulin therapy prevents the progression of diabetic microvascular complications in Japanese patients with non-insulin-dependent diabetes mellitus: a randomized prospective 6-year study. *Diabetes Res Clin Pract*, 1995; Vol. 28: pp. 103–17.
Comments: A summary of the results of the Kumamoto Trial.

The Diabetes Control and Complications Trial Research Group. The effect of intensive treatment of diabetes on the development and progression of long-term complications in insulin-dependent diabetes mellitus. *NEJM*, 1993; Vol. 329: pp. 977–86.
Comments: A summary of the results of the DCCT research group.

Lewis EJ, Hunsicker LG, Bain RP, et al. The effect of angiotensin-converting-enzyme inhibition on diabetic nephropathy. The Collaborative Study Group. *NEJM*, 1993; Vol. 329: pp. 1456–62.
Comments: A summary of the results of the Collaborative Study Group.

The Diabetic Retinopathy Vitrectomy Study Research Group. Early vitrectomy for severe proliferative diabetic retinopathy in eyes with useful vision. Results of a randomized trial—Diabetic Retinopathy Vitrectomy Study Report 3. *Ophthalmology*, 1988; Vol. 95: pp. 1307–20.
Comments: A summary of the results of the Diabetic Retinopathy Vitrectomy Study Report 3.

Klein R, Klein BE, Moss SE, et al. Glycosylated hemoglobin predicts the incidence and progression of diabetic retinopathy. *JAMA*, 1988; Vol. 260: pp. 2864–71.
Comments: A summary of the results of the Wisconsin Study.

Early Treatment Diabetic Retinopathy Study Research Group. Photocoagulation for diabetic macular edema. Early Treatment Diabetic Retinopathy Study report number 1. *Arch Ophthalmol*, 1985; Vol. 103: pp. 1796–806.
Comments: A summary of the results of the ETDRS research group.

The Diabetic Retinopathy Study Research Group. Photocoagulation treatment of proliferative diabetic retinopathy. Clinical application of Diabetic Retinopathy Study (DRS) findings, DRS Report Number 8. *Ophthalmology*, 1981; Vol. 88: pp. 583–600.
Comments: A summary of the results of the DRS research group.

KEY STUDIES IN DIABETES CARE: EFFICACY OF THERAPIES

Christopher D. Saudek, MD, and Rita Rastogi Kalyani, MD, MHS

MEDICAL THERAPIES FOR TYPE 1 AND TYPE 2 DIABETES

- **Metformin (The Multicenter Metformin Study Group, 1995):** randomized trial comparing effect of metformin versus placebo in 289 patients with type 2 diabetes who were moderately obese. After 29 weeks, the metformin group had lower fasting plasma glucose (189 mg/dl vs 244 mg/dl) and hemoglobin A1c (7.1% vs 8.6%) compared to placebo. Combination therapy with glyburide compared to glyburide alone resulted in lower fasting plasma glucose (187 mg/dl vs 261 mg/dl) and HbA1c (7.1% vs 8.7%). However, 18% had hypoglycemia in the combination group, compared to only 2% with metformin alone and 3% with glyburide alone (DeFronzo).
- **Metformin (United Kingdom Prospective Diabetes Study 34, 1998):** UKPDS 34 studied the effect of intensive glycemic control with metformin in newly diagnosed,

overweight people with type 2 diabetes. 1704 patients who were hyperglycemic after 3 months of diet alone were randomly continued on "conventional" management mainly with diet alone or metformin, sulfonylureas, or insulin. Metformin reduced any diabetes-related endpoint (p = 0.0034), all-cause mortality (p = 0.021), and stroke (p = 0.032). In an unexpected and unexplained result, early addition of metformin in the sulfonylurea-treated group increased diabetes-related deaths (p = 0.039), although there was no overall association of metformin plus sulfonylurea with increased death risk. Conclusion was that metformin may be the first-line therapy of choice (UKPDS 34).

- **Sulfonylureas (The University Group Diabetes Program, 1970):** an early and much-debated study of new-onset type 2 diabetes, the UGDP randomized patients to treatment with a first-generation sulfonylurea (SU) (tolbutamide), phenformin, or insulin. Found deaths from lactic acidosis in the phenformin group, and slightly but significantly more deaths from cardiovascular disease in the SU group. Serious critiques were leveled regarding methods and conclusions, for instance, by A. R. Feinstein. The UGDP finding of adverse effects of SU have not been confirmed or widely accepted, but continue to prompt a black box warning in the package insert. SUs have been used safely in myriad studies since (Meinert).

- **Glyburide (Nathan et al., 1988):** randomized 31 patients with type 2 diabetes previously inadequately controlled on diet alone to once daily NPH insulin or glyburide. Baseline HbA1c ~10% in both groups. After 9 months, HbA1c dropped similarly in both groups by ~3%.

- **Acarbose (Essen Study, 1994):** randomized 96 patients with type 2 diabetes and dietary failure to acarbose versus glibenclamide versus placebo. After 24 weeks, mean HbA1c dropped by 1.1% with acarbose and 0.9% with glibenclamide compared to placebo. Acarbose also showed lower postprandial insulin increase (Hoffman).

- **Troglitazone (Nolan et al., 1994):** an early description of how thiazolidinediones (TZDs) (troglitazone in this case) work by reducing insulin resistance in 18 obese patients with either normal or impaired glucose tolerance. While troglitazone is no longer available due to adverse hepatic effects, this mechanism is a class effect for TZDs.

- **Pioglitazone (Pioglitazone 001 Study Group, 2000):** randomized 408 patients to placebo or four different doses of pioglitazone monotherapy. HbA1c decreased on average between 1%–1.6% on the three highest doses of pioglitazone (15–45 mg daily) after 26 weeks compared to placebo. Improvements in fasting glucose were observed after two 2 weeks therapy, and were maximal at 10–14 weeks but maintained until study completion (−39 to −65 mg/dl vs placebo). The improvement in glycemic control was greatest in those who were treatment naive (HbA1c difference from placebo of −2.55%) (Aronoff).

- **Pioglitazone (PROspective pioglitAzone Clinical Trial in macroVascular Events, 2005):** in the PROActive trial, 5238 patients with type 2 diabetes and evidence of macrovascular disease were randomized to pioglitazone versus placebo. After an average follow-up of 34.5 months, the primary composite endpoint of all-cause mortality, nonfatal myocardial infarction, acute coronary syndrome, endovascular or surgical intervention in the coronary or leg arteries, and amputation above the ankles was not significantly different between groups. However, the composite secondary endpoint of all-cause mortality, nonfatal myocardial infarction and stroke was 16% lower in the pioglitazone group (p = 0.027) (Dormandy).

- **Pioglitazone (Pioglitazone Effect on Regression of Intravascular Sonographic Coronary Obstruction Prospective Evaluation Trial, 2008):** the PERISCOPE Trial performed coronary intravascular ultrasonography (IVUS) on 543 patients with coronary disease and type 2 diabetes. Patients were then randomized to receive glimepiride (a sulfonylurea) or pioglitazone (a thiazolidinedione) followed by repeat intravascular ultrasound (IVUS) in 360 patients after 18 months. Percent atheroma volume increased 0.73% (95% CI, 0.33%–1.12%) with glimepiride and decreased 0.16% (95% CI, −0.57%–0.25%) with pioglitazone (p = 0.002). Using this extremely fine measurement, the conclusion was that pioglitazone was more favorable than SU in slowing progression of coronary atherosclerosis (Nissen).
- **Pioglitazone versus rosiglitazone effects on lipids (Goldberg et al., 2005):** subjects with type 2 diabetes and dyslipidemia, not previously on insulin or lipid-lowering agents, were treated with pioglitazone (n = 400) or rosiglitazone (n = 402) for 12 weeks. Triglyceride levels fell by 51 (7.8 mg/dl) with pioglitazone, but increased by 13.1 (7.8 mg/dl) with rosiglitazone (p < 0.001 between treatments). Pioglitazone also increased HDL cholesterol (5.2 [0.5 mg/dl] vs 2.4 [0.5 mg/dl]; p < 0.001) and increased LDL cholesterol less (12 [1.6 mg/dl] vs 21 [1.6 mg/dl]; p < 0.001). LDL particle concentration was reduced and LDL particle size was increased more with pioglitazone (p = 0.005), both considered favorable changes, suggesting that pioglitazone and rosiglitazone have significantly different effects on plasma lipids (pioglitazone being more favorable).
- **Rosiglitazone (Nissen et al., 2007):** a meta-analysis of 42 published and unpublished, small and large studies, which found that use of rosiglitazone was associated with a significant increase in deaths from myocardial infarction (odds ratio = 1.43, 95% CI 1.03–1.98; p = 0.03) and an increase in death from cardiovascular disease that had borderline significance (odds ratio = 1.64, 95% CI 0.98–2.74; p = 0.06). Immediately controversial.
- **Rosiglitazone (Rosiglitazone Evaluated for Cardiovascular Outcomes in oRal agent Combination therapy for type 2 Diabetes, 2009):** RECORD is a large (n = 4447 patients) randomized trial of the cardiovascular events following addition of rosiglitazone to metformin or sulfonylurea therapy in type 2 diabetes. After 5.5 years, the study found that rosiglitazone treatment was associated with a significant increase in body weight (~4 kg), an increased risk of heart failure (hazard ratio 2.10, 95% CI 1.35–3.27) and overall bone fractures (relative risk 1.57, 95% CI 1.26–1.97), mainly among women and primarily in upper and lower limb fractures. However, no overall increase in cardiovascular morbidity or mortality was found in this study (Home). Concerns over the open-blind study design have led to the FDA's readjudication of the results, suggesting increased risk of myocardial infarction in the rosiglitazone group (Psaty).
- **Rosiglitazone (Nissen et al., 2010):** an updated meta-analysis of 56 trials of rosiglitazone at least 24 weeks in duration. Found that rosiglitazone significantly increased risk of myocardial infarction (odds ratio = 1.39, excluding RECORD trial, 95% CI 1.02–1.89, p = 0.04) but not cardiovascular mortality (odds ratio = 1.03, 95% CI 0.78–1.36, p = 0.86).
- **Comparative efficacy of oral agents (A Diabetes Outcome Progression Trial, 2006):** the ADOPT study (n = 4360) evaluated longevity of glycemic control with several oral agents in type 2 diabetes over 5 years. Monotherapy failure was defined

as fasting plasma glucose of >180 mg/dl. Glyburide had the most significant early hypoglycemic effect but the highest failure rate (34%) at 5 years. 15% failed rosiglitazone, and 21% failed metformin. Rosiglitazone was associated with more weight gain and edema, and an increased rate of new fractures (Kahn).

- **Sitagliptin (Study 021 Group, 2006):** a safety and efficacy trial of sitagliptin as monotherapy in type 2 diabetes. Randomized 741 patients to sitagliptin (100 or 200 mg) or placebo. After 24 weeks, overall significant reductions in A1c in sitagliptin group (100 or 200 mg) of −0.79 and −0.94%, respectively, compared to placebo. A1c-lowering effects greatest when baseline A1c >9% (∼−1.50%). Sitagliptin was weight neutral, with similar incidence of hypoglycemia and slightly higher GI side effects compared to placebo (Aschner).

- **Exenetide versus insulin glargine (Barnett et al., 2007):** an early open-label comparison of exenatide (an incretin mimetic) versus insulin glargine in 138 persons with type 2 diabetes who had failed oral agents. Found that exenatide had similar glycemic efficacy after 16 weeks (∼38% had HbA1c <7%), but exenatide had more weight reduction (difference of −2.2 kg between groups, p < 0.001), as well as a higher incidence of gastrointestinal side effects (42.6% vs 3.1% with nausea).

- **Inhaled insulin (Skyler et al., 2007):** a safety and efficacy trial of inhaled insulin in 580 adults with type 1 diabetes, showing efficacy and safety over 2 years, although a small decrease in FEV1 during the first 3 months that was not progressive thereafter and cough was noted. Inhaled insulin was marketed briefly and then removed from the market, because it was not well accepted and did not sell. Subsequently, the FDA announced a worrisome finding: While there were few deaths among study participants, there was an imbalance of deaths due to lung cancer in those taking inhaled insulin.

MEDICAL THERAPIES FOR GESTATIONAL DIABETES

- **Glyburide (Langer et al., 2000):** randomized 404 women with singleton pregnancy and gestational diabetes requiring treatment to receive glyburide or insulin between 11–33 weeks gestation. Mean concentrations of glucose before treatment ∼115 mg/dl and after treatment ∼105 mg/dl in both groups. No significant differences in macrosomia, hypoglycemia, lung complications, fetal anomalies, or requirement for neonatal intensive care between infants in both groups. Suggested that glyburide could be a clinically effective alternative to insulin in management of gestational diabetes. However, later studies suggested that although glyburide may be as effective as insulin, it may be associated with increased incidence of preeclampsia and phototherapy, and these risks require further study (Jacobson).

- **Metformin (Moore et al., 2010):** randomized 149 patients with gestational diabetes inadequately controlled on diet to metformin versus glyburide. Failure to achieve adequate glycemic control was significantly higher in metformin group (35%) versus glyburide group (16%), requiring insulin.

SURGICAL THERAPIES FOR DIABETES AND RELATED COMPLICATIONS

- **Islet transplantation (Shapiro et al., 1975):** the first demonstration that islet transplantation is feasible. Seven patients with type 1 diabetes who had history of severe metabolic instability and hypoglycemia were transplanted with 2–3 donor pancreases, and managed with a steroid-free regimen of sirolimus, tacrolimus, and daclizumab. After 1 year, insulin independence was achieved in all 7 patients, though longer-term follow-up showed some deterioration. The positive results on insulin independence were thought to be due to advances in the islet isolation techniques and the steroid-free immunosuppressive regimen.

- **Islet transplantation (Edmonton protocol, 2006):** an expanded, international trial of the Edmonton Protocol for islet transplantation in 36 patients with type 1 diabetes. After 1 year, 16 patients (44%) had insulin independence and adequate glycemic control, 10 patients (28%) had partial function, and 10 patients (28%) had complete graft loss. At 2 years, 5 of the 16 subjects (31%) who were free of insulin at 1 year remained insulin independent. The authors concluded that insulin independence after islet transplantation is possible but not usually sustained; however, protection from severe hypoglycemia and improved HbA1c are benefits of persistent islet function (Shapiro).

- **Implantable insulin pump (Department of Veteran Affairs Implantable Insulin Pump Study Group, 1996):** randomized 171 male patients with type 2 diabetes on insulin therapy to implantable insulin pump (IIP) versus multiple daily insulin injections (MDI). After 1 year, similar decline in blood glucose levels (~8 mmol/L) and hemoglobin A1c was observed. IIP had significantly reduced glucose fluctuations, mild clinical hypoglycemia and weight gain, while improving quality of life. However, 25% of patients had insulin underdelivery due to insulin microprecipitates within the implantable insulin pump (Saudek).

- **Gastric banding (University Obesity Research Center, Australia, 2008):** one of the few randomized trials of laparoscopic adjustable gastric banding (bariatric surgery) for type 2 diabetes. Of 60 obese patients enrolled, 73% in the surgery group had remission of type 2 diabetes versus only 13% in the lifestyle modification group (relative risk 5.5, 95% CI 2.2–14.0). The benefit was directly related to weight loss; in the surgical group, mean weight was reduced by 20.7% versus 1.7% in lifestyle modification group (Dixon).

- **Bariatric surgery (Adams et al., 2007):** long-term mortality after the most common bariatric surgery procedure, gastric bypass (n = 9949), compared to a retrospectively evaluated control group of obese patients (n = 9628), was reduced by 40% (p < 0.001), particularly deaths from diabetes, heart disease, and cancer after 7 years. However, the rate of deaths from accidents and suicides were 58% higher (p = 0.04) in the surgery versus control group.

- **Bariatric surgery (Swedish Obesity Subjects study, 2007):** the SOS study followed 4047 obese subjects for up to 11 years of whom 2010 underwent bariatric surgery and 2037 received conventional treatment. Weight loss was ± 2% in the conventional group for up to 15 years compared to the surgical group after 1–2 years and 10 years, respectively, as follows: gastric bypass (32%, 25%), vertical-banded gastroplasty (25%, 16%), banding (20%, 14%). The sex, age, and risk factor adjusted mortality rate was 29% lower in the surgically versus conventionally treated group (p = 0.01) (Sj).

- **Bariatric surgery (Longitudinal Assessment of Bariatric Surgery Consortium, 2009):** the LABS consortium report evaluated safety of bariatric surgery in 4776 patients, about three-quarters with Roux-en-Y gastric bypass, the rest with adjustable gastric banding. Overall, 4.3% had at least one major adverse outcome, and 30-day death rate was 0.3%. Extreme obesity was associated with an increased risk of adverse outcomes (Flum).

- **Cardiac bypass surgery (The Bypass Angioplasty Revascularization Investigation, 1996):** the BARI trial compared the efficacy of coronary-artery bypass grafting (CABG) with percutaneous transluminal coronary angioplasty (PTCA) in 1829 patients with multivessel disease. There was no significant difference in mortality between the two groups after an average follow-up of 5.4 years. However, when the analysis was restricted to persons with diabetes (n = 353), a subgroup that had not been prespecified, survival was significantly better in the CABG compared to the PTCA group (80.6% vs 65.5%, p = 0.003). The study put into question the use of PTCA in people with diabetes, with the caveat that PTCA methods are constantly improving (BARI investigators).
- **Cardiac bypass surgery (The Bypass Angioplasty Revascularization Investigation 2 Diabetes Trial, 2009):** the BARI 2D study enrolled 2368 people with type 2 diabetes and stable ischemic heart disease. They were randomly assigned to either prompt intervention with revascularization (CABG) or percutaneous coronary intervention (PCI), versus optimization of medical therapy. The type of prompt intervention was selected according to severity of the disease. With an average 5-year follow-up, optimal medical intervention resulted in no difference in deaths or major cardiovascular events compared to prompt revascularization, unless the patient was selected for CABG (had more severe disease), in which case CABG had significantly lower rate of major cardiovascular events than medical management (22.4% vs 30.5%, p = 0.01) (Frye).

EXPERT OPINION

- Note that studies describing the relative efficacy of various insulin regimens were not included in this list.
- Trials of drug efficacy may be subject to publication bias; however, several prominent medical journals now require that clinical trials be registered in a public database from the start, reducing the possibility that only positive results will be published.
- Relatively greater glucose-lowering effects may be observed when HbA1c is higher (i.e., >9%) at baseline or in treatment-naive patients.
- The rosiglitazone versus pioglitazone controversy has been particularly active. For perspective, there are clear, known side effects of both these thiazolidinediones: they each cause fluid retention, an increased incidence of congestive heart failure, weight gain, and increased fracture rate. One head-to-head study (Goldberg et al., see p. 31). found a significantly better lipid profile for pioglitazone. The controversy is about whether rosiglitazone also causes more CVD than does pioglitazone. The evidence is mainly from the Nissen meta-analyses (see p. 31). A panel convened by the FDA announced in September 2010 that rosiglitazone will stay on the market, but severely restricted its use.
- Surgical therapies are primarily available for complications of diabetes (e.g., obesity, cardiovascular disease), but novel curative treatments such as islet transplantation for type 1 diabetes are being investigated.

REFERENCES

Psaty BM, Prentice RL. Minimizing bias in randomized trials: the importance of blinding. *JAMA*, 2010; Vol. 304: pp. 793–4.

Comments: A commentary on bias in clinical trials, specifically addressing the RECORD trial.

Moore LE, Clokey D, Rappaport VJ, et al. Metformin compared with glyburide in gestational diabetes: a randomized controlled trial. *Obstet Gynecol*, 2010; Vol. 115: pp. 55–9.

Comments: An original study comparing metformin versus glyburide for treatment of gestational diabetes.

Nissen SE, Wolski K. Rosiglitazone revisited: an updated meta-analysis of risk for myocardial infarction and cardiovascular mortality. *Arch Intern Med*, 2010; Jun 28 [Epub ahead of print].
  Comments: Updated meta-analysis of 52 trials.

BARI 2D Study Group, Frye RL, August P, et al. A randomized trial of therapies for type 2 diabetes and coronary artery disease. *NEJM*, 2009; Vol. 360: pp. 2503–15.
  Comments: A summary of results from the BARI 2D Study Group.

Home PD, Pocock SJ, Beck-Nielsen H, et al. Rosiglitazone evaluated for cardiovascular outcomes in oral agent combination therapy for type 2 diabetes (RECORD): a multicentre, randomised, open-label trial. *Lancet*, 2009; Vol. 373: pp. 2125–35.
  Comments: A summary of the results of the RECORD Study.

Longitudinal Assessment of Bariatric Surgery (LABS) Consortium, Flum DR, Belle SH, et al. Perioperative safety in the longitudinal assessment of bariatric surgery. *NEJM*, 2009; Vol. 361: pp. 445–54.
  Comments: Results from a study of bariatric surgery from the LABS Consortium.

Dixon JB, O'Brien PE, Playfair J, et al. Adjustable gastric banding and conventional therapy for type 2 diabetes: a randomized controlled trial. *JAMA*, 2008; Vol. 299: pp. 316–23.
  Comments: Results from the University Obesity Research Center.

Nissen SE, Nicholls SJ, Wolski K, et al. Comparison of pioglitazone vs glimepiride on progression of coronary atherosclerosis in patients with type 2 diabetes: the PERISCOPE randomized controlled trial. *JAMA*; 2008; Vol. 299: pp. 1561–73.
  Comments: A summary of the results of the PERISCOPE Study.

Adams TD, Gress RE, Smith SC, et al. Long-term mortality after gastric bypass surgery. *NEJM*, 2007; Vol. 357: pp. 753–61.
  Comments: Results of a study examining gastric bypass surgery long-term mortality.

Barnett AH, Burger J, Johns D, et al. Tolerability and efficacy of exenatide and titrated insulin glargine in adult patients with type 2 diabetes previously uncontrolled with metformin or a sulfonylurea: a multinational, randomized, open-label, two-period, crossover noninferiority trial. *Clin Ther*, 2007; Vol. 29: pp. 2333–48.
  Comments: Results of a study of exenetide versus insulin glargine.

Nissen SE, Wolski K. Effect of rosiglitazone on the risk of myocardial infarction and death from cardiovascular causes. *NEJM*, 2007; Vol. 356: pp. 2457–71.
  Comments: Meta-analysis of rosiglitazone on cardiovascular outcomes.

Sjöström L, Narbro K, Sjöström CD, et al. Effects of bariatric surgery on mortality in Swedish obese subjects. *NEJM*, 2007; Vol. 357: pp. 741–52.
  Comments: A summary of results from the Swedish Obesity Subjects study.

Skyler JS, Jovanovic L, Klioze S, et al. Two-year safety and efficacy of inhaled human insulin (Exubera) in adult patients with type 1 diabetes. *Diabetes Care*, 2007; Vol. 30: pp. 579–85.
  Comments: Safety study of the effects of inhaled insulin in adult patients with type 1 DM.

Aschner P, Kipnes MS, Lunceford JK, et al. Effect of the dipeptidyl peptidase-4 inhibitor sitagliptin as monotherapy on glycemic control in patients with type 2 diabetes. *Diabetes Care*, 2006; Vol. 29: pp. 2632–7.
  Comments: An early study of sitagliptin as monotherapy for T2DM patients.

Kahn SE, Haffner SM, Heise MA, et al. Glycemic durability of rosiglitazone, metformin, or glyburide monotherapy. *NEJM*, 2006; Vol. 355: pp. 2427–43.
  Comments: A summary of the results from the ADOPT study.

Shapiro AM, Rocordi C, Hering BJ, et al. International trial of the Edmonton protocol for islet transplantation. *NEJM*, 2006; Vol. 355: pp. 1318–30.

Dormandy JA, Charbonnel B, Eckland DJ, et al. Secondary prevention of macrovascular events in patients with type 2 diabetes in the PROactive Study (PROspective pioglitAzone Clinical Trial In macroVascular Events): a randomised controlled trial. *Lancet*, 2005; Vol. 366: pp. 1279–89.
  Comments: A summary of the results of the PROactive Study.

Goldberg RB, Kendall DM, Deeg MA, et al. A comparison of lipid and glycemic effects of pioglitazone and rosiglitazone in patients with type 2 diabetes and dyslipidemia. *Diabetes Care*, 2005; Vol. 28: pp. 1547–54.
  Comments: A study comparing effects of pioglitazone versus rosiglitazone on lipids.

Jacobson GF, Ramos GA, Ching JY, et al. Comparison of glyburide and insulin for the management of gestational diabetes in a large managed care organization. *Am J Obstet Gynecol*, 2005; Vol. 193: pp. 118–24.
  Comments: A study examining glyburide for treatment of gestational diabetes.

Aronoff S, Rosenblatt S, Braithwaite S, et al. Pioglitazone hydrochloride monotherapy improves glycemic control in the treatment of patients with type 2 diabetes: a 6-month randomized placebo-controlled dose-response study. The Pioglitazone 001 Study Group. *Diabetes Care*, 2000; Vol. 23: pp. 1605–11.
  Comments: A summary of results of the Pioglitazone 001 Study Group.

Langer O, Conway DL, Berkus MD, et al. A comparison of glyburide and insulin in women with gestational diabetes mellitus. *NEJM*, 2000; Vol. 343: pp. 1134–8.
  Comments: A study examining glyburide for treatment of gestational diabetes.

Shapiro AM, Lakey JR, Ryan EA, et al. Islet transplantation in seven patients with type 1 diabetes mellitus using a glucocorticoid-free immunosuppressive regimen. *NEJM*, 2000; Vol. 343: pp. 230–8.
  Comments: A summary of the results of a study of islet transplantation.

UK Prospective Diabetes Study (UKPDS) Group. Effect of intensive blood-glucose control with metformin on complications in overweight patients with type 2 diabetes (UKPDS 34). *Lancet*, 1998; Vol. 352: pp. 854–65.
  Comments: A summary of the results of the UKPDS Group 34 Study.

The Bypass Angioplasty Revascularization Investigation (BARI) Investigators. Comparison of coronary bypass surgery with angioplasty in patients with multivessel disease. *NEJM*, 1996; Vol. 335: pp. 217–25.
  Comments: A summary of the results of The Bypass Angioplasty Revascularization Investigation.

Saudek CD, Duckworth WC, Giobbie-Hurder A, et al. Implantable insulin pump vs multiple-dose insulin for non-insulin-dependent diabetes mellitus: a randomized clinical trial. Department of Veterans Affairs Implantable Insulin Pump Study Group. *JAMA*, 1996; Vol. 276: pp. 1322–7.
  Comments: Department of Veteran Affairs Implantable Insulin Pump Study Group.

DeFronzo RA, Goodman AM. Efficacy of metformin in patients with non-insulin-dependent diabetes mellitus. The Multicenter Metformin Study Group. *NEJM*, 1995; Vol. 333: pp. 541–9.
  Comments: A summary of the results of The Multicenter Metformin Study Group.

Hoffmann J, Spengler M. Efficacy of 24-week monotherapy with acarbose, glibenclamide, or placebo in NIDDM patients. The Essen Study. *Diabetes Care*, 1994; Vol. 17: pp. 561–6.
  Comments: A summary of the results of the Essen Study.

Nolan JJ, Ludvik B, Beerdsen P, et al. Improvement in glucose tolerance and insulin resistance in obese subjects treated with troglitazone. *NEJM*, 1994; Vol. 331: pp. 1188–93.
  Comments: A study of troglitazone benefits on insulin resistance.

Nathan DM, Roussell A, Godine JE. Glyburide or insulin for metabolic control in non-insulin-dependent diabetes mellitus. A randomized, double-blind study. *Ann Intern Med*, 1988; Vol. 108: pp. 334–40.
  Comments: A study examining efficacy of glyburide on glycemic control.

Meinert CL, Knatterud GL, Prout TE, et al. A study of the effects of hypoglycemic agents on vascular complications in patients with adult-onset diabetes. II. Mortality results. *Diabetes*, 1970; Vol. 19: pp. 789–830.
  Comments: A summary of the results of a study from the University Group Diabetes Program.

SECTION 2
MANAGEMENT

DIABETIC KETOACIDOSIS (DKA)

Rita Rastogi Kalyani, MD, MHS

DEFINITION

- A metabolic acidosis characterized by the triad of hyperglycemia (glucose >250 mg/dl), metabolic acidosis (arterial pH ≤7.3, serum bicarbonate ≤18 mEq/L) and moderate ketonuria or ketonemia.
- Most, but not all, patients have type 1 diabetes.
- Patients with type 2 diabetes also susceptible during acute illness (especially of African American or Hispanic descent) referred to as "ketosis-prone type 2 diabetes," likely due to greater relative insulinopenia (Linfoot).

EPIDEMIOLOGY

- Most patients 18–44 years (56%); two-thirds have type 1 diabetes and one-third have type 2 diabetes (Kitabchi; Wang).
- Mortality rates <1% in adults, >5% in elderly, but most common cause of death in children and adolescents with type 1 diabetes (CDC).
- Infection most common precipitant.
- Other common causes: myocardial infarction, pancreatitis, failure of insulin delivery from pump, nonadherence, psychological factors, drugs (e.g., steroids, thiazides).
- Often the presenting manifestation in new-onset type 1 diabetes.
- 35% increase in number of hospitalizations over a decade with DKA as discharge diagnosis, rising from 93,000 (1995) to 120,000 (2005) discharges in the US (CDC).
- More than one-third of hospitalizations are repeat DKA admissions (CDC).
- Average length of stay declined from 7.9 days in 1980 to 3.6 days in 2005 (CDC).
- No significant differences by age, sex, ethnicity in emergency room visits for DKA, although trend towards increased DKA visits among blacks, perhaps due to ketosis-prone diabetes (Ginde).
- DKA episodes represent 1 out of every 4 dollars spent on medical care for patients with type I diabetes (Javor). Cost of avoidable hospitalizations due to short-term uncontrolled diabetes including DKA is $2.8 billion USD (Kim).

DIAGNOSIS

- Can develop rapidly, in less than 24 hours, especially if an insulin pump stops delivery for any reason.
- Perform a thorough physical examination looking for evidence of deep, rapid breathing (Kussmaul respiration), dehydration, volume depletion, and an underlying precipitant.
- Arterial blood gas to assess acidosis and respiratory compensation; venous pH can be used after initial draw by adding 0.03 to venous pH value.
- Serum and urine ketones to identify ketosis as cause of acidosis. Caveat: positive ketones can occur with fasting (bicarbonate usually not <18 mEq/L) or alcohol (glucose rarely >200 mg/dl); false positive ketones with captopril, sulfhydryl drugs.

- Further laboratory tests include complete blood cell count (WBC frequently >10,000 mm³), electrolytes, blood urea nitrogen, creatinine, transaminases, amylase, lipase, cardiac enzymes, lactate, plasma osmolality, toxicology screen, urinalysis.
- Correct serum sodium by adding 1.6 mEq/L to the measured Na⁺ for each 100 mg/dl glucose above 100 mg/dl; elevated corrected Na⁺ reflects dehydration.
- Hyperkalemia and hyperphosphatemia may exist despite actual total body depletion due to extracellular shifts associated with insulin deficiency.
- High anion gap reflects degree of acidosis and hydration, calculated as: $Na^+ - (Cl^- + HCO3^-)$ (mEq/L). Use uncorrected Na⁺. Normal anion gap (AG) = serum albumin × 3. High AG >10–12 mEq/L.
- Calculated osmolality should be compared with measured osmolality to exclude unmeasured osmoles (ethanol, methanol) if toxic ingestion suspected; serum osmolality (mOsm/L) = $2(Na^+ + K^+)$ (mEq/L) + Glucose (mg/dl)/18 + BUN (mg/dl)/2.8.
- Electrocardiogram, chest X-ray, and urine, sputum, or blood cultures should also be considered.

SIGNS AND SYMPTOMS

- **Signs:** poor skin turgor, dry mucous membranes, absence of axillary sweat, tachycardia, orthostatic hypotension, Kussmaul respirations (rapid and deep breathing as respiratory compensation for metabolic acidosis), fruity breath odor from ketonemia, emesis and abdominal guarding, guaiac-positive stools resulting from hemorrhagic gastritis.
- **Symptoms:** polyuria, polydipsia, weight loss, dehydration, weakness, fatigue, nausea, vomiting, "air hunger", abdominal pain, fatigue, stupor, coma, seizures.
- Altered mental status (usually when serum osmolality ≥360 mOsm/L), hypotension, and severe comorbidities identifies those at highest risk for a bad outcome.
- See Table 2-1 for risk stratification of DKA.

TABLE 2-1. RISK STRATIFICATION OF DKA (GLUCOSE >250 mg/dl)

	Mild	Moderate	Severe
Arterial pH	7.25–7.30	7.00–7.24	<7.00
Serum bicarbonate (mEq/L)	15–18	10–15	<10
Urine ketone	Positive	Positive	Positive
Serum ketone	Positive	Positive	Positive
Effective serum osmolality	Variable	Variable	Variable
Anion gap	>10	>12	>12
Mental status	Alert	Alert/drowsy	Stupor/coma

Source: Kitabchi AE, Nyenwe EA. Hyperglycemic crises in diabetes mellitus: diabetic ketoacidosis and hyperglycemic hyperosmolar state. *Endocrinol Metab Clin North Am,* 2006; Vol. 35(4): pp. 725–51, viii. Reprinted with permission from Elsevier.

CLINICAL TREATMENT

Fluid Therapy

- Goal is to expand intravascular, interstitial, and intracellular volume and restore renal perfusion.
- Fluid replacement should correct estimated deficits in 24 hours. Average fluid deficit 6 L.
- Potassium replacement must be initiated concurrently with fluid therapy if K+ <5.2 mEq/L.
- In absence of cardiac compromise, isotonic saline (0.9% NaCl) infused at 15–20 ml*kg body weight^{-1}*h^{-1} or 1–1.5 L during first hour and then continued at this rate for severe dehydration.
- Normal or elevated corrected sodium: 0.45% NaCl infused at 250–500 ml/h after first hour depending on hydration status for mild dehydration.
- Low corrected serum sodium: 0.9% NaCl at 250–500 ml/h after first hour depending on hydration status for mild dehydration.
- Measure improvement by monitoring blood pressure, fluid input/output, laboratory values, physical examination.
- In patients with cardiac or renal compromise, monitor more carefully to avoid iatrogenic volume overload.
- Hyperglycemia (glucose >250 mg/dl) corrected faster than ketoacidosis (pH >7.30, bicarbonate >18 mEq/L); mean duration 6 hours versus 12 hours.
- Once plasma glucose ≤200 mg/dl, change to 5% dextrose with 0.45% NaCl at 125–250 ml/hr to allow continued insulin therapy until ketonemia is resolved.

Insulin Therapy

- Insulin therapy effective in DKA regardless of route (intravenous, subcutaneous)
- Continuous intravenous infusion of regular insulin preferred due to short half-life and easy titration; glucose should be checked every hour while on IV insulin infusion using glucometer and at least every 2–4 hours by laboratory testing. Rapid-acting analogs such as lispro, aspart, and glulisine insulin may be as effective during the acute treatment of DKA but require further investigation (Kitabchi; Umpierrez).
- Either 0.1 U/kg body weight as IV bolus followed by 0.1 U/kg/hr IV continuous insulin infusion or 0.14 U/kg body weight/hr without bolus.
- If glucose does not fall by 50–75 mg/dl in first hour, increase insulin infusion until steady glucose decline achieved. Alternatively, if glucose does not fall by 10% in first hour, give IV bolus of 0.14 U/kg and resume previous treatment.
- When glucose falls below 200 mg/dl, reduce regular insulin infusion to 0.02–0.05 U/kg/hr IV, or give rapid-acting insulin 0.1 U/kg subcutaneously to maintain glucose between 125–200 mg/dl until ketosis resolved.
- In patients with mild DKA, subcutaneous rapid-acting insulin in nonintensive care settings may be as safe and effective as intravenous insulin therapy.
- Resolution of ketoacidosis includes blood glucose <200 mg/dl, and two of the following: serum bicarbonate >15 mEq/L, pH >7.3, or calculated anion gap <12 mEq/L.
- To transition to subcutaneous insulin after resolution, give overlap of at least 1–2 hours between discontinuation of IV insulin and administration of subcutaneous insulin. Human insulin (NPH and regular) regimens are usually given in two or three doses per day. Basal-bolus regimens with basal (glargine and detemir) and rapid-acting (lispro,

aspart, or glulisine) insulin analogs may be more physiologic in patients with type 1 diabetes.

- In patients who were previously well controlled on insulin, resume previous regimen; in insulin-naive patients, total insulin dosage should be 0.5–0.8 U/kg/day divided in multiple doses with dose modifications based on insulin needs during hospitalization (see Type 1 Diabetes: Insulin Treatment, p. 155).

Correction of Electrolyte Imbalances

- **Potassium:** First establish adequate renal function (urine output >50 ml/hr). If K^+ <3.3 mEq/L, hold insulin and give 20–30 mEq/hr until K^+ >3.3 mEq/L. If K^+ >5.2 mEq/L, do not give K^+ but check serum K^+ every 2 hours. If K^+ between 3.3–5.2 mEq/L, give 20–30 mEq K^+ in each liter of IV fluid to keep K^+ between 4–5 mEq/L.
- **Bicarbonate:** If pH ≥6.9, do not supplement with bicarbonate. If pH <6.9, give 100 mmol bicarbonate in 400 mmol water + 20 mEq KCl and infuse for 2 hours; repeat every 2 hours until pH >7.
- **Phosphate:** In patients with cardiac dysfunction, anemia, respiratory compromise or serum phosphate <1.0 mg/dl, 20–30 mEq potassium phosphate in replacement fluids may be considered (maximum tolerated rate 4.5 mmol/hr or 1.5 ml/h).
- **Magnesium:** Often depleted, replace to maintain goal of >2 mg/dl and help with resolution of hypokalemia.
- Serum electrolyte panel including BUN and creatinine should be checked every 2–4 hours to monitor electrolyte imbalances and resolution of anion gap.

Complications

- Common: hypoglycemia and hypokalemia due to overtreatment with insulin and bicarbonate.
- Hyperchloremic non-anion gap acidosis can be seen in recovery phase and is self-limited.
- Cerebral edema occurs in 0.3%–1.0% of DKA episodes in children, rare in adults, and associated with high mortality rate. Symptoms include headache, seizures, sphincter incontinence, pupillary changes, high blood pressure, low heart rate, respiratory depression, and deterioration in consciousness. Preventive measures include gradual reduction of plasma osmolarity and glucose, and avoiding aggressive hydration. Treatment includes mannitol and mechanical ventilation.

FOLLOW-UP

- In patients with ketosis-prone type 2 diabetes, 40% still noninsulin dependent at 10 years (Mauvais-Jarvis).

EXPERT OPINION

- Hypokalemia is the most frequent cause of death during treatment of DKA; pay close attention to potassium replacement.
- Fluid therapy will decrease blood glucose, but insulin therapy is necessary for resolution of ketonemia. Correction of electrolyte imbalances is especially important to preserve cardiac, neurologic, and respiratory function.
- Patients often need to be monitored on general medicine floor or intensive care unit until DKA is resolved.
- Euglycemic DKA (glucose ≤250 mg/dl) could be due to many factors, including insulin injection en route to hospital or antecedent food restriction.

MANAGEMENT

- DKA and hyperosmotic states often overlap, with some degree of both hyperosmolarity and ketoacidosis.
- Nausea, vomiting, diffuse abdominal pain, often with elevated WBC and liver enzymes, are more frequent in patients with DKA (>50%) than in hyperosmolar hyperglycemic state.
- Since IV insulin disappears from blood with a half-life of <6 minutes, subcutaneously delivered insulin must be given before stopping IV insulin, to avoid relapse into DKA.
- Most cases of DKA can be prevented with better healthcare access, patient education (especially sick day management), and early contact with a healthcare provider.
- Home glucose ketone monitoring may guide insulin therapy at home and possibly prevent hospitalization.
- Explore possible economic reasons for self-discontinuation of insulin therapy, especially among minority populations, and help provide resources to overcome barriers.

BASIS FOR RECOMMENDATIONS

Kitabchi AE, Umpierrez GE, Miles JM, et al. Hyperglycemic crises in adult patients with diabetes. *Diabetes Care*, 2009; Vol. 32: pp. 1335–43.

    Comments: ADA consensus statement for management of DKA and HHS.

OTHER REFERENCES

Umpierrez GE, Jones S, Smiley D, et al. Insulin analogs versus human insulin in the treatment of patients with diabetic ketoacidosis: a randomized controlled trial. *Diabetes Care*, 2009; Vol. 32: pp. 1164–9.

    Comments: Regular and glulisine insulin are equally effective during the acute treatment of DKA.

Kitabchi AE, Umpierrez GE, Fisher JN, et al. Thirty years of personal experience in hyperglycemic crises: diabetic ketoacidosis and hyperglycemic hyperosmolar state. *J Clin Endocrinol Metab*, 2008; Vol. 93: pp. 1541–52.

    Comments: Summarizes prospective studies on the management and pathophysiology of DKA.

Wang ZH, Kihl-Selstam E, Eriksson JW. Ketoacidosis occurs in both Type 1 and Type 2 diabetes—a population-based study from Northern Sweden. *Diabet Med*, 2008; Vol. 25: pp. 867–70.

    Comments: Contrasts clinical presentation of DKA in type 1 and type 2 diabetes; type 2 diabetes accounted for one-third of all cases.

Kitabchi AE, Nyenwe EA. Hyperglycemic crises in diabetes mellitus: diabetic ketoacidosis and hyperglycemic hyperosmolar state. *Endocrinol Metab Clin North Am*, 2006; Vol. 35: pp. 725–51, viii.

    Comments: Comprehensive technical review of DKA and HHS.

Ginde AA, Pelletier AJ, Camargo CA. National study of U.S. emergency department visits with diabetic ketoacidosis, 1993–2003. *Diabetes Care*, 2006; Vol. 29: pp. 2117–9.

    Comments: Describes number of emergency room visits for DKA and demographic trends.

Centers for Disease Control and Prevention (CDC). Diabetes Data and Trends. *http://www.cdc.gov/diabetes/statistics/hospitalization_national.htm*. Accessed February 23, 2011.

    Comments: Describes US trends for diabetes hospitalizations from 1980–2006, including DKA.

Linfoot P, Bergstrom C, Ipp E. Pathophysiology of ketoacidosis in Type 2 diabetes mellitus. *Diabet Med*, 2005; Vol. 22: pp. 1414–9.

    Comments: Explores possible explanations for DKA in type 2 diabetes including free fatty acids, growth hormone and suppression of insulin. Individuals with ketosis-prone type 2 diabetes had greater insulinopenia compared to those with nonketosis-prone type 2 diabetes.

Mauvais-Jarvis F, Sobngwi E, Porcher R, et al. Ketosis-prone type 2 diabetes in patients of sub-Saharan African origin: clinical pathophysiology and natural history of beta-cell dysfunction and insulin resistance. *Diabetes*, 2004; Vol. 53: pp. 645–53.

Comments: Describes probability of remission and need for long-term insulin among African patients with ketosis-prone type 2 diabetes.

Javor KA, Kotsanos JG, McDonald RC, et al. Diabetic ketoacidosis charges relative to medical charges of adult patients with type I diabetes. *Diabetes Care,* 1997; Vol. 20: pp. 349–54.

Comments: The direct medical care charges associated with DKA episodes represented 28.1% of the direct medical care charges for a cohort of 228 patients with type I diabetes. The average charge per DKA episode was $6444.

Centers for Disease Control and Prevention (CDC). Hospitalizations for diabetic ketoacidosis—Washington State, 1987–1989. *MMWR,* 1992; Vol. 41: pp. 837–9.

Comments: Summarizes surveillance of DKA hospitalizations among Washington State residents from 1987 through 1989.

HYPEROSMOLAR HYPERGLYCEMIC STATE (HHS)

Vanessa Walker Harris, MD, and Rita Rastogi Kalyani, MD, MHS

DEFINITION

- Characterized by severe hyperglycemia, hyperosmolality, and dehydration in the absence of significant ketoacidosis (plasma glucose >600 mg/dl, arterial pH >7.30, serum bicarbonate >18 mEq/L, effective serum osmolality >320 mOsm/kg) (Kitabchi).
- Initiated by osmotic diuresis due to hyperglycemia. Maintained by insulin levels sufficient to prevent lipolysis and subsequent ketogenesis, but inadequate to appropriately reduce blood glucose levels (Stoner).
- Can be associated with proinflammatory state, reversed by effective hydration and insulin treatment (Kitabchi).
- Usually seen in patients with type 2 diabetes (T2DM), in whom it may be the initial presentation. Rarely occurs in children or patients with type 1 diabetes (Stoner; Nugent).

EPIDEMIOLOGY

- Mortality rates 5%–20%; significantly higher >70 years of age. Early mortality (<72 hrs) more common and likely due to sepsis, shock, or underlying illness. Late mortality (>72 hrs) usually due to thromboembolic events or the effects of therapy (Kitabchi; Trence; Magee; Nugent).
- Infection (e.g., pneumonia, urinary tract infection) most common precipitating factor. Other common causes: medication noncompliance, undiagnosed diabetes, myocardial infarction, pancreatitis, cerebrovascular accident, medications (calcium channel blockers, thiazide diuretics, atypical antipsychotics), and drug use (alcohol, cocaine). Endocrine causes include thyrotoxicosis, Cushing's syndrome, and acromegaly.
- In children, long-term steroid use and gastroenteritis common causes (Kitabchi; Stoner; Trence).
- Underlying medical illnesses that compromise access to water or promote release of counterregulatory hormones (i.e., catecholamines, glucagon, cortisol, growth hormone) can result in severe dehydration and predispose to HHS (Kitabchi).
- Mean age of presentation 57–69 years.
- Common in nursing home residents (28%) (Delaney; Nugent).

MANAGEMENT

DIAGNOSIS

- Usually evolves over several days to weeks.
- Thorough history and physical examination, looking for signs (below), and an underlying precipitant (listed previously).
- Plasma glucose (>600 mg/dl), electrolytes with calculated anion gap (serum bicarbonate >18 mEq/L), osmolality (>320 mOsm/kg), arterial blood gas to assess acidosis (pH >7.30), serum and urinary ketones to identify ketosis (may be present from dehydration).
- Corrected serum sodium calculated by adding 1.6 mEq/L to the measured Na^+ for each 100 mg/dl of glucose above 100 mg/dl. Elevated corrected serum sodium reflects dehydration, and the value can be used to calculate free water deficit: Total Body Water (TBW) × [(Current (corrected) serum Na/Desired serum Na) −1], where TBW is weight (kg) * % water (varies by gender and age; % water ~60%). Example: TBW = 0.6 × 70 kg man = 42, Corrected Serum Sodium = 160 mEq/L; Free Water Deficit = 42 × [160/140 −1] = 6 L.
- Additional laboratory: blood urea nitrogen (mean 65 mg/dl); serum creatinine (mean 3 mg/dl); blood count with differential (leukocytosis may be present even in the absence of infection); electrocardiogram; chest X-ray; toxicology; transaminases (abnormal in up to one-third of patients with uncontrolled diabetes); lipase and amylase (elevations may suggest pancreatitis); creatine kinase (abnormal in up to two-thirds of patients) and urine, sputum, or blood cultures to exclude infection.
- Anion gap is calculated as $Na-(Cl^- + HCO3^-)$ (mEq/L). Use uncorrected Na^+. Normal anion gap = serum albumin × 3. About 50% of patients have mild anion gap acidosis (Stoner; Magee).
- Effective serum osmolarity reflects tonicity and is calculated as (2 × Na mEq/L) + Glucose (mg/dl)/18 + BUN (mg/dl)/2.8. Note that serum Na is the main contributor to osmolarity.
- Serum levels of potassium, magnesium, and phosphate are typically normal or elevated despite actual total body depletion due to shifts from the intracellular to the extracellular space due to insulin deficiency (Stoner; Magee).
- Prerenal azotemia (elevated BUN out of proportion to elevated creatinine) often present.
- Elevated creatine kinase usually due to dehydration, but need to consider rhabdomyolysis.

SIGNS AND SYMPTOMS

- **Signs:** poor skin turgor; dry mucous membranes; cool extremities; tachycardia; hypotension; low-grade fever or hypothermia; tachypnea; abdominal distention (possibly due to gastroparesis induced by hypertonicity); focal neurologic signs such as seizures, hemianopia, hemiparesis, aphasia, myoclonus, dysphagia (Kitabchi; Stoner; Magee).
- **Symptoms:** polyuria, polydipsia, weakness, weight loss, visual disturbance, leg cramps, nausea, vomiting, and abdominal pain (less common in HHS and may suggest intraabdominal pathology), lethargy, confusion, stupor, coma (occurs with effective serum osmolality >350 mOsm/L) (Kitabchi; Stoner; Magee).
- The presence of coma or hypotension is associated with poor prognosis. Mortality increases with increasing age and with higher levels of serum osmolality (Nugent).
- See Table 2-2 for diagnostic criteria.

TABLE 2-2. DIAGNOSTIC CRITERIA FOR HHS

Arterial pH	>7.30
Serum bicarbonate (mEq/L)	>18
Urine ketones	Small
Serum ketones	Small
Effective serum osmolality	>320 mOsm/kg
Anion gap	Variable
Mental status	Stupor/coma if >~360 mOsm/kg

Source: Kitabchi AE, Umpierrez GE, Miles JM, Fisher JN. Hyperglycemic crises in adult patients with diabetes. *Diabetes Care*, 2009; Vol. 32(7): pp. 1335–43. Reproduced with permission of The American Diabetes Association.

CLINICAL TREATMENT

Fluid Therapy

- Goal to expand intravascular, interstitial, and intracellular volume and restore renal perfusion (Kitabchi).
- On average, fluid deficits 100–200 ml/kg, 20%–25% of body water, 12% of body weight, or approximately 9 L. One-half of the calculated deficit should be replaced in the first 18–24 hours, and the remainder over the next 24 hours (Kitabchi; Trence; Stoner).
- In absence of cardiac compromise, isotonic saline (0.9% NaCL) infused at 15–20 ml*kg body wt-1*h-1 or 1–1.5 L during the first hour (Kitabchi).
- Normal or elevated corrected serum sodium: 0.45% NaCl infused at 250–500 ml/h after the first hour (Kitabchi).
- Low corrected sodium: 0.9% NaCl at 250–500 ml/h after the first hour (Kitabchi).
- Successful fluid replacement assessed by hemodynamic monitoring, measuring fluid input/output, laboratory values, and clinical examination (Kitabchi).
- In patients with cardiac or renal compromise, monitor serum osmolality and clinical exam more frequently to avoid iatrogenic volume overload (Kitabchi).
- Fluids alone can decrease serum glucose levels by 80–200 mg/dl/hour. Once serum glucose <300 mg/dl, change fluid to 5% dextrose with 0.45% NaCl to prevent cerebral edema from too rapid correction of hyperosmolality (Delaney; Stoner; Trence).

Insulin Therapy

- Adequate fluids must be given before initiation of insulin; otherwise hypotension, vascular collapse, or death can occur due to intracellular shifting of water (Stoner; Kitabchi; Delaney; Trence).
- Continuous intravenous infusion of regular insulin is preferred due to its short half-life and easy titration; capillary blood glucose should be checked by glucometer every hour while on IV insulin infusion and plasma glucose at least every 2–4 hours (Stoner; Kitabchi).
- Give an initial bolus of 0.1 units/kg, followed by a continuous insulin infusion of 0.1 units/kg/hr or 0.14 units/kg continuous insulin infusion without bolus (Stoner; Kitabchi).

MANAGEMENT

- If glucose level does not fall by 50–75 mg/dl/hr, then increase the insulin infusion rate until a steady glucose decline is achieved (Stoner; Kitabchi).
- When plasma glucose <300 mg/dl, decrease insulin infusion to 0.02–0.05 units/kg/hr to keep glucose between 250–300 mg/dl until patient mentally alert (Kitabchi, Stoner).
- Once hyperosmolar state resolves and patient able to eat, initiate subcutaneous insulin. To transition to subcutaneous insulin, allow an overlap of 1–2 hours between administration of subcutaneous insulin and discontinuation of the intravenous insulin drip. If patient NPO, continue IV insulin (Stoner; Kitabchi).
- In insulin-naive patients, total daily dosage should be 0.5–0.8 units/kg divided into multiple doses (Kitabchi).
- Some patients can be controlled on small doses of subcutaneous insulin and may be later transitioned to oral hypoglycemic agents upon discharge (Delaney; Stoner; Kitabchi).

Correction of Electrolyte Imbalances

- Potassium: establish adequate renal function (urine output >50 ml/hr). If K^+ >5.2 mEq, do not give K^+, but check serum K^+ every 2 hrs. If K^+ is 3.3–5.2 mEq/L, give 20–30 mEq K^+ in each liter of IV fluid for goal serum K^+ 4–5 mEq/L. If K^+ <3 mEq/L, hold insulin and give 20–30 mEq/hr until K^+ >3.3 mEq/L (Kitabchi; Stoner; Delaney).
- Phosphate and calcium: no controlled data to suggest improved outcomes with phosphate replacement. Consider replacement with potassium phosphate if serum phosphate level <1 mEq/L and muscle weakness is a concern. Monitor serum calcium carefully due to risk of severe, symptomatic hypocalcemia (Delaney; Stoner).
- Magnesium: often depleted in uncontrolled diabetes. Replace to maintain goal >2 mEq/dl. Correcting hypomagnesemia will aid in resolution of hypokalemia (Stoner).
- Bicarbonate: No indication for repletion with bicarbonate unless lactic acidosis results in pH <7 (Magee).
- Serum electrolyte panel including BUN and creatinine should be checked every 2–4 hours to monitor electrolyte imbalances (Kitabchi).

COMPLICATIONS

- Common: hypoglycemia, hypokalemia, inadequate volume replacement, sudden large volume shifts, premature discontinuance of insulin therapy (Delaney).
- Vascular occlusions (mesenteric ischemia, myocardial infarction, disseminated intravascular coagulopathy) occur due to increased viscosity and hypercoagulability. Treat with full-dose heparin or low-molecular-weight heparin if there is clinical evidence of thrombosis (Magee; Stoner).
- Atraumatic rhabdomyolysis with or without acute tubular necrosis may occur in patients with decompensated diabetes and is associated with increased mortality (Magee; Stoner).
- Cerebral edema and acute respiratory distress syndrome due to overhydration are rare but often fatal in children and young adults. Treatment of cerebral edema includes intravenous mannitol, mechanical ventilation, and intravenous dexamethasone (Stoner).

FOLLOW-UP

- Patient education focused on encouraging adherence to blood glucose monitoring and compliance with prescribed medications coupled with adequate follow-up to establish a durable diabetes management regimen (Delaney; Stoner; Kitabchi).

- Sick day management education to encourage early contact with healthcare providers; review of blood glucose goals and appropriate use of insulin; and starting liquid diet containing carbohydrates and salt when nauseated (Kitabchi; Stoner; Trence).
- Review with nursing home staff the importance of adequate fluid intake and close monitoring of hydration status in patients with diabetes (Trence; Stoner).
- Avoid medications that interfere with effectiveness of insulin (Delaney).

EXPERT OPINION

- Compared to diabetic ketoacidosis: mortality rates are considerably higher; symptoms develop over a longer period of time; usually less ketosis and greater hyperglycemia.
- Suspect a mixed syndrome of DKA and HHS in patients with pH <7.3, ketonemia, osmolarity >320 mOsm/L (Delaney; Magee).
- Severe anion gap metabolic acidosis should prompt consideration of lactic acidosis or other non-HHS entities (Trence; Stoner).
- Abdominal distention, abdominal pain, nausea, or vomiting that persist after rehydration may be related to an acute intraabdominal process (Stoner; Magee).
- Focal neurologic signs such as seizures, hemiparesis, lethargy, coma often resolve with correction of fluid deficit and hyperglycemia (Stoner; Magee).
- Patients with hemodynamic instability, compromised airway, obtundation, or acute abdominal symptoms should be managed in the intensive care unit (Stoner; Magee).
- Mental status changes occur only with severe hyperosmolarity; coma usually only if osmolarity >360. Suspect other causes, e.g., stroke, if change in mental status with less severe hyperosmolarity.

MANAGEMENT

BASIS FOR RECOMMENDATIONS

Kitabchi AE, Umpierrez GE, Miles JM, et al. Hyperglycemic crises in adult patients with diabetes. *Diabetes Care*, 2009; Vol. 32: pp. 1335–43.

> **Comments:** Consensus statement outlining precipitating factors and recommendations for the diagnosis, treatment, and prevention of DKA and HHS.

OTHER REFERENCES

Nugent BW. Hyperosmolar hyperglycemic state. *Emerg Med Clin North Am*, 2005; Vol. 23: pp. 629–48, vii.

> **Comments:** Discussion of the emergency department management of HHS.

Stoner GD. Hyperosmolar hyperglycemic state. *Am Fam Physician*, 2005; Vol. 71: pp. 1723–30.

> **Comments:** Discussion of precipitating factors, diagnosis, and treatment of HHS.

Magee MF, Bhatt BA. Management of decompensated diabetes. Diabetic ketoacidosis and hyperglycemic hyperosmolar syndrome. *Crit Care Clin*, 2001; Vol. 17: pp. 75–106.

> **Comments:** Discussion of the management of DKA and HHS.

Trence DL, Hirsch IB. Hyperglycemic crises in diabetes mellitus type 2. *Endocrinol Metab Clin North Am*, 2001; Vol. 30: pp. 817–31.

> **Comments:** Focuses on management of decompensated diabetes, specifically HHS and DKA.

Delaney MF, Zisman A, Kettyle WM. Diabetic ketoacidosis and hyperglycemic hyperosmolar nonketotic syndrome. *Endocrinol Metab Clin North Am*, 2000; Vol. 29: pp. 683–705, v.

> **Comments:** Details the pathophysiology, clinical management, and prevention of DKA and HHS.

General Principles

DAWN PHENOMENON

Shivam Champaneri, MD, and Rita Rastogi Kalyani, MD, MHS

Definition
- The tendency for blood glucose to rise between 4 AM and 8 AM.
- To be clinically relevant, should have an increase of blood glucose by >10 mg/dl or an increased insulin requirement of 20% during these hours (Carroll).

Epidemiology
- Estimates of frequency range from 29%–91% in type 1 diabetes (Perriello; Koivisto; Edge; Havlin; Bending; Bolli), 6%–89% in type 2 (Carroll; Atiea; Havlin; Bolli). Overall, about 55% of patients likely experience the dawn phenomenon (Carroll).
- Mechanism: impaired insulin sensitivity in muscle and liver from nocturnal secretion of growth hormone. Growth hormone deficient patients do not have the dawn phenomenon. Dawn phenomenon is not inhibited by suppression of cortisol or catecholamines, suggesting that these hormones do not significantly contribute (Edge; Carroll).
- Poor glucose control is associated with higher magnitude and prevalence of the dawn phenomenon; in type 1 diabetes, longer duration associated with less dawn phenomenon (Perriello); however, in type 2 diabetes, longer duration, with worsening beta-cell function, hyperglycemia, and need for insulin therapy all contribute to more dawn phenomenon.

Diagnosis
- Blood glucose measurements at bedtime (10–11 PM) and early morning (2, 4, and 8 AM) should be obtained. Dawn phenomenon shows an abrupt increase between 4 AM and 8 AM, whereas waning of exogenous insulin effect shows gradual rise between 2 AM and 8 AM (see Table 2-3).
- No currently recognized role for obtaining growth hormone or IGF-1 levels in diagnosis.

Signs and Symptoms
- Signs and symptoms depend on the degree of early morning hyperglycemia.
- The following table illustrates the differentiation of dawn phenomenon from waning effect of exogenous insulin.

TABLE 2-3. DIFFERENTIAL DIAGNOSIS OF DAWN PHENOMENON (GLUCOSE IN MG/DL)

	10 PM	2 AM	4 AM	8 AM
Dawn phenomenon	100	110	135	250
Waning of insulin	100	160	220	270
Courtesy of Shivam Champaneri.

CLINICAL TREATMENT

Type 1 Diabetes

- The dawn phenomenon contributes to worse glucose control: in one study (Atiea), mean A1c was 9.5% in those with dawn phenomenon versus 8.4% without.
- Treatment may include intensifying insulin therapy to improve overall glycemic control (Perriello).
- Increasing bedtime basal insulin can be effective unless it causes nocturnal hypoglycemia.
- With insulin pump therapy, increase basal rate by at least 20% specifically in the predawn hours.
- Avoid late night snacking, unless appropriate quick-acting insulin is given.

Type 2 Diabetes

- Adjust diet content (decrease carbohydrates) and timing of the evening meal so that the glucose level at bedtime is 70–110 mg/dl.
- If dietary modification is not enough, consider an intermediate or long-acting sulfonylurea at evening meal.
- Basal insulin is indicated if the dawn phenomenon continues.
- For patients with type 2 diabetes on insulin, treatment similar to type 1 diabetes.

FOLLOW-UP

- Continued monitoring of early morning blood glucose levels while therapy is being modified to assess efficacy and continued need for dietary or pharmacologic adjustments.

EXPERT OPINION

- Insulin glargine and detemir, with their slower duration of action, cause less nocturnal hypoglycemia than NPH insulin.
- Antecedant nocturnal hypoglycemia causing morning hyperglycemia has been called the "Somogyi effect," but evidence suggests that nocturnal hypoglycemia is *not* a cause of significant morning hyperglycemia (Tordjman).

REFERENCES

Carroll MF, Schade DS. The dawn phenomenon revisited: implications for diabetes therapy. *Endocr Pract*, 2005; Vol. 11: pp. 55–64.

  Comments: This article is an excellent review of the literature that summarizes data on prevalence, pathogenesis, and management of the dawn phenomenon.

Sheehan JP. Fasting hyperglycemia: etiology, diagnosis, and treatment. *Diabetes Technol Ther*, 2004; Vol. 6: pp. 525–33.

  Comments: This is a review of causes and treatment of morning hyperglycemia amongst type 1 and type 2 diabetes patients.

Masharani U, Karam JH. Diabetes mellitus and hypoglycemia. In: Tierney LMJ, McPhee SJ, Papadakis MA, eds. *2002 Current Medical Diagnosis and Treatment: Adult Ambulatory and In-Patient Management*. New York: McGraw-Hill; 2002: pp. 1203–1250.

  Comments: This is a textbook chapter summarizing diabetes and its management in the outpatient setting, including handling the dawn phenomenon.

Carroll MF, Hardy KJ, Burge MR, et al. Frequency of the dawn phenomenon in type 2 diabetes: implications for diabetes therapy. *Diabetes Technol Ther*, 2002; Vol. 4: pp. 595–605.

  Comments: This study of 16 type 2 diabetes found that most patients failed to secrete growth hormone during insulin-induced hypoglycemia and noted rare occurrence of the dawn phenomenon.

Bolli GB, Perriello G, Fanelli CG, et al. Nocturnal blood glucose control in type I diabetes mellitus. *Diabetes Care*, 1993; Vol.16 Suppl 3: pp.71–89.

MANAGEMENT

Comments: This is a review of dawn phenomenon and Somogyi effect in type 1 diabetes patients and the limitations of certain insulin treatment modalities.

Atiea JA, Luzio S, Owens DR. The dawn phenomenon and diabetes control in treated NIDDM and IDDM patients. *Diabetes Res Clin Pract*, 1992; Vol. 16: pp. 183–90.
Comments: This study found that poorly controlled diabetic patients had higher morning hour glucose rises compared to well-controlled patients.

Perriello G, De Feo P, Torlone E, et al. The dawn phenomenon in type 1 (insulin-dependent) diabetes mellitus: magnitude, frequency, variability, and dependency on glucose counterregulation and insulin sensitivity. *Diabetologia*, 1991; Vol. 34: pp. 21–8.
Comments: This study of 114 type 1 diabetes patients found 101 patients had an increase in insulin requirement in the morning hours, and it correlated inversely with the duration of diabetes.

Bolli GB, Perriello G. Impact of activated glucose counterregulation on insulin requirements in insulin-dependent diabetes mellitus. *Horm Metab Res Suppl*, 1990; Vol. 24: pp. 87–96.
Comments: This is a review of the role of counterregulatory states in insulin-dependent diabetes for dawn phenomenon and Somogyi effect.

Edge JA, Matthews DR, Dunger DB. The dawn phenomenon is related to overnight growth hormone release in adolescent diabetics. *Clin Endocrinol* (Oxford, UK), 1990; Vol. 33: pp. 729–37.
Comments: 26 diabetic adolescents were studied in insulin clamp settings with the finding of an increase in insulin infusion rate in the early morning hours with correlation with mean overnight growth hormone concentration. With growth hormone blockade, insulin requirements in the early morning diminished.

Atiea JA, Vora JP, Owens DR, et al. Non-insulin-dependent diabetic patients (NIDDMs) do not demonstrate the dawn phenomenon at presentation. *Diabetes Res Clin Pract*, 1988; Vol. 5: pp. 37–44.
Comments: This study of 17 newly diagnosed type 2 diabetes patients and 11 patients after 1 year of treatment noted that no dawn phenomenon was noted in new patients, but a significant rise in glucose was observed in patients having been treated for one year.

Atiea JA, Ryder RR, Vora J, et al. Dawn phenomenon: its frequency in non-insulin-dependent diabetic patients on conventional therapy. *Diabetes Care*, 1987; Vol. 10: pp. 461–5.
Comments: 19 type 2 diabetes patients were studied with 17 noted to have a dawn rise of plasma glucose with a noted rise in insulin during those hours in both diet alone treated and diet plus oral agents.

Havlin CE, Cryer PE. Nocturnal hypoglycemia does not commonly result in major morning hyperglycemia in patients with diabetes mellitus. *Diabetes Care*, 1987; Vol. 10: pp. 141–7.
Comments: This study of 75 diabetes patients noted that the dawn phenomenon was present in only a third of patients, and nocturnal hypoglycemia did not commonly result in major morning hyperglycemia (Somogyi phenomenon).

Tordjman KM, Havlin CE, Levandoski LA, et al. Failure of nocturnal hypoglycemia to cause fasting hyperglycemia in patients with insulin-dependent diabetes mellitus. *NEJM*, 1987; Vol. 317: pp. 1552–9.
Comments: A clinical trial inducing nocturnal hypoglycemia under controlled circumstances did not find that it was associated with morning hyperglycemia.

Koivisto VA, Yki-Järvinen H, Helve E, et al. Pathogenesis and prevention of the dawn phenomenon in diabetic patients treated with CSII. *Diabetes*, 1986; Vol. 35: pp. 78–82.
Comments: This study of 12 type 1 diabetes patients treated with continuous subcutaneous insulin infusion and noted increase in insulin requirement in the early morning hours with higher growth hormone levels compared to controls.

Bending JJ, Pickup JC, Collins AC, et al. Rarity of a marked "dawn phenomenon" in diabetic subjects treated by continuous subcutaneous insulin infusion. *Diabetes Care*, 1985; Vol. 8: pp. 28–33.
Comments: In studying 41 insulin-dependent diabetes patients treated with insulin pumps, marked dawn phenomenon was rare when a single adequate basal infusion rate was used.

Bolli GB, Gerich JE. The "dawn phenomenon"—a common occurrence in both non-insulin-dependent and insulin-dependent diabetes mellitus. *NEJM,* 1984; Vol. 310: pp. 746–50.

Comments: Among 20 insulin-dependent diabetes patients and 13 non-insulin-dependent diabetes patients, 76% were noted to have an increase in insulin requirements in the early morning hours amongst both groups.

Schmidt MI, Hadji-Georgopoulos A, Rendell M, et al. The dawn phenomenon, an early morning glucose rise: implications for diabetic intraday blood glucose variation. *Diabetes Care,* 1982; Vol. 4: pp. 579–85.

Comments: This is the first description of the dawn phenomenon.

HYPOGLYCEMIA: PREVENTION AND TREATMENT

Ari Eckman, MD, and Sherita Hill Golden, MD, MHS

DEFINITION

- Blood glucose level ≤70 mg/dl (3.9 mmol/L).
- Clinically, hypoglycemia is suggested by typical symptoms (tremulousness, diaphoresis, tachycardia, or mental status change) that is corrected by carbohydrate intake.
- Most often, hypoglycemia is caused by too much insulin or oral hypoglycemic agent, or not enough food intake.

EPIDEMIOLOGY

- In patients receiving intensive therapy, risk of severe hypoglycemia is increased more than threefold.
- Average patient with type 1 diabetes suffers two episodes of symptomatic hypoglycemia per week and one episode of temporarily disabling hypoglycemia per year.
- In the Diabetes Control and Complications Trial (DCCT), more patients in intensively treated group had at least one episode of severe hypoglycemia (65% vs 35% in the control group), with overall rates of 61 and 19 per 100 patient-years, respectively.
- Risk factors: (1) type 1 diabetes which has not only insulin deficiency but also usually deficient glucagon response; (2) history of hypoglycemia, hypoglycemia unawareness, or both; (3) aggressive glycemic therapy with lower glycemic goals; (4) recent moderate or intensive exercise; (5) irregular dietary intake; (6) sleep; and (7) renal failure.

DIAGNOSIS

- Documented by Whipple's triad: symptoms consistent with hypoglycemia, a low plasma glucose concentration, and relief of symptoms when plasma glucose concentration raised.
  - **Severe hypoglycemia:** Requires assistance of another person to administer carbohydrate, glucagon, or other resuscitative actions. May develop sufficient neuroglycopenia to induce seizure or coma.
  - **Documented symptomatic hypoglycemia:** Typical symptoms of hypoglycemia accompanied by a measured plasma glucose (PG) concentration ≤70 mg/dl (3.9 mmol/l).
  - **Asymptomatic hypoglycemia:** No symptoms of hypoglycemia but with a measured PG <70 mg/dl (3.9 mmol/l).

MANAGEMENT

- **Probable symptomatic hypoglycemia:** Symptoms of hypoglycemia not accompanied by a plasma glucose determination (but presumably caused by a PG ≤70 mg/dl [3.9 mmol/l]). Treating symptoms suggestive of hypoglycemia with oral carbohydrate without a test of plasma glucose.
- **Relative hypoglycemia:** Typical symptoms of hypoglycemia, interpreted as hypoglycemia, but with measured PG >70 mg/dl (3.9 mmol/l). Patients with chronically poor glycemic control can experience symptoms of hypoglycemia at PG levels >70 mg/dl (3.9 mmol/l) as PG concentrations decline toward that level. Probably poses no direct harm.
- **Hypoglycemia unawareness:** Reduced sympathoadrenal and symptomatic response to low PG as a result of recurrent hypoglycemia

SIGNS AND SYMPTOMS

- Can be nonspecific.
- As glucose levels fall, autonomic (adrenergic) symptoms occur initially, followed by neuroglycopenic symptoms (mental status changes) as glucose values decline further.
- **Signs:** diaphoresis and pallor are common; tachycardia and systolic blood pressures mildly raised, and neuroglycopenic manifestations often observable.
- **Adrenergic (autonomic) symptoms:** palpitations, anxiety, tremor, hunger, sensation of warmth, nausea, and sweating
- **Neuroglycopenic symptoms:** fatigue, dizziness, headache, visual disturbances, drowsiness, difficulty speaking, inability to concentrate, abnormal behavior, loss of memory, difficulty thinking and/or frank confusion, seizure, coma, and even death.
- Occasionally, transient neurological deficits occur. Permanent neurological damage rare.
- If patient has hypoglycemia unawareness, may be asymptomatic.

CLINICAL TREATMENT

Prevention

- Prevention of hypoglycemia preferable to its treatment (Cryer).
- Patient's close friends or relatives should be aware of prevention strategies.
- Aggressive therapy, including (1) patient education, (2) frequent self-monitoring blood glucose (SMBG), (3) flexible insulin and other drug regimens, (4) individualized glycemic goals, and (5) ongoing professional guidance and support.
- Consider both conventional risk factors and those indicative of compromised glucose counterregulation.
- Review SMBG record to estimate frequency of hypoglycemia and adequacy of counterregulation, particularly before starting intensive insulin therapy or if there is previous history of hypoglycemic episodes.
- Consider less aggressive goals for A1c values in patients with severe hypoglycemia or with significant impairment in recovery from hypoglycemia, particularly in those with hypoglycemia unawareness.
- Continually reevaluate with patient the benefits of improved blood glucose control balanced against the risks of hypoglycemia.
- Medic-alert bracelet to facilitate rapid treatment in emergency settings.
- Hypoglycemia is the limiting factor in reducing A1c too aggressively.

Treatment of Asymptomatic and Symptomatic Hypoglycemic Episodes

- Patients should have fast-acting carbohydrate (glucose tablets, hard candy, glucose paste, or sweetened fruit juice) available at all times.
- Self-monitored blood glucose ≤70 mg/dl (3.9 mmol/L)—reasonable to self-treat (eat a glucose tablet or carbohydrate-containing juice, soft drinks, milk, candy, other snacks, or a meal).
- Recommended dose of glucose in adults is 20 grams (6-oz cup of orange juice or cola or 4-oz cup of grape juice).
- Clinical improvement should occur in 15–20 minutes.
- Since glycemic response to oral glucose lasts only about 2 hours, a more substantial snack or a meal should be taken shortly after initial treatment.
- Patients should be advised to monitor blood glucose levels serially after self-treating an episode of hypoglycemia to determine individual response to carbohydrate ingested.

Treatment of Severe Hypoglycemic Episodes

- Train friends or relatives to recognize and treat hypoglycemia.
- Friends and family should know never to put anything in the mouth of a person who is not able to sit up and ingest the food or drink. No cake paste, sugar, etc., in an unresponsive person.
- If patient cannot eat or drink safely, use injectable glucagon.
- Glucagon: Subcutaneous or intramuscular injection of 0.5–1.0 mg used to treat patient who is unable to eat/drink. Usually recovery of consciousness within 10–15 minutes; may cause marked nausea and hyperglycemia 60–90 minutes later. Only one dose of glucagon should be administered within a 24-hour period.
- Check glucagon kit regularly; replace when beyond its expiration date.
- In medical setting (emergency department, office, hospital), 25 cc of 50% glucose (dextrose) intravenously will have immediate response.
- Subsequent glucose infusion (or food, if patient is able to eat) often needed, depending upon the cause of hypoglycemia.
- Food should be provided orally as soon as patient able to ingest it safely.
- Hospitalization for prolonged treatment and observation may be necessary.

FOLLOW-UP

- In patients with clinical hypoglycemia unawareness, a 2- to 3-week period of diligent avoidance of hypoglycemia advisable to allow return of awareness of hypoglycemia (Cryer).
- Establish somewhat higher glucose targets in the short term.
- More frequent self-monitoring of blood glucose, especially before driving or other dangerous activities.
- With severe hypoglycemia, particularly at night or with unawareness, consider continuous glucose monitoring (see p. 565).

EXPERT OPINION

- Hypoglycemia establishes the lower limit of blood glucose control. It is unpleasant, potentially dangerous, and can (rarely) be fatal.
- Minimize the frequency and severity of hypoglycemia, avoiding especially nocturnal hypoglycemia.
- Replace insulin in a physiologic fashion to compensate for compromised glucose counterregulation.

MANAGEMENT

- To avoid overcorrection of hypoglycemia, with rebound hyperglycemia, wait 15–20 minutes before further treatment.
- A low A1c (i.e., <5.5%) may indicate unrecognized hypoglycemic events, especially between meals or overnight, and may indicate need for closer monitoring.

REFERENCES

Cryer PE, Axelrod L, Grossman AB, et al. Evaluation and management of adult hypoglycemic disorders: an Endocrine Society Clinical Practice Guideline. *J Clin Endocrinol Metab,* 2009; Vol. 94: pp. 709–28.
    Comments: Provides guidelines for evaluation and management of adults with hypoglycemic disorders, including those with diabetes mellitus.

Workgroup on Hypoglycemia, American Diabetes Association. Defining and reporting hypoglycemia in diabetes: a report from the American Diabetes Association Workgroup on Hypoglycemia. *Diabetes Care,* 2005; Vol. 28: pp. 1245–9.
    Comments: Important discussion on definition and classification of hypoglycemic episodes.

Cryer PE Diverse causes of hypoglycemia-associated autonomic failure in diabetes. *NEJM,* 2004; Vol. 350: pp. 2272–9.
    Comments: Discusses clinical problem of hypoglycemia in diabetes.

Cryer PE, Davis SN, Shamoon H. Hypoglycemia in diabetes. *Diabetes Care,* 2003; Vol. 26: pp. 1902–12.
    Comments: Excellent discussion on benefits and approach to managing and preventing hypoglycemic unawareness.

The Diabetes Control and Complications Trial Research Group. Hypoglycemia in the Diabetes Control and Complications Trial. *Diabetes,* 1997; Vol. 46: pp. 271–86.
    Comments: 65% of patients in the intensive group versus 35% of patients in conventional group had at least one episode of severe hypoglycemia; overall rates of severe hypoglycemia were 61.2 per 100 patient-years versus 18.7 per 100 patient-years in the intensive and conventional treatment groups, respectively, with a relative risk (RR) of 3.28. The relative risk for coma and/or seizure was 3.02 for intensive therapy.

The Diabetes Control and Complications Trial Research Group. The effect of intensive treatment of diabetes on the development and progression of long-term complications in insulin-dependent diabetes mellitus. *NEJM,* 1993; Vol. 329: pp. 977–86.
    Comments: In the Diabetes Control and Complications Trial, there was a progressive increase in the incidence of severe hypoglycemic episodes (per 100 patient-years) at lower attained hemoglobin A1c values during intensive insulin therapy in patients with type 1 diabetes.

HYPOGLYCEMIA: NOCTURNAL

Ari Eckman, MD, and Christopher D. Saudek, MD

DEFINITION

- Low blood sugar (≤70 mg/dl [3.9 mmol/l]) during sleep.
- Suspected if symptoms occur but low blood glucose not documented; definite if symptoms occur *and* low blood glucose documented; severe if assistance of another person is needed.

EPIDEMIOLOGY

- In the Diabetes Control and Complications Trial (DCCT), 43% of all hypoglycemic episodes and 55% of severe episodes occurred during sleep.
- Also in DCCT, severe hypoglycemic episodes were three times more likely in patients on intensive insulin therapy than in those on conventional therapy.

- Common, especially in patients with type 1 diabetes, when blood glucose is most variable (Yale).
- Often episodes occur without symptoms and go unrecognized; majority of episodes in type 1 diabetes occur during late sleep (3 AM–7 AM) (Amin).

DIAGNOSIS

- Risk factors include: slow clearance of insulin or oral antihyperglycemic agents (e.g., liver or kidney disease); use of intermediate-acting (NPH) insulin at suppertime; missed meal; unplanned exercise; alcohol; infection; decreased gluconeogenic substrate (e.g., from cachexia); long-acting sulfonylureas, insulin, or insulin combined with oral antihyperglycemic agents; history of hypoglycemia, hypoglycemia unawareness, or both; age.
- Most convincingly diagnosed if Whipple's triad documented: symptoms compatible with hypoglycemia, low blood glucose concentration recorded, and resolution of these symptoms after correcting blood glucose.

SIGNS AND SYMPTOMS

- **Signs:** pallor and diaphoresis; increased heart rate and systolic blood pressure; hypothermia; in severe episodes, unarousable, transient focal neurological deficits (e.g., diplopia, hemiparesis), or seizures. Partner may note altered breathing, irritable sleep.
- **Symptoms:** episodes range from asymptomatic to severe; can, rarely, be fatal. Patients often awaken due to bad dreams, sweating.
- Neurogenic symptoms: adrenergic (catecholamine-mediated)—tremulousness, palpitations, and anxiety/arousal; cholinergic—sweating, hunger, and paresthesias.
- May also be asymptomatic, due to hypoglycemia unawareness, or because cognition is suppressed during sleep.

CLINICAL TREATMENT

- Key to treatment is early recognition.
- **Do not administer anything by mouth (such as juice) if the patient cannot sit up and eat/drink. This may cause aspiration.**
- In awake individual, prefer 15–20 grams of fast-acting carbohydrate (e.g., glucose-containing drink, cookies, candy, glucose tablets).
- Repeat self-monitored blood glucose in 15–20 min if symptoms not improved or the monitored blood glucose remains low.
- Since glycemic response to oral glucose is transient (<2 h), eat snack or meal shortly after plasma glucose concentration is raised.
- Avoid foods high in fat, which delay glucose absorption.
- Intramuscular glucagon administration (1 mg, may be administered by a nonprofessional) or intravenous glucose (25 cc of 50% dextrose, administered by a healthcare professional) is required if the patient is unable to sit up and drink liquid.
- Nausea and vomiting are common side effects of glucagon.
- For hospitalized patients, document absence of nocturnal hypoglycemia before patient discharged.

FOLLOW-UP

- Change treatment regimen in order to prevent subsequent episodes of nocturnal hypoglycemia, reducing nighttime dose of insulin or oral hypoglycemic agent, or instituting a small bedtime snack.

MANAGEMENT

- Provide education to patient and family about risks and risk-reduction strategies.
- Plan meals and exercise carefully.
- Avoid NPH insulin at suppertime, or short-/fast-acting insulin at bedtime, as insulin levels will peak during sleep.
- Use fast-acting insulin analogs (instead of regular insulin) at dinnertime.
- If insulin administered at bedtime, long-acting insulin preferred.
- Try moving long-acting insulin analog to morning, instead of bedtime, if nocturnal hypoglycemia persists.
- Avoid excess alcohol intake.
- Carefully and consistently perform self-monitoring blood glucose (SMBG), including in middle of night to avoid nocturnal hypoglycemia.
- Reinforce that a change in routine (e.g., change in time zone, holidays, vacation) may increase risk for nocturnal hypoglycemia.
- Continuous glucose monitoring may be useful for patients with hypoglycemic unawareness and frequent nocturnal hypoglycemia.

EXPERT OPINION

- Nocturnal hypoglycemia remains significant barrier to intensive therapy needed to avoid long-term complications of diabetes.
- Though rarely fatal, nocturnal hypoglycemia accounted for half of all unexpected deaths of people with type 1 diabetes in a study from the United Kingdom (Tattersall). Should therefore be taken seriously.
- Frequent episodes of nocturnal hypoglycemia can exacerbate hypoglycemia unawareness.
- Choosing a more carefully fine-tuned insulin regimen or use of an insulin pump can lower nocturnal hypoglycemia risk without compromising glycemic control.
- Though often called the "Somogyi phenomenon," nocturnal hypoglycemia is *not* a cause of significant morning or subsequent day hyperglycemia (unless overtreated) (Tordjman; Hirsch).
- A common vicious cycle, however, is to become hypoglycemic at night, overtreat the hypoglycemia, and start the day hyperglycemic.

REFERENCES

Brunton SA. Nocturnal hypoglycemia: answering the challenge with long-acting insulin analogs. *MedGenMed*, 2007; Vol. 9: p. 38.
  Comments: Discusses prevalence, causes, and consequences of nocturnal hypoglycemia; detection and prevention strategies including use of long-acting insulin analogs, offering more physiologic and predictable time-action profiles than traditional human basal insulin, associated with a lower risk for nocturnal hypoglycemia than NPH without sacrificing glycemic control.

Workgroup on Hypoglycemia, American Diabetes Association. Defining and reporting hypoglycemia in diabetes: a report from the American Diabetes Association Workgroup on Hypoglycemia. *Diabetes Care*, 2005; Vol. 28: pp. 1245–9.
  Comments: Important discussion on defining and classification of hypoglycemic episodes.

Allen KV, Frier BM. Nocturnal hypoglycemia: clinical manifestations and therapeutic strategies toward prevention. *Endocr Pract*, 2004; Vol. 9: pp. 530–43.
  Comments: Almost 50% of all episodes of severe hypoglycemia occur at night during sleep. Recurrent exposure to nocturnal hypoglycemia may impair cognitive function; other substantial long-term morbidity includes the development of acquired hypoglycemia syndromes, such as impaired awareness of hypoglycemia.

Gabriely I, Shamoon H. Hypoglycemia in diabetes: common, often unrecognized. *Cleve Clin J Med*, 2004; Vol. 71: pp. 335–42.

Comments: Hypoglycemic episodes often go unrecognized, and over time, patients with diabetes may lose ability to sense hypoglycemia, increasing their risk.

Yale JF. Nocturnal hypoglycemia in patients with insulin-treated diabetes. *Diabetes Res Clin Pract*, 2004; Vol. 65 Suppl 1: pp. S41–6.
Comments: Nocturnal hypoglycemia is a frequent event among patients with type 1 diabetes, while severe hypoglycemic episodes are approximately three times more likely in patients on intensive insulin therapy than in those on conventional therapy.

Cryer PE, Davis SN, Shamoon H. Hypoglycemia in diabetes. *Diabetes Care*, 2003; Vol. 26: pp. 1902–12.
Comments: Discusses signs, symptoms, and clinical risk factors for hypoglycemia.

Amin R, Ross K, Acerini CL, et al. Hypoglycemia prevalence in prepubertal children with type 1 diabetes on standard insulin regimen: use of continuous glucose monitoring system. *Diabetes Care*, 2003; Vol. 26: pp. 662–7.
Comments: Hypoglycemia was more common at night compared with daytime (18.81% vs 4.4%, p < 0.001); 78% and 43% of subjects showed hypoglycemia on at least one night and two or more nights, respectively. Nocturnal episodes were prolonged (median 3.3 h) and asymptomatic (91% of episodes). Prevalence was greater between 4 AM and 7:30 AM.

Cryer PE. *Hypoglycemia: Pathophysiology, Diagnosis and Treatment*. New York: Oxford University Press; 1997.
Comments: Textbook describing the diagnosis and treatment of hypoglycemia.

Tattersall RB, Gill GV. Unexplained deaths of type 1 diabetic patients. *Diabet Med*, 1991; Vol. 8: pp. 49–58.
Comments: A report from the UK indicating that about half of unexpected deaths in type 1 diabetes were compatible with nocturnal hypoglycemia.

The DCCT Research Group. Epidemiology of severe hypoglycemia in the diabetes control and complications trial. *Am J Med*, 1991; Vol. 90: pp. 450–9.
Comments: In the DCCT, intensive treatment of IDDM increased the frequency of severe hypoglycemia relative to conventional therapy. Severe hypoglycemia occurred more often during sleep (55%); 43% of all episodes occurred between midnight and 8 AM.

Hirsch IB, Smith LJ, Havlin CE, et al. Failure of nocturnal hypoglycemia to cause daytime hyperglycemia in patients with IDDM. *Diabetes Care*, 1990; Vol. 13: pp. 133–42.
Comments: Demonstration that induced nocturnal hypoglycemia does not increase hyperglycemia throughout the following day.

Tordjman KM, Havlin CE, Levandoski LA, et al. Failure of nocturnal hypoglycemia to cause fasting hyperglycemia in patients with insulin-dependent diabetes mellitus. *NEJM*, 1987; Vol. 317: pp. 1552–9.
Comments: Demonstration that induced nocturnal hypoglycemia does not increase fasting blood glucose.

HYPOGLYCEMIA: POSTPRANDIAL

Ari Eckman, MD, and Christopher D. Saudek, MD

DEFINITION
- Symptomatic hypoglycemia due to low blood glucose (≤70 mg/dl) occurring within 2–5 h after food intake, in the absence of hypoglycemic medications.
- Also referred to as reactive hypoglycemia.
- Highly disputed and controversial entity.

EPIDEMIOLOGY
- 10% of normal subjects have a blood glucose concentration <50 mg/dl 4–6 hours following oral glucose tolerance test.

- An unproven observation is that patients with prediabetes or early, mild type 2 diabetes, may have postprandial hypoglycemia due to delayed but exaggerated insulin secretion.
- Postprandial hypoglycemia is more common in very lean people, or after extreme weight reduction.
- Prevalence and incidence figures are virtually impossible to determine since symptoms are nonspecific and blood glucose is rarely measured during symptoms.
- Can be seen after bariatric surgery, due to dumping syndrome or beta-cell hyperplasia.

DIAGNOSIS

- Whipple's triad: symptoms compatible with hypoglycemia, documentation of low blood glucose concentration, and resolution of symptoms after treating the hypoglycemia.
- After an overnight fast, administer type of food intake thought to induce hypoglycemia. Hold all nonessential medications. Observe patient for signs and symptoms of hypoglycemia, with written log. Avoid treatment, if possible, until test completed.
- Measure plasma glucose, before ingestion and every 30 minutes up to 300 minutes after eating meal. Some experts recommend also sending insulin, C-peptide, and proinsulin for analysis if plasma glucose <60 mg/dl (3.3 mmol/L) (Cryer).
- Mixed meal tests (10 kcal/kg, 45% carbohydrate, 15% protein, and 40% fat) have been used for diagnosis but standards for interpretation have not been established.
- Oral glucose tolerance test is not usually recommended (Cryer), but may be helpful in prediabetes or early diabetes.
- Factitious hypoglycemia should always be considered and may be excluded with a detailed medication history and screening for sulfonylureas in urine.
- Insulin autoantibodies may be helpful in selected populations where these antibodies are more prevalent (i.e., Asian).

SIGNS AND SYMPTOMS

- **Autonomic symptoms:** sweating, palpitations, shaking, hunger, anxiety, weakness, tremor, or perspiration.
- Rarely if ever a cause of mental status changes or death.
- **Neuroglycopenic symptoms:** confusion, drowsiness, speech difficulty are probably not due to postprandial hypoglycemia.

CLINICAL TREATMENT

- Diet is main treatment, and can be a simple diagnostic as well as therapeutic modality.
- Patient should ingest a small carbohydrate-containing snack (15–30 gm) anticipating the time symptoms usually occur (such as late morning or mid-afternoon). This will keep blood glucose from going low and if effective, it is easy to implement and consistent with the diagnosis of postprandial hypoglycemia (Brun).
- Avoid high carbohydrate meals, rapidly absorbable sugars, and drinks rich in glucose or sucrose.
- Avoid drinks combining sugar with alcohol, especially in fasting state.
- Some experts recommend, without proven efficacy, adding protein or soluble dietary fibers to meals, to slow gastric emptying and reduce insulin response.

- If symptoms persist, a number of medications have been tried: (1) alpha-glucosidase inhibitors (acarbose, miglitol) to delay starch and sucrose digestion or (2) metformin, 500–850 mg orally, taken with meals.
- In exceptional cases, the somatostatin analogue octreotide has been used.
- Diazoxide is not recommended due to side effects including water retention, hypertrichosis, and digestive disorders.

FOLLOW-UP
- Encourage dietary management as long as patient experiences symptoms.
- Not a progressive disorder.
- Rarely, if ever, a cause of mental status changes or death.
- Usually responds well to dietary modification.
- Medication may be needed in extreme cases.

EXPERT OPINION
- As indicated previously, postprandial hypoglycemia is a controversial entity, difficult to prove, and of unclear mechanism. Most experts question whether it is a real disease.
- Since the adrenergic symptoms are identical to those of simple anxiety and caused by the same hormones (catecholamines), underlying anxiety, depression, or psychiatric illness may be misattributed to hypoglycemia.
- Must rule out fasting hypoglycemia, which is an important diagnosis to establish (see p. 51).
- Blood glucose frequently dips below baseline, and normal counterregulatory hormones (epinephrine, glucagon) bring glucose back to baseline. The controversy is whether, or how often, this process causes symptoms.
- For most patients, simple dietary treatment alone is sufficient.

REFERENCES

Cryer PE, Axelrod L, Grossman AB, et al. Evaluation and management of adult hypoglycemic disorders: an Endocrine Society Clinical Practice Guideline. *J Clin Endocrinol Metab,* 2009; Vol. 94: pp. 709–28.
   Comments: Recent guidelines provided for evaluation of reactive hypoglycemia.

Brun JF, Fedou C, Mercier J. Postprandial reactive hypoglycemia. *Diabetes Metab,* 2000; Vol. 26: pp. 337–51.
   Comments: Important to add small meals at the middle of morning and afternoon, when glycemia would start to decrease. If composition of the meal is adequate, fall in blood glucose can be prevented.

Ozgen AG, Hamulu F, Bayraktar F, et al. Long-term treatment with acarbose for the treatment of reactive hypoglycemia. *Eat Weight Disord,* 1998; Vol. 3: pp. 136–40.
   Comments: Study showing that acarbose may be of value in preventing and treating reactive hypoglycemia by reducing early hyperglycemic stimulus to insulin secretion.

Hofeldt FD. Reactive hypoglycemia. *Endocrinol Metab Clin North Am,* 1989; Vol. 18: pp. 185–201.
   Comments: Most patients with symptoms following meals have another diagnosis other than reactive hypoglycemia, including neuropsychiatric disease.

Lev-Ran A, Anderson RW. The diagnosis of postprandial hypoglycemia. *Diabetes,* 1981; Vol. 30: pp. 996–9.
   Comments: Many patients with postprandial adrenergic symptoms had similar symptoms following placebo administration in place of glucose.

MANAGEMENT

OUTPATIENT MANAGEMENT OF DIABETES AND ACUTE ILLNESS

Nisa M. Maruthur, MD, MHS

DEFINITION

- Acute changes in medical condition that can cause either hyperglycemia (including diabetic ketoacidosis [DKA] and hyperosmolar hyperglycemic state [HHS]) or hypoglycemia.
- **Hyperglycemia** may be due to stress of illness, failure to take adequate insulin or other diabetic medication, dehydration, or excess sweet liquid intake.
- **Hypoglycemia** may be caused by decreased oral caloric intake, decreased endogenous glucose production (e.g., adrenal crisis or liver failure), increased glucose utilization (e.g., infection), or decreased insulin clearance (e.g., renal failure).

EPIDEMIOLOGY

- Infection is the most common cause of DKA and HHS.
- Other important acute changes in medical condition that can cause hyperglycemic states include trauma, stroke, myocardial infarction, alcohol abuse, and pancreatitis.
- Patients with diabetes mellitus (DM) are more likely to require hospitalization for acute illnesses such as infections.

DIAGNOSIS

- Glucose should be monitored more frequently with any acute illness.
- Evaluation of urine or blood for ketones should be considered in patients at risk for DKA.
- Consider medications used to treat acute illness (corticosteroids, thiazide diuretics, sympathomimetics, and atypical antipsychotic agents), which can also precipitate hyperglycemia.
- Certain antibiotics (e.g., quinolones) can cause both hyper- and hypoglycemia.

SIGNS AND SYMPTOMS

- Evaluate for signs and symptoms of DKA (see p. 38), HHS (see p. 43), and hypoglycemia (see p. 51).

CLINICAL TREATMENT

- Pronounced hyperglycemia may require a change in outpatient treatment plan, such as increased short-acting insulin.
- Inability to maintain oral intake, vomiting, or alteration of mental status: refer to an emergency department for evaluation of DKA and HHS.
- In general, diabetes medications (including insulin) should be continued during acute illness, but dosage may need adjustment.
- Monitor blood glucose every 4 hours during acute illness, and adjust medications based on results.
- Encourage patients to call their healthcare provider earlier, rather than later, when ill.
- Short- or rapid-acting insulin can be substituted for long-acting insulin during acute illness.
- Encourage antipyretics for fever.

- Maintain oral intake as much as possible and supplement with caloric beverages and salt.
- Self-monitoring of urine and blood ketones is available and can be used in conjunction with frequent blood glucose monitoring during acute illness.

EXPERT OPINION

- Alteration in outpatient treatment plan due to hyperglycemia or hypoglycemia is individualized based on patient's history of response to illness (e.g., history of ketosis) and current regimen (e.g., diet or insulin).
- Timely outpatient or emergency department visits may be necessary to address glycemic control and avoid ketoacidosis both during and after acute illness.
- Physicians should have a lower threshold for referral to the emergency department and potential hospitalization for patients with diabetes and acute illness.

REFERENCES

American Diabetes Association. Standards of medical care in diabetes—2011. *Diabetes Care,* 2011; Vol. 34 Suppl 1: pp. S11–61.
  Comments: Standards of medical care recommended by the American Diabetes Association.

Aspinall SL, Good CB, Jiang R, et al. Severe dysglycemia with the fluoroquinolones: a class effect? *Clin Infect Dis,* 2009; Vol. 49: pp. 402–8.
  Comments: VA study of over 1.2 million patients evaluating the effect of quinolone antibiotics on hyper- and hypoglycemia.

Weber C, Kocher S, Neeser K, et al. Prevention of diabetic ketoacidosis and self-monitoring of ketone bodies: an overview. *Curr Med Res Opin,* 2009; Vol. 25: pp. 1197–207.
  Comments: Review of self-monitoring of ketones for preventing ketoacidosis in insulin-dependent diabetes.

Kitabchi AE, Umpierrez GE, Miles JM, et al. Hyperglycemic crises in adult patients with diabetes. *Diabetes Care,* 2009; Vol. 32: pp. 1335–43.
  Comments: American Diabetes Association consensus statement, which includes discussion of sick day management.

Kitabchi AE, Umpierrez GE, Murphy MB, et al. Hyperglycemic crises in diabetes. *Diabetes Care,* 2004; Vol. 27 Suppl 1: pp. S94–102.
  Comments: American Diabetes Association position statement on the management of diabetic ketoacidosis and hyperosmolar hyperglycemic state.

American Diabetes Association, American Psychiatric Association, American Association of Clinical Endocrinologists, et al. Consensus development conference on antipsychotic drugs and obesity and diabetes. *Diabetes Care,* 2004; Vol. 27: pp. 596–601.
  Comments: Consensus statement concluding that clozapine and olanzapine increase risk of diabetes.

Cryer PE, Davis SN, Shamoon H. Hypoglycemia in diabetes. *Diabetes Care,* 2003; Vol. 26: pp. 1902–12.
  Comments: Unstructured review of hypoglycemia including detailed description of pathophysiology.

ROUTINE PREVENTIVE CARE

Nisa M. Maruthur, MD, MHS

DEFINITION

- Interventions for prevention of diabetes-associated comorbidities including microvascular (retinopathy, nephropathy, neuropathy) and macrovascular (cardiovascular disease) complications, infectious diseases, periodontal disease, and cancer.

MANAGEMENT

EPIDEMIOLOGY

- Modification of multiple risk factors (glycemic control, high blood pressure, dyslipidemia, aspirin therapy, and smoking cessation) decreases mortality by 46%, cardiovascular disease death and events by 57% and 59%, respectively, and microvascular complications by 55% relative to conventional therapy among individuals with diabetes (Gaede).
- Influenza and pneumococcal pneumonia are associated with higher mortality rates in diabetes.
- Periodontal disease frequently complicates diabetes and may worsen glycemic control.
- Diabetes is associated with increased risk of cancer, including that for breast cancer (RR 1.2) and colon cancer (RR 1.3), and is associated with increased all-cause mortality in cancer patients (RR 1.4).

DIAGNOSIS

- **Hemoglobin A1c:** every 3 months if therapy is changed or patient not yet at goal. Every 6 months in patients with stable control.
- **Self-monitoring of blood glucose:** at least 3 times a day for individuals on multiple insulin injections or insulin pump therapy; less frequently for other patients to help guide therapy.
- **Continuous glucose monitoring:** may be useful in brittle diabetes.
- **Blood pressure:** each routine diabetes visit.
- **Fasting lipid profile:** at least annually.
- **Urine albumin excretion:** annually (i.e., spot urine albumin-to-creatinine ratio) for individuals with type 1 diabetes >5 years duration and with type 2 diabetes beginning at diagnosis.
- **Serum creatinine:** annually to estimate glomerular filtration rate.
- **Ophthalmologic evaluation:** annually beginning 5 years after type 1 diagnosis and at initial type 2 diagnosis.
- **Foot examination:** annually for (1) distal symmetric polyneuropathy: pinprick sensation, vibration sense, Achilles reflexes, monofilament testing; (2) peripheral arterial disease: evaluation for claudication, examination of distal pulses (i.e., dorsalis pedis or posterior tibial).
- **Autonomic neuropathy evaluation:** annually by history and physical.
- **Depression, anxiety, and dementia: screen** at routine diabetes visits, especially if concerned about adherence or self-management.
- **Age-appropriate cancer screening:** per United States Preventive Services Task Force (*http://www.ahrq.gov/CLINIC/uspstfix.htm*).
- **Estimated 10-year cardiovascular disease (CVD) risk:** evaluate at routine visits (see Cardiovascular Disease Screening and Management, p. 178).

SIGNS AND SYMPTOMS

- **HEENT:** hearing loss, visual acuity, diplopia, scotomata, blurry vision, dizziness, lightheadedness.
- **Cardiovascular:** chest pain, exercise intolerance, heart palpitations, numbness, tingling, weakness, intermittent claudication.
- **Pulmonary:** shortness of breath, orthopnea, daytime somnolence or fatigue.
- **GI:** constipation, nausea, abdominal pain.
- **GU:** erectile dysfunction, bladder dysfunction, urinary tract infections, incontinence, frothy urine.

- **Extremities:** foot ulcers, hand/foot pain, numbness, tingling.
- **Orthostatic hypotension:** decrease in systolic blood pressure of more than 20 mmHg or decrease in diastolic blood pressure of more than 10 mmHg upon standing from seated position; this may indicate autonomic dysfunction but may be related to medication (e.g., diuretics) as well (JNC 7).
- **Psychiatric:** mood changes, changes in energy level.

CLINICAL TREATMENT

- **Glycemic control** (goal A1c <7% ADA; <6.5% IDF): to decrease risk of microvascular and macrovascular complications of diabetes. Medications should be intensively escalated until goal A1c reached (see Type 2 Diabetes: Sequencing Therapies, p. 170, and Type 1 Diabetes: Insulin Treatment, p. 155).
- **Lifestyle recommendations:** (1) physical activity (see Physical Activity and Exercise, p. 103): hyper- or hypoglycemia, diabetic retinopathy, and diabetic neuropathy may limit physical activity; and (2) diet. Weight loss of 7–10% recommended (see Nutrition: Overview in Diabetes, p. 89).
- **Lipid control** (goal LDL-cholesterol <100 mg/dl, or <70 mg/dl in patients at very high risk for coronary events): regardless of lipid profile, HMG CoA reductase inhibitors (statins) recommended if patient has known cardiovascular disease or is >40 years of age and has >1 risk factor for cardiovascular disease.
- **Hypertension** (goal blood pressure <130/80): measurements above this value warrant further evaluation and management.
- **ACE inhibitor:** recommended for patients with: (1) known cardiovascular disease; (2) micro- or macroalbuminuria (ACE inhibitor or ARB acceptable).
- **Beta-blocker:** recommended for patients with prior myocardial infarction for at least 2 years after event.
- **Smoking cessation:** for cardiovascular disease prevention, offer treatment to facilitate smoking cessation. Counsel patients following the 5 A's model: Ask, Advise, Assess, Assist, Arrange. Pharmacologic agents include nicotine replacement, bupropion, and varenicline (*www.surgeongeneral.gov/tobacco*).
- **Aspirin** (75–162 mg/day): for primary or secondary prevention of cardiovascular disease. Primary prevention indication: 10-year cardiovascular disease (CVD) risk >10% in the absence of elevated risk of bleeding (typically, men >50 years, women >60 years) with an additional risk factor (hypertension, family history, dyslipidemia, microalbuminuria, family history of premature CVD, or smoking). Consideration of aspirin in those without CVD but at intermediate 10-year risk (5%–10%). Aspirin is not recommended for primary prevention for low-risk patients without CVD (e.g., no risk factors, 10-year risk <5%). Secondary prevention indications: patients with CVD. Consider clopidogrel if aspirin allergy present.
- **Foot care:** referral to podiatrist if patient smokes, has neurologic deficit, or prior foot disease.
- **Vaccinations:** pneumococcal and influenza vaccinations as recommended.

FOLLOW-UP

- Patients should be seen at least every 3 months for a diabetes-specific visit. This interval can be extended in the setting of stable control (especially for diet- or well-controlled type 2 diabetes).

MANAGEMENT

EXPERT OPINION

- Routine care of the patient with diabetes should be multidisciplinary and include the patient, family members, physicians, nurses, dieticians, and other healthcare professionals in the management plan.
- Routine preventive care, when effectively implemented, can delay the development of complications and preserve quality-of-life for individuals with diabetes.
- Recommendations have been updated to narrow the group of patients with diabetes for whom aspirin for primary prevention of CVD is recommended, now based on estimated CVD risk (Pignone). Multiple CVD risk prediction tools specifically for diabetes are available as described in the American Diabetes Association (ADA) position statement (1. *http://www.dtu.ox.ac.uk/riskengine/index.php*, 2. *http://www.aricnews. net/riskcalc/html/RC1.html*, 3. *http://www.diabetes.org/living-with-diabetes/ complications/diabetes-phd/*).

BASIS FOR RECOMMENDATIONS

American Diabetes Association. Standards of medical care in diabetes—2011. *Diabetes Care,* 2011; Vol. 34 Suppl 1: pp. S11–61.

    Comments: Summary of American Diabetes Association recommendations for routine preventive care.

OTHER REFERENCES

Pignone M, Alberts MJ, Colwell JA, et al. Aspirin for primary prevention of cardiovascular events in people with diabetes: a position statement of the American Diabetes Association, a scientific statement of the American Heart Association, and an expert consensus document of the American College of Cardiology Foundation. *Diabetes Care,* 2010; Vol. 33: pp. 1395–402.

    Comments: Statement from American Diabetes Association, American Heart Association, and American College of Cardiology Foundation on the use of aspirin for primary prevention in diabetes.

Gaede P, Lund-Andersen H, Parving HH, et al. Effect of a multifactorial intervention on mortality in type 2 diabetes. *NEJM,* 2008; Vol. 358: pp. 580–91.

    Comments: Observational follow-up of the Steno-2 Trial participants (patients with diabetes and microalbuminuria) showing benefit of control of multiple risk factors in preventing death, cardiovascular morbidity, and mortality and microvascular complications.

Demmer RT, Jacobs DR, Desvarieux M. Periodontal disease and incident type 2 diabetes: results from the First National Health and Nutrition Examination Survey and its epidemiologic follow-up study. *Diabetes Care,* 2008; Vol. 31: pp. 1373–9.

    Comments: Study based on National Health and Nutritional Examination Survey evaluating the relationship between periodontal disease and diabetes risk.

Barone BB, Yeh HC, Snyder CF, et al. Long-term all-cause mortality in cancer patients with preexisting diabetes mellitus: a systematic review and meta-analysis. *JAMA,* 2008; Vol. 300: pp. 2754–64.

    Comments: Meta-analysis establishing link between diabetes and all-cause mortality in cancer patients.

Patel A, ADVANCE Collaborative Group, MacMahon S, et al. Effects of a fixed combination of perindopril and indapamide on macrovascular and microvascular outcomes in patients with type 2 diabetes mellitus (the ADVANCE trial): a randomised controlled trial. *Lancet,* 2007; Vol. 370: pp. 829–40.

    Comments: Results of blood-pressure lowering regimen (perindopril + indapamide) from the ADVANCE Trial, a factorial trial, which evaluated the effect of blood pressure-lowering and glycemic control on vascular disease in diabetes.

Larsson SC, Mantzoros CS, Wolk A. Diabetes mellitus and risk of breast cancer: a meta-analysis. *Int J Cancer,* 2007; Vol. 121: pp. 856–62.

    Comments: Meta-analysis of observational studies evaluating the relationship between obesity and breast cancer risk.

Mealey BL, Oates TW, American Academy of Periodontology. Diabetes mellitus and periodontal diseases. *J Periodontol,* 2006; Vol. 77: pp. 1289–303.

Comments: Review (unstructured) commissioned by the American Academy of Periodontology describing the bidirectional relationship between periodontal disease and diabetes.

Larsson SC, Orsini N, Wolk A. Diabetes mellitus and risk of colorectal cancer: a meta-analysis. *J Natl Cancer Inst,* 2005; Vol. 97: pp. 1679–87.

Comments: Meta-analysis of observational studies evaluating the relationship between obesity and colon cancer risk.

US Dept of Health and Human Services. *The seventh report of the Joint National Committee on Prevention, Detection, Evaluation, and Treatment of High Blood Pressure.* NIH Publication No. 04-5230, August 2004.

Comments: Report of epidemiology, diagnosis, and management of hypertension.

Gaede P, Vedel P, Larsen N, et al. Multifactorial intervention and cardiovascular disease in patients with type 2 diabetes. *NEJM,* 2003; Vol. 348: pp. 383–93.

Comments: Main results of Steno-2 Trial in which modification of multiple risk factors reduced risk of macro- and microvascular complications in patients with type 2 diabetes and microalbuminuria.

Smith SA, Poland GA. Use of influenza and pneumococcal vaccines in people with diabetes. *Diabetes Care,* 2000; Vol. 23: pp. 95–108.

Comments: Technical review from the American Diabetes Association reviewing the epidemiology and response to vaccinations for influenza and pneumococcal pneumonia in diabetes.

UK Prospective Diabetes Study Group. Tight blood pressure control and risk of macrovascular and microvascular complications in type 2 diabetes: UKPDS 38. *BMJ,* 1998; Vol. 317: pp. 703–13.

Comments: Randomized trial (UK Prospective Diabetes Study Group 38) showing benefit of tight compared to less tight blood pressure control on diabetes complications.

VACCINATION GUIDELINES FOR DIABETES

Nisa M. Maruthur, MD, MHS

DEFINITION

- Guidelines based on the Advisory Committee on Immunization Practices (ACIP) recommendations for the control of communicable diseases that can be prevented by vaccination.

EPIDEMIOLOGY

- Patients with diabetes have comorbid factors such as age and other chronic diseases that increase morbidity and mortality from infection.
- Influenza and pneumococcal infection associated with high death rates in those with diabetes (Smith).
- For those with diabetes, influenza vaccination associated with 54% reduction in hospitalizations and 58% reduction in deaths (Looijmans-Van). Similar clinical outcomes are unfortunately not available for the pneumococcal vaccine.
- Annual influenza vaccination may decrease cardiovascular disease morbidity and mortality (Davis).
- Prevalence of pneumococcal vaccination among patients with diabetes may be as low as 38% in the United States (Resnick), and national estimates of influenza vaccination in the general population (>65 years of age) range from 33% to 75% (Kilmer).

CLINICAL TREATMENT

Treatment

- Age-specific adult immunization schedule recommended per Centers for Disease Control and Prevention (for specific schedules see: *http://www.cdc.gov/mmwr/PDF/wk/mm5753-Immunization.pdf*).

Influenza—Diabetes-Specific Treatment Recommendations

- Annual vaccination.
- Two versions of the influenza vaccine: injectable (inactivated) and inhaled (live). Either type is safe in diabetes. Both forms can cause mild symptoms, but not an influenza infection. Side effects of the inactivated injection: erythema, swelling, and pain at injection site. Both types of vaccine can cause upper respiratory infection-type symptoms (e.g., fever, myalgias). More serious (but rare) risks include life-threatening allergic reactions and Guillain-Barre Syndrome (seen with inactivated swine flu vaccine in 1970s) (*http://www.cdc.gov/vaccines/vac-gen/side-effects.htm#flu*).
- Annual influenza vaccine typically becomes available in October each year.

Streptococcal Pneumonia—Diabetes-Specific Treatment Recommendations

- Before age 65, single vaccination with pneumococcal polysaccharide vaccine.
- After age 65 and no previous pneumococcal vaccine, single vaccination with pneumococcal polysaccharide vaccine (repeat vaccine not necessary).
- If vaccinated before age 65 and greater than 5 years since vaccination, administer second vaccination.

EXPERT OPINION

- Primary care clinics should consider vaccine implementation strategies to ensure appropriate adherence to vaccination schedules.
- It should be noted that the vaccine for pneumonia can only prevent pneumonia caused by *Streptococcus pneumoniae*.
- People with diabetes should routinely receive seasonal flu vaccine and vaccine for pneumonia as stated previously.
- The CDC provides destination-specific recommendations for vaccinations on its website (*http://wwwnc.cdc.gov/travel/destinations/list.aspx*).

REFERENCES

MMWR Adult Schedule, CDC 2009 Centers for Disease Control and Prevention. Recommended adult immunization schedule—United States, 2009. *MMWR,* 2009; Vol. 57: pp. Q1–4.

    Comments: Centers for Disease Control and Prevention vaccination guidelines, 2009. Approved by Advisory Committee on Immunization Practices, the American Academy of Family Physicians, the American College of Obstetricians and Gynecologists, and the American College of Physicians.

Fiore AE, Shay DK, Broder K, et al. Prevention and control of seasonal influenza with vaccines: recommendations of the Advisory Committee on Immunization Practices (ACIP), 2009. *MMWR Recomm Rep,* 2009; Vol. 58: pp. 1–52.

    Comments: Updated review of influenza vaccination from Centers for Disease Control and Prevention.

Kilmer G, Roberts H, Hughes E, et al. Surveillance of certain health behaviors and conditions among states and selected local areas—Behavioral Risk Factor Surveillance System (BRFSS), United States, 2006. *MMWR Surveill Summ,* 2008; Vol. 57: pp. 1–188.

    Comments: Provides national estimates of influenza vaccination in the general population (in addition to other health behaviors).

Looijmans-Van den Akker I, Verheij TJ, Buskens E, et al. Clinical effectiveness of first and repeat influenza vaccination in adult and elderly diabetic patients. *Diabetes Care,* 2006; Vol. 29: pp. 1771–6.

Comments: Nested-case control study from PRISMA (Prospective, Randomized Trial on Intensive Self-Monitoring Blood Glucose Management Added Value in Non-Insulin Treated Type 2 Diabetes Mellitus Patients) conducted in the Netherlands to evaluate the effect of influenza vaccination on hospitalization and death in patients with diabetes.

Davis MM, Taubert K, Benin AL, et al. Influenza vaccination as secondary prevention for cardiovascular disease: a science advisory from the American Heart Association and the American College of Cardiology. *J Am Coll Cardiol,* 2006; Vol. 48: pp. 1498–502.

Comments: Science advisory from AHA/ACC regarding influenza vaccination for secondary prevention of CVD.

Resnick HE, Foster GL, Bardsley J, et al. Achievement of American Diabetes Association clinical practice recommendations among U.S. adults with diabetes, 1999–2002: the National Health and Nutrition Examination Survey. *Diabetes Care,* 2006; Vol. 29: pp. 531–7.

Comments: Study of patients with diabetes meeting general clinical recommendations (from 1999–2002: The National Health and Nutrition Examination Survey).

Smith SA, Poland GA. Use of influenza and pneumococcal vaccines in people with diabetes. *Diabetes Care,* 2000; Vol. 23: pp. 95–108.

Comments: Technical review from the American Diabetes Association of influenza and pneumococcal pneumonia epidemiology and response to vaccination in diabetes.

MANAGEMENT

Hospital and Surgical Management

HOSPITAL MANAGEMENT OF DIABETES

Joanne Dintzis, CRNP, CDE, and Sherita Hill Golden, MD, MHS

DEFINITION

- Goal of inpatient management: achieving a level of glycemic control that will improve patient outcomes, while reducing the risk of either hypoglycemia or iatrogenic hyperglycemia (e.g., diabetic ketoacidosis).
- In critically ill patients, 2009 AACE/ADA recommendations: intravenous (IV) insulin infusion to control hyperglycemia targeting 140–180 mg/dl (target <110 mg/dl is no longer recommended) (Moghissi).
- In noncritically ill patients, 2009 AACE/ADA recommendations: premeal target <140 mg/dl, random BG <180 mg/dl; if BG <100, consider reassessing insulin regimen; if BG <70, regimen should be less intensified.

EPIDEMIOLOGY

- Inpatient hyperglycemia is associated with increased: infection, impaired wound healing, renal failure, risk of organ failure following transplant, and overall mortality.
- Medical conditions that cause glucose instability: infection, renal failure, malnutrition, advanced age, steroids and other medications that impair glucose homeostasis.
- Carbohydrate administration by tube feedings, parenteral nutrition, and intravenous dextrose solutions frequently cause hyperglycemia.
- Disruptions in nutrition are common due to nothing by mouth (NPO) orders, anorexia, or feeding intolerance, putting patients at risk for hypoglycemia.

CLINICAL TREATMENT

Oral and Antidiabetic Agents

- There are numerous contraindications to use of oral agents during acute illness (Figure 2-1).
- The general recommendation is to discontinue oral agents during hospitalization.

FIGURE 2-1. CONTRAINDICATIONS TO ORAL AGENTS

> **Contraindications/Precautions For Use of Oral Agents in the Hospital Setting:** Note that many of the contraindications can develop unexpectedly during acute illness. For this reason, the general recommendation is to discontinue oral agents during hospitalization.
>
> **METFORMIN:** Contraindications: (1) serum creatinine levels >1.5 mg/dl (males), >1.4 mg/dl (females). (2) Congestive heart failure requiring pharmacologic treatment. (3) Metabolic acidosis, including DKA. (4) Hypoperfusion. (5) For studies involving iodinated contrast materials, discontinue at the time of or prior to the procedure, and withhold for 48 hours subsequent to the procedure. Restart only after renal function has been re-evaluated and found to be normal. Cautions: advanced age.

FIGURE 2-1. CONTRAINDICATIONS TO ORAL AGENTS *(CONT.)*

SULFONYLUREAS: Contraindications: DKA, NPO status. Cautions: risk of prolonged/severe hypoglycemia. Long action with varied duration of action in different individuals, particularly high risk in renal or hepatic impairment, elderly.

TZDs: Contraindications: CHF. Cautions: Can increase intravascular volume, predisposing to CHF. Associate with fractures. Rosiglitazone, but probably not pioglitazone, associated with an increased risk of myocardial infarction. Do not use if baseline ALT >2.5× upper limit of normal. Slow onset of effect (6 weeks).

Courtesy of Joanne Dintzis and Sherita Hill Golden.

Intravenous IV Insulin Infusions

- Use IV insulin infusion to control hyperglycemia in critically ill patients, and all patients with DKA or hyperglycemic hyperosmolar state (HHS).
- Consider IV insulin perioperatively, especially in those destabilized by high-dose steroid pulses, or with hyperglycemia nonresponsive to subcutaneous (SQ) therapy.
- Administer IV insulin using validated written or computerized protocols that allow for predefined (often hourly) adjustments in the insulin infusion rate based on glycemic fluctuations and insulin dose.

Subcutaneous (SQ) Insulin Injections

- For noncritically ill patients: Scheduled SQ insulin injections are recommended previously sliding scale correction alone, because of proven efficacy and decreased risk of both hyper- and hypoglycemia.
- Physiologic insulin dosing is recommended, including basal, nutritional, and correctional components, based on the concept of total daily dose (TDD) of insulin (Figures 2-2 and 2-3).
- For insulin-deficient patients (type 1 diabetes, post-total pancreatectomy, or type 2 diabetes treated at home with insulin >5 years): use basal insulin at all times, even if not receiving nutrition, to prevent ketosis.
- The basal component of insulin is typically 40%–50% of the TDD of insulin; for patients who are NPO, eating poorly, or have hypoglycemia, consider 20%–40% reduction in basal dose.
- Insulin-deficient patients, if eating, require nutritional insulin, typically 10%–20% of the TTD; hold nutritional insulin if the patient is NPO or does not consume at least 50% of their carbohydrates.
- With new-onset hyperglycemia, or type 2 diabetes managed with diet or oral agents at home: place initially on correctional insulin alone (rapid acting, by sliding scale, see Figure 2-4); however, prolonged therapy with sliding scale insulin alone is not recommended.
- Consider adding basal and/or nutritional insulin if patient requires >20 units of correctional insulin per 24 hours, or if hyperglycemia persists despite correction.
- If hyperglycemia continues, total the doses of correctional insulin over the previous 24 hours to gauge the next day's regimen. Add 50% of the correctional total to the current basal dose; add 15% of the correctional total to current mealtime nutritional doses.
- If hypoglycemia occurs, decrease the total daily dose by 20%. Consider switching to a less aggressive correctional scale.

MANAGEMENT

FIGURE 2-2. METHODS FOR DETERMINING TOTAL DAILY DOSE (TDD) OF INSULIN*

Home regimen	Total of SQ insulin received over past 24 hours in hospital	Extrapolation of 24-hour total of IV insulin received	Weight-based calculation (while inpatient, recommended only for type 1 patients new to insulin)
Total the doses of all insulin types routinely taken at home e.g., • All NPH plus all Regular insulin doses • All mixed insulin doses (70/30, 75/25) • All long-acting (glargine or detemir) plus all rapid-acting (aspart or lispro)	Can be pulled from patient's medical record	Extrapolated from a stable 6-hour period on IV infusion	0.3–0.5 × patient's weight in kilograms

*Recommendations use the concept of total daily dose (TDD) of insulin. TDD includes the total amount of basal plus nutritional plus correctional insulin received over 24 hours. Courtesy of Joanne Dintzis and Sherita Hill Golden.

FIGURE 2-3. COMPONENTS OF PHYSIOLOGICAL INSULIN DOSING

Basal Insulin	Nutritional Insulin (prandial or mealtime)	Correctional Insulin
Timing Scheduled dose: Covers hour to hour insulin needs and suppresses hepatic glucose production	Scheduled dose: Covers ingested carbohydrate	PRN: "as needed" for blood glucose >150 mg/dl corrects for hyperglycemia
Types • Long-acting insulin, delivered daily • Intermediate-acting insulin, delivered twice	• Rapid-acting insulin • Short-acting insulin	• Rapid-acting insulin • Short-acting insulin
Calculations 40% to 50% of TDD	TDD minus basal insulin dose • Split to cover meals • Can give with breakfast, lunch, and dinner if patient eats at least 50% of carbohydrate foods on tray	• Graded scale based on suspected insulin activity • Administer in combination with nutritional dose if patient is eating • If patient requires correctional insulin regularly, adjust basal and prandial doses

Courtesy of Joanne Dintzis and Sherita Hill Golden.

FIGURE 2-4. DOSING FOR CORRECTIONAL SCALE INSULIN

	Low-Dose Algorithm for Patients Requiring <40 units of Insulin/Day		Medium-Dose Algorithm for Patients Requiring 40–80 units of Insulin/Day		High-Dose Algorithm for Patients Requiring >80 units of Insulin/Day	
	Glucose	Correctional Insulin	Glucose	Correctional Insulin	Glucose	Correctional Insulin
Mealtime	0–60 mg/dl	Treat per hypoglycemia protocol	0–60 mg/dl	Treat per hypoglycemia protocol	0–60 mg/dl	Treat per hypoglycemia protocol
	61–120 mg/dl	0 unit	61–120 mg/dl	0 unit	61–120 mg/dl	0 unit
	121–170 mg/dl	1 unit	121–150 mg/dl	1 unit	121–160 mg/dl	2 units
	171–220 mg/dl	2 units	151–180 mg/dl	2 units	161–200 mg/dl	4 units
	221–270 mg/dl	3 units	181–210 mg/dl	3 units	201–240 mg/dl	6 units
	271–320 mg/dl	4 units	211–240 mg/dl	4 units	241–280 mg/dl	8 units
	>320 mg/dl	5 units and NHO	241–270 mg/dl	5 units	281–320 mg/dl	10 units
			271–300 mg/dl	6 units	>320 mg/dl	12 units and NHO*
			301–330 mg/dl	7 units		
			>330 mg/dl	8 units and NHO		
Bedtime	0–60 mg/dl	treat per hypoglycemia protocol	0–60 mg/dl	Treat per hypoglycemia protocol	0–60 mg/dl	treat per hypoglycemia protocol
	61–250 mg/dl	0 units	61–250 mg/dl	0 units	61–250 mg/dl	0 units
	251–300 mg/dl	1 unit	251–280 mg/dl	2 units	251–290 mg/dl	4 units
	301–350 mg/dl	2 units	281–310 mg/dl	3 units	291–350 mg/dl	5 units
	>350 mg/dl	3 units and NHO	311–350 mg/dl	4 units	>350 mg/dl	6 units and NHO
			>350 mg/dl	5 units and NHO		

Note: Bedtime correctional insulin scales are more conservative (i.e., glucose target of 250 mg/dl or more)

*NHO stands for notify house officer

Courtesy of Joanne Dintzis and Sherita Hill Golden.

Subcutaneous External Insulin Pumps

- Patients using insulin pumps at home may have mental status changes that can impede safe self-management of pump due to pain medication, sleep deprivation, medically induced delirium, and severe physiological stress.
- For safe insulin pump therapy during a hospital stay, establish a systematic approach to screening patients for contraindications, clear and detailed guidelines for staff to follow in case of pump failure, and the availability of knowledgeable personnel.
- Institution policies should specifically define safety practices and responsibilities of the patient, nurse, prescriber, and pharmacy.
- Patient self-monitoring, insulin administration, and documentation are always observed by the nurse and confirmed in the medical record.

Nutritional Considerations

- Hospitalization frequently disrupts nutrition in unexpected ways: for example, NPO for unexpected procedures, malfunction of feeding tubes, malfunction of lines delivering parenteral nutrition. For these events, a basal/nutritional/correctional insulin regimen can increase patient safety.
- Nutritional insulin is scheduled and dosed to maintain euglycemia during absorption of carbohydrates; if the carbohydrate source is disrupted, the nutritional insulin component is held, thereby reducing the risk of hypoglycemia.
- *Patients eating meals or on bolus tube feeds:* Rapid-acting insulin analogs provide better coverage of absorbed carbohydrate than does regular insulin, improving glycemic control and reducing the risk of insulin "stacking" between breakfast and lunch doses, thereby reducing the risk of mid-afternoon hypoglycemia (Figure 2-5).
- *NPO status:* If a patient is made NPO, consider basal insulin dose reduction (e.g., 20%–40%); hold nutritional insulin and continue correctional insulin.
- *Continuous tube feeds:* The glycemic response to continuous enteral nutrition is exaggerated compared to that of discrete meals; nutritional insulin can be provided as a fixed dose of short- or rapid-acting insulin every 4–6 hours to reach glycemic targets, and allow the insulin to be held if the tube feed is disrupted, reducing the risk of hypoglycemia. Insulin-deficient patients will also continue to receive SQ basal insulin and correctional insulin (Gottschlich).
- *Continuous parenteral nutrition:* The glycemic response to parenteral nutrition is exaggerated compared to discrete meals. Insulin can be added to the parenteral nutrition formulation, delivering nutritional insulin in concert with incoming carbohydrates. If the parenteral source is disrupted, nutritional insulin automatically stops, reducing the risk of hypoglycemia. Insulin-deficient patients will also continue to receive SQ basal insulin and correctional insulin (Gottschlich).
- *Cycled nutrition regimens (enteral or parenteral):* Highly individualized, and will benefit from the expertise of endocrinology or specialists in parenteral/enteral support.

Patient Education

- For significant changes in regimen during the inpatient stay, written discharge instructions include follow-up within 1 month; instructions for monitoring blood sugars via glucose meter, bringing glucose log to follow-up appointment; and instructions to call healthcare provider immediately for any blood sugar <70 mg/dl, >300 mg/dl, or 4 consecutive readings >200 mg/dl.

FIGURE 2-5. SUBCUTANEOUS INSULIN FOR PATIENTS EATING MEALS OR ON BOLUS TUBE FEEDS

Examples	Type of Diabetes	Insulin Components Recommended	Basal	Nutritional	Correctional
Insulin-deficient patients	• Type 1 diabetes • Post-total pancreatectomy • Type 2 diabetes on insulin at home >5 years • Treated at home with nutritional insulin (including BID mixes or BID NPH/R regimens)	• Basal • Nutritional • Correctional	• If using long-acting insulin, give 40% of total daily dose (TDD) every 4 hours. Administer at same time every day. • If using intermediate-acting insulin, give 20% of total daily dose with breakfast, 20% of total daily dose at bedtime.	Take 60% of TDD. Divide by number of meals to determine amount needed to cover each meal. Give this amount of insulin as rapid-acting insulin with each meal. OR Utilize an insulin-to-carbohydrate ratio to determine nutritional dose if patient was using this method at home.	Order MEALtime and BEDtime rapid-acting correctional scales. BEDtime scales have more conservative targets (i.e., <250 mg/dl). Choose scale based on TDD: <40 units TDD = LOW dose 41–80 units TDD = MEDIUM dose <80 units TDD = HIGH dose

(Continued)

MANAGEMENT

FIGURE 2-5. SUBCUTANEOUS INSULIN FOR PATIENTS EATING MEALS OR ON BOLUS TUBE FEEDS *(CONT.)*

Examples	Type of Diabetes	Insulin Components Recommended	Basal	Nutritional	Correctional
Non-insulin-deficient patients	• Type 2 diabetes NOT on insulin at home • Acute hyperglycemia, no prior diabetes history	For initial therapy: • Correctional only • Basal and nutritional insulin can be added as needed after assessing daily blood glucose (BG) patterns	To determine need, review daily: • BG patterns (for consistent elevations) • Amount of correctional insulin required in 24 hours • If patient has required >20 units correction within 24 hours and hyperglycemia persists, add basal insulin at 40% of TDD (total of all types of insulin over past 24 hours).	To determine need, review BG daily. If hyperglycemia persists after addition of basal insulin, and BG elevations increase through the day, consider adding nutritional insulin.	Start with LOW dose MEALtime and BEDtime as part correctional scales. Evaluate after 24 hours. If hyperglycemia persists, consider: • switching to a more aggressive correction dose, using TDD as a guideline. • adding basal insulin.

Courtesy of Joanne Dintzis and Sherita Hill Golden.

FIGURE 2-6. ELEMENTS TO REVIEW AND ADDRESS BEFORE DISCHARGE

1. Level of understanding related to the diagnosis of diabetes
2. Monitoring a. technique b. when to test c. BG targets d. obtaining supplies
3. Hypoglycemia awareness a. signs/symptoms b. treatment c. driving safety d. notifying provider
4. Appointment with healthcare provider who will be responsible for diabetes care after discharge a. when to call the healthcare provider (i.e., notification parameters for BG) b. how to access an education program
5. Information on consistent eating patterns/basics of meal plan
6. When and how to take BG-lowering medications a. oral agents b. insulin
7. Sick day management
8. Proper use and disposal of needles and syringes

Courtesy of Joanne Dintzis and Sherita Hill Golden.

- The following areas should be reviewed and addressed before discharge (Figure 2-6):
  - Level of understanding related to the diagnosis of diabetes
  - Monitoring: techniques, when to test, BG targets, obtaining supplies
  - Hypoglycemia awareness: signs/symptoms, treatment, driving safety, notifying provider
  - Consistent eating patterns, basics of meal plan
  - When and how to take BG-lowering medications: oral agents, insulin
  - Sick day management
  - Proper use and disposal of needles and syringes

FOLLOW-UP
- Transition to home regimen: see Figure 2-7 for transition back to home regimen for patients on insulin during hospitalization.
- Clear communication with outpatient providers is essential for ensuring safe and successful transition to outpatient glycemic management.

EXPERT OPINION
- Insulin is the treatment that provides the greatest flexibility, but also has the highest risk of potential medication errors and adverse events, including hypoglycemia.
- Inpatient insulin management requires ongoing assessment and adjustment. Consider factors that influence insulin requirements such as steroid dose changes; nutritional

MANAGEMENT

FIGURE 2-7. TRANSITIONING BACK TO HOME REGIMEN FOR PATIENTS ON INSULIN DURING HOSPITALIZATION

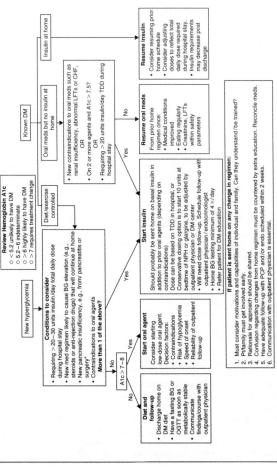

Review Hemoglobin A1c
○ < 5.2 unlikely to have DM
○ 5.2–6 indeterminate
○ > 6 highly likely to have DM
○ > 7 requires treatment change

New hyperglycemia

Known DM

Conditions to consider
- Requiring > 20–30 units insulin/day total daily dose during hospital stay
- New med regimen likely to cause BG elevation (e.g., steroids or anti-rejection drugs) that will continue at home
- New pancreatic insufficiency, e.g., from pancreatitis or surgery*
- Contraindications to oral agents
More than 1 of the above?

Diet/exercise controlled

Oral meds but no insulin at home
- New contraindications to oral meds such as renal insufficiency, abnormal LFTs or CHF,
OR
- On 2 or more agents and A1c > 7.5?
OR
- Requiring > 20 units insulin/day TDD during hospital stay

Insulin at home

A1c > 7–8

No → **Diet and follow-up**
- Discharge home on DM diet
- Have a fasting BG or OGTT as soon as metabolically stable
- Communicate findings/course with outpatient physician

Yes → **Start oral agent**
Consider starting low-dose oral agent.
Decision factors:
- Risk of hypoglycemia
- Contraindications
- Speed of onset
- Reliability of outpatient follow-up

Start insulin
Should probably be sent home on basal insulin in addition to prior oral agents (depending on contraindications)
- Dose can be based on TDD in hospital, or
- Conservative dosing option is to start 10 units at bedtime of NPH or glargine, to be adjusted by outpatient physician or DM center
- Will need close follow-up. Schedule follow-up with outpatient physician / endocrinologist
- Home BG testing minimum of 4 ×/day
- Refer patient for DM education

Resume oral meds
From prior home regimen once:
- Medical conditions improved
- Eating regularly
- Creatinine, LFTs within safety parameters

Yes

No

Resume insulin
- Consider resuming prior home schedule
- Consider adjusting doses to reflect total daily dose required during hospital stay. Insulin requirements may decrease post discharge

If patient is sent home on any change in regimen:
1. Must consider motivations and capabilities of individual and family. Can they understand / be trained?
2. Pt/family must get involved early.
3. Rationale for approach should be shared.
4. Confusion regarding changes from home regimen must be countered by extra education. Reconcile meds.
5. Have adequate follow-up with PCP and/or endo scheduled within 2 weeks.
6. Communication with outpatient physician is essential.

*Note: Any patient following TOTAL pancreatectomy, or with newly diagnosed type 1 DM will always require basal/nutritional/and correctional insulin on discharge.
Courtesy of Joanne Dintzis and Sherita Hill Golden.

status; renal status changes; onset of and recovery from fevers, infections, and/or surgical stress; and changes in activity level.

- Challenges include rapid changes in insulin requirements during acute illness and unpredictable nutrition disruptions.
- Higher glucose ranges may be acceptable in critically ill patients, patients with severe comorbidities, or in settings where frequent glucose monitoring is not possible.
- Intensive glycemic control to a target of 80–110 mg/dl has not yielded consistent improvement in mortality in clinical trials, and some studies reported an increased mortality risk with targets in the 80–100 mg/dl range (Finfer; Griesdale).
- Recurrent hypoglycemia may lead to increased mortality and long-term cognitive deficits resulting in recently updated targets for hospitalized patients.
- Recent guidelines recommend not using intensive insulin therapy in hospitalized patients (Qaseem).
- Because of the need to educate and monitor a large interdisciplinary team in new and complex insulin treatment modalities, safe achievement of goals requires administrative support for a sustained, systematic, and interdisciplinary effort.

REFERENCES

Qaseem A, Humphrey LL, Chou R, et al. Use of intensive insulin therapy for the management of glycemic control in hospitalized patients: a clinical practice guideline from the American College of Physicians. *Ann Intern Med,* 2011; 154: pp. 260–7.

   Comments: Recently released guidelines from the ACP.

Moghissi ES, Korytkowski MT, DiNardi M, et al. American Association of Clinical Endocrinologists and American Diabetes Association consensus statement on inpatient glycemic control. *Endocrine Practice,* 2009; Vol. 15(4): pp. 1–17.

   Comments: Guidelines from the AACE and ADA.

Griesdale DE, de Souza RJ, van Dam RM, et al. Intensive insulin therapy and mortality among critically ill patients: a meta-analysis including NICE-SUGAR study data. *CMAJ,* 2009; Vol. 180: pp. 799–800.

   Comments: Meta-analysis of randomized trials demonstrating differential effects of tight glucose control between medical vs surgical ICUs.

NICE-SUGAR Study Investigators, Finfer S, Chittock DR, et al. Intensive versus conventional glucose control in critically ill patients. *NEJM,* 2009; Vol. 360: pp. 1283–97.

   Comments: Results of a large, international, randomized trial demonstrating increased mortality with intensive glucose control in ICU settings.

Michele M Gottschlich, editor in chief. The A.S.P.E.N. Nutritional Support Core Curriculum. American Society for Parenteral and Enteral Nutrition (A.S.P.E.N.): Silver Spring; MD; 2007.

   Comments: Recommendations related to glycemic control during parenteral and enteral nutrition.

Combes JR, Cousins D, Kercher LL, Rich V, et al. American Society of Health-System Pharmacists' professional practice recommendations for safe use of insulin in hospitals, 2004. Available at American Society of Health-System Pharmacists website: *http://www.ashp.org/s_ashp/docs/files/Safe_Use_of_Insulin.pdf* (accessed 1/12/2010).

   Comments: A comprehensive and systematic list of best practice recommendations for safe and effective insulin use in hospitals.

Clement S, Braithwaite SS, Magee MF, et al. Management of diabetes and hyperglycemia in hospitals. *Diabetes Care,* 2004; Vol. 27: pp. 553–91.

   Comments: A comprehensive review of evidence related to management of hyperglycemia in hospitals, including focus on approaches to subcutaneous insulin use as well as IV insulin infusion.

van den Berghe G, Wouters P, Weekers F, et al. Intensive insulin therapy in the critically ill patients. *NEJM,* 2001; Vol. 345: pp. 1359–67.

   Comments: Landmark study demonstrating reduced mortality with improved glycemic control in a SICU.

MANAGEMENT

PERIOPERATIVE CARE OF DIABETES

Mary Huizinga, MD, MPH

DEFINITION

- Perioperative care of people with diabetes involves preoperative assessment and modification of usual antidiabetic medications, and intraoperative and postoperative management.

EPIDEMIOLOGY

- Patients with diabetes have an estimated 50% lifetime risk of undergoing surgery.
- Patients with diabetes are at increased risk of complications due to the complexity of care, increased risk of infections, complications and comorbidities, and possible asymptomatic coronary artery disease (CAD).

CLINICAL TREATMENT

Preoperative Evaluation

- Diabetes assessment includes current medications; baseline glycemic control (blood glucose ranges, A1c level within last 3 months); history of diabetic ketoacidosis; long-term complications (retinopathy, nephropathy, neuropathy); history of hypoglycemia (awareness, frequency, severity).
- If diabetic control is poor, consider postponing elective surgery.
- Medication needs will change in the perioperative and postoperative period; preoperative time is a good time to plan for these changes.
- **Cardiovascular:** thorough history and physical and EKG. If symptoms of CAD are present, consider cardiac stress test prior to elective surgery.
- **Pulmonary:** With obesity, consider obstructive sleep apnea (OSA). Treatment of OSA for a minimum of 2 weeks is needed to decrease potential operative risk. If OSA is diagnosed, may require extubation to CPAP. Other pulmonary considerations include chronic obstructive pulmonary disease and asthma.
- **Nephropathy:** Document GFR and stage of chronic kidney disease if present, as this may affect dosage of medications.
- **Hypertension:** Consider medications prior to surgery. Do **not** hold beta-blockers prior to surgery but do stop other antihypertensives the morning of surgery.
- **Antiplatelet therapy:** Hold aspirin for 7 days prior to surgery. The management of long-term antithrombotic therapy depends on the patients risk of thromboembolism and the type of surgery to be performed. The American College of Chest Physicians recommends that patients at high risk of thromboembolism (e.g., mechanical heart valve) should be bridged from coumadin to heparin; however, those with low risk may stop antithrombotic therapy for 5 days before surgery. If the INR in those who stopped antithrombotic therapy remains elevated, oral vitamin K should be used to normalize INR. Antithrombotic therapy should resume 12–24 hours after surgery.

Perioperative Management

- Some evidence suggests that better baseline glycemic control is associated with a reduction in postoperative infections.
- The ADA recommends that fasting blood glucose <140 mg/dl and random blood glucose <180 mg/dl for non-critically ill hospitalized patients.

- Patients with type 2 diabetes on diet alone usually do not require therapy before surgery, but fast-acting insulin by sliding scale according to blood glucose may be used to treat hyperglycemia perioperatively.
- Patients on oral agents should continue their normal therapy until the morning of surgery when medications are held. Most will not require additional therapy, but may be given sliding scale insulin if needed perioperatively.
- Insulin-requiring patients can continue their subcutaneous insulin, usually reducing long-acting insulin by one-half the evening preoperatively to prevent hypoglycemia. The morning of surgery, hold short-acting insulin and administer one-half to two-thirds of basal insulin. People with type 1 diabetes must receive basal insulin to prevent ketoacidosis. Fast-acting insulin may be given to control hyperglycemia during surgery. Administer IV fluids containing 5% dextrose at 75–125 cc/hour (3.75–6.25 grams of glucose/hour) to avoid catabolic effects of starvation and avoid hypoglycemia. Alternatively, insulin may be given by continuous IV infusion intraoperatively.
- Potassium may be added (10–20 mEg/L) to fluid infusion in patients with normal renal function and normal preoperative serum potassium.
- Longer, complex operations require more intensive management, often with a glucose-insulin-potassium fluid infusion.

Postoperative Management

- Follow general principles of hospital management (see p. 68), especially for patients on insulin at baseline, and inpatient glycemic targets postoperatively.
- Immediately postoperatively, blood glucose monitoring should occur at least 4 times a day (before meals and at bedtime). More frequent monitoring is needed if the patient is on an insulin infusion.
- Once patients are eating well, restart oral agents. However, hold metformin until confident of normal renal and hepatic function and lack of congestive heart failure. Also, avoid thiazolidinediones in patients with congestive heart failure or impaired liver function; avoid sulfonylureas with severe renal impairment. Restart sulfonylureas at reduced dosage if patient is consuming fewer calories, to prevent hypoglycemia.

Clinical Treatment

- Surgery and general anesthesia are associated with a neuroendocrine response that can lead to hyperglycemia and ketosis.
- First goal is to maintain fluid/electrolyte balance and prevent marked hyperglycemia, ketoacidosis, hyperosmolar hyperglycemic state, and hypoglycemia.
- Second goal is to promote wound healing and minimize postoperative catabolism by maintaining reasonable glycemic control.

EXPERT OPINION

- Immediate metabolic status (glycemia, ketosis) as well as established complications of diabetes increase surgical risk.
- Elective surgery allows for a more thorough preoperative evaluation and management than urgent surgery.
- With emergency surgery, manage hyperglycemia with IV or subcutaneous fast-acting insulin, and hypoglycemia with 5% or 10% IV dextrose infusions. Be aware of stopping/reversing

MANAGEMENT

anticoagulation; stopping metformin; and taking previously administered long-acting insulin into account.

- With elective surgery, evaluate as previously, and prepare patient as well as possible for surgery.

REFERENCES

Moghissi ES, Korytkowski MT, DiNardo M, et al. American Association of Clinical Endocrinologists and American Diabetes Association consensus statement on inpatient glycemic control. *Diabetes Care,* 2009; Vol. 32: pp. 1119–31.

    Comments: Consensus statement from AACE and ADA of inpatient glycemic control with review of epidemiology of diabetes and hospitalizations.

Griesdale DE, de Souza RJ, van Dam RM, et al. Intensive insulin therapy and mortality among critically ill patients: a meta-analysis including NICE-SUGAR study data. *CMAJ,* 2009; Vol. 180: pp. 821–7.

    Comments: Systematic review and meta-analysis of intensive insulin therapy and mortality among critically ill patients; shows significantly increased risk of hypoglycemia and no mortality benefit, however, may be beneficial in patients in surgical ICU.

NICE-SUGAR Study Investigators, Finfer S, Chittock DR, et al. Intensive versus conventional glucose control in critically ill patients. *NEJM,* 2009; Vol. 360: pp. 1283–97.

    Comments: NICE-SUGAR is the largest randomized controlled trial of intensive glucose management in ICU patients; intensive glucose management was found to increase mortality.

Douketis JD, Berger PB, Dunn AS, et al. The perioperative management of antithrombotic therapy: American College of Chest Physicians evidence-based clinical practice guidelines (8th edition). *Chest,* 2008; Vol. 133: pp. 299S–339S.

    Comments: American College of Chest Physicians Guidelines for the perioperative management of antithrombotic therapy.

Rodbard HW, Blonde L, Braithwaite SS, et al. American Association of Clinical Endocrinologists medical guidelines for clinical practice for the management of diabetes mellitus. *Endocr Pract,* 2007; Vol. 13 Suppl 1: pp. 1–68.

    Comments: AACE medical guidelines for clinical management of diabetes.

Fleisher LA, Beckman JA, Brown KA, et al. ACC/AHA 2007 guidelines on perioperative cardiovascular evaluation and care for noncardiac surgery: a report of the American College of Cardiology/American Heart Association Task Force on Practice Guidelines (Writing Committee to Revise the 2002 Guidelines on Perioperative Cardiovascular Evaluation for Noncardiac Surgery). Developed in collaboration with the American Society of Echocardiography, American Society of Nuclear Cardiology, Heart Rhythm Society, Society of Cardiovascular Anesthesiologists, Society for Cardiovascular Angiography and Interventions, Society for Vascular Medicine and Biology, and Society for Vascular Surgery. *Circulation,* 2007; Vol. 116: pp. e418–99.

    Comments: ACC and AHA guidelines on perioperative cardiac evaluation for noncardiac surgery.

Dronge AS, Perkal MF, Kancir S, et al. Long-term glycemic control and postoperative infectious complications. *Arch Surg,* 2006; Vol. 141: pp. 375–80; discussion 380.

    Comments: Retrospective cohort from the VA National Surgical Quality Improvement Program; found that A1c level was significantly associated with postoperative infections.

Van den Berghe G, Wilmer A, Hermans G, et al. Intensive insulin therapy in the medical ICU. *NEJM,* 2006; Vol. 354: pp. 449–61.

    Comments: Randomized controlled trial of intensive glycemic management in medical ICU patients found intensive management reduced morbidity but not mortality.

Gross JB, Bachenberg KL, Benumof JL, et al. Practice guidelines for the perioperative management of patients with obstructive sleep apnea: a report by the American Society of Anesthesiologists Task Force on perioperative management of patients with obstructive sleep apnea. *Anesthesiology,* 2006; Vol. 104: pp. 1081–93; quiz 1117–8.

Comments: American Society of Anesthesiologists statement on perioperative management of obstructive sleep apnea.

Clement S, Braithwaite SS, Magee MF, et al. Management of diabetes and hyperglycemia in hospitals. *Diabetes Care,* 2004; Vol. 27: pp. 553–91.

Comments: Review article written by ADA Professional Practice Committee.

Marks JB. Perioperative management of diabetes. *Am Fam Physician,* 2003; Vol. 67: pp. 93–100.

Comments: Clinically oriented review of perioperative management of diabetes.

van den Berghe G, Wouters P, Weekers F, et al. Intensive insulin therapy in the critically ill patients. *NEJM,* 2001; Vol. 345: pp. 1359–67.

Comments: Randomized controlled trial of intensive glycemic management in surgical ICU patients found that intensive management reduced morbidity and mortality.

POSTPANCREATECTOMY DIABETES

Joanne Dintzis, CRNP, CDE, and Sherita Golden, MD, MHS

MANAGEMENT

DEFINITION

- Endocrine pancreatic insufficiency occurring after surgical resection of the pancreas.
- Associated with development of new-onset diabetes, exacerbation of preexisting diabetes, or progression of preexisting glucose intolerance to overt diabetes.
- Important factors include amount of pancreatic parenchymal tissue removed, resection versus "sparing" of adjacent organs, preoperative pancreatic function, peripheral insulin resistance, preoperative diabetes, and postoperative changes in nutrition.

EPIDEMIOLOGY

- Pancreatic resections in the United States have increased overall 15.0% in the last decade, with a 27% increase in resections for benign pancreatic disease alone.
- Indications for pancreatic surgery include malignancies (curative or palliative resection), chronic pancreatitis (palliation, drainage of pseudocysts, or repair of obstruction or fistulas), and acute necrotizing pancreatitis (necrosectomy or lavage-pseudocyst drainage).

CLINICAL TREATMENT

General Considerations

- Postoperatively, insulin requirements are affected by nutritional disruptions due to ileus, pancreatic leak, or chyle leak. Also consider preoperative malnutrition, as well as parenteral nutrition required during periods of bowel or pancreatic rest.
- In setting glycemic goals with pancreatic malignancy, consider overall prognosis and nutritional instability from chemotherapy or radiation therapy. Higher glycemic targets may be indicated in these settings.

Total Pancreatectomy

- Total pancreatectomy results in total insulin deficiency and near-absent glucagon production.
- All patients will require exogenous basal and correctional insulin to treat hyperglycemia and mealtime rapid- or short-acting insulin to cover ingested carbohydrates once diet is consistent.

- Initial insulin requirements during immediate postoperative fasting period are usually low, possibly due to the lack of glucagon production causing less hepatic gluconeogenesis.
- IV insulin infusion along with a low level of IV dextrose while patient is NPO provides the greatest flexibility.
- Because of the exaggerated sensitivity to insulin postoperatively, transition from IV to SQ insulin regimens utilizing conservative doses.

Partial Pancreatectomy

- **Near-total pancreatectomy:** ~95% is removed, may be offered to patients with intractable pain from pancreatitis. Postoperatively, ~60%–75% of patients require insulin.
- **Proximal pancreatectomy:** most commonly the "classic Whipple" or pancreaticoduodenectomy; head of the pancreas, duodenum, distal stomach (often), common bile duct, and gallbladder are removed. Recent refinements may preserve the pylorus and/or duodenum. May have leaks from the pancreaticojejunostomy, other perioperative events, or delayed gastric emptying. New-onset diabetes in ~20%–50%.
- **Distal pancreatectomy:** for disease processes in the tail. Spleen may be removed and the flow of pancreatic secretions not normally interrupted. Diabetes in ~3%–30%.
- **Middle pancreatectomy:** preserves pancreatic parenchyma, reducing the risk of exocrine and endocrine insufficiency. Less diabetes but higher rates of fistulas and pancreatic leaks.
- During hospital stay, closely monitor glycemia as diet is advanced and implement insulin therapy if needed.
- Prior diabetes regimens will likely need to be increased after pancreatic surgery, often requiring insulin.
- Rarely, removal of diseased tissue and subsequent reduced inflammation brings improved glycemic control.

FOLLOW-UP

- Gastrointestinal disturbances are common and sometimes prolonged, often requiring pancreatic enzymes. Gastric emptying can be delayed, and nausea and diarrhea can occur.
- Oral intake may be irregular and sporadic for several months making insulin management challenging.
- Additional changes in nutrition and insulin requirements can occur during chemotherapy in cancer patients.
- After total and distal pancreatectomy, patients are at increased risk for rapid development of hypoglycemia due to deficiency of glucagon-secreting alpha cells.
- For total pancreatectomy patients, include basal and correctional insulin, with nutritional insulin once food intake is stabilized and consistent.
- Partial pancreatectomy patients show wide variability in postoperative insulin requirements. A preoperative A1c >6% can be predictive of patients who will require postoperative insulin therapy.
- Insulin requirements may be erratic for several months after surgery, until healing has progressed, perioperative inflammation has resolved, and nutritional intake has normalized. During this period of instability, more conservative glycemic targets may be indicated.
- Patients on insulin need outpatient follow-up with an endocrinologist and/or diabetes educator, no longer than 1 month post discharge.

- For insulin-treated patients, include on discharge syringes/vials, insulin pens/needles, and glucagon emergency kits.
- All patients with blood glucose elevations postoperatively should receive a glucose meter, prescriptions for glucose testing strips and instructions to monitor their blood glucose regularly until follow-up with their primary care provider within 1 month of hospital discharge.
- Discharge instructions include contact healthcare provider for blood glucose <70 mg/dl, glucose >300 mg/dl, or 3 consecutive glucose readings >250 mg/dl.

EXPERT OPINION

- Inpatient consults should be initiated as soon as possible postpancreatectomy with a dietician and diabetes care team.
- Patient instruction, including hands-on practice with insulin self-administration and blood glucose monitoring, should begin as early as possible and continue with frequent reinforcement and practice throughout the hospital stay.
- After pancreatectomy, patients are under severe physical and emotional stress. This may impact their ability to understand and retain safety-related instructions.
- Patients with total pancreatectomy especially will require close outpatient diabetes education follow-up, having become rapidly and totally insulin-deficient in the context of simultaneous glucagon deficiency, often leading to brittle diabetes.

REFERENCES

Teh SH, Diggs BS, Deveney CW, and Sheppard BC. Patient and hospital characteristics on the variance of perioperative outcomes for pancreatic resection in the United States. *Arch of Surg,* 2009; Vol. 144(8): pp. 713–21.
   Comments: This article describes the effect of patient and hospital characteristics on perioperative outcomes (in-hospital mortality, perioperative complications, and mortality following a major complication) for pancreatic resection in the United States.

Irani JL, Ashley SW, Brooks DC, Osteen RT, et al. Distal pancreatectomy is not associated with increased perioperative morbidity when performed as part of a multivisceral resection. *J Gastroint Surg,* 2008; Vol. 12: pp. 2177–2182.
   Comments: This article evaluates the indications for and the outcomes from distal pancreatectomy.

King J, Kazanjian K, Matsumoto J, Reber HA, et al. Distal pancreatetomy: incidence of postoperative diabetes. *J. Gastrointest Surg,* 2008; Vol. 12(9): pp. 1548–1553.
   Comments: This article describes the rate of clinically apparent new-onset diabetes in 125 patients after distal pancreatetomy.

Riediger H, Adam U, Fischeer E, Keck T, et al. Long-term outcome after resection for chronic pancreatitis in 224 patients. *Gastoint Surg,* 2007; Vol. 11(8): pp. 949–59.
   Comments: The focus of this article is on long-term outcome after pancreatic surgery for chronic pancreatitis. Morbidities examined include pain, exocrine/endocrine pancreatic function, and control of organ complications in 224 patients with a median follow-up period of 54 months.

Hamilton L, Jeyarajah DR. Hemoglobin A1c can be helpful in predicting progression to diabetes after Whipple procedure. *HBP* (Oxford, UK*),* 2007; Vol. 9(1): pp. 26–8.
   Comments: This article from the official journal of the Hepato Pancreato Biliary Association reports results of a small-scale study that utilizes preoperative A1c levels to predict progression to diabetes post pancreatic surgery.

Crippa S, Bassi C, Warshaw AL, Falconi M, et al. Middle pancreatectomy: indications, short- and long-term operative outcomes. *Ann of Surg,* 2007; Vol. 246(1): pp. 69–76.

MANAGEMENT

Comments: This article evaluates the indications, perioperative and long-term outcomes of a large cohort of patients who underwent middle pancreatectomy.

Jethwa P, Sodergren M, Lala A, Webber JAC, et al. Diabetic control after total pancreatectomy. *Digest Liver Dis,* 2006; Vol. 38(6): pp. 415–419.

Comments: This article describes a retrospective analysis of patients undergoing total pancreatectomy from a single institution over a 15-year time frame, comparing data of diabetic control.

Kahl S, Malfertheiner P. Exocrine and endocrine pancreatic insufficiency after pancreatic surgery. *Best Pract Res Clin Gastroenterol,* 2004; Vol. 18(5): pp. 947–955.

Comments: This article provides an overview of indications for pancreatic surgery and effects on exocrine and endocrine function following surgery.

Hutchins RR, Hart RS, Pacifico M, Bradley NJ, Williamson RC. Long-term results of distal pancreatectomy for chronic pancreatitis in 90 patients. *Ann Surg,* 2002; Vol. 236(5): pp. 612–8.

Comments: This article describes the indications for total pancreatectomy for chronic pancreatitis, and evaluates the risks, functional loss, and outcome of the procedure in 90 patients.

Slezak LA, Anderson DK. Pancreatic resection: effects on glucose metabolism. *World J Surg,* 2001; Vol. 25: pp. 452–460.

Comments: This article describes the characteristics of the endocrine abnormalities that develop postsurgical resection of the pancreas

BARIATRIC SURGERY

Octavia Pickett-Blakely, MD, MHS, and Mary Huizinga, MD, MPH

DEFINITION

- A frequently done, effective surgical intervention for obese individuals to reduce weight and improve obesity-related comorbidities such as diabetes. Results in weight loss by restriction of overall nutrient intake, malabsorption of nutrients, and/or a combination of restriction and malabsorption.
- **Laparoscopic adjustable gastric band:** restrictive procedure that inserts a band around the proximal stomach; the band is connected to a subcutaneous port used to adjust the amount of gastric restriction provided by the band.
- **Laparoscopic sleeve gastrectomy:** restrictive procedure that removes large portion of the greater curvature of the stomach leaving a stomach "sleeve" along the lesser curvature. Can be done as the first part of a duodenal switch or as a stand-alone procedure.
- **Roux-en-Y gastric bypass:** combination restrictive and malabsorptive procedure that creates a small gastric pouch by separating the proximal and distal stomach; the proximal gastric pouch is anastomosed to a loop of jejunum ("Roux limb"), while the bypassed distal stomach and proximal small bowel ("Y limb") is anastomosed distally to the jejunum.
- **Biliopancreatic diversion (BPD) with or without duodenal switch:** combination restrictive and malabsorptive procedure that creates a laparoscopic sleeve gastrectomy with remaining stomach either (1) attached to lower portion of smaller intenstine (BPD) or (2) attached to upper small intestine with creation of separate biliary loop, both of which connect to common channel of lower smaller intestine (duodenal switch).

EPIDEMIOLOGY

- Up to 55% of all patients diagnosed with diabetes are obese (CDC).
- Of an estimated 225,000 bariatric surgeries performed per annum, 15%–30% have diabetes (CDC).
- Bariatric surgery can result in the resolution of type 2 diabetes in 48%–98% of cases depending on the type of surgery performed (Segal; Vetter).
- Diabetes-related mortality and all-cause mortality is significantly decreased after gastric bypass (Christou; Segal).

DIAGNOSIS

- Eligibility for bariatric surgery is established according to National Institutes of Health guidelines: BMI ≥40 kg/m² or a BMI ≥35 kg/m² with an obesity-related comorbidity such as diabetes, hypertension, obstructive sleep apnea, obesity hypoventilation syndrome, Pickwickian syndrome, severe urinary incontinence, hyperlipidemia, debilitating osteoarthritis, nonalcoholic fatty liver disease, coronary artery disease, gastroesophageal reflux disease, and pseudotumor cerebri (NIH consensus conference).
- In February 2011, the FDA approved use of laparoscopic adjustable gastric banding for BMI ≥30 kg/m² with an obesity-related comorbidity in response to a study presented by the manufacturer that showed significant weight loss after the surgery for persons who were mildly obese.
- Specific coverage guidelines vary by insurance carrier (e.g., documentation of a failed trial of diet and exercise and performance of surgery at an American Society for Bariatric Surgery designated Center of Excellence).

CLINICAL TREATMENT

Glycemic Control in Immediate Postoperative Period (Days 0–3)

- Insulin-requiring patients often require significantly lower doses of insulin and oral hypoglycemic agents postoperatively due to decreased oral intake.
- With Roux-en-Y or BPD procedures, hyperglycemia may improve dramatically within several days, well before significant weight loss.
- Advance oral intake according to institution- or provider-specific protocols. Most diets begin with clear liquids and advance to full liquids or pureed foods that are high in protein and low in fat and carbohydrates.
- A combination of basal and rapid-acting prandial insulin is preferred to keep fasting blood glucose levels between 80–110 mg/dl and postprandial glucose levels below 180 mg/dl.
- Some patients only require mealtime insulin during this time period due to irregular intake and decreasing insulin requirements.
- Doses of oral agents should be withheld or adjusted in noninsulin-requiring patients. Specifically, secretagogues should be discontinued in the immediate postoperative period.

Glycemic Control in the Outpatient Setting

- Oral intake is advanced further from full liquids and pureed foods ultimately to a regular diet (small, frequent meals) consisting of high-protein, low-fat, and low-carbohydrate meals.
- In patients with type 2 diabetes, home preprandial and fasting blood glucose measurements should be performed periodically.

MANAGEMENT

- The use of insulin and/or oral agents is dictated by the patient's home glucose measurements and often (in up to 76% of patients) declines within 1 year of bariatric surgery.
- Most patients will be off insulin and oral agents by 3 months postoperatively.

Micronutrient Deficiencies

- Post-bariatric surgery patients are at risk for a variety of micronutrient deficiencies including: B12, iron, calcium, vitamin D, folate, B1, and others.
- All patients receiving bariatric surgery should be started on a multivitamin with iron and calcium citrate with vitamin D after bariatric surgery.
- Patients should be monitored regularly for micronutrient deficiencies. The frequency depends on the type of surgery. Patients undergoing laparoscopic adjustable band should be monitored annually, gastric bypass require monitoring every 3–6 months, and bilopancreatic diversion patients should be monitored every 3–6 months.
- Although calcium is absorbed throughout the small intestine and colon, calcium-containing foods (e.g., milk, cheese) may provoke bloating, cramping, and diarrhea in post-bariatric patients, placing them at risk for deficiency. Calcium citrate with vitamin D is the recommended form of calcium because of increased absorption.
- Oral B12 is often not sufficient to replete B12 deficiencies. B12 should be administered in sublingual, intranasal, or intramuscular forms given that oral B12 is not absorbed due the anatomical disruption of B12 and intrinsic factor binding in gastric bypass and other malabsorptive surgeries (bilopancreatic diversion/duodenal switch).
- Iron absorption is impaired in gastric bypass and other malabsorptive surgeries due to bypass of the duodenum (the site of iron absorption). Some patients may require intravenous iron therapy.
- Folate deficiency may occur as a result of B12 deficiency, impaired intestinal absorption, or inadequate oral intake. Folate supplementation is recommended in patients after bariatric surgery.
- B1 deficiency can arise in the setting of inadequate oral intake, or impaired intestinal absorption, and may result in Wernicke-Korsakoff syndrome. B1 is usually a component of most multivitamin preparations, but deficient individuals can be treated with intramuscular injections.
- Vitamin D deficiency can result from decreased oral intake, and impaired absorption due to poor mixing of vitamin D with bile salts. Daily oral supplementation is recommended.

Complications

- **Medical:** electrolyte abnormalities.
- Dumping syndrome (hyperinsulinemic hypoglycemia approximately 30 minutes postprandially resulting from rapid gastric emptying). Acarbose may help to treat symptoms.
- Nesidioblastosis (hyperinsulemic hypoglycemia greater than 1 hour postprandially resulting from pancreatic beta cell hyperfunction) remains controversial (Service).
- Weight regain.
- Gallstones.
- Loose skin after weight loss.
- Laparoscopic adjustable band: vomiting, pain, dysphagia, reflux.
- **Surgical:** Roux-en-Y gastric bypass or BPD: anastamotic leak, marginal ulceration, stomal stenosis.

- Laparoscopic adjustable band or sleeve gastrectomy: band malfunction (slippage, erosion, infection), leakage, hemorrhage, fistula.

FOLLOW-UP

- Follow-up in bariatric surgery patients depends on the comorbidities and the type of surgery performed. Note potential complications previously.
- Diabetes recurrence can be as high as 43% after Roux-en-Y gastric bypass (associated with lower preoperative BMI, failed weight loss, weight regain, and high postoperative blood glucose) (Vetter).
- Hemoglobin A1c monitoring should be continued in the postoperative period.
- Weight loss depends on the type of operation performed. Expected average weight loss in the first 1–2 years after surgery is 45%–85% and 29%–87% for Roux-en-Y gastric bypass and laparoscopic adjustable band surgery, respectively (Buchwald).

EXPERT OPINION

- There is often a significant decline in postoperative requirements for insulin or oral agents due to improved insulin sensitivity postoperatively. Glucose tolerance may normalize.
- Maintain a high index of suspicion for micronutrient deficiencies.
- Bariatric surgery is covered by many insurance carriers (e.g., Medicaid), but specific coverage guidelines are carrier dependent.
- Bariatric surgery enforces a new relationship to food: Patients cannot eat the amount of food they previously consumed.
- Recent findings include an increased incidence of postoperative, long-term hyperinsulinemic hypoglycemia associated with pancreatic beta-cell hyperplasia (nesidioblastosis); however, these findings remain controversial.

MANAGEMENT

REFERENCES

Segal JB, Clark JM, Shore AD, et al. Prompt reduction in use of medications for comorbid conditions after bariatric surgery. *Obes Surg*, 2009; Vol. 19: pp. 1646–56.
   Comments: Bariatric surgery can resolve type 2 diabetes.

Vetter ML, Cardillo S, Rickels MR, et al. Narrative review: effect of bariatric surgery on type 2 diabetes mellitus. *Ann Intern Med*, 2009; Vol. 150: pp. 94–103.
   Comments: This systematic review reports on the effect of bariatric surgery on T2DM.

Christou NV. Impact of obesity and bariatric surgery on survival. *World J Surg*, 2009; Vol. 33: pp. 2022–7.
   Comments: Bariatric surgery reduces the relative risk of death in morbidly obese patients.

Mechanick JI, Kushner RF, Sugerman HJ, et al. American Association of Clinical Endocrinologists, The Obesity Society, and American Society for Metabolic and Bariatric Surgery medical guidelines for clinical practice for the perioperative nutritional, metabolic, and nonsurgical support of the bariatric surgery patient. *Obesity* (Silver Spring, MD), 2009; Vol. 17 Suppl 1: pp. S1–70.
   Comments: Guidelines published for the perioperative management of bariatric surgery patients.

Dixon JB, O'Brien PE, Playfair J, et al. Adjustable gastric banding and conventional therapy for type 2 diabetes: a randomized controlled trial. *JAMA*, 2008; Vol. 299: pp. 316–23.
   Comments: Laparoscopic adjustable band surgery is superior to conventional diabetes therapy for the remission of diabetes and weight loss.

Adams TD, Gress RE, Smith SC, et al. Long-term mortality after gastric bypass surgery. *NEJM*, 2007; Vol. 357: pp. 753–61.
   Comments: This article reviews how mortality is decreased after gastric bypass surgery.

Service GJ, Thompson GB, Service FJ, et al. Hyperinsulinemic hypoglycemia with nesidioblastosis after gastric-bypass surgery. *NEJM*, 2005; Vol. 353: pp. 249–54.

Comments: Nesidioblastosis is an uncommon phenomenon in bariatric surgery patients associated with hyperinsulinemic hypoglycemia.

Centers for Disease Control and Prevention (CDC) Prevalence of overweight and obesity among adults with diagnosed diabetes—United States, 1988–1994 and 1999–2002. *MMWR,* 2004; Vol. 53: pp. 1066–8.

Comments: This article reports on the epidemiology of obesity in the diabetic population.

Buchwald H, Avidor Y, Braunwald E, et al. Bariatric surgery: a systematic review and meta-analysis. *JAMA,* 2004; Vol. 292: pp. 1724–37.

Comments: This systematic review reports on the efficacy of bariatric surgery for weight loss.

Consensus Development Conference Panel. NIH conference. Gastrointestinal surgery for severe obesity. *Ann Intern Med,* 1991; Vol. 115: pp. 956–61.

Comments: NIH consensus panel recommendations that bariatric surgery be considered for carefully selected, morbidly obese patients with acceptable operative risks.

Lifestyle and Education

NUTRITION: OVERVIEW IN DIABETES

Christopher D. Saudek, MD, and Emily Loghmani, MS, RD, LDN, CDE

DEFINITION

- An individualized meal plan, integrated with oral diabetes medications or insulin, is the basis of all therapy for diabetes.
- Experts avoid the term "diet," which may carry negative connotations, and prefer more generally to promote a healthy meal plan and regular physical activity.
- A well-developed meal plan is *not* a single one-size-fits-all handout.
- The meal plan will help promote a healthy weight, reach HbA1c goals while avoiding hypoglycemia, improve lipid levels, promote healthy blood pressure, and provide a good quality of life.
- The meal plan is developed by the process of medical nutrition therapy (MNT). This includes assessment of eating habits and diabetes knowledge, identification and negotiation of nutrition goals, nutrition education and intervention, ongoing monitoring and evaluation of outcomes.

CLINICAL TREATMENT

General Guidelines

- Individualize the nutrition meal plan based on age, type of diabetes, comorbidities, cardiovascular risk factors, patient preferences, and cultural and personal circumstances (Franz).
- Consider energy requirements, macronutrients (carbohydrates, fats, proteins), vitamins, and minerals.
- Refer to a registered dietician familiar with diabetes whenever possible, preferably for more than one visit.
- Choose a meal planning method that matches patient's needs and ability: healthy food choices, portion control, carbohydrate awareness, and carbohydrate counting or exchanges.

Goals of Diabetes Nutrition (American Diabetes Association)

- Achieve target blood glucose levels while minimizing episodes of hypoglycemia and hyperglycemia.
- Promote lipid and blood pressure levels that reduce the risk of cardiovascular disease.
- Promote normal growth and development in children and adolescents and a healthy weight in adults.
- Prevent, delay, or reduce chronic complications of diabetes.
- Adjust nutrition guidelines to match the patient's needs, preferences, and lifestyle.

Specific Nutrition Recommendations (American Diabetes Association)

- Choose carbohydrates from whole grains, fruit, vegetables, and low-fat milk and yogurt.
- Track total carbohydrate, but be aware that source and type may also affect postprandial blood glucose levels.
- Reduce total fat, saturated fat and cholesterol, and avoid trans-fats. Use more mono- and polyunsaturated fats.

MANAGEMENT

- Choose lean meats, poultry, fish, and other lower fat proteins.
- Increase fiber intake with whole grains, dried peas and beans, and more fruit and vegetables.
- Eat foods that are lower in sodium if patient has high blood pressure.
- May use sugar substitutes approved by the FDA.

Diabetes Nutrition for Prediabetes (Impaired Fasting Glucose or Impaired Glucose Tolerance)

- If overweight, promote lifestyle intervention with increased physical activity (150 minutes/week) and 5%–10% weight loss (Diabetes Prevention Program).
- Refer to a structured, individualized weight management program that promotes reduced calorie intake, increased physical activity, and frequent follow-up visits.
- Reduce excessive carbohydrate intake.
- See Prediabetes or Categories of Increased Risk for Diabetes, p. 117.

Diabetes Nutrition for Gestational Diabetes

- Adjust energy and carbohydrate intake to achieve appropriate weight gain, target blood glucose levels, and absence of maternal ketosis.
- Provide nutrients necessary for maternal and fetal health.
- Monitor blood glucose levels at fasting and 1–2 hours after eating.
- Add exogenous insulin if target blood glucoses are not achieved by diet alone.
- Encourage physical activity to improve glucose tolerance.
- Encourage breastfeeding.
- Promote lifestyle changes to prevent progression to type 2 diabetes.
- See Gestational Diabetes Mellitus, p. 121.

FOLLOW-UP

- Initial: Includes nutrition assessment, basic nutrition education with meal planning guidelines and, if relevant, education about prevention/treatment of hypoglycemia.
- Follow-up: Frequency and length of visits depends on the complexity of the case and the success of treatment.

EXPERT OPINION

- The central importance of good nutrition as an integral part of diabetes management cannot be overemphasized.
- Individualization is the key.
- In general, the goals of treating type 2 diabetes include weight control (Klein), whereas the goals of treating type 1 diabetes include careful carbohydrate awareness to match insulin doses and activity (American Diabetes Association, 2010).
- Sustainability of a meal plan is pivotal to succes: the extreme, restrictive diet will never be as successful as the more moderate, healthy, and sustainable meal plan.

REFERENCES

American Diabetes Association. Standards of medical care in diabetes—2011. *Diabetes Care,* 2011; Vol. 34 Suppl 1: pp. S11–61.

    Comments: Discusses standards of care for prevention, treatment, and management of diabetes, with a section on type 1 diabetes.

American Dietetic Association. *International Dietetics and Nutrition Terminology (IDNT) Reference Manual, Standardized Language for the Nutrition Care Process,* 2nd edition. Chicago: American Dietetic Association; 2009.

Comments: Provides listings of standardized language to be used at each stage of the nutrition care process after critical evaluation of nutrition assessment data and information; helps with provision of more focused nutrition care and evaluation of outcomes by a registered dietician.

American Diabetes Association, Bantle JP, Wylie-Rosett J, et al. Nutrition recommendations and interventions for diabetes: a position statement of the American Diabetes Association. *Diabetes Care*, 2008; Vol. 31 Suppl 1: pp. S61–78.
Comments: Summarizes nutritional management for the prevention and treatment of diabetes.

Klein S, Sheard NF, Pi-Sunyer X, et al. Weight management through lifestyle modification for the prevention and management of type 2 diabetes: rationale and strategies. A statement of the American Diabetes Association, the North American Association for the Study of Obesity, and the American Society for Clinical Nutrition. *Am J Clin Nutr*, 2004; Vol. 80: pp. 257–63.
Comments: Reviews the use of lifestyle modifications to reduce energy intake and increase physical activity in overweight/obese patients with type 2 diabetes.

Franz MJ, Bantle JP, Beebe CA, Brunzell JD, et al. Evidence-based nutrition principles and recommendations for the treatment and prevention of diabetes and related complications. *Diabetes Care*, 2002; Vol. 25: pp. 148–198.
Comments: Summarizes the research and clinical evidence to support nutrition recommendations for diabetes; also defines medical nutrition therapy.

The Diabetes Prevention Program Research Group, Knowler WC, Barrett-Connor E, Fowler SE, et al. Reduction in the incidence of type 2 diabetes with lifestyle intervention or metformin. *NEJM*, 2002; Vol. 346: pp. 393–403.
Comments: Documents the safety and effectiveness of three treatment groups for the prevention of diabetes in a diverse population of high-risk individuals.

MANAGEMENT

NUTRITION FOR TYPE 1 DIABETES

Emily Loghmani MS, RD, LDN, CDE, and Christopher D. Saudek, MD

DEFINITION
- The nutrition plan for type 1 diabetes (T1DM) integrates food choices and physical activity with insulin therapy to achieve normal growth, appropriate body weight, optimal control of blood glucose, and other risk factors, while avoiding hypoglycemia.
- Base food intake on age, sex, stage of growth, food preferences, and usual eating, activity, school and work schedule.
- Use food intake guidelines to help achieve and maintain healthy blood glucoses, lipid levels, and blood pressure to prevent, reduce, or delay complications.
- Provide medical nutrition therapy (MNT) that emphasizes age and developmentally appropriate guidelines (Silverstein).

CLINICAL TREATMENT
Medical Nutrition Therapy (MNT)
- Assess growth and body mass index related to age, sex, and activity level to determine energy needs.
- Promote normal growth and development in children and adolescents with adequate nutrition.
- Achieve and/or maintain healthy weight in adults.
- Teach carbohydrate (carb) counting, or carb awareness to match the level of detail the patient can handle (Gillespie).
- Choose goal of consistent carb intake for patients on fixed insulin doses or variable carb intake based on insulin-to-carb ratios for patients on intensive insulin regimens or insulin pump therapy.

- Patient can assess blood glucose response to snacks and meals by self-monitoring (SMBG).
- Patient should adjust carb intake for exercise. Example: Add 10–15 grams carb per hour of extra activity or reduce insulin in anticipating activity. Amount of carb required preexercise depends on intensity and duration of exercise.
- To avoid symptomatic hypoglycemia, patient ingests 15 grams quick-acting carb when blood glucose level is <70 mg/dl or dropping quickly and rechecks 15–20 minutes later. For children <5 years of age, provide treatment when blood glucose level is <100 mg/dl.
- To further reduce the risk of hypoglycemia, limit alcohol intake and consume alcohol with food.

Key Nutrition Recommendations for Type 1 Diabetes

- Patients on intensified insulin regimens should count anticipated carb intake and adjust fast-acting insulin (nutritional dose) based on insulin-to-carb ratio. Example: Determine if patient needs 1 unit (U) per 15 g carb (average); 1 U per 10 g (less insulin-sensitive); or 1 U per 20 g (more insulin-sensitive).
- May use the "Rule of 500": 500/total daily dose (TDD) = insulin:carb ratio. Example: if TDD is 50 U, 500/50 = 1 U per 10 g carb.
- In addition to the nutritional dose, patients on intensified insulin regimens check blood glucose by SMBG and add correctional dose. Example 1 U per 40 mg/dl over 120 mg/dl; 1 U per 50 over 120 (more insulin-sensitive); or 1 U per 30 over 120 mg/dl (less insulin-sensitive).
- Can calculate correctional dose with the "Rule of 1800": 1800/total daily dose = correction ratio. Example: if TDD is 30 U, 1800/30 = 1 U per 60 mg/dl over target level.
- Patients on fixed insulin doses, for whom carb counting may be difficult, should be taught carb awareness or size of 15-g carb portions. In this case, goal is to keep carb portions consistent, meal to meal, and not adjust insulin dose based blood glucose.
- Target glycemia above which correctional dose is added varies with the age of the patient and goals for reduction of hypoglycemia (American Diabetes Association).
- High fat content in a meal will prolong the absorption of carbs, sometimes causing late hyperglycemia.
- "Smart pumps" will use the above calculations to suggest an insulin dose. BE AWARE that the conversions programmed into the pump by the healthcare professional determine the recommendations of the smart pump.

Meal Planning

- Individualize distribution of carb, protein, and fat based on nutrition assessment.
- Monitor total amount of carbs, more importantly than the source, at the meal or snack.
- Provide 3 meals and 1–3 snacks/day as needed based on the age of the patient and usual eating, activity, school and work schedule.
- Control protein and fat intake, as well as carbs to maintain healthy weight and control blood lipids.
- Adherence to a meal plan, a consistent snacking pattern, timely adjustments for hyperglycemia, and appropriate treatment of hypoglycemia are associated with better glucose control (Delahanty, 1993).

FOLLOW-UP

- Initial: Nutrition assessment and basic survival nutrition education with carbohydrate counting/awareness and prevention/treatment of hypoglycemia at diagnosis.
- Ongoing: Review and evaluate regularly, usually every 3 months.

- Intensive, topic-specific: For certain circumstances, such as change to intensive insulin regimens, initiation of insulin pump therapy, post-discharge diet after hospitalization for diabetic ketoacidosis or severe hypoglycemia, or pregnancy.

EXPERT OPINION

- Carb awareness is essential in treating T1DM, so that patient knows the effect of the meal on blood glucose and can better match food intake to insulin doses.
- Carb *restriction*, on the other hand is *not* recommended. Better glycemic control is established by providing 40%–55% of total caloric intake as carb, and adjusting insulin to "cover" this carb (Delahanty, 2009).
- Accurate carb counting promotes better glycemic control and more flexibility of lifestyle, with flexible insulin adjustments according to carb intake and blood glucose.
- Sugar-containing foods raise blood glucose, gram for gram, about equal to the same load of complex carbs (Loghmani), but must be substituted for other carbs, adequately covered with insulin, limited to occasional use, and not simply added to the meal.
- Glycemic index is sometimes helpful for the sophisticated patient, but more often we recommend that patients learn which foods raise their blood glucose too high and avoid them.

REFERENCES

American Diabetes Association. Standards of medical care in diabetes—2011. *Diabetes Care,* 2011; Vol. 34 Suppl 1: pp. S11–61.

    Comments: This American Diabetes Association statement addresses how medical nutrition therapy is in an integral component of care with a section devoted to type 1 diabetes.

American Diabetes Association Diabetes. Care in the school and day care setting. *Diabetes Care,* 2009; Vol. 32 Suppl 1: pp. S68–72.

    Comments: This American Diabetes Association statement provides practical advice on the management of type 1 diabetes at school and in day care.

Delahanty LM, Nathan DM, Lachin JM, et al. Association of diet with glycated hemoglobin during intensive treatment of type 1 diabetes in the Diabetes Control and Complications Trial. *Am J Clin Nutr,* 2009; Vol. 89: pp. 518–24.

    Comments: The paper reports how dietary composition is related to subsequent A1c levels in DCCT in the intensive treatment group. Poorer control perhaps due to insulin resistance was related to higher saturated fat intake but not the amount of carbohydrate intake.

Silverstein J, Klingensmith G, Copeland K, et al. Care of children and adolescents with type 1 diabetes: a statement of the American Diabetes Association. *Diabetes Care,* 2005; Vol. 28: pp. 186–212.

    Comments: This American Diabetes Association statement provides age-appropriate recommendations for the management of children and adolescents with type 1 diabetes.

Brand-Miller J, Hayne S, Petocz P, et al. Low-glycemic index diets in the management of diabetes: a meta-analysis of randomized controlled trials. *Diabetes Care,* 2003; Vol. 26: pp. 2261–7.

    Comments: This research suggests that the use of foods with a low glycemic index may help promote a small reduction in glycemic control.

Gillespie SJ, Kulkarni KD, Daly AE. Using carbohydrate counting in diabetes clinical practice. *J Am Diet Assoc,* 1998; Vol. 98: pp. 897–905.

    Comments: This paper discusses carbohydrate counting as a meal planning approach with practical suggestions for teaching different levels of complexity (i.e., basic, intermediate, and advanced) to match what the patient can handle.

Delahanty LM, Halford BN. The role of diet behaviors in achieving improved glycemic control in intensively treated patients in the Diabetes Control and Complications Trial. *Diabetes Care,* 1993; Vol. 16: pp. 1453–8.

MANAGEMENT

Comments: This paper reports how dietary behaviors (e.g., treatment of hypoglycemia, consistency of meals), were related to glycemic control (A1c levels) in the DCCT.

Loghmani E, Rickard K, Washburne L, et al. Glycemic response to sucrose-containing mixed meals in diets of children of with insulin-dependent diabetes mellitus. *J Pediatr,* 1991; Vol. 119: pp. 531–7.

Comments: This study reports no additional hyperglycemia when sucrose-containing foods are substituted for complex carbohydrates in healthy meals for children with type 1 diabetes. Sucrose-free diet contained 2% of total calories from sucrose versus 10% for the sucrose-containing diet.

NUTRITION: CARBOHYDRATE COUNTING

Emily Loghmani, MS, RD, LDN, CDE, and Christopher D. Saudek, MD

DEFINITION

- A method for estimating carbohydrate (carb) intake, either in total grams of carb or in 15-g servings.
- Important because carb is the primary nutrient affecting postprandial blood glucose levels (Sheard).
- For people with diabetes on oral medications or fixed insulin doses, carb counting promotes consistent carb intake; for weight loss, helps control overall calories; for those using insulin:carb ratios, helps match premeal insulin dose to amount of carb eaten.
- Carb counting allows flexibility in food choices and helps promote glycemic control (Chiesa).
- Other methods for estimating carb intake are the exchange system and experience-based estimations (Wheeler 2008a).

CLINICAL TREATMENT

Practical Tips for Carb Counting

- Carbs include starch, fiber, sugar alcohols (such as sorbitol), and/or simple sugar (such as sucrose or fructose, either natural or added) (Wheeler 2008b).
- 1 carb serving is defined as 15 grams of carbohydrates.
- Using exchanges, the starch/grain, fruit, and dairy groups all contain carb.
- 1 carb serving = 1 starch/grain or 1 fruit, or 1 dairy, each having 15 grams of carb.
- Healthy meals include carb from whole grains, dried beans and legumes, low-fat dairy products, and fruit.
- Recommended Dietary Allowance for carb is at least 130 g/day (8–9 servings) for adults and children, 45% to 65% of energy (IOM, 2005).
- For weight loss: women need 30–45 grams/meal (2–3 servings), 15 grams/snack; men need 45–60 grams/meal (3–4 servings), 15–30 grams/snack.
- Read food labels for the manufacturer's serving size and total grams of carb/serving; adjust based on amount eaten. The "serving" listed on the nutrition label reflects the amount of the food normally eaten, *not* necessarily a 15-gram carb serving.
- The listed serving (amount usually eaten) therefore does not necessarily equal a carb serving (15 g).
- Labels may be misleading. For instance, a package that is normally eaten at one time may be listed with "2 servings"; e.g., a candy bar with 2 servings of 150 calories each has 300 calories for the whole bar.

Examples of 15 Grams Carb (Choose Your Foods: Exchange Lists for Diabetes)
- **Starch/grain group:** 1/4 large bagel, 1 slice bread, one 6-inch tortilla, 3/4 cup unsweetened cold cereal, 1/2 cup cooked cereal, 1/3 cup pasta, 1/3 cup rice, 1 cup soup, 1/2 cup corn, 1/2 cup mashed potatoes, 5 crackers, 3 cups popcorn, 3/4 oz potato/tortilla chips, 1/2 cup cooked beans or lentils
- **Fruit group:** 1 small fresh fruit, 1/2 banana, 1/2 canned fruit in light syrup, 2 tbsp dried fruit, 17 small grapes, 1 cup melon, 3/4–1 cup berries
- **Dairy group:** 1 cup white milk, 1/2 cup chocolate milk, 1 cup soy milk, 1 cup plain yogurt
- **Sweets:** 2-inch square piece of cake or brownie without icing, 2 small cookies, 5 vanilla wafers, 1/2 cup sugar-free pudding, 1 tbsp sugar or honey, 1/2 cup plain ice cream, 1/4 cup sherbet/sorbet
- **Combination foods:** 1/2 cup casserole, 1/2 sandwich, 1 cup meat stew with vegetables, 1 small taco

Levels of Carb Counting (Gillespie)
- Individual patients may have different levels of knowledge and practice, from general carb awareness to careful carb counting or even consideration of glycemic index.
- **Carb awareness:**
  1. Know which foods contain carbohydrates.
  2. Choose healthy, consistent portion sizes.
  3. Avoid sweets and sweetened beverages.
- **Basic Carb Counting:**
  1. Promotes consistency of carb intake.
  2. Understand effect of food, medication, and physical activity on blood glucose levels and identify patterns.
  3. Use food labels and carb-counting resources to obtain carb information.
  4. Estimate the number of servings (or half-servings) in food to be ingested.
- **Advanced Carb Counting:**
  1. In addition to above, adds precision to actual grams ingested.
  2. Calculate grams of carb more accurately (e.g., +/–5 g) rather than just as servings.
  3. Know and quantitate less obvious sources of carb (nonstarchy vegetables, dairy products, etc.).
  4. Use insulin-to-carbohydrate ratio to calculate dose of fast-acting insulin.
  5. Adjust for foods high in fat or fiber.
  6. Adjust for individual glycemic index (GI).
  7. Be aware that high fat intake slows absorption of carbohydrate.

Clinical Treatment
- Glycemic index (GI) may provide additional benefit over tracking total carb alone, but research has shown mixed results (Sheard).

EXPERT OPINION
- Monitoring carb intake is a key strategy in meeting glycemic goals (American Diabetes Association).
- For type 1 diabetes, the goal is to match premeal insulin to carb intake, premeal blood glucose level, and exercise.

MANAGEMENT

- For type 2 diabetes, the goal is to fit carb intake into a generally healthy, often hypocaloric, meal plan.
- Carb counting can help patients monitor overall food intake for both consistency and weight loss.
- There are many published and online sources of reliable information describing the carb content of various foods. Examples: Choose Your Foods: Exchange Lists for Diabetes, Diabetes Carbohydrate and Fat Gram Guide, *http://www.calorieking.com*, *http://www.acaloriecounter.com*.
- Levels of carb counting must be tailored to the individual, his/her readiness to learn, ability with numbers, and many other factors.
- It is useless to try to teach advanced carb counting to someone unwilling or unable to learn it.
- Levels of carb counting can be improved gradually.
- Many people *wrongly* think that carb restriction is the recommended approach to managing diabetes.
- In our practice, we rarely address GI as such. While scientifically sound, many factors influence the postprandial response to carb, such as amount ingested ("glycemic load"), type of carb, speed of absorption, fat and protein content of the meal, degree of processing, cooking method, etc. Frequently, an experiential approach is more practical. Individuals can test blood glucose 2 hours after eating and learn which foods raise their blood glucose to a surprisingly high level.

REFERENCES

Holzmeister, LA. *Diabetes Carbohydrate and Fat Gram Guide*, 4th edition. Alexandria, VA: American Diabetes Association; 2010.
Comments: Provides complete nutrition information, including grams of carb, for over 8000 foods and menu items.

American Diabetes Association. Standards of medical care in diabetes—2011. *Diabetes Care,* 2011; Vol. 34 Suppl 1: pp. S11–61.
Comments: Reviews recommended medical nutrition therapy for type 1 and type 2 diabetes, including carbohydrate intake.

Wheeler ML, Daly A, Evert A, Franz MJ, et al. Choose your foods: exchange lists for diabetes, 6th edition, 2008: Description and guidelines for use. *J Am Diet Assoc,* 2008a; Vol. 108: pp. 883–888.
Comments: Provides evidence base for nutrition recommendations and revisions in the basic nutrition education booklet for diabetes.

Wheeler ML, Pi-Sunyer FX. Carbohydrate issues: type and amount. *J Am Diet Assoc,* 2008b; Vol. 108: pp. S34–9.
Comments: Reviews how type and amount of different carbohydrates influence postprandial glucose levels and overall glycemic control.

American Diabetes Association and American Dietetic Association. *Choose Your Foods: Exchange Lists for Diabetes,* 6th edition. Alexandria, VA: American Diabetes Association and American Dietetic Association; 2008.
Comments: Basic nutrition education booklet for healthy eating for people with diabetes; provides information and portion sizes for foods that contain carbohydrate, protein, and fat.

Chiesa G, Piscopo MA, Rigamonti A, et al. Insulin therapy and carbohydrate counting. *Acta Biomed,* 2005; Vol. 76 Suppl 3: pp. 44–8.
Comments: Reviews data on how carb counting benefits diabetes management.

Institute of Medicine, Food, and Nutrition Board. *Dietary reference intakes for energy, carbohydrate, fiber, fat, fatty acids, cholesterol, protein, and amino acids.* Washington, DC: The National Academies Press; 2005.

Comments: A series of reports that presents dietary reference values for the intake of nutrients by Americans and Canadians, including the role of various nutrients in the body and dietary intake data.

Sheard NF, Clark NG, Brand-Miller JC, et al. Dietary carbohydrate (amount and type) in the prevention and management of diabetes: a statement by the American Diabetes Association. *Diabetes Care,* 2004; Vol. 27: pp. 2266–71.

Comments: Discusses the role of carbohydrates on blood glucose levels, including influence of type and amount, glycemic index, and glycemic load.

Gillespie SJ, Kulkarni KD, Daly AE. Using carbohydrate counting in diabetes clinical practice. *J Am Diet Assoc,* 1998; Vol. 98: pp. 897–905.

Comments: Provides historical background and information about the use of carbohydrate counting for planning meals and snacks, with description of step-wise approach to developing skills.

NUTRITION FOR TYPE 2 DIABETES

Emily Loghmani, MS, RD, LDN, CDE, and Christopher D. Saudek, MD

MANAGEMENT

DEFINITION
- A sound nutrition program is the basis of preventing and managing type 2 diabetes (T2DM).
- The nutrition plan for T2DM usually emphasizes weight control and control of cardiovascular disease (CVD) risk factors.
- Medical Nutrition Therapy (MNT) includes development of a specific nutrition plan by a qualified nutritionist.

EPIDEMIOLOGY
- 80%–90% of people in the US with T2DM are overweight or obese.
- In the US, 16% of people with T2DM are treated without pharmacologic intervention (i.e., diet-controlled), 57% with oral agents alone, 14% with insulin alone, and 13% combined oral agents and insulin.
- The average lag time between the onset and the diagnosis of T2DM in the US is estimated to be 7 years.

CLINICAL TREATMENT
Medical Nutrition Therapy (American Diabetes Association)
- Assess weight and body mass index relative to age, sex, and activity level to determine energy goal.
- In overweight/obese patients, promote weight loss to reduce insulin resistance (Table 2-4).
- Individualize the distribution of carbohydrate, protein, and fat to improve glucose levels, lipids, and blood pressure.
- Reduce total fat and saturated fat intake and avoid trans-fat.
- Teach healthy eating, carbohydrate awareness, or carbohydrate counting to match medication/insulin and level of detail the patient can handle.
- Individualize meal plans to allow for social and cultural influences, eating habits, and readiness to change.
- Promote regular physical activity.

TABLE 2-4. THE DIABETES PREVENTION PROGRAM RECOMMENDATIONS FOR TOTAL CALORIES AND GRAMS OF FAT PER DAY, FOR WEIGHT LOSS

Initial Body Weight	Recommendation	Fat
120–170 lb	1200 calories	33 g
175–215 lb	1500 calories	42 g
220–245 lb	1800 calories	50 g
>250 lb	2000 calories	55 g

Adapted from Wing R, Gillis B. The Diabetes Prevention Program's Lifestyle Change Program: Section 5: Overview of Strategies to Achieve the Weight Loss Goal. Pittsburgh, PA: University of Pittsburgh; 1996:5-3.

Matching Nutrition to Pharmacologic Therapy

- Certain pharmacologic therapies (insulin, sulfonylureas, metaglinides, exenatide, pramlintide) can cause hypoglycemia. A nutrition plan includes regular meals and a hypoglycemia treatment plan.
- Metformin, exenatide, and pramlintide can cause nausea, less if taken with meals.
- Glucosidase inhibitors, pramlintide, and exenatide, by slowing carbohydrate absorption and gastric emptying, can interfere with treatment of hypoglycemia. Sugar-containing liquid may be recommended if needed.
- Weight gain is a common side effect of thiazolidinediones and insulin, and a less prominent effect of sulfonylurea use. Recommend careful adherence to low-calorie meal plan.

Clinical Treatment

- Calories DO count: each diet is as effective in the long run as the resulting caloric deficit (Bravata).
- Caloric deficit of ~3500 calories less than weight-maintenance needs, over any time, will reduce body weight by about 1 pound. However, other factors affect long-term weight change, and this 3500-calorie deficit per pound relationship is attenuated over the long term (Katan).
- No consensus on whether restricting carbohydrate or fat is most effective (Sacks; Gardner). Some evidence that the Mediterranean diet is effective for weight loss and improved glycemic control (Shai) (see Nutrition: Popular Diets in Diabetes, p. 100).
- Severe restriction of carbohydrates (Atkins diet and others) induces early diuresis (rapid weight loss but not loss of adiposity), and mild ketosis, which limits appetite (Hession).
- Severe fat restriction (Pritikin diet and others) reduces the most calorically dense macronutrients.
- Sustainability of a nutrition plan is important, particularly transitioning patients from a significantly hypocaloric to weight maintenance diet, avoiding weight regain.
- Unbalanced diets (very low carb or very low fat) are hardest to sustain.

- Lipids are improved by diets low in saturated and trans-fats, and high in fiber.
- Hypertension is often improved by diets low in sodium.
- Moderate weight loss (7% of body weight) is highly effective both in preventing and in treating type 2 diabetes.

FOLLOW-UP

- MNT requires multiple visits, with repeated instruction and reinforcement.
- Frequency of follow-up is individualized.
- Group therapy, with peer support and peer pressure, is often effective.

EXPERT OPINION

- Individualization of MNT is the key.
- We recommend balanced macronutrient (fat, carb, protein) intake, although some people do well with more extreme restriction of fat or carbohydrate.
- Blood glucose control improves almost immediately with hypocaloric diet.
- Insulin resistance diminishes as weight loss continues.
- Nonnutritive (0 calorie) beverages do not affect weight, although effect on appetite is controversial (Mattes), whereas high-fructose corn syrup drinks are a cause of significant caloric intake (Ludwig).
- We recommend consideration of bariatric surgery for severely obese people (BMI >40) who have not responded to nutritional management and have significant comorbidities (Buchwald).
- Nutrition plans must address not only diabetes but the common comorbidities and cardiovascular risk factors—obesity, heart disease, hypertension.
- Concentrated sweets (cake, candy, cookies, etc.) are at best "empty" calories, providing little nutrition and high caloric content.

REFERENCES

Katan MB, Ludwig DS. Extra calories cause weight gain—but how much? *JAMA*, 2010; Vol. 303: pp. 65–6.
  Comments: A carefully reasoned consideration of the factors that regulate body weight gain in addition to the starting figure that 3500-calorie deficit equals about 1 pound.

Sacks FM, Bray GA, Carey VJ, et al. Comparison of weight-loss diets with different compositions of fat, protein, and carbohydrates. *NEJM*, 2009; Vol. 360: pp. 859–73.
  Comments: 811 overweight adults assigned to one of four reduced-calorie diets that varied in fat, protein, and carbohydrate for 2 years. All diets promoted weight loss regardless of macronutrient composition.

Hession M, Rolland C, Kulkarni U, et al. Systematic review of randomized controlled trials of low-carbohydrate vs. low-fat/low-calorie diets in the management of obesity and its comorbidities. *Obes Rev*, 2009; Vol. 10: pp. 36–50.
  Comments: Review of 13 studies that compared low-carbohydrate/high-protein and low-fat/high-carbohydrate diets. Data suggest that low-carbohydrate diets promote more weight loss at 6 months and similar weight loss at 12 months compared to low-fat diets.

Mattes RD, Popkin BM. Nonnutritive sweetener consumption in humans: effects on appetite and food intake and their putative mechanisms. *Am J Clin Nutr*, 2009; Vol. 89: pp. 1–14.
  Comments: Comprehensive review of nonnutritive sweeteners including safety and influence on appetite, energy intake, and body weight.

Ludwig DS. Artificially sweetened beverages: cause for concern. *JAMA*, 2009; Vol. 302: pp. 2477–8.
  Comments: A discussion of the contribution of high fructose corn syrup (HFCS) to caloric intake, and the argument for taxing sweetened beverages.

Buchwald H, Estok R, Fahrback K, et al. Weight and type 2 diabetes after bariatric surgery: systematic review and meta-analysis. *Am J Med*, 2009; Vol. 122: pp. 248–256.

MANAGEMENT

Comments: Systematic review of 621 studies from 1990 to 2006 that document resolution of type 2 diabetes in 78% and improvement in 87% of patients undergoing bariatric surgery.

American Diabetes Association. Standards of medical care in diabetes—2011. *Diabetes Care,* 2011; Vol. 34 Suppl 1: pp. S11–61.

Comments: This statement by the American Diabetes Association discusses medical nutrition therapy and its role in preventing and managing diabetes complications.

Shai I, Schwarzfuchs D, Henkin Y, et al. Weight loss with a low-carbohydrate, Mediterranean, or low-fat diet. *NEJM,* 2008; Vol. 359: pp. 229–41.

Comments: 322 obese subjects, randomized to low-fat calorie restricted, Mediterranean calorie restricted, or low-carbohydrate unrestricted diets. Concluded that Mediterranean was most effective in glycemic control, and low-carb diets more effective in lipid control. Both more effective than low-fat in weight control.

Gardner CD, Kiazand A, Alhassan S, et al. Comparison of the Atkins, Zone, Ornish, and LEARN diets for change in weight and related risk factors among overweight premenopausal women: the A TO Z Weight Loss Study: a randomized trial. *JAMA,* 2007; Vol. 297: pp. 969–77.

Comments: 311 obese women randomized to Atkins, Zone, Ornish and LEARN diets for 12 months. Authors concluded that the Atkins diet promoted greater weight loss and more favorable metabolic effects.

Bravata DM, Sanders L, Huang J, et al. Efficacy and safety of low-carbohydrate diets: a systematic review. *JAMA,* 2003; Vol. 289: pp. 1837–50.

Comments: Review of 107 reduced carbohydrate diets of varying content and duration. Authors concluded that main determinants of weight loss were duration of diet and decreased caloric intake, not carbohydrate content.

Diabetes Prevention Program (DPP) Research Group. The Diabetes Prevention Program (DPP): description of lifestyle intervention. *Diabetes Care,* 2002; Vol. 25: pp. 2165–71.

Comments: Description of the successful lifestyle intervention for participants in the Diabetes Prevention Program. Goals of weight loss and physical activity were achieved with lifestyle coaches, frequent follow-up, behavioral strategies, supervised activity, individualization, and support.

NUTRITION: POPULAR DIETS IN DIABETES

Simeon Margolis, MD, PhD

DEFINITION

- Many weight-loss diets have been promoted over the years and are usually popular for only a short time.
- Some diets specifically restrict calories, but most are aimed at reducing caloric intake indirectly by placing restrictions on the percentages of fat, protein, and carbohydrates in the diet.
- Other popular diets aim to control blood glucose and/or reduce cardiovascular risk, usually in conjunction with pharmacotherapy.

CLINICAL TREATMENT

Weight-Loss Diets

- New weight-loss diets pop up constantly; many reach best-seller lists.
- Most recent fad diets do not restrict calories per se, but restrict a given foodstuff.
- Atkins: 20% carbohydrates (C), 50% fat (F), 30% protein (P).
- South Beach and Zone: 40% C, 30% F, 30% P.
- Weight Watchers: 40% C, 40% F, 20% P, and calorie restriction.

Diets to Control Blood Glucose and/or Risk Factors for Cardiovascular Disease (CVD)

- American Diabetes Association (ADA) diet aims to achieve and maintain: (1) blood glucose as close to normal as safely possible; (2) a lipid and lipoprotein profile to reduce CVD; (3) blood pressure normal or as close to normal as possible (American Diabetes Association).
- ADA nutritional recommendations: (1) restrict calories if needed to approach normal weight; (2) balanced diet of 50% C, 30% F, 20% P ($<$7% saturated fat, $<$200 mg cholesterol per day) (American Diabetes Association).
- The Pritikin Weight Loss Breakthrough: about 10% of calories from fat. Very low-fat diets raise triglycerides and lower HDL cholesterol (Lichtenstein).
- Ornish diet: 70% C, 10% F, 20% P, and other lifestyle measures for regression of coronary atherosclerosis.
- Mediterranean diet: includes a high consumption of fruits, vegetables, bread, wheat, cereals, potatoes, beans, nuts, seeds, and olive oil, with limited intake of red meats and eggs; yields a higher intake of monounsaturated fatty acids (Martinez).
- DASH diet: emphasizes fruits, vegetables, and low-fat dairy products. The diet includes whole grains, poultry, fish, and nuts; contains only small amounts of red meat, sweets, and sugar-containing beverages; and has decreased amounts of saturated fat and cholesterol (Appel; Liese).
- National Cholesterol Education Program (NCEP) and American Heart Association (AHA) diets similar to ADA diet.
- AHA and ADA recommend eating fish at least twice a week or possibly taking fish oil supplements (Wang).
- Low glycemic index (GI) and low glycemic load diets: GI of a food is the increase in the blood glucose area over 2 hours after ingestion of a specific amount of that food (usually a 50-g carbohydrate portion) divided by the glucose response to a similar amount of reference food (usually glucose or white bread). For example, low GI = kidney beans; high GI = mashed potatoes. Glycemic load calculated by multiplying the glycemic index of the constituent foods by the amounts of carbohydrate in each food (Brand-Miller).
- Low-protein diet for chronic kidney disease (Robertson).

FOLLOW-UP

- Long-term weight loss the same with Atkins, South Beach, Zone, Ornish as with more conventional diets: about 6 kg at 6 months, 3.3 kg at 2 years (Sacks).
- Very low-fat diets do not lower cholesterol any more than a diet containing about 25% of calories as fat; but they also decrease HDL cholesterol and raise triglycerides.
- DASH diet lowers blood pressure (Appel) and may prevent development of type 2 diabetes.
- Mediterranean diet improves lipid pattern and may prevent type 2 diabetes (Martinez).
- NCEP diet improves LDL cholesterol.
- Low glycemic index diet improves postprandial glucose; longer term benefits uncertain (Brand-Miller).
- Low-protein diet may prevent progression of kidney disease (Robertson).

EXPERT OPINION

- Even relatively small amounts of weight loss, for example 7% of body weight, can significantly improve glycemic control.

MANAGEMENT

- Calories do count. Diets that restrict a major food stuff (e.g., Atkins restricts carbohydrate) achieve weight loss because total caloric intake is also decreased.
- Different diets affect the speed of short-term weight loss, but weight loss outcomes are similar regardless of the diet; in the end, no single diet has been proven especially advantageous (Sacks).
- Unbalanced diets or severe calorie-restricted diets can be difficult to maintain.
- Over time, most people regain weight lost on weight-loss diets.
- **Expert's choice:** follow the ADA dietary recommendations with additional sodium restriction (i.e., no added salt [<3–4 g/day]).

REFERENCES

Sacks FM, Bray GA, Carey VJ, et al. Comparison of weight-loss diets with different compositions of fat, protein, and carbohydrates. *NEJM,* 2009; Vol. 360: pp. 859–73.
  Comments: Over a 2-year period, overweight adults lost similar amounts of weight whether they followed low-fat, low-carbohydrate, or high-protein diets.

Liese AD, Nichols M, Sun X, et al. Adherence to the DASH Diet is inversely associated with incidence of type 2 diabetes: the insulin resistance atherosclerosis study. *Diabetes Care,* 2009; Vol. 32: pp. 1434–6.
  Comments: Adherence to a DASH-like diet was associated with a decrease in the development of type 2 diabetes among whites but not blacks or Hispanics.

American Diabetes Association, Bantle JP, Wylie-Rosett J, et al. Nutrition recommendations and interventions for diabetes: a position statement of the American Diabetes Association. *Diabetes Care,* 2008; Vol. 31 Suppl 1: pp. S61–78.
  Comments: Nutritional recommendations by American Diabetes Association.

Martínez-González MA, de la Fuente-Arrillaga C, Nunez-Cordoba JM, et al. Adherence to Mediterranean diet and risk of developing diabetes: prospective cohort study. *BMJ,* 2008; Vol. 336: pp. 1348–51.
  Comments: Adherence to a Mediterranean diet was associated with a lower risk of developing type 2 diabetes.

Tinker LF, Bonds DE, Margolis KL, et al. Low-fat dietary pattern and risk of treated diabetes mellitus in postmenopausal women: the Women's Health Initiative randomized controlled dietary modification trial. *Arch Intern Med,* 2008; Vol. 168: pp. 1500–11.
  Comments: A low-fat dietary pattern among generally healthy postmenopausal women showed no evidence of reducing diabetes risk after 8.1 years.

Robertson L, Waugh N, Robertson A. Protein restriction for diabetic renal disease. *Cochrane Database Syst Rev,* 2007; CD002181.
  Comments: Reducing protein intake appears to slightly slow progression to renal failure but the differences were not statistically significant.

Appel LJ, Brands MW, Daniels SR, et al. Dietary approaches to prevent and treat hypertension: a scientific statement from the American Heart Association. *Hypertension,* 2006; Vol. 47: pp. 296–308.
  Comments: DASH diet recommended to control hypertension.

Wang C, Harris WS, Chung M, et al. Fatty acids from fish or fish-oil supplements, but not alpha-linolenic acid, benefit cardiovascular disease outcomes in primary- and secondary-prevention studies: a systematic review. *Am J Clin Nutr,* 2006; Vol. 84: pp. 5–17.
  Comments: Omega-3 fatty acids from fish or fish oil supplements, but not from alpha-linolenic acid, are beneficial for cardiovascular disease outcomes.

Dansinger ML, Gleason JA, Griffith JL, et al. Comparison of the Atkins, Ornish, Weight Watchers, and Zone diets for weight loss and heart disease risk reduction: a randomized trial. *JAMA,* 2005; Vol. 293: pp. 43–53.
  Comments: Each popular weight-loss diet modestly reduced body weight and several cardiac risk factors at 1 year. Overall dietary adherence rates were similar and low for all diets.

Brand-Miller J, Hayne S, Petocz P, et al. Low-glycemic index diets in the management of diabetes: a meta-analysis of randomized controlled trials. *Diabetes Care,* 2003; Vol. 26: pp. 2261–7.

Comments: Choosing low glycemic index (GI) foods in place of conventional or high GI foods has a small but clinically useful effect on medium-term glycemic control in patients with diabetes.

Lichtenstein AH, Van Horn L. Very low fat diets. *Circulation*, 1998; Vol. 98: pp. 935–9.

Comments: Very low-fat diets do not lower cholesterol more than diets containing 25% fat. They also raise triglycerides and lower HDL cholesterol.

PHYSICAL ACTIVITY AND EXERCISE

Mariana Lazo, MD, ScM, PhD, and Mary Huizinga, MD, MPH

DEFINITION

- Physical activity and exercise: bodily movements produced by the contraction of skeletal muscle that require energy expenditure beyond resting energy expenditure and improve one or more components of physical fitness.
- Physical fitness: includes cardiorespiratory fitness, muscular fitness, and flexibility (see below).
- Classification of physical intensity: light (35%–54% maximum heart rate); moderate (55%–69% maximum heart rate); high (70%–89% maximum heart rate).
- Maximum heart rate = 220 − age, preferably determined by graded exercise testing (GXT).

EPIDEMIOLOGY

- Physical activity is an important element in the prevention and management of type 2 diabetes.
- Many beneficial effects of exercise, alone and in combination with diet, in diabetes (Thomas; Wasserman).
- **Glycemic control:** average A1c reduction of −0.3% to −0.8% after exercise training for ≥6 months (Snowling; Church; Balducci), within the range to promote significant reductions in microvascular, macrovascular, and nonvascular complications (UKPDS).
- **Body composition:** exercise reduces body mass (average −5%), waist circumference (−2 to −3 cm) and body fat (average −15%). Resistance training with or without aerobic activity also increases lean body mass (Snowling; Church).
- **Risk factor control:** improvement in hypertension (average reduction SBP −4 to −6 mmHg, DBP −2 to 6 mmHg), hyperlipidemia (triglycerides −26.6 mg/dl on average, LDL −9.6 mg/dl, HDL + 3.7 to 5.0 mg/dl on average), and obesity (Marwick; Snowling; Balducci).
- **Cardiovascular benefits:** maximum oxygen consumption (VO2 max), vascular structure and function (endothelial dysfunction and vascular distensibility), myocardial function and CAD (coronary artery disease) risk and mortality (Desai; Stewart; Church).
- **Psychological effects:** improves quality-of-life and depression symptoms (Williamson).

CLINICAL TREATMENT

Patient Evaluation Needed Before Recommending an Exercise Program

- **Cardiac risk:** ADA recommendation to consider ECG stress testing in individuals at high risk for CAD about to undergo moderate- to high-intensity exercise with age >40 years or age >30 years and (1) type 1 or 2 diabetes >10 years; (2) additional risk factor for CAD (hypertension, smoking, dyslipidemia); or (3) presence of microvascular complications (retinopathy or nephropathy). Also in any of the following regardless of age: (1) known or suspected CAD, stroke, and/or peripheral vascular disease; (2) autonomic neuropathy; or (3) advanced nephropathy with renal failure.

- AHA/ACC recommends GXT if one of the following criteria exists: (1) CAD and no stress test within past 2 years; (2): symptoms of chest discomfort or dyspnea; (3) clinical or laboratory evidence of peripheral artery disease (PAD) or cerebrovascular disease; (4) ECG evidence of infarction or ischemia; (5) objective of vigorous exercise program.
- **Noncardiac factors:** Hypoglycemia risk factors include recurrent low glucose measurements, longer duration of diabetes, lower BMI, impaired hypoglycemia unawareness, insulin treatment and insulin secretagogues (e.g., sulfonylureas and meglitinides). Consider hypoglycemia preventive measures before exercise (see Hypoglycemia: Prevention and Treatment, p. 51).
- Peripheral arterial disease and foot care: Presence of PAD requires individualized supervised exercise program, and foot injury prevention strategies such as limiting exercise to walking speed, aquatic exercise or recumbent cycle ergometry, proper footwear, and regular inspection of the feet.
- Microvascular disease: Aerobic exercise or activities that result in a Valsalva maneuver is contraindicated in presence of proliferative retinopathy.
- Severe peripheral neuropathy: increased risk of foot damage with exercise.
- Risk of skin ulceration and development of charcot joint.

ADA/AHA Guidelines for Prescribing an Exercise Program

- **General:** Middle-aged patients may be deconditioned, with limited strength and flexibility and other comorbidities (e.g., obesity, osteoarthritis) that hinder engagement in any activity. Set an achievable goal—short with frequent periods of brisk activity instead of a single 30-minute session. Combination of aerobic with resistance training will increase endurance. Progressive increments: if sedentary, initiate at low level and gradually increase.
- **Frequency:** Minimum 3 days/week with no more than 2 consecutive days between bouts of aerobic exercise and at least 2–3 times weekly of resistance exercise on nonconsecutive days; more frequent exercise training maximizes both acute glucose-lowering effect and CAD benefits.
- **Intensity:** Moderate-intensity exercise has positive effects. Corresponds to approximately 40%–60% of maximum aerobic capacity. Recommend vigorous-intensity exercise if tolerated and no contraindications.
- **Education:** Instruct patients to identify atypical symptoms of ischemia, and adjust medications based on self-monitoring of blood glucose. Proper foot care and nutrition before exercise. Diabetes identification bracelet or shoe tag if needed.
- **Warm-up:** 5–10 min aerobic activity at low intensity and 5–10 min muscle stretching and cool down periods.
- **Hydration:** Before and during exercise, frequently, and in amounts sufficient to compensate for losses.
- **Session duration:** 150 min/week of moderate-intensity exercise or 90 min/week of high-intensity exercise each week. Each session should be minimum 10 minutes. Because of improved adherence and similar efficacy, 3 short sessions of 10 minutes may be preferable to a single 30-minute session in some individuals (Jakicic).

- **Program duration:** Acute and chronic improvements in insulin resistance with physical acticity. Changes in body composition usually require longer. Ideally, changes in lifestyle should be permanent.
- **Type:** *Aerobic exercise:* Rhythmic, repeated, and continuous movements of the same large muscle groups for at least 10 min at a time (e.g., walking, bicycling, jogging, and swimming). Increases cardiorespiratory fitness and energy expenditure. *Resistance exercise:* Activities that use muscular strength to move a weight or work against a resistive load (e.g., weight lifting and exercise using weight machines). Increases muscular fitness and whole body glucose utilization. Includes 5–10 exercises involving the major muscles groups (upper body, lower body, core) and completion of 1–4 sets of 10–15 repetitions to near fatigue; slow progression over time to heavier weights that can only be lifted 8–10 times. Both types of exercise are important in diabetes; combination may offer greatest health benefits although milder forms (i.e., yoga) have mixed results.

Special Considerations for Patients with Insulin-Treated Diabetes

- **Metabolic control before exercise:** Avoid physical activity if fasting glucose >250 mg/dl and urinary ketones present; use caution if glucose is high even if no ketones. Ingest additional carbohydrate if glucose levels <100 mg/dl.
- **Blood glucose monitoring before and after exercise:** Identify when changes in insulin or food intake are necessary. Learn the glycemic response to different exercises. This varies from patient to patient.
- **Reduction of insulin dose:** Often need to reduce dose of rapid- or short-acting insulin taken before exercise. 50% reduction is a common starting place. Titrate insulin reduction for each patient and for different types of exercise. Intense aerobic activity may require greater insulin reduction than resistance training. Persons on insulin and insulin secretagogues may be at higher risk of hypoglycemia and advised to supplement with carbohydrate as needed.
- **Food intake:** For unplanned activity, increase carbohydrate consumption to avoid hypoglycemia. Have readily available carbohydrates during and after physical activity. Reduction of rapid or short-acting insulin is preferable to additional carbohydrate intake for planned activity.
- **Hypoglycemia:** Stop physical activity if hypoglycemic symptoms develop during exercise. Be aware of delayed hypoglycemic effect, 6–12 hours after exercise.
- **Hyperglycemia:** In some patients, glucose may rise during resistance or intense aerobic exercise due to increased catecholamines but not as common.

Prevention of Type 2 Diabetes

- At least 2.5 hours/week of moderate to vigorous physical activity should be undertaken in high-risk adults to prevent type 2 diabetes.
- Higher physical activity levels may also reduce risk of developing gestational diabetes.
- The Diabetes Prevention Program demonstrated 58% reduced risk of developing diabetes in persons with prediabetes who underwent an intensive lifestyle program (see Key Studies in Diabetes Care: Prevention and Glycemic Control, p. 12).

FOLLOW-UP

- Factors affecting adherence: perceived barriers and benefits, self-efficacy, motivation, social support, access, provider support, presence of depression or anxiety.
- Factors effective in improving long-term adherence: ongoing individual or group counseling, exercise consultation, group support, and telephone counseling.

MANAGEMENT

EXPERT OPINION

- Beneficial effects of exercise in diabetes are well documented and include metabolic effects, risk factor control, cardiovascular benefits, and psychological effects.
- Exercise prescription includes assessment of preexercise cardiac and noncardiac risks, and a detailed program (duration, frequency, intensity, and type of exercise).
- Encourage a combination of aerobic and resistance training.
- Aim to have at least 3 nonconsecutive days/week of training, minimum of 150 minutes/week of moderate-intensity exercise or 90 minutes/week of high-intensity exercise, and individual sessions lasting 10 minutes or more or aerobic exercise. Recommendations for resistance exercise are 2–3 times per week.
- Presence of known cardiovascular disease is not an absolute contraindication to exercise but may necessitate a supervised cardiac rehabilitation program.
- Exercise training may even be undertaken during dialysis sessions.
- Persons with uncontrolled proliferative retinopathy should avoid activities that increase intraocular pressure and hemorrhage risk.
- Moderate walking will likely not increase risk of ulcerative disease in persons with peripheral neuropathy.
- Focus on developing self-efficacy in physical activity programs.
- Encourage long-term exercise programs to achieve maximal benefits.

BASIS FOR RECOMMENDATIONS

Colberg SR, Sigal RJ, Fernhall B, et al. Exercise and type 2 diabetes: the American College of Sports Medicine and the American Diabetes Association: joint position statement executive summary. *Diabetes Care*, 2010; Vol. 33: pp. 2692–6.

    Comments: American Diabetes Association and American College of Sports Medicine joint position statement on exercise and type 2 diabetes.

Marwick TH, Hordern MD, Miller T, et al. Exercise training for type 2 diabetes mellitus: impact on cardiovascular risk: a scientific statement from the American Heart Association. *Circulation*, 2009; Vol. 119: pp. 3244–62.

    Comments: Most recent scientific statement of this topic from the American Heart Association.

OTHER REFERENCES

Balducci S, Zanuso S, Nicolucci A, et al. Effect of an intensive exercise intervention strategy on modifiable cardiovascular risk factors in subjects with type 2 diabetes mellitus: a randomized controlled trial: the Italian Diabetes and Exercise Study (IDES). *Arch Intern Med*, 2010; Vol. 170: pp. 1794–>803.

    Comments: Describes the metabolic benefits of supervised combination exercise training versus control group over 1 year in diabetes.

Church TS, Blair SN, Cocreham S, et al. Effects of aerobic and resistance training on hemoglobin A1c levels in patients with type 2 diabetes: a randomized controlled trial. *JAMA*, 2010; Vol. 304: pp. 2253–62.

    Comments: This randomized controlled study found that combination aerobic and resistance training over 9 months was more beneficial than either alone in reducing HbA1c (−0.3%, p=0.03).

Weltman NY, Saliba SA, Barrett EJ, et al. The use of exercise in the management of type 1 and type 2 diabetes. *Clin Sports Med*, 2009; Vol. 28: pp. 423–39.

    Comments: Provides a summary of the recommendations from the American College of Sport Medicine.

Williamson DA, Rejeski J, Lang W, et al. Impact of a weight management program on health-related quality of life in overweight adults with type 2 diabetes. *Arch Intern Med*, 2009; Vol. 169: pp. 163–71.

    Comments: Describes improvements in quality of life and depression scores in the Look AHEAD study that were mediated by enhanced physical fitness.

Snowling NJ, Hopkins WG, Effects of different modes of exercise training on glucose control and risk factors for complications in type 2 diabetic patients: a meta-analysis. *Diabetes Care*, 2006; Vol. 29: pp. 2518–27.

Comments: Meta-analysis demonstrating the effects of exercise on A1c and other measures of glucose control and risk factors.

Thomas DE, Elliott EJ, Naughton GA. Exercise for type 2 diabetes mellitus. *Cochrane Database Syst Rev*, 2006; Vol. 3: CD002968.
Comments: Systematic review of trials testing the effects of exercise in people with T2DM.

Zinman B, Ruderman N, Campaigne BN, et al. Physical activity/exercise and diabetes. *Diabetes Care*, 2004; Vol. 27 Suppl 1: pp. S58–62.
Comments: Summary of ADA recommendations of Physical Activity and Diabetes based on technical reviews. Covers type 1 and type 2 diabetes recommendations.

Sigal RJ, Kenny GP, Wasserman DH, et al. Physical activity/exercise and type 2 diabetes. *Diabetes Care*, 2004; Vol. 27: pp. 2518–39.
Comments: Most comprehensive review of the literature on the role of exercise and Type 2 diabetes.

Desai MY, Nasir K, Rumberger JA, et al. Relation of degree of physical activity to coronary artery calcium score in asymptomatic individuals with multiple metabolic risk factors. *Am J Cardiol*, 2004; Vol. 94: pp. 729–32.
Comments: Large observational study demonstrating that individuals who engage in physical activity are less likely to present with atherosclerosis.

Stewart KJ. Exercise training and the cardiovascular consequences of type 2 diabetes and hypertension: plausible mechanisms for improving cardiovascular health. *JAMA*, 2002; Vol. 288: pp. 1622–31.
Comments: Well-conducted narrative review of the current evidence of the benefits of exercise training beyond the glycemic control and blood pressure reduction.

UK Prospective Diabetes Study (UKPDS) Group. Intensive blood-glucose control with sulphonylureas or insulin compared with conventional treatment and risk of complications in patients with type 2 diabetes (UKPDS 33). *Lancet*, 1998; Vol. 352: pp. 837–53.
Comments: This study helped to determine clinically meaningful reductions in A1c, setting a reference value for RCT of therapies for T2DM.

Jakicic JM, Wing RR, Butler BA, et al. Prescribing exercise in multiple short bouts versus one continuous bout: effects on adherence, cardiorespiratory fitness, and weight loss in overweight women. *Int J Obes Relat Metab Disord*, 1995; Vol. 19: pp. 893–901.
Comments: Early RCT that supports the benefit of prescribing short bouts of exercise among people with obesity.

Wasserman DH, Zinman B. Exercise in individuals with IDDM. *Diabetes Care*, 1994; Vol. 17: pp. 924–37.
Comments: Evidence of effect of exercise in T1DM.

PATIENT EDUCATION: OVERVIEW IN DIABETES

Nancyellen Brennan, CRNP, CDE, and Rita Rastogi Kalyani, MD, MHS

DEFINITION
- Ongoing process through which people with diabetes obtain the knowledge, attitudes, and skills necessary to make daily decisions about their medications, physical activity, meal plan, and other psychosocial challenges that impact their blood glucose levels, cardiovascular risk factors, and quality of life.
- Includes evidence-based clinical knowledge, behavior strategies, and educational theory.

MANAGEMENT

EPIDEMIOLOGY

- Clinical measures improved by diabetes education: Hemoglobin A1c (1.9% reduction over 4–6 months), blood pressure (5 mmHg reduction over 4–6 months), weight loss (1.6 kg over 12–14 months) (Duke).
- Provided primarily by nurse educators and dieticians, also by pharmacists, clinicians, and community health workers.

CLINICAL TREATMENT

Guiding Principles

- The following general principles provide a framework for how to approach all patients; can be used as needed.
- **Empowerment:** facilitating and supporting the patient's capacity to make informed decisions about their own care. The approach is patient-centered, not authoritarian.
- **Adult learning:** patients learn best if they: (1) believe the information is important to them; (2) address the impact of past experiences that help or hinder learning; (3) have control over the learning experience.
- Determine what the patient knows about diabetes, what they want to learn, and their learning style.
- **Transtheoretical model of health behavior change:** patients are at different stages of readiness to change and need specific interventions to move to the action stage. Help the patient choose realistic goals based on their readiness to change.
- **Health belief model:** helps to predict or explain health behaviors based on attitudes and beliefs of individuals with respect to: (1) their susceptibility to the disease; (2) the severity of disease and its complications; (3) the perceived benefits and costs; (4) confidence in their ability to make a change (self-efficacy). The approach is to: (1) explore the patient's views on how serious their diabetes is and how they think it will affect them; (2) identify the risks and benefits of self-care; and (3) evaluate their level of confidence.

Interventions

- **Goal setting:** (1) define goals in collaboration with the patient; (2) be specific (What steps will you take to lose weight?), measurable (How often will you do this?), and realistic (On a scale of 1 to 10, how likely are you to follow this plan?). Examples of goals: I will walk 3 times a week for 15 minutes. I will stop eating snacks after dinner.
- **Problem solving:** brainstorm options, pick the best option, and evaluate the effectiveness of the option. This can be used to help patients set their goals.
- **Motivational interviewing:** a directive, patient-centered style of counseling that uses reflective listening and explores ambivalence to help patients change difficult behaviors. (1) Reflective listening helps patients clarify behaviors they want to change and lets them know you have heard what they said. (2) Identifying ambivalence about the change helps patients change their behaviors. (3) A patient-centered style helps patients define a goal that has a greater chance for success.
- The first two interventions can be used during an office visit and require minimal training. Motivational interviewing takes more time and training.

FOLLOW-UP

- **Frequency:** Diabetes education is not effective if done only once. It requires follow-up and reinforcement. Frequency, timing, and location of follow-up will vary.
- **Immediate follow-up:** Teach by answering patients' questions: What questions do you have today about your diabetes? What worries you most about your diabetes? What

would you like to learn today about your diabetes? Tell me one thing you want to make sure we address today.
- **Evaluate goals:** What's working? What isn't working? What problems are you having with your plan? Who can help and support you? Where can you get help?
- **Set new goals:** What would you like to work on for your next visit?
- **Celebrate success:** Always look for and celebrate attainment of goals, no matter how small.

EXPERT OPINION
- Providers are responsible not only for making recommendations but also for ensuring that patients are optimally educated about the goals of their diabetes care with individualized strategies to attain them.
- Patients are responsible for the execution of recommendations on a day-to-day basis.
- **Listen more, talk less:** patients know what works for them. The task is to help THEM come up with their own solutions, giving information as needed, and supporting their efforts.
- **Build on success:** What has worked for you in the past? How did you lose weight the last time?

BASIS FOR RECOMMENDATIONS

Anderson RM, Funnell MM. Patient empowerment: Myths and misconceptions. *Patient Educ Couns,* 2009; Vol. 79: pp. 277–82.
  Comments: Excellent discussion of the use and misuse of empowerment.

Bodenheimer T, Handley MA. Goal-setting for behavior change in primary care: an exploration and status report. *Patient Educ Couns,* 2009; Vol. 76: pp. 174–80.
  Comments: Review of the literature on goal setting. It does not look at outcomes. Goal setting was performed by clinicians during the visit, nonclinicians after a visit, or computer-based programs.

Duke SA, Colagiuri S, Colagiuri R. Individual patient education for people with type 2 diabetes mellitus. *Cochrane Database Syst Rev,* 2009.
  Comments: This systematic review suggests a benefit of individual education on glycemic control when compared with usual care in a subgroup of those with a baseline HbA1c greater than 8%. In the small number of studies comparing group and individual education, there was an equal impact on HbA1c at 12–18 months.

Russell SS. An overview of adult-learning processes. *Urol Nurs,* 2006; Vol. 26: pp. 349–52, 370.
  Comments: Description of the adult learning theory in clinical practice.

Deakin TA, McShane CE, Cade JE, Williams R. Group based training for self-management strategies in people with type 2 diabetes mellitus. *Cochrane Database of Systematic Reviews,* 2005.
  Comments: Adults with type 2 diabetes who have participated in group based training programs show improved diabetes control (fasting blood glucose and glycated hemoglobin) and knowledge of diabetes in the short (4–6 months) and longer-term (12–14 months). There is some evidence that group based education programs may increase self-empowerment, quality of life, self-management skills, and treatment satisfaction.

Miller WR, Rollnick S. *Motivational Interviewing: Preparing People to Change Addictive Behavior.* New York: The Guilford Press; 2002.
  Comments: This is the original publication on motivation interviewing—it describes the process in detail.

Prochaska JO, Velicer WF. The transtheoretical model of health behavior change. *Am J Health Promot,* 1997; Vol. 12: pp. 38–48.
  Comments: Description and use of the transtheoretical model.

OTHER REFERENCES

Hill-Briggs F, Gemmell L. Problem solving in diabetes self-management and control: a systematic review of the literature. *Diabetes Educ,* 2007; Vol. 33: pp. 1032–50; discussion 1051–2.

MANAGEMENT

Comments: Review of the literature of 52 studies on problem solving, individual and group sessions by nonclinicians. 37% of the studies showed an improvement in A1c.

Hill-Briggs F. Problem solving. In: *The Art and Science of Diabetes Self-Management Education: A Desk Reference for Healthcare Professionals.* Chicago: American Associates of Diabetes Educators; 2006; pp. 731–759.
   Comments: Good summary of how to do problem solving with patients.

Rosenstock IM. Understanding and enhancing patient compliance with diabetic regimens. *Diabetes Care,* 1985; Vol. 8: pp. 610–6.
   Comments: Discussion of health belief model and self efficacy as a concept for supporting behavior change.

American Diabetes Association. *http://www.diabetes.org/.*
   Comments: American Diabetes Association website has information for health professionals and patients, such as type 1, type 2, prediabetes, nutrition, and different age groups, and some information is available in Spanish. The site is somewhat difficult to navigate. You can cut and paste paragraphs to design your own patient handouts.

American Dietetic Association. *http://www.eatright.org.*
   Comments: This website has one-page handouts on over 50 topics related to nutrition, which can be downloaded (not as PDF file). The handouts sponsored by food companies are biased; read carefully before using. The handouts authored by the association are better.

National Diabetes Education Program. *http://www.ndep.nih.gov/.*
   Comments: This website has over 100 brochures and one-page handouts for patients and health professionals. The publications can be downloaded as PDF files or purchased from them for a low price. It covers a wide range of topics, including age, ethnicity, work place, and school issues, in 21 languages. Easy to navigate.

National Institute of Diabetes and Digestive and Kidney Diseases. *http://www.diabetes.niddk.nih.gov.*
   Comments: This website has information on over 100 topics related to diabetes and complications. You can cut and paste to make your own handouts. They have an "easy-to-read" series. Easy to navigate.

PATIENT EDUCATION: CURRICULUM TOPICS IN DIABETES

Nancyellen Brennan, CRNP, CDE, and Rita Rastogi Kalyani, MD, MHS

DEFINITION
- Coordinated set of information and educational experiences, which include learning outcomes and effective teaching strategies.
- DSME (Diabetes Self-Management Education) is a structured and continuous process of learning the knowledge and skills necessary for successful management of diabetes.
- In the US, a Certified Diabetes Educator (CDE) is a healthcare professional who has specialized training in diabetes education, completed 1000 hours of patient education in diabetes, and passed a standardized examination. Other countries are just beginning to develop their own CDE programs.

EPIDEMIOLOGY
- 57% of adults in the US attended DSME provided in outpatient clinical settings in 2007 (CDC).
- Taught by nurses, dieticians, pharmacists, doctors, and counselors who have had instruction in diabetes management, preferably a CDE.
- Emphasizes practical problem-solving skills, collaborative care, and strategies that sustain self-management

CLINICAL TREATMENT

Survival Skills—Information Newly Diagnosed Patients Need to Know

- Survival skills adapted from Inpatient Management Guidelines for People with Diabetes.
  - How and when to take medications: review timing (before or after meals), most common side effects; if taking insulin, review injection technique, storage, needle disposal.
  - How and when to monitor blood glucose or urine: how to use a glucometer or urine dipstick, write down results for clinician visit.
  - Basics regarding meal planning: "healthy eating," categories of carbohydrate foods (handouts with pictures is very helpful), emphasize regularity and consistency of carbohydrate intake.
  - How to treat hypoglycemia: review symptoms, management; carry treatment (e.g., orange juice or sugar tablets) at all times.
  - Sick day management: risk of hyperglycemia (or hypoglycemia) and need to change doses of insulin, monitor glucose frequently, urine test for ketones.
  - Date and time of follow-up with clinician.
  - Information on how to obtain further diabetes education.
  - When to call for medical advice.

More Advanced Diabetes Self-Management Education (American Diabetes Association)

- **Diabetes:** how it is diagnosed, basic disease mechanisms, risk factor management, and treatment options
- **Nutrition:** describe carbohydrate-containing foods, distribution of carbohydrates using the plate method, reading labels; will need carbohydrate counting if taking insulin with meals
- **Physical activity:** aerobic versus resistance exercise, frequency recommended, how to adapt to physical limitations
- **Medications:** mode of action, side effects, how and when to take, proper storage
- **Glucose monitoring:** how to perform blood or urine testing, record results, and use them to adjust food intake and activity; interpretation and use of hemoglobin A1c
- **Preventive screening strategies:** including particular tests recommended and frequency
- **Preventing, detecting, and treating acute complications** (DKA, hypoglycemia, hyperosmolar hyperglycemic syndrome): symptoms, treatment, when to seek medical attention
- **Preventing, detecting, and treating chronic complications** (retinopathy, nephropathy, neuropathy, and cardiovascular disease): symptoms, treatment, when to seek medical attention
- **Developing personal strategies to address psychosocial issues and concerns:** lack of support and depression can be addressed in support groups including family or church members, social workers, or counselors.
- **Developing personal strategies to promote health and behavior change:** goal setting to clarify the change desired, peer support, and support groups can help maintain changes, family support for help with healthy meal planning, transportation to appointments, and maintaining needed medication.

MANAGEMENT

FOLLOW-UP

- Evaluate personal goals such as increasing frequency of exercise or limiting unhealthy snacks. If not achieved, reevaluate; if achieved, set new ones but no more than two goals at a time.
- For learning content, give one-page handout on a topic of interest or answer patient questions.

EXPERT OPINION

- Understanding diabetes helps patients and their families learn how to manage it successfully.
- Information can be overwhelming; cover topics on a need-to-know basis or in short 1- to 2-hour hour segments.
- Use visual aids (pictures, models) to make it interactive and fun or group activities (games, skits).
- Provide individual education if patients have unique needs (physical, learning, or social limitations); otherwise, group education is valuable for support and sharing ideas. Support groups can also have an educational component.

BASIS FOR RECOMMENDATIONS

Duke S-AS, Colagiuri S, Colagiuri R. Individual patient education for people with type 2 diabetes mellitus. *Cochrane Database of Systematic Reviews*, 2009; Vol. 21: CD005268.
   Comments: Review of the value of individual education.

Funnell M, Brown T, Childs B, Haas L, et al. National Standards for Diabetes Self-Management Education. *Diabetes Care*, 2008; pp. S97–104.
   Comments: Summary of ADA standards for education.

Centers for Disease Control and Prevention. Age-Adjusted Percentage of Ever Attended Diabetes Self-Management Class for Adults >18 Years with Diabetes, United States, 2000–2007. Behavior Risk Factor Surveillance System; 2007. *http://www.cdc.gov/diabetes/statistics/preventive/fY_class.htm*,
   Comments: Graph depicting adults attending DSMT.

Deakin TA, McShane CE, Cade JE, Williams R. Group-based training for self management strategies in people with Type 2 diabetes mellitus. *Cochrane Database of Systematic Reviews*, 2005; Vol. 18: CD003417.
   Comments: Review of the value of group education.

American Healthways. Inpatient Management Guidelines for People with Diabetes; 2004. *http://www.healthways.com/WorkArea/showcontent.aspx?id=322*.
   Comments: List of survival skills on p. 10.

International Diabetes Federation. Consultative Section on Education International Standards for Diabetes Education. Brussels: International Diabetes Federation; 2003.
   Comments: Summary of International Diabetes Federation standard for diabetes education; very similar to ADA standards.

International Diabetes Federation Consultative Section on Education. *http://www.idf.org/Diabetes_Education*.
   Comments: IDF diabetes curriculum—ready to use with PowerPoint slides, notes, and curriculum.

OTHER REFERENCES

American Diabetes Association. *http://www.diabetes.org/living-with-diabetes/treatment-and-care/blood-glucose-control/blood-glucose-meters.html*.
   Comments: One-page patient handout on blood glucose meters.

American Diabetes Association. *http://www.diabetes.org/living-with-diabetes/treatment-and-care/blood-glucose-control/hypoglycemia-low-blood.html*.
   Comments: Patient handout on hypoglycemia.

American Diabetes Association. *http://www.diabetes.org/living-with-diabetes/treatment-and-care/who-is-on-your-healthcare-team/when-youre-sick.html.*

Comments: Patient handout on sick day management.

American Diabetes Association. *http://www.diabetes.org/living-with-diabetes/treatment-and-care/who-is-on-your-healthcare-team/visiting-your-health-care.html.*

Comments: Patient handout on visiting the doctor.

PATIENT EDUCATION: OVERCOMING BARRIERS IN DIABETES

Nancyellen Brennan, CRNP, CDE, and Rita Rastogi Kalyani, MD, MHS

DEFINITION
- Any condition that interferes with a patient's ability to learn about or manage his or her diabetes.
- Barriers can be related to the patient, provider, or environment.

EPIDEMIOLOGY
- People with inadequate health literacy are twice as likely to have poor glycemic control and retinopathy (Schillinger).
- Diabetes-related numeracy is a strong predictor of A1c and may help explain racial disparities in glycemic control (Osborn; Cavanaugh).
- Half of patients taking insulin reported they would be more likely to take their injections regularly if another product was available to reduce the pain (Rubin).
- 41% of patients with diabetes report poor psychological well-being, which affected diabetes care (Peyrot).
- Depression is a common comorbidity among persons with diabetes that affects diabetes care.

CLINICAL TREATMENT
Overcoming Patient Barriers
- **Literacy:** (1) use picture-based handouts, repetition, short teaching sessions covering one topic at a time, written instructions to share with literate caregiver or family member; (2) ask patient how he or she likes to learn (e.g., reading, videos, music, games, or skits). Vanderbilt Diabetes Literacy and Numeracy Education Toolkit (DLNET) is a good resource.
- **Cultural:** (1) important to know health beliefs, foods, complementary and alternative medicines that are culture-based; (2) include members from target culture in planning of educational tools; (3) provide cultural sensitivity training for all staff.
- **Physical Impairments:** (1) vision: large print or audio tools, computer aides; (2) hearing: written material, bring a friend or family member, computer-assisted learning; (3) manual dexterity: observe glucometer use and insulin injection technique, choose meters that are easier to use, use insulin pens or prefilled syringes.
- **Pain:** (1) short sessions, repetition; (2) pain medication may interfere with ability to pay attention; (3) discomfort of pricking blood for glucometer testing can be minimized by alternating fingers.
- **Emotional:** (1) shock, anger, denial and feeling overwhelmed are common; let the patient talk for a few minutes at the beginning of the visit and use reflective listening. (2) Screen patients for depression. (3) Stressful living conditions (e.g., crime, financial problems, alcohol, verbal and sexual abuse, or neglect); consider referral to mental health and/or social work.

MANAGEMENT

- **Health beliefs:** patients do not see the importance of learning about diabetes because they do not understand the risks associated with an asymptomatic disease; discuss during the visit or refer for education.
- **Social stigma:** patients may feel reluctant to share their illness with others for fear of discrimination which hinders their ability to optimally self-manage their diabetes; encourage patients to talk about their concerns; support groups may be helpful.
- **Lack of social support:** Help patients identify their support system. Family and friends may not always be helpful; other forms of social support include internet-based or telephone peer support and volunteer organizations (e.g, church, diabetes associations, or service groups).
- **Socially disadvantaged:** patients may especially benefit from literacy interventions, participatory decision making, and social support.

Overcoming Clinical Barriers
- Diabetes educators may have more time than physicians for assessment and teaching.
- Minimize perceived or actual differences in teaching content and philosophy (e.g., targets for metabolic control) between doctor and diabetes educator; educational curriculum or patient handouts should be developed as a team.
- Patients are more likely to attend education sessions if they are recommended to attend by their doctor.

Overcoming Health System Barriers
- **Lack of certified diabetes educators:** not enough to meet patients' need. Solutions: train clinic staff or laypeople from churches, diabetes association; hang posters or show videos in the waiting room; hand out single topic written materials related to patients' questions or concerns; initiate group medical visits, which include education (Deitrick).
- **Logistical:** inconvenient time or place and lack of transportation. Solutions: extended hours, diabetes clinics where the patient can see the doctor and diabetes educator the same day; teaching in the community (i.e., churches, women's or men's groups, schools).
- **Lack of community resources:** cannot get medications due to cost or transportation; no one to help with insulin administration; poor eating due to lack of help with food shopping or preparation. Solutions: help the patient identify and recruit neighbors, relatives, or church members who can help with these tasks; make a list of volunteer organizations in the community who can help.

Overcoming Barriers to Starting Insulin
- **Fear of needles:** demonstrate injection technique; use ultrafine needles, pen injectors.
- **Fear of hypoglycemia:** emphasize incidence of serious hypoglycemia is low if administered appropriately.
- **Fear of weight gain:** reinforce healthy eating and physical activity.
- **Feeling of failure:** emphasize the progressive nature of the disease and that majority of people with diabetes will eventually need insulin.

FOLLOW-UP
- Review knowledge and skills: Is the patient remembering and acting on the information you are giving him or her?
- Continue to explore barriers: What is making it difficult for you to . . . take your medicine? . . . monitor your blood sugar?

EXPERT OPINION

- Addressing barriers to patient education are especially important for patients who are not meeting glycemic targets despite optimization of medical therapy.
- Consider individual teaching and frequent follow-up for patients with significant barriers.
- Patients often hear conflicting information on diabetes; coordinate with your team to develop consistent messages about diabetes care.
- A supportive provider–patient relationship is key to successful learning and health behavior change.

BASIS FOR RECOMMENDATIONS

American Association of Diabetes Educators. AADE position statement. Cultural sensitivity and diabetes education: recommendations for diabetes educators. *Diabetes Educ*, 2007; Vol. 33: pp. 41–44.

> **Comments:** Position statement by American Association of Diabetes Educators, includes definition and ways to incorporate cultural sensitivity into your practice.

OTHER REFERENCES

Peyrot M, Rubin RR, Funnell MM, et al. Access to diabetes self-management education: results of national surveys of patients, educators, and physicians. *Diabetes Educ*, 2009; Vol. 35: pp. 246–8, 252–6, 258–63.

> **Comments:** Interview of 1169 patients, 1871 diabetes educators, and 629 doctors to determine perceived barriers to receiving DSME.

Osborn CY, Cavanaugh K, Wallston KA, et al. Diabetes numeracy: an overlooked factor in understanding racial disparities in glycemic control. *Diabetes Care*, 2009; Vol. 32: pp. 1614–9.

> **Comments:** Cross-sectional study examining the mediating effect of health literacy and numeracy on the relationship between African American race and glycemic control.

Cavanaugh K, Wallston KA, Gebretsadik T, et al. Addressing literacy and numeracy to improve diabetes care: two randomized controlled trials. *Diabetes Care*, 2009; Vol. 32: pp. 2149–55.

> **Comments:** Randomized controlled trials evaluating the impact of providing literacy- and numeracy-sensitive teaching in a diabetes care program on A1c and other diabetes outcomes.

Rubin RR, Peyrot M, Kruger DF, et al. Barriers to insulin injection therapy: patient and health care provider perspectives. *Diabetes Educ*, 2009; Vol. 35: pp. 1014–22.

> **Comments:** A survey of patient and provider perspectives on barriers to insulin injection therapy.

Funnell MM, Brown TL, Childs BP, et al. National standards for diabetes self-management education. *Diabetes Care*, 2009; Vol. 32 Suppl 1: pp. S87–94.

> **Comments:** Guidelines designed to define quality diabetes self-management education and to assist diabetes educators to provide evidence-based education.

Brown AF. Patient, system and clinician level interventions to address disparities in diabetes care. *Curr Diabetes Rev*, 2007; Vol. 3: pp. 244–8.

> **Comments:** Discusses evidence on interventions at the individual, provider, healthcare system, and community levels that have the potential to reduce diabetes disparities.

Marrero DG. Overcoming patient barriers to initiating insulin therapy in type 2 diabetes mellitus. *Clin Cornerstone*, 2007; Vol. 8: pp. 33–40, discussion 41-3.

> **Comments:** Reviews the importance of starting insulin early and how to overcome patient's resistance to starting insulin.

Peyrot M, Rubin RR, Lauritzen T, et al. Psychosocial problems and barriers to improved diabetes management: results of the Cross-National Diabetes Attitudes, Wishes and Needs (DAWN) Study. *Diabet Med*, 2005; Vol. 22: pp. 1379–85.

> **Comments:** Cross-sectional study looking at the patient- and provider-reported psychosocial problems and barriers to effective self-care.

MANAGEMENT

Deitrick L, Swavely D, Merkle LN, et al. Group medical visits for patients with type 2 diabetes: patient and physician perspectives. *Abstr Academy Health Meet,* 2005; Vol. 22: abstract no. 4077.
Comments: Description of the successful use of group medical visits for diabetes education.

Schillinger D, Grumbach P, Piette J. Association of Health Literacy with Diabetes Outcomes. *JAMA,* 2002; Vol. 288: p. 475.
Comments: Cross-sectional study showing that inadequate health literacy is independently associated with poorer glycemic control and higher rates of retinopathy.

Vanderbilt University Diabetes Research and Training Center Diabetes Literacy and Numeracy Education Toolkit (DLNET). *http://www.mc.vanderbilt.edu/diabetes/drtc/preventionandcontrol/tools.php.*
Comments: 24 modules covering diabetes topics for those with low health literacy. Can be used as needed over multiple visits.

Prediabetes

PREDIABETES OR CATEGORIES OF INCREASED RISK FOR DIABETES

Rachel Derr, MD, PhD

DEFINITION
- Impaired fasting glucose (IFG) and impaired glucose tolerance (IGT) are intermediate states of abnormal glucose homeostasis between normal and overt diabetes.
- Prediabetes is a designation including either IFG, IGT, or both.
- Documentation of IFG requires only a fasting plasma glucose. Documentation of IGT requires a 75-g oral glucose tolerance test.
- A hemoglobin A1c of 5.7%–6.4% identifies individuals in "categories of high risk for diabetes" (ADA Standards of Medical Care in Diabetes).
- See Table 2-5 for exact definitions.

TABLE 2-5. DIAGNOSTIC CRITERIA FOR ABNORMAL GLUCOSE STATES

State	Fasting Glucose (mg/dl)	2-hour Glucose (mg/dl) during a 75-g OGTT	A1c (%)
Normal	<100	<140	<5.7
Isolated Impaired Fasting Glucose*	100–125	<140	–
Isolated Impaired Glucose Tolerance	<100	140–199	–
Combined IFG and IGT	100–125	140–199	–
Prediabetes or Categories of Increased Risk**	100–125	140–199	5.7–6.4
Diabetes**	≥126	≥200	>6.5

*The WHO and IDF recommend that Impaired Fasting Glucose be 110–125 mg/dl.
**At least one criterion needs to be satisfied for diagnosis.
Courtesy of Rachel Derr.

EPIDEMIOLOGY

- In the US during years 2005–2006, for people aged ≥20 years, crude prevalence of IFG was 25.7% and IGT was 13.8%; ~30% had either (Nathan; Cowie).
- 10-year incidence of IFG = 14% and IGT = 48%, in subjects with an average age of 57 years at baseline (Meigs).
- Presence of either or both abnormalities confers high risk for developing type 2 diabetes (approximately 25% in 3–5 years and up to 70% over lifetime) and modestly increased risk of cardiovascular disease (HR 1.1–1.4) (Nathan).
- Risk factors same as for diabetes.

DIAGNOSIS

- Screen individuals >45 years of age or in adults of any age with BMI ≥25 mg/kg² and additional diabetes risk factors (see Type 2 Diabetes: Genetic Risk Factors, p. 168, and Type 2 Diabetes: Environmental Risk Factors and Screening, p. 165) to identify risk for future diabetes (ADA Standards of Medical Care in Diabetes).
- Usually no overt symptoms.
- Fasting plasma glucose after a minimum 8-hour fast and adequate carbohydrate intake in preceding days.
- 75-gram 2-hour oral glucose tolerance test (OGTT): the gold-standard method for diagnosis of prediabetes, but can be time-consuming.
- A1c: new criterion for "categories of increased risk for diabetes" includes HbA1c 5.7%–6.4%.
- For all these tests, risk is continuous, increasing at higher ends of the range.

CLINICAL TREATMENT

Standard of Care (According to the American Diabetes Association)

- Moderate-intensity exercise (30 minutes daily), weight loss (5%–10% of body weight) according to the Diabetes Prevention Program (DPP) protocol, and smoking cessation.
- Metformin, to be considered for individuals with both IFG and IGT and any of the following: age <60 yo, BMI ≥35 mg/m², family history of DM, high triglycerides, reduced HDL, hypertension, A1c >6.0%.
- Other medications studied (thiazolidinediones, acarbose) may also be effective for preventing DM, but not uniformly recommended secondary to cost/adverse effects.

Prognosis After Treatment (Randomized Controlled Trials)

- DPP (3234 patients): progression from IFG or IGT to DM over 3 years occurred in 29% of the control group versus 14% of the intensive lifestyle group (58% relative reduction), and 22% of the metformin group (31% relative reduction); metformin was most effective in younger patients with BMI ≥35 kg/m² (Knowler).
- Finnish Diabetes Prevention Study (522 patients): progression from IGT to DM over 4 years occurred in 23% of the control group versus only 11% of the weight-reduction/exercise group (58% reduction) (Tuomilehto).
- In the Da Qing study (557 patients): progression from IGT to DM over 6 years occurred in 67.7% of the control group versus 46% in the diet and exercise group (31% reduction) (Pan)
- DPPOS found sustained long-term benefits of the lifestyle intervention, with 34% reduction in diabetes incidence up to 10 years later (Knowler). These results were similar to other long-term follow up studies of lifestyle interventions in persons with

prediabetes including the Finnish Diabetes Prevention study (43% reduction at 7 years) (Lindstrom) and Da Qing study (43% reduction at 20 years) (Li).

FOLLOW-UP

- At least annual follow-up for weight-loss counseling and measurement of fasting glucose and serum lipids.
- If on metformin, twice yearly follow-up with A1c measurement.
- Patients with prediabetes do not appear to be at increased risk for retinopathy or nephropathy, but risk is higher for neuropathy and macrovascular complications, so consider screening for these.

EXPERT OPINION

- Isolated impaired fasting glucose (IFG) indicates predominantly hepatic insulin resistance; isolated impaired glucose tolerance (IGT) indicates predominantly (peripheral) muscle insulin resistance.
- Diagnosing prediabetes early allows patients the opportunity to make changes to prevent or delay the onset of type 2 diabetes.
- Randomized trials show that successful lifestyle changes and moderate weight loss are more effective than medication for preventing DM, likely cost-effective, and benefits persist over the long-term.
- Lifestyle interventions are hard to implement, and weight reduction is difficult to maintain. Therefore, consider metformin if adequate weight loss is not observed after 6 months.

BASIS FOR RECOMMENDATIONS

American Diabetes Association. Standards of medical care in diabetes—2011. *Diabetes Care,* 2011; Vol. 34 Suppl 1: pp. S11–61.

Comments: Screening, diagnosing, and management recommendations for favorably affecting health outcomes of patients with diabetes.

International Expert Committee International Expert Committee report on the role of the A1c assay in the diagnosis of diabetes. *Diabetes Care,* 2009; Vol. 32: pp. 1327–34.

Comments: Consensus view from the 2008 committee that proposes the use of the A1c assay for the diagnosis of prediabetes and diabetes, suggests appropriate cut-points, and argues that A1c testing has many advantages over plasma glucose testing.

Nathan DM, Davidson MB, DeFronzo RA, et al. Impaired fasting glucose and impaired glucose tolerance: implications for care. *Diabetes Care,* 2007; Vol. 30: pp. 753–9.

Comments: Summary of the ADA consensus position on prediabetic states in 2006, addressing the definition, pathogenesis, natural history, consequences, and treatment of IFG and IGT.

Knowler WC, Barrett-Connor E, Fowler SE, et al. Reduction in the incidence of type 2 diabetes with lifestyle intervention or metformin. *NEJM,* 2002; Vol. 346: pp. 393–403.

Comments: Landmark RCT showing the beneficial effects of lifestyle changes and metformin on prevention of type 2 diabetes among subjects with baseline IFG and IGT.

OTHER REFERENCES

Cowie CC, Rust KF, Ford ES, et al. Full accounting of diabetes and pre-diabetes in the U.S. population in 1988–1994 and 2005–2006. *Diabetes Care,* 2009; Vol. 32: pp. 287–94.

Comments: Using data from National Health and Nutrition Examination Survey in 1988–2004 and 2005–2006, provides estimates for prevalence of diabetes and prediabetes in the US using glucose criteria.

MANAGEMENT

Knowler WC, Fowler SE, Hamman RF, et al. 10-year follow-up of diabetes incidence and weight loss in the Diabetes Prevention Program Outcomes Study. *Lancet*, 2009; Vol. 374: pp. 1677–86.
Comments: A summary of the results of the DPPOS follow-up study.

Li G, Zhang P, Wang J, et al. The long-term effect of lifestyle interventions to prevent diabetes in the China Da Qing Diabetes Prevention Study: a 20-year follow-up study. *Lancet*, 2008; Vol. 371: pp. 1783–9.
Comments: A summary of the results of the Da Qing follow-up study.

Lindström J, Ilanne-Parikka P, Peltonen M, et al. Sustained reduction in the incidence of type 2 diabetes by lifestyle intervention: follow-up of the Finnish Diabetes Prevention Study. *Lancet*, 2006; Vol. 368: pp. 1673–9.
Comments: A summary of the results of the Finnish Diabetes Prevention follow-up study.

World Health Organization and International Diabetes Federation. Definition and diagnosis of diabetes mellitus and intermediate hyperglycemia: Report of WHO/IDF consultation. World Health Organization; 2006.
Comments: Describes the WHO/IDF criteria for diabetes, IGT, and IFG.

Meigs JB, Muller DC, Nathan DM, et al. The natural history of progression from normal glucose tolerance to type 2 diabetes in the Baltimore Longitudinal Study of Aging. *Diabetes*, 2003; Vol. 52: pp. 1475–84.
Comments: Characterizes the natural history of progression from normal glucose tolerance to IFG/IGT to type 2 diabetes using data from >20 years of biennial oral glucose tolerance tests performed in a large cohort.

Tuomilehto J, Lindstrom J, Eriksson JG, et al. Prevention of type 2 diabetes mellitus by changes in lifestyle among subjects with impaired glucose tolerance. *NEJM*, 2001; Vol. 344: pp. 1343–50.
Comments: First large RCT showing that type 2 diabetes can be effectively prevented by changes in lifestyle among subjects with baseline IGT.

Pan XR, Li GW, Hu YH, et al. Effects of diet and exercise in preventing NIDDM in people with impaired glucose tolerance. The Da Qing IGT and Diabetes Study. *Diabetes Care*, 1997; Vol. 20: pp. 537–44.
Comments: A summary of the results of the Da Qing IGT and Diabetes Study.

Pregnancy

GESTATIONAL DIABETES MELLITUS

Wanda K. Nicholson, MD, MPH, MBA

DEFINITION

- Gestational diabetes mellitus (GDM) defined as glucose intolerance first identified during pregnancy, distinct from type 1 (T1DM) and type 2 diabetes mellitus (T2DM), which are initially diagnosed outside of pregnancy.

EPIDEMIOLOGY

- GDM is the most common metabolic disease of pregnancy.
- GDM affects an estimated 170,000 (1%–14%) pregnancies each year in the United States, depending on the diagnostic criteria used and characteristics of the population (Jovanovic).
- 30%–50% of women with GDM will have recurrent GDM in a future pregnancy (Bellamy; Kim).
- Of particular concern, 20%–50% of women with GDM will develop T2DM in the 5–10 years after delivery (Jovanovic).
- Recent meta-analysis reports that GDM corresponds to a 7.4-fold increased risk for developing T2DM (Bellamy).

DIAGNOSIS

- At first prenatal visit, women at high risk of GDM (severe obesity, previous delivery of large-for-gestational age infant, glycosuria, PCOS, personal history of GDM, or a strong family history of diabetes) should undergo standard diagnostic testing for diabetes. If abnormal, consider these individuals to have "overt" (not gestational) diabetes. If normal, retest between 24–28 weeks (ADA Standards of Medical Care 2011).
- New ADA guidelines (2011) recommend to perform a 75-gram oral glucose tolerance test (OGTT), with plasma glucose measurement fasting and at 1 and 2h at 24–28 weeks in *all* women not known to have diabetes.
- OGTT should be performed in the morning after an overnight fast of at least 8 hours.
- The diagnosis of GDM is made when any *one* of the following plasma glucose values are exceeded: fasting >92 mg/dl (5.1 mmol/l), 1h >180 mg/dl (10.0 mmol/l), or 2h >153 mg/dl (8.5 mmol/l).
- Former criteria for the diagnosis of GDM (i.e., Carpenter and Coustan) were based on having at least *two* abnormal values on 3-hour 100-gram OGTT after failing a 1-hour 50-gram OGTT; the two step screening for GDM is no longer recommended.

SIGNS AND SYMPTOMS

- Classic signs and symptoms of hyperglycemia (such as polyuria, polydypsia, blurry vision, vaginal yeast infections) reflect blood glucose generally over 180 mg/dl. GDM, however, is frequently asymptomatic.
- Common symptoms during pregnancy include increased urination and are not necessarily related to hyperglycemia.

MANAGEMENT

CLINICAL TREATMENT
Glucose Control
- Tight glycemic control is the primary goal, similar to targets in pregnant women with previous history of diabetes.
- Generally accepted goals for blood glucose levels during pregnancy are shown in Table 2-6.

TABLE 2-6. GLUCOSE VALUES FOR ADEQUACY OF CONTROL

Fasting	60–90 (or 95) mg/dl
Premeal	60–100 mg/dl
1 hour postprandial (after meal)	<140 mg/dl
2 hours postprandial	<120 mg/dl
Bedtime	<120 mg/dl
2:00–6:00 AM	60–120 mg/dl

Source: ACOG Committee on Practice Bulletins. ACOG Practice Bulletin. Clinical management guidelines for obstetrician-gynecologists. Number 60, March 2005. Pregestational diabetes mellitus. *Obstet Gynecol,* 2005; Vol. 105(3): pp. 675-85. Reproduced with permission of Lippincott Williams & Wilkins.

Non-Pharmacologic Management
- The most important objective in managing GDM is to control maternal glycemia as close to normal as possible in order to reduce the chance of fetal loss, maternal and neonatal complications.
- Obese women diagnosed with GDM should be started on a 30 kcal/kg/day American Diabetes Association (ADA) diet.
- Carbohydrates should be restricted to 40%–50% of diet.
- Daily low-to-moderate intensity physical activity is recommended.

Pharmacologic Management
- Should be initiated if dietary therapy alone fails. Insulin is considered the primary therapy.
- Currently, the ADA and the American College of Obstetricians and Gynecologists do not endorse the routine use of oral antihyperglycemic agents during pregnancy, and such therapy has not been approved by the US Food and Drug Administration for treatment of GDM.
  - However, glyburide and metformin are still used for pharmacologic management in practice, although insulin is preferred.
  - Metformin (Glucophage) primarily used up to 14 weeks in women with PCOS, shown to be safe throughout pregnancy in an efficacy trial (Rowan).
  - No difference in maternal or neonatal outcomes with glyburide or metformin compared with insulin (Rowan, Nicholson, Langer, Moore).
- See Pregnancy and Diabetes on p. 124 for further information on insulin treatment.

FOLLOW-UP

- Can usually stop pharmacologic therapy for GDM after delivery as insulin sensitivity markedly improves postpartum.
- About 75% of women with GDM normalize glucose tolerance postpartum, but will have an increased risk of later T2DM.
- ACOG and ADA recommend screening for diabetes at 6–12 wks postpartum.
- If normal, assess glycemic status every 3 years.
- Recent systematic review shows low sensitivity of fasting blood glucose as postpartum screening test for type 2 DM (Bennett).

EXPERT OPINION

- Pregnancy always confers insulin resistance. Women with normal insulin secretion overcome this by increasing insulin output.
- If a woman develops GDM, it signals subnormal insulin reserve.
- Occasionally, T1DM presents during pregnancy, and the woman remains insulin-dependent postpartum, with unstable glycemia suggestive of T1DM.
- Large observational studies have reported associations between mild elevations in maternal glucose levels even in the non-diabetic range with maternal, perinatal, and neonatal outcomes which have prompted recent changes in the diagnosis of GDM (Metzger).
- New 2011 ADA criteria for diagnosis of GDM no longer suggest use of 50-gram screening OGTT, followed by 100-gram diagnostic OGTT in high-risk women only; instead 75-gram OGTT alone is sufficient for both screening and diagnosis and is to be performed in all pregnant women. These new criteria will significantly increase the prevalence of GDM, primarily because only one abnormal value, not two, is sufficient to make the diagnosis.

BASIS FOR RECOMMENDATIONS

American Diabetes Association. Standards of medical care in diabetes—2011. *Diabetes Care*, 2011; Vol. 34 Suppl 1: pp. S11–61.
  Comments: Describes new America Diabetes Association guidelines on diagnosis and treatment of GDM.

OTHER REFERENCES

Bellamy L, Casas JP, Hingorani AD, et al. Type 2 diabetes mellitus after gestational diabetes: a systematic review and meta-analysis. *Lancet*, 2009; Vol. 373: pp. 1773–9.
  Comments: Systematic review and pooled estimates of development of type 2 diabetes after gestational diabetes.

Nicholson W, Bolen S, Witkop CT, et al. Benefits and risks of oral diabetes agents compared with insulin in women with gestational diabetes: a systematic review. *Obstet Gynecol*, 2009; Vol. 18: pp. 193–205.
  Comments: Systematic review of 4 RCTs and 5 observational studies on the effectiveness and safety of metformin and glyburide compared to insulin among women with gestational diabetes.

Bennett WL, Bolen S, Wilson LM, et al. Performance characteristics of postpartum screening tests for type 2 diabetes mellitus in women with a history of gestational diabetes mellitus: a systematic review. *J Womens Health* (Larchmont, NY), 2009; Vol. 18: pp. 979–87.
  Comments: Systematic review of 11 studies comparing sensitivity and specificity of fasting blood glucose to 75-g 2-hour OGTT.

Metzger BE, Lowe LP, Dyer AR, et al. Hyperglycemia and adverse pregnancy outcomes. *N Engl J Med*, 2008; Vol. 358: pp. 1991–2002.
  Comments: A large study (~25,000 pregnant women) that found a strong, continuous association of maternal glucose levels within the nondiabetic range with increased birth weight and increased cord-blood serum C-peptide levels. Prompted recent changes in ADA guidelines for diagnosis of GDM.

MANAGEMENT

Rowan JA, Hague WM, Gao W, et al. Metformin versus insulin for the treatment of gestational diabetes. *NEJM,* 2008; Vol. 358: pp. 2003–15.

Comments: Randomized clinical trial of 754 women with gestational diabetes at 20–33 weeks gestation in Australia and New Zealand.

Kim C, Berger DK, Chamany S. Recurrence of gestational diabetes mellitus: a systematic review. *Diabetes Care,* 2007; Vol. 30: pp. 1314–9.

Comments: Systematic review and pooled estimates of development of recurrence of gestational diabetes.

Jovanovic L, Pettitt DJ. Gestational diabetes mellitus. *JAMA,* 2001; Vol. 286: pp. 2516–8.

Comments: Review article of epidemiology of gestational diabetes.

Langer O, Conway DL, Berkus MD, et al. A comparison of glyburide and insulin in women with gestational diabetes mellitus. *NEJM,* 2000; Vol. 343: pp. 1134–8.

Comments: Randomized clinical trial of 404 women with gestational diabetes in the United States.

PREGNANCY AND DIABETES

Wanda K. Nicholson, MD, MPH, MBA

DEFINITION
- Diabetic pregnancy refers to both pregestational and gestational diabetes.
- Pregestational diabetes: diabetes diagnosed before a woman conceives.
- Gestational diabetes (GDM): diabetes diagnosed after the onset of pregnancy.

EPIDEMIOLOGY
- Pregestational diabetes (including both type 1 and type 2) affects 1% of all pregnancies (Lawrence).
- Epidemiology of GDM described elsewhere.
- In type 1 diabetes, duration of diabetes significant predictor of caesearian delivery. Chronic hypertension associated with prematurity and perinatal mortality (Gonzalez).
- In type 2 diabetes, higher A1c in first trimester significant predictor of congenital malformations and perinatal mortality; higher A1c in third trimester related to prematurity. Macrosomia associated with higher rates of caesearian delivery (Gonzalez).

DIAGNOSIS
- For diagnosis of pregestational diabetes, see Diagnosis and Classification of Diabetes, p. 5.
- For diagnosis of GDM, see Gestational Diabetes Mellitus, p. 121.

CLINICAL TREATMENT
Glucose Goals in Diabetic Pregnancy
- Extremely "tight" blood glucose control is targeted during pregnancy, in order to minimize the risk of neonatal congenital abnormalities (related to hyperglycemia in first trimester), fetal macrosomia (related to hyperglycemia in last 2 trimesters), prematurity and perinatal mortality.
- Targets shown in Table 2-6 (see Gestational Diabetes Mellitus, p. 121). Using self-monitoring, mean fasting glucose levels target 100 mg/dl. Goal hemoglobin A1c <6%.
- Check HbA1c monthly, although SMBG more useful for immediate care.

Evaluation and Assessment of Diabetic Pregnancy

- **Laboratory and diagnostic testing:** check comprehensive metabolic panel, thyroid function tests, electrocardiogram after pregnancy confirmed.
- **Retinopathy screening:** refer to ophthalmology if not evaluated in past year.
- **Renal function:** assess with spot or 24-hour urine protein and creatinine clearance.
- **Ultrasound evaluations:** early ultrasound for dating and estimated due date; anatomical ultrasound (18–22 weeks); and serial ultrasounds around 28–32 weeks and 34–36 weeks gestation to access fetal growth percentiles.
- **Fetal echo:** at 18–22 weeks to assess fetal cardiac structure; at 34–36 weeks, ultrasound evaluation of the fetal cardiac interventricular septum may also be performed. An increase in size may indicate poor glucose control.
- **Fetal surveillance:** beginning at 32–34 weeks gestation, should be conducted at appropriate intervals and can include a combination of fetal movement counting, nonstress test, contraction stress test, and biophysical profile. Twice weekly fetal surveillance has been widely adopted beginning at 32–34 weeks gestation, but can be individualized.
- **Doppler velocimetry of the umbilical artery:** useful in monitoring pregnancies with poor fetal growth.

Dietary and Pharmacologic Management of Glycemia in Pregnancy

- In GDM, dietary control may be adequate with appropriate carbohydrate restriction. A diet consisting of 40%–50% carbohydrate is recommended. A nutritionist may help with calorie and carbohydrate counting; women with normal weight require up to 30–35 kcal/kg/day. Women with mild gestational diabetes (i.e., an abnormal result on an oral glucose-tolerance test but a fasting glucose level below 95 mg per deciliter [5.3 mmol per liter]) may do well on diet control alone.
- Oral hypoglycemic agents, including glyburide (FDA category C) and metformin (FDA category B), can be considered in GDM, but insulin is considered the primary therapy and preferred if hyperglycemia persists with diet alone.
- Insulin can be delivered through subcutaneous administration or insulin pump (for type 1 diabetes).
- Regular, lispro, aspart, and NPH insulins are all FDA Category B; insulin glargine, detemir, and glulisine are all FDA Category C.
- Administer short- or rapid-acting insulins (regular, lispro, and aspart) before meals to reduce postmeal hyperglycemia.
- Give regular insulin ~30 minutes before eating. Give lispro and aspart immediately before eating.
- Lispro and aspart are very fast acting, so hypoglycemia can occur if food is not ingested shortly after their administration. Use caution especially if patient is vomiting frequently or has morning sickness.
- Long- and intermediate-acting insulins (NPH, glargine, detemir) are used once or twice daily.
- Insulin requirements usually increase during pregnancy, especially during the third trimester, but decline soon after delivery; patients usually require lower insulin doses if at all following childbirth and with breastfeeding.
- Preferred insulin injection site is abdomen, with no evidence that it will harm the baby.

MANAGEMENT

Management of Delivery in Diabetic Pregnancy

- Control maternal glucose during labor with intravenous regular insulin to keep glucose levels less than 120 mg/dl.
- Delivery of pregnancies complicated by diabetes can occur safely at 39 weeks gestation.
- Earlier delivery, particularly in pregnancies complicated by diabetic vascular changes, can occur but only after amniocentesis has been performed to confirm fetal lung maturity.
- Although ultrasound is often used to assess fetal weight and rule out macrosomia before delivery, it has not proven to be more effective than clinician evaluation.
- Cesarean delivery should be considered if the estimated fetal weight is greater than 4500 g in women with diabetes.
- Induction of labor in pregnancies for suspected macrosomia does not reduce birth trauma and may increase the risk of cesarean delivery.

Complications of Diabetic Pregnancy

- Maternal complications during pregnancy may occur more frequently, but are similar to diabetic complications in nonpregnant women.
- Diabetes increases the risk of cesarean delivery and postoperative complications.
- Shoulder dystocia three times higher compared to nondiabetic pregnancy.
- Risk of preeclampsia 13%–14% higher during diabetic pregnancy.
- Polyhydramnios more common in diabetic pregnancy.
- Maternal hyperglycemia can lead to miscarriage or premature labor and delivery.
- Maternal hyperglycemia can also lead to vascular disease including the development of hypertension, kidney disease, stroke, and worsening diabetic retinopathy in the mother.
- Maternal hyperglycemia contributes to poor or delayed fetal lung maturity in the infant.
- Accelerated growth of the fetus with uncontrolled maternal hyperglycemia can lead to a large-for-gestational age infant. Macrosomia, defined as an infant >4500 grams, occurs in up to 10% of diabetic pregnancies. Even mild hyperglycemia increases birth weight (Landon).
- In the infant: neonatal hypoglycemia/seizures, hypocalcemia, hyperbilirubinemia, polycythemia occur more frequently; also increased risk of congenital abnormalities, perinatal mortality, and intrauterine growth retardation (with coexisting maternal vascular disease).

FOLLOW-UP

- Women with gestational diabetes should be informed about their risk of developing subsequent diabetes and undergo appropriate preventive screening.

EXPERT OPINION

- Preconception care should include A1c as close to 7 as possible and evaluation for medications that are commonly used to treat diabetes and its complications, since they may be contraindicated during pregnancy, including statins, ACE inhibitors, ARBs, and most noninsulin diabetes therapies.
- *Diabetic retinopathy* may progress during pregnancy and should be evaluated by an ophthalmologist before and during pregnancy.
- Emerging evidence shows that a fetus exposed to maternal hyperglycemia during development undergoes alterations in metabolism ("fetal programming"), which predispose the infant to childhood obesity and diabetes.

BASIS FOR RECOMMENDATIONS

American Diabetes Association. Preconception care of women with diabetes. *Diabetes Care,* 2004; Vol. 27 Suppl 1: pp. S76–8.

    Comments: Outlines the American Diabetes Association guidelines on preconception care in women with diabetes.

OTHER REFERENCES

Landon MB, Spong CY, Thom E, et al. A multicenter, randomized trial of treatment for mild gestational diabetes. *NEJM,* 2009; Vol. 361: pp. 1339–48.

    Comments: A randomized clinical trial indicating that even mild elevation in mean glucose, within range of impaired glucose tolerance, is associated with larger birth weight. Study also found that treatment of mild gestational diabetes mellitus did not significantly reduce the frequency of a composite outcome (stillbirth, perinatal disease, neonatal complications).

Lawrence JM, Contreras R, Chen W, et al. Trends in the prevalence of preexisting diabetes and gestational diabetes mellitus among a racially/ethnically diverse population of pregnant women, 1999–2005. *Diabetes Care,* 2008; Vol. 31: pp. 899–904.

    Comments: Epidemiology of pregestational and gestational diabetes.

Gonzalez-Gzonzalez NL, Ramirez O, Mozas J, et al. Factors influencing pregnancy outcome in women with type 2 versus type 1 diabetes mellitus. *Acta Obstet Gynecol Scand,* 2008; Vol. 87: pp. 43–9.

    Comments: Describes factors associated with adverse perinatal outcomes in women with type 1 and type 2 diabetes.

MANAGEMENT

DRIVING WITH DIABETES

Rita Rastogi Kalyani, MD, MHS

DEFINITION
- The vast majority of people with diabetes drive regularly and safely.
- Driving by patients with diabetes may, however, be impaired by three factors: hypoglycemia, diabetes complications, and hyperglycemia.
- Hypoglycemia unawareness may pose an increased threat to driving.

EPIDEMIOLOGY
- Only 0.4%–3% of fatal motor vehicle accidents (MVAs) are caused by medical conditions (Grattan). Epilepsy most common medical condition (38%), followed by insulin-treated diabetes (18%), and acute myocardial infarction (8%); no cause in 21% of cases.
- MVA rates are variably reported as being similar, higher or lower among persons with insulin-treated diabetes compared to their counterparts (Cox; Mathieson).
- Among US persons with type 1 diabetes, 31% admitted to driving in hypoglycemic stupor during past 2 years; 28% experienced hypoglycemia while driving during past 6 months. In persons with type 2 diabetes, figures were lower (8% and 6%, respectively) (Cox).
- Hypoglycemia unawareness may lead to undetected hypoglycemia while driving and affects approximately 25% of patients with type 1 diabetes; incidence in type 2 diabetes is lower (Johnson; Zammit).
- Among drivers with diabetes, insulin-treated diabetes and diabetes duration >5 years both associated with higher injury risk (Koepsell).
- Hospital admission rates of drivers with insulin-treated diabetes versus those without diabetes is slightly increased (de Klerk; Kennedy).
- In survey of 68,770 drivers by National Highway Traffic Safety Administration, drivers with diabetes (and other metabolic conditions) and an unrestricted driving license had 1.44 times higher risk of at-fault accidents.
- Retinopathy associated with decreased vision; treatment with laser coagulation may also reduce peripheral vision (Pearson). Peripheral neuropathy may interfere with operation of vehicle.
- Cognitive dysfunction may interfere with driving ability; associated with acute and possibly chronic hyperglycemia (Cox), tight glycemic control, and acute hypoglycemia.
- Older drivers may represent a subset of individuals at higher risk for MVAs (McCoy), but older women with diabetes are more likely to give up driving than older women without diabetes (Forrest).

SIGNS AND SYMPTOMS
- Driving associated with increased metabolic demand in persons with diabetes, manifesting as increased heart rate, more autonomic symptoms, and trend toward greater epinephrine release (Cox).

CLINICAL TREATMENT

Hypoglycemia and Blood Glucose Awareness Training

- Persons with type 1 diabetes may not correctly judge when their blood glucose is too low; in one study, subjects stated they would drive 38%–47% of the time when their actual blood glucose was <40 mg/dl (2.2 mmol/l) (Clarke).
- Hypoglycemia unawareness associated with increased likelihood of driving while hypoglycemic (Stork).
- Hypoglycemia induced by hyperinsulinemic clamp in persons with type 1 diabetes is used during driving simulation studies to examine effects on performance (Cox).
- Moderate hypoglycemia <50 mg/dl (2.6 mmol/l) associated with reduced driving performance (swerving, spinning, time over midline, time off the road) and more compensatory slow driving; only 50% of patients said they would not drive under similar conditions in real life.
- When subjects given opportunity to self-treat symptoms of hypoglycemia or discontinue driving in simulation studies, only 32% of patients took corrective action although 79% detected moderate hypoglycemia.
- However, real-life driving conditions are more complex and control group not included in these studies.
- Blood glucose awareness training programs teach patients to more accurately estimate blood glucose levels; MVA rates significantly lower in educated versus uneducated persons with diabetes (Cox; Broers).

Avoidance of Hypoglycemia While Driving

- Always keep carbohydrate in vehicle.
- Self-monitoring of blood glucose equipment (i.e., glucometer) should be available in vehicle.
- Consider testing blood glucose before driving, especially in patients with hypoglycemia unawareness.
- Stop driving at the very first symptom of possible hypoglycemia and do not resume driving until blood glucose is proven to be in safe range.
- Patient education to emphasize potential deterioration in driving performance when blood glucose <70 mg/dl (4 mmol/l).
- Licensing authority and motor insurance company should be informed if hypoglycemia while driving occurs; patient compliance with statutory requirements generally good (Graveling).

Legal Restrictions

- Current legal restrictions regarding diabetes and driving privileges vary widely; most laws are prompted by potential risks of hypoglycemia, though some may, unfortunately, be prompted by a limited understanding of diabetes and its complications.
- Laws should balance individual interests of patient with general traffic safety.
- In US, many states have restrictive licensing programs for persons with diabetes.
- In California, mandatory for doctors to report unexpected loss of consciousness from hypoglycemia, usually resulting in revocation of driver's license.
- In most other states, such reporting is voluntary.
- Insulin-treated individuals are automatically denied an interstate commercial driving license with few exceptions; however, waivers have been granted in 39 out of 50 states in last decade (Stork).

MANAGEMENT

- In Europe, restrictions range from more frequent medical examinations to denial of driving privileges for people with diabetes.

EXPERT OPINION

- MVAs directly caused by diabetes are rare.
- There are many people with diabetes who can and do drive safely, but some who cannot.
- Absence of severe hypoglycemia (change in mental status) for the previous 3 years, and presence of hypoglycemia awareness indicate good chance of driving safely.
- Hypoglycemia during driving does occur, however, especially in persons with insulin-treated diabetes, causing what is a slightly increased risk of MVAs.
- Risk factors for MVA include recent severe hypoglycemia (mental status change), hypoglycemia unawareness, older age (with more rapid decline in cognitive function).
- Our recommendation is that each person be considered and evaluated individually, rather than setting blanket policies that unfairly discriminate against people with diabetes.
- Further research is still needed to better describe the association between diabetes and MVAs.

BASIS FOR RECOMMENDATIONS

Stork AD, van Haeften TW, Veneman TF. Diabetes and driving: desired data, research methods and their pitfalls, current knowledge, and future research. *Diabetes Care*, 2006; Vol. 29: pp. 1942–9.

> **Comments:** Most up-to-date review on the current knowledge regarding diabetes and driving, along with recommendations for future research directions.

OTHER REFERENCES

Stork AD, van Haeften TW, Veneman TF. The decision not to drive during hypoglycemia in patients with type 1 and type 2 diabetes according to hypoglycemia awareness. *Diabetes Care,* 2007; Vol. 30: pp. 2822–6.

> **Comments:** Individuals with hypoglycemia unawareness are more likely to drive.

Zammitt NN, Frier BM. Hypoglycemia in type 2 diabetes: pathophysiology, frequency, and effects of different treatment modalities. *Diabetes Care,* 2005; Vol. 28: pp. 2948–61.

> **Comments:** Describes epidemiology of hypoglycemia in type 2 diabetes.

Broers S, van Vliet KP, le Cessie S, et al. Blood glucose awareness training in Dutch type 1 diabetes patients: one-year follow-up. *Neth J Med*, 2005; Vol. 63: pp. 164–9.

> **Comments:** Dutch study describing beneficial effects of blood glucose awareness training; educated versus uneducated patients less likely to be involved in accidents (0.6 vs 0.2 accidents per patient per year, $p = 0.04$).

Cox DJ, Kovatchev BP, Gonder-Frederick LA, et al. Relationships between hyperglycemia and cognitive performance among adults with type 1 and type 2 diabetes. *Diabetes Care*, 2005; Vol. 28: pp. 71–7.

> **Comments:** Cognitive dysfunction associated with hyperglycemia in adults with diabetes.

Graveling AJ, Warren RE, Frier BM. Hypoglycaemia and driving in people with insulin-treated diabetes: adherence to recommendations for avoidance. *Diabet Med*, 2004; Vol. 21: pp. 1014–9.

> **Comments:** Describes how well individuals with diabetes adhere to guidelines for avoiding hypoglycemia while driving.

Cox DJ, Penberthy JK, Zrebiec J, et al. Diabetes and driving mishaps: frequency and correlations from a multinational survey. *Diabetes Care,* 2003; Vol. 26: pp. 2329–34.

> **Comments:** Describes the frequency of driving injury in persons with diabetes using data from a large, multinational survey. In US, 31% admitted to driving in hypoglycemic stupor in past 2 years and 28% experienced hypoglycemia while driving in past 6 months. Type 1 diabetic drivers reported more crashes than type 2 diabetic drivers and nondiabetic spouses (19% vs 12% vs 8%, $p < 0.001$).

Johnson ES, Koepsell TD, Reiber G, et al. Increasing incidence of serious hypoglycemia in insulin users. *J Clin Epidemiol,* 2002; Vol. 55: pp. 253–9.

Comments: Describes epidemiology of hypoglycemia in insulin-treated diabetes.

Kennedy RL, Henry J, Chapman AJ, et al. Accidents in patients with insulin-treated diabetes: increased risk of low-impact falls but not motor vehicle crashes—a prospective register-based study. *J Trauma,* 2002; Vol. 52: pp. 660–6.

Comments: Suggests that accident rates not significantly different between adults with insulin-treated diabetes (44.4 per 100,000 people per year) compared to the general population (34.4); relative risk = 1.29, nonsignificant.

Cox DJ, Gonder-Frederick LA, Kovatchev BP, et al. The metabolic demands of driving for drivers with type 1 diabetes mellitus. *Diabetes Metab Res Rev,* 2002; Vol. 18: pp. 381–5.

Comments: Patients with type 1 diabetes divided into 2 groups: watching a driving video or actually driving a simulator during constant insulin/dextrose infusion to maintain euglycemia. Actual driving associated with significantly higher dextrose infusion rate, more autonomic symptoms, increased heart rate, trend toward greater epinephrine release, and significantly more frequent hypoglycemic self-treatment.

Cox DJ, Gonder-Frederick L, Polonsky W, et al. Blood glucose awareness training (BGAT-2): long-term benefits. *Diabetes Care,* 2001; Vol. 24: pp. 637–42.

Comments: Describes beneficial impact of blood glucose awareness training on accident rates. After 4 years, 6.8 accidents/million miles driven in educated group versus 29.8 in control group.

National Highway Traffic Safety Administration. Medical conditions and driver crash risk: do license restrictions affect public safety? *Ann Emerg Med,* 2000; Vol. 36: pp. 164–5.

Comments: National Highway Traffic Safety Administration's investigation on impact of restricted driving licenses on accident rate in persons with different medical conditions, including diabetes.

Cox DJ, Gonder-Frederick LA, Kovatchev BP, et al. Progressive hypoglycemia's impact on driving simulation performance. Occurrence, awareness and correction. *Diabetes Care,* 2000; Vol. 23: pp. 163–70.

Comments: In driving simulation study, the authors examined the impact of progressive hypoglycemia on driving performance. Diminished driving performance was seen at all glucose levels (4.0–3.3, 3.3–2.8, <2.8 mmol/l). Only 32% took corrective action, although 79% detected hypoglycemia <2.8 mmol/l.

Clarke WL, Cox DJ, Gonder-Frederick LA, et al. Hypoglycemia and the decision to drive a motor vehicle by persons with diabetes. *JAMA,* 1999; Vol. 282: pp. 750–4.

Comments: Persons with diabetes may not accurately judge when they are hypoglycemic.

Pearson AR, Tanner V, Keightley SJ, et al. What effect does laser photocoagulation have on driving visual fields in diabetics? *Eye* (London), 1998; Vol. 12 (Pt 1): pp. 64–8.

Comments: Summary of laser treatment's effects on peripheral vision in patients with diabetic retinopathy.

Mathiesen B, Borch-Johnsen K. Diabetes and accident insurance. A 3-year follow-up of 7599 insured diabetic individuals. *Diabetes Care,* 1997; Vol. 20: pp. 1781–4.

Comments: Danish Diabetes Association reported that risk of any accident significantly lower in those with diabetes (0.7 per 1000 persons) compared with two control groups (4.5 and 5.5, respectively).

Forrest KY, Bunker CH, Songer TJ, et al. Driving patterns and medical conditions in older women. *J Am Geriatr Soc,* 1997; Vol. 45: pp. 1214–8.

Comments: Older women with diabetes are significantly more likely to give up driving compared to those without diabetes (odds ratio 2.53, 95% CI 1.57–4.07).

Koepsell TD, Wolf ME, McCloskey L, et al. Medical conditions and motor vehicle collision injuries in older adults. *J Am Geriatr Soc,* 1994; Vol. 42: pp. 695–700.

Comments: Authors reported a 2.6-fold increased risk of driving injury in older drivers with diabetes, especially for insulin-treated patients and diabetes duration >5 years.

MANAGEMENT

McCoy GF, Johnston RA, Duthie RB. Injury to the elderly in road traffic accidents. *J Trauma*, 1989; Vol. 29: pp. 494–7.
   Comments: In general, older adults are more likely to sustain driving injuries than younger adults.

de Klerk NH, Armstrong BK. Admission to hospital for road trauma in patients with diabetes mellitus. *J Epidemiol Community Health*, 1983; Vol. 37: pp. 232–7.
   Comments: Describes higher rate of hospital admissions for driving-related trauma among persons with diabetes in men <55 years, both as pedestrians and drivers.

Grattan E, Jeffcoate GO. Medical factors and road accidents. *BMJ*, 1968; Vol. 1: pp. 75–9.
   Comments: Describes relatively low frequency of accidents caused by medical conditions.

EMPLOYMENT AND DISCRIMINATION

Christopher D. Saudek, MD

DEFINITION
- Employment discrimination is when a person is unreasonably denied a job, terminated from employment, or kept from promotion on the basis of his or her medical condition.
- A person with diabetes may be discriminated against if he or she is not offered employment opportunities that he or she is able to perform.
- Legal definitions of employment discrimination vary from state to state and country to country, and can be complex.
- An experienced lawyer may be needed to evaluate the strength of a case involving employment discrimination.

EPIDEMIOLOGY
- No reliable statistics exist to describe the extent of job discrimination against people with diabetes.
- Discrimination may be subtle, as employers may not specify that diabetes is the reason a person is not hired, not promoted, or terminated; or it may be overt, if the employer has a fixed policy against employing people with diabetes or people who take insulin.
- Employers in the US may fear that hiring a person with diabetes will adversely affect the cost of employer-based health insurance.
- Discrimination may occur in individual, isolated circumstances or as a broad, blanket employer policy.
- Unfair and potentially illegal discrimination in employment practices may occur because employers misunderstand diabetes, including its management and treatment.

DIAGNOSIS
- In the US, the Americans with Disabilities Act (ADA) protects people with disabilities. Due to successful amendments effective starting in 2009, virtually all people with diabetes are considered to have a "disability" and therefore covered by the ADA.
- The ADA requires that an employer make "reasonable accommodations" to help people with disabilities.
- In the case of diabetes, reasonable accommodations may include, for example, allowing a person to carry a snack, or to measure his or her own blood glucose level while on the job.
- As above, an experienced lawyer may be needed to advise on what is truly employment discrimination.

SIGNS AND SYMPTOMS

- Any employer with a blanket policy of not hiring people with diabetes may be guilty of employment discrimination.
- A potential employer cannot ask about a person's health history, including whether or not the person has diabetes, before making a job offer, but an offer may be contingent upon passing a medical history and examination.
- Failure to make reasonable accommodations in the workplace for a person with diabetes may be employment discrimination.

CLINICAL TREATMENT

- Healthcare professionals are frequently asked to evaluate a person with diabetes for employment.
- The medical evaluation for employment should consider: Does the person have long-term complications that would significantly impair job performance? Does he or she have a recent history of severe hypoglycemia? What are the job requirements? Is the individual able to perform the job despite having diabetes?
- Healthcare professionals may be in a position to advise employers about the benefits of treating people with diabetes fairly.
- When advising employers, some key points may be that (1) people with diabetes can and have been successful in virtually all types of work; (2) people with diabetes are often more health/safety conscious and personally careful or reliable than the average employee; (3) the main risk—severe hypoglycemia—occurs only in some people who take certain medications and are prone to hypoglycemia.
- Sometimes, healthcare professionals will be in a position to advise people with diabetes about seeking employment.
- In advising people with diabetes, it is important not to be too pessimistic or restrictive. While there are some employers (such as the military) that categorically will not hire people with diabetes, most will and should.
- People with diabetes do not need to tell potential employers about their health history (including having diabetes) until they have been offered a job and are having a preemployment physical examination.
- In unusual cases, healthcare professionals may need to help people with diabetes get further legal assistance if discrimination occurs. Diabetes organizations such as the American Diabetes Association can often be of assistance.

EXPERT OPINION

- The healthcare professional's first obligation is to the patient. This is compatible with simultaneously protecting public safety and the legitimate interests of an employer.
- The healthcare professional should promote safety in the workplace and a productive work force.
- Employers are often happy to be educated about diabetes and willing to hire and promote people with diabetes when they understand the facts.
- In protecting people with diabetes from employment discrimination, the first principle is that each person deserves individual consideration. Not every person is able to do every job (e.g., severe retinopathy may prohibit work requiring fine eyesight); but blanket policies against diabetes are potentially discriminatory and illegal.

MANAGEMENT

- Helping employers make reasonable accommodations for the person with diabetes, and helping the person with diabetes have reasonable expectations, is the optimal role of the healthcare professional.
- Severe hypoglycemia (requiring another person's assistance) is the real potential danger in certain high-stress employment situations, not whether hyperglycemia is well controlled.
- On the whole, people with diabetes can be outstanding employees in the vast majority of employment positions.

BASIS FOR RECOMMENDATIONS

American Diabetes Association. Diabetes and employment. *Diabetes Care,* 2009; Vol. 32, Suppl 1: pp. S80–4.

> **Comments:** The American Diabetes Association's policy statement, with good advice for healthcare professionals on all aspects of evaluating individuals.

Specific Populations or Subtypes

CHILDREN AND TYPE 2 DIABETES

Ali Mohamadi, MD, and David W. Cooke, MD

DEFINITION

- Type 2 diabetes mellitus (T2DM) is a disease that used to be seen in adults only, hence the previous name "adult onset diabetes."
- However, it is now well recognized that T2DM also occurs in children younger than 19 years old, and in increasing incidence.
- The pathophysiology of T2DM in children is similar to that seen in adults.

EPIDEMIOLOGY

- The prevalence of T2DM in children has increased dramatically in recent decades, with an estimated 10-fold increase in the incidence from 1982 to 1994 (Dabaela).
- T2DM now accounts for approximately 15% of new-onset diabetes in non-Hispanic white children over 9 years of age, and more than half of such cases in minority youth (Dabelea).
- T2DM remains extremely rare in prepubertal children but incidence is as high as 11.8 per 100,000 person years in children 10–19 years old (Dabelea).
- Obesity, which causes insulin resistance, is the strongest modifiable risk factor for T2DM in children 10–19 years old; the increased incidence of T2DM is related to the increased prevalence of obesity in children.
- In children with increased insulin resistance, endogenous sex hormone production during puberty may accelerate progression to T2DM among adolescents.
- There is a strong genetic component to the risk of T2DM in children, with multiple family members often affected.

DIAGNOSIS

- The American Academy of Pediatrics and American Diabetes Association recommend screening all obese children with additional risk factors for T2DM such as positive family history, nonwhite race, and acanthosis nigricans on physical examination.
- The diagnostic criteria for diabetes in children is the same as those for adults.
- Because T2DM occurs rarely in prepubertal children, do not screen children until they reach puberty or 10 years old.

SIGNS AND SYMPTOMS

- Identify asymptomatic T2DM by routinely screening high-risk children for glucosuria or hyperglycemia, hyperglycemia being more sensitive.
- Vaginal or penile moniliasis or nocturia suggests T2DM.
- Some children present with classic diabetes symptoms: polyuria, polydipsia, polyphagia, weight loss.
- Up to 33% of children have ketonuria at diagnosis, and 5%–25% of children with T2DM present in ketoacidosis (including coma).
- Although rare, children with T2DM have presented with hyperosmolar hyperglycemic state.

- In patients whose phenotypes and family history are not classic for T1DM, T2DM, or MODY, measure autoantibodies and/or screen for gene mutations to distinguish subtype.

CLINICAL TREATMENT

- Therapeutic options for T2DM include three categories: (1) lifestyle modification, (2) oral agents, and (3) insulin therapy.
- In the absence of ketosis or ketoacidosis, or marked hyperglycemia at diagnosis, lifestyle modification (diet and exercise) should be the initial approach for youth with T2DM.
- Weight loss goal is 5%–7% of body weight; exercise goal is 20–30 minutes of vigorous exercise per day.
- Children with T2DM who fail to achieve normal glucose control after 3–6 months of attempting lifestyle modification, or those with hemoglobin A1c (HbA1c) >8% at diagnosis, should be treated pharmacologically.
- Limited evidence guides the use of medications, and the natural history of childhood T2DM is not fully known.
- Only insulin and metformin are approved for use in children by the US Food and Drug Administration (FDA).
- If a child presents in diabetic ketoacidosis or if the child's HbA1c at diagnosis is >9%, insulin is indicated.
- Goals of therapy: normalize blood glucose levels and minimize the risk of long-term complications.
- Target for HbA1c is <7%–8% or as close to normal as possible without significant hypoglycemia.
- Metformin dose is 500 mg twice a day, up to 1000 mg twice a day; metformin should be taken with meals, and started at 500 mg once a day for 5–7 days before increasing to 500 mg twice a day in order to minimize gastrointestinal side effects.

FOLLOW-UP

- Measure HbA1c every three months; a HbA1c >7%–8% indicates a need to intensify treatment.
- Screen for dyslipidemia every 2 years. LDL >160 mg/dl indicates a need for medication for postpubertal children.
- Screen blood pressure quarterly, with aggressive treatment of hypertension (goal <95th percentile for age and sex).
- Annual urine microalbumin testing (spot microalbumin/creatinine) with treatment of persistent microalbuminuria with angiotensin converting enzyme inhibitors or angiotensin receptor blocking agents.
- Dilated retinal examination by an ophthalmologist at the time of diagnosis and annually thereafter.

EXPERT OPINION

- Though formal ADA guidelines exist for A1c targets in type 1 diabetes among children (A1c <8% for ages 6–12 years; A1c <7.5% for ages 13–18 years), the A1c targets for type 2 diabetes in children are not as clearly defined.
- It may be reasonable to adopt similar A1c goals as in adults. One study found that ADA targets for adults (A1c <7%) are suboptimally achieved in pediatric patients with T2DM (Valent).

- HbA1c goal is thus individualized: some children can safely be <6.5%–7%; others have unacceptable hypoglycemia with these targets.
- Pediatric primary care providers must be familiar with T2DM and must be prepared to diagnose and initiate treatment.
- Gaps remain in the knowledge about natural history of T2DM in children and about the optimal treatment of pediatric patients that develop the disease.
- Given the likely life-long risk accumulation, treat based on the best available data and seek evidence to develop optimal therapies.

BASIS FOR RECOMMENDATIONS

American Academy of Pediatrics and American Diabetes Association. Type 2 diabetes in children and adolescents. *Pediatrics*, 2000; Vol. 105: pp. 671–80.

    Comments: Consensus statement of AAP and ADA providing guidelines for screening for T2DM in children.

OTHER REFERENCES

American Diabetes Association. Standards of medical care in diabetes—2011. *Diabetes Care*, 2011; Vol. 34 Suppl 1: pp. S11–61.

    Comments: Outlines standards of medical care for adults and children with diabetes.

Valent D, Pestak K, Otis M, et al. Type 2 diabetes in the pediatric population: are we meeting ADA clinical guidelines in Ohio? *Clin Pediatr* (Philadelphia), 2010; Vol. 49: pp. 316–22.

    Comments: Suggests that adherence to ADA clinical guidelines for pediatric patients with type 2 diabetes is not good. Authors recommend that specific evidence-based guidelines be developed for children with type 2 diabetes.

Grant RW, Moore AF, Florez JC. Genetic architecture of type 2 diabetes: recent progress and clinical implications. *Diabetes Care*, 2009; Vol. 32: pp. 1107–14.

    Comments: 2009 review of recently identified genes implicated in T2DM and potential clinical applications of new genetic knowledge to risk prediction, pharmacologic management, and patient behavior.

Writing Group for the SEARCH for Diabetes in Youth Study Group, Dabelea D, Bell RA, et al. Incidence of diabetes in youth in the United States. *JAMA*, 2007; Vol. 297: pp. 2716–24.

    Comments: Landmark population-based study providing data on the incidence of DM among US youth according to racial/ethnic background and DM type.

Fourtner SH, Weinzimer SA, Levitt Katz LE. Hyperglycemic hyperosmolar non-ketotic syndrome in children with type 2 diabetes. *Pediatr Diabetes*, 2005; Vol. 6: pp. 129–35.

    Comments: Large retrospective chart review providing information on typical clinical course and sequelae of hyperglycemic hyperosmolar nonketotic syndrome in children with T2DM.

Expert Committee on the Diagnosis and Classification of Diabetes Mellitus. Report of the expert committee on the diagnosis and classification of diabetes mellitus. *Diabetes Care*, 2003; Vol. 26 Suppl 1: pp. S5–20.

    Comments: Report of international expert committee establishing current standards for definition and description of diabetes, classification of the disease, diagnostic criteria, and testing for diabetes.

MANAGEMENT

MATURITY ONSET DIABETES OF THE YOUNG (MODY)

Ali Mohamadi, MD, and David W. Cooke, MD

DEFINITION

- Maturity onset diabetes of youth (MODY) is a monogenic form of early-onset diabetes mellitus (DM), which usually develops in childhood, adolescence, or young adulthood.
- It is characterized by nonketotic DM, autosomal dominant transmission, onset before the age of 25 years of age, and pancreatic beta-cell dysfunction.

EPIDEMIOLOGY

- Up to 5% of patients with antibody-negative DM have been found to have a MODY gene defect (Owen).
- Molecular genetic studies of MODY families find that it is not a single entity, but a clinically and genetically heterogeneous disease.
- Mutations in eight genes have now been identified as causing MODY.
- MODY2 is caused by a defect in the gene encoding for the enzyme glucokinase (GCK), while MODY8 is caused by mutations in the gene for carboxy ester lipase (CEL).
- MODY1 and MODY3–7 are caused by gene defects in a number of transcription factors: Hepatocyte nuclear factor-4 alpha (HNF-4 alpha/MODY1), hepatocyte nuclear factor-1 alpha (HNF-1 alpha/MODY3—most common, accounting for 20%–75% of MODY cases); pancreatic duodenal homeobox 1 (PDX1/MODY4), hepatocyte nuclear factor 1 beta (HNF-1 beta/MODY 5), neurogenic differentiation factor 1 (Neuro D1-beta 2/MODY6), and Krüppel-like factor 11 (KLF11/MODY7).

DIAGNOSIS

- At least five major diagnostic criteria for MODY are usually accepted. These include:
  - Hyperglycemia usually diagnosed before age 25 years in at least one and ideally two family members.
  - Autosomal-dominant pattern of inheritance, with a vertical transmission of diabetes through at least three generations, and a similar phenotype shared by diabetic family members.
  - Absence of insulin therapy at least 5 years after diagnosis or significant C-peptide levels even in a patient on insulin treatment.
  - Insulin levels often in the normal range, though inappropriately low for the degree of hyperglycemia, suggesting a primary defect in beta-cell function.
  - Normal body habitus, with generally low incidence of overweight or obesity.
- Notably, since mild hyperglycemia may not cause the classic symptoms of DM, the diagnosis may not be made until adulthood.

SIGNS AND SYMPTOMS

- Most common clinical presentation of MODY is mild, asymptomatic hyperglycemia in nonobese individuals.
- Onset may be hastened by factors affecting insulin sensitivity, such as acute illness or infection, onset of puberty, or pregnancy.
- Clinical features differ among the various MODY subtypes and depend upon the affected gene.
  - **MODY1** (HNF-4 alpha) and **MODY3** (HNF-1 alpha): Mild–moderate fasting and postprandial plasma glucose (PG) concentrations that increase over time due to progressive decrease in insulin secretion.
  - **MODY2** (Glucokinase): Mild fasting hyperglycemia due to impaired glucose tolerance. Less than 50% of carriers have overt DM, and diabetic-associated complications are rare.
  - **MODY4** (PDX1): Phenotypes ranging from impaired glucose tolerance to overt DM; homozygous or compound heterozygous mutations of PDX1 are associated with pancreatic agenesis.
  - **MODY5** (HNF-1 beta): Overt DM in association with renal cysts.

- **MODY6** (NeuroD1-beta 2): Rare, with phenotype characterized by obesity and insulin resistance.
- **MODY7** (KFL11): Very rare; phenotype ranges from impaired glucose tolerance or impaired fasting glucose to overt DM.
- **MODY8** (CEL): Very rare; associated with both exocrine and endocrine pancreatic deficiency and with demyelinating peripheral neuropathy.

CLINICAL TREATMENT

- Treatment depends upon the MODY subtype and underlying genetic defect.
    - **MODY1** (HNF-4 alpha) and **MODY3** (HNF-1 alpha): Oral hypoglycemic agents may be effective early in disease; patients often require insulin therapy as endogenous insulin secretion decreases.
    - **MODY2** (Glucokinase): Diet and exercise, with sulfonylureas to be considered for treatment failure with conservative measures.
    - **MODY4** (PDX1): Oral hypoglycemic agents may be considered, although most require insulin therapy.
    - **MODY5** (HNF-1 beta): Insulin therapy.
    - **MODY6** (NeuroD1-beta 2): Oral hypoglycemic agents or insulin therapy.
    - **MODY7** (KFL11): Oral hypoglycemic agents or insulin therapy.
    - **MODY8** (CEL): Pancreatic enzyme replacement and insulin therapy.

FOLLOW-UP

- As with other causes of DM, follow-up at regular intervals, and routine management of diabetes.
- Preventing, screening for, and managing complications of DM as for all people with DM.
- Since certain MODY subtypes have worsening hyperglycemia over time, be vigilant about changing treatment as needed for glycemic control.

EXPERT OPINION

- With currently available testing of MODY genes, can identify family members who have inherited the specific mutation affecting their family prior to onset of hyperglycemia.
- If a child does carry the mutation, periodic testing for abnormalities of carbohydrate metabolism is recommended.
- Larger scale genetic and epidemiological studies will be needed to determine whether monogenic diabetes genes also contribute to the genetic risk of other forms of DM (such as type 2).

REFERENCES

Vaxillaire M, D P, Bonnefond A, Froguel P. Breakthroughs in monogenic diabetes genetics: from pediatric forms to young adulthood diabetes. *Pediatr Endocrinol Rev,* 2009; Vol. 6: pp. 405–17.

   Comments: Review describing genetic and molecular mechanisms underlying the clinical features of MODY, and how new genetic and biological insights led to novel pharmacogenomic approaches.

Vaxillaire M, Froguel P. Monogenic diabetes in the young, pharmacogenetics and relevance to multifactorial forms of type 2 diabetes. *Endocr Rev,* 2008; Vol. 29: pp. 254–64.

   Comments: Review of updating advances in research on genetics of MODY and explaining how these genes may play a role in multifactorial forms of T2DM.

Winckler W, Weedon MN, Graham RR, et al. Evaluation of common variants in the six known maturity-onset diabetes of the young (MODY) genes for association with type 2 diabetes. *Diabetes,* 2007; Vol. 56: pp. 685–93.

   Comments: Study determining patterns of common sequence variation in the genes encoding MODY subtypes; concluded common variants contribute modestly to T2DM.

MANAGEMENT

Slingerland AS. Monogenic diabetes in children and young adults: challenges for researcher, clinician and patient. *Rev Endocr Metab Disord,* 2006; Vol. 7: pp. 171–85.

    Comments: Article detailing genes and mutations involved in insulin synthesis, secretion, and resistance. Provides guidance for genetic testing for MODY and other forms of monogenic diabetes.

Owen KR, Stride A, Ellard S, et al. Etiological investigation of diabetes in young adults presenting with apparent type 2 diabetes. *Diabetes Care,* 2003; Vol. 26: pp. 2088–93.

    Comments: Describes the changing diagnostic approach to the growing population of youth and young adults who present with hyperglycemia but lack clinical and biochemical findings pathognomonic of type 1 diabetes.

Fajans SS, Bell GI, Polonsky KS. Molecular mechanisms and clinical pathophysiology of maturity-onset diabetes of the young. *NEJM,* 2001; Vol. 345: pp. 971–80.

    Comments: Key review of genetics, pathophysiology, and treatment of MODY subtypes.

MITOCHONDRIAL DIABETES

Ali Mohamadi, MD, and David W. Cooke, MD

DEFINITION

- Specific, known mutations in the mitochondrial genome (mtDNA) can cause diabetes mellitus (DM).
- Distinguishing clinical feature of mitochondrial diabetes: association with other symptoms, including deafness, neurological disorders, cardiac failure, and renal failure.
- These mutations can be large deletions, duplications, or point mutations.

EPIDEMIOLOGY

- Mitochondrial mutations account for 0.5%–2.8% of patients with diabetes.
- Genes for mtDNA are inherited maternally, making a positive maternal history an important feature of mitochondrial diabetes.
- Spontaneous (not inherited) mutations in mtDNA have also been described.
- Higher prevalence of mitochondrial diabetes among Asians (up to 1.5% among the entire Japanese population).
- DM can occur in isolation among patients with mtDNA disorders, but is more frequently associated with a number of characteristic comorbidities (see below).

DIAGNOSIS

- Should always be considered in patients with DM associated with deafness, myopathy, cerebellar ataxia, or other unusual neurological features.
- Increased suspicion when strong familial clustering of diabetes and maternal transmission.
- Onset before the age of 40 years and lean habitus is characteristic of mitochondrial diabetes (similar to the more common type 1 diabetes).
- Distinguished from maturity onset diabetes of the young (MODY) by maternal transmission and comorbidities.
- Impaired hearing is detected by audiometry and with decreased perception of frequencies above 5 kHz.
- Diagnosis is confirmed by genetic analysis for mutations in mtDNA.
- Point substitution at nucleotide position 3243 (A to G) in the mtDNA-encoded *tRNALeu(UUR)* gene is the most common mtDNA mutation associated with DM.
- A3243G mutation results in a phenotype similar to type 1 diabetes mellitus and includes impaired insulin secretion, altered glucose metabolism in muscle, and increased gluconeogenesis due to overproduction of lactate.

- Mitochondrial diabetes as a result of the A3243G mutation presents at a mean age of 38 years and has nearly 100% penetrance.

SIGNS AND SYMPTOMS

- Although only mothers can pass on mitochondrial conditions to their children, either males or females may be affected.
- Presentation may resemble type 1 (T1DM) or type 2 diabetes (T2DM) depending on the severity of insulinopenia.
- Substantial fraction of A3243G carriers will develop a type 1-like phenotype.
- Insulinopenia is progressive in nature, and most patients require insulin treatment shortly after the onset of diabetes.
- Hearing impairment generally precedes the onset of DM by several years.
- Changes in retinal pigmentation also present in many carriers of the A3243G mutation.
- Other comorbidities include gastrointestinal abnormalities (dysphagia, dysmotility, gastroesophageal reflux), cardiomyopathy, and renal dysfunction.
- Other associated syndromes: MELAS (mitochondrial encephalomyopathy with lactic acidosis and stroke-like episodes); Kearns-Sayre syndrome (external ophthalmoplegia, retinopathy, and cardiac conduction abnormalities); and MERRF syndrome (myoclonus, epilepsy, with ragged red fibers).

CLINICAL TREATMENT

- Because of progressive insulin deficiency, exogenous insulin is the mainstay of treatment.
- The less-common T2DM-like phenotype can be initially treated with dietary changes or sulfonylurea drugs.
- Metformin is contraindicated because of the risk for lactic acidosis.
- Coenzyme Q10 and carnitine have been used in treatment of patients with mitochondrial myopathies (Maassen).

FOLLOW-UP

- Follow-up treatment and screening for complications of DM should proceed as for patients with either T1DM or T2DM.
- Since a large proportion of patients with mitochondrial diabetes present with other comorbidities, follow-up should be coordinated with the appropriate specialists.

EXPERT OPINION

- Studies suggest that T2DM is more common among patients with affected mothers; it is becoming increasingly clear some of these patients may instead carry mtDNA mutations.
- Accurate diagnosis of mitochondrial diabetes prompts the search for other comorbidities associated with mtDNA mutations.
- Although the variable phenotype makes genetic counseling difficult, diagnosis of mitochondrial diabetes in the patient implicates other at-risk maternal relatives; those family members with clinical findings suggestive of a mitochondrial disorder should be screened.

REFERENCES

Pagel-Langenickel I, Bao J, Pang L, et al. The role of mitochondria in the pathophysiology of skeletal muscle insulin resistance. *Endocr Rev,* 2010; Vol. 31: pp. 25–51.

Comments: Analyzes the data regarding skeletal muscle mitochondrial biology in the pathogenesis of insulin resistance.

Ma Y, Fang F, Yang Y, et al. The study of mitochondrial A3243G mutation in different samples. *Mitochondrion,* 2009; Vol. 9: pp. 139–43.

MANAGEMENT

Comments: Comparison of the mutation ratio of A3243G in blood, urine, hair follicle, and saliva samples in patients with A3243G mutations and their maternal relatives to determine which sample type (urine) is most appropriate for detection of the patients and carriers.

Scaglia F, Hsu CH, Kwon H, et al. Molecular bases of hearing loss in multi-systemic mitochondrial cytopathy. *Genet Med*, 2006; Vol. 8: pp. 641–52.

Comments: Evaluation of the clinical features and molecular bases of hearing loss associated with multisystemic mitochondrial cytopathy

Finsterer J. Genetic, pathogenetic, and phenotypic implications of the mitochondrial A3243G tRNALeu(UUR) mutation. *Acta Neurol Scand*, 2007; Vol. 116: pp. 1–14.

Comments: Comprehensive review of the mitochondrial A3243G *tRNALeu(UUR)* mutation, the most common cause of mitochondrial DM.

Maassen JA, T Hart LM, Van Essen E, et al. Mitochondrial diabetes: molecular mechanisms and clinical presentation. *Diabetes*, 2004; Vol. 53 Suppl 1: pp. S103–9.

Comments: Review of clinical characteristics of mitochondrial diabetes and its molecular diagnosis, also discussing recent developments in the pathophysiological and molecular mechanisms leading to diabetes.

LATENT AUTOIMMUNE DIABETES IN ADULTS (LADA)

Ari Eckman, MD, and Christopher D. Saudek, MD

DEFINITION

- Latent autoimmunie diabetes in adults (LADA) is a slowly developing type 1 diabetes, often misdiagnosed as type 2 diabetes, that progresses relatively quickly to insulin dependence as pancreatic beta-cell failure progresses.
- Also called "slowly progressing insulin-dependent diabetes," "type 2 diabetes with islet autoantibodies," and "type 1.5 diabetes."

EPIDEMIOLOGY

- In the UK Prospective Diabetes Study (UKPDS), approximately 10% of patients who appeared to have type 2 diabetes actually had antibodies to glutamic acid decarboxylase (GAD) and progressed to insulin dependency (Turner; Stenström).
- Among patients <35 yrs of age, frequency of antibody positivity increased to 25% (Turner, Stenström).
- Like classic type 1 diabetes, may have personal or family history of other autoimmune diseases (e.g., autoimmune thyroid disease, pernicious anemia, celiac disease, vitiligo).
- Often do not have family history of diabetes.
- Glycemic control stronger risk factor for cardiovascular disease in LADA patients than in patients with type 2 diabetes, possibly related to lower prevalence of the metabolic syndrome seen in LADA patients (Isomaa).

DIAGNOSIS

- Based on three criteria: adult age at diagnosis; presence of diabetes-associated autoantibodies; delay from diagnosis (at least 6 months) in the need for insulin therapy to manage hyperglycemia.
- Positive tests for glutamic acid decarboxylase autoantibodies (anti-GAD), islet cell autoantibodies (anti-ICA), and tyrosine phosphatase autoantibodies (anti-IA2 or anti-ICA512) predictive of insulin dependency within 3 years (Turner).

- Anti-GAD most sensitive antibody marker: sensitivity 85%.
- Antiinsulin autoantibodies more common among patients with classic type 1 diabetes than in patients with LADA.
- Associated with increased frequency of HLA DR3 (28%), DR4 (27%), and DR3/DR4 (22%) (Ola).
- HLA-DR4-DQ8 antigens: associated with more destructive progression of beta cells, more widespread among patients with classic type 1 diabetes than among those with LADA.

SIGNS AND SYMPTOMS

- Insidious onset of hyperglycemia.
- Lack of acute hyperglycemic crisis (such as diabetes ketoacidosis [DKA]).
- Typically normal to slightly overweight body habitus.
- Usually lack overt signs of insulin resistance as seen in classic type 2 diabetes such as acanthosis nigricans (darkening of the skin in body folds) or acrochordons (skin tags).
- Reduced frequency of metabolic syndrome as compared to type 2 diabetes.
- C-peptide levels may be low/normal (Fielding).

CLINICAL TREATMENT

- Insulin therapy treatment of choice; treat as type 1 diabetes.
- Control hyperglycemia and other risk factors for complications.
- Obese LADA patients benefit from restriction in calories consumed and increased levels of physical activity.
- If overweight, consider metformin for insulin resistance.
- Thiazolidinediones may improve secretory function of beta cells.
- Sulphonylurea treatment may deplete already low reserves of endogenous insulin and should be avoided (Maruyama).
- Unclear whether early insulin therapy contributes to the preservation of beta-cell function (Maruyama).
- Early insulin therapy associated with better glycemic control and less complications.

FOLLOW-UP

- Majority of patients become insulin dependent within 6 years of diagnosis (Fourlanos).
- Frequency of retinopathy and nephropathy in LADA similar to that in type 2 diabetes and dependent on same risk factors, particularly hyperglycemia.
- Neuropathy uncommon initially but increases with duration of disease.
- Prevalence of retinopathy, coronary heart disease (CHD), and cardiovascular mortality similar between LADA and type 2 diabetes.

EXPERT OPINION

- LADA is a form of autoimmune diabetes, genetically and immunologically like type 1 diabetes but with more gradual onset in an adult age group.
- Autoimmune system leads to pancreatic beta cell destruction much more slowly than in classic type 1 diabetes.
- LADA is adult-onset diabetes that lacks classic features of type 2 diabetes such as obesity or a good response to oral agents.
- The pitfall in missing the diagnosis of LADA is not using insulin early or intensively enough.

MANAGEMENT

REFERENCES

Appel SJ, Wadas TM, Rosenthal RS, et al. Latent autoimmune diabetes of adulthood (LADA): an often misdiagnosed type of diabetes mellitus. *J Am Acad Nurse Pract*, 2009; Vol. 21: pp. 156–9.

Comments: LADA is a common and often underrecognized form of diabetes whose clinical presentation falls somewhere between that of type 1 DM and type 2 DM. From a pathophysiological perspective, it is more closely related to type 1 DM. Often misdiagnosed and treated as type 2 DM.

Fielding AM, Brophy S, Davies H, et al. Latent autoimmune diabetes in adults: increased awareness will aid diagnosis. *Ann Clin Biochem*, 2007; Vol. 44: pp. 321–3.

Comments: High titres of serum glutamic acid decarboxylase (GAD) antibodies act as a marker for LADA. Serum C-peptide concentrations are also lower in autoimmune diabetic patients. Early insulin treatment may prevent pancreatic beta-cell failure.

Ola TO, Gigante A, Leslie RD. Latent autoimmune diabetes of adults (LADA). *Nutr Metab Cardiovasc Dis*, 2006; Vol. 16: pp. 163–7.

Comments: Associated with increased frequency of HLA DR3 (28%), DR4 (27%), and DR3/DR4 (22%).

Fourlanos S, Perry C, Stein MS, et al. A clinical screening tool identifies autoimmune diabetes in adults. *Diabetes Care*, 2006; Vol. 29: pp. 970–5.

Comments: Study aimed to develop clinical screening tool to identify adults at high risk of LADA who require islet antibody testing.

Leslie RD, Williams R, Pozzilli P. Clinical review: Type 1 diabetes and latent autoimmune diabetes in adults: one end of the rainbow. *J Clin Endocrinol Metab*, 2006; Vol. 91: pp. 1654–9.

Comments: Explores pathogenic and clinical spectrum of type 1 diabetes, including a form of adult onset autoimmune diabetes referred to as LADA.

Stenström G, Gottsäter A, Bakhtadze E, et al. Latent autoimmune diabetes in adults: definition, prevalence, beta-cell function, and treatment. *Diabetes*, 2005; Vol. 54 Suppl 2: pp. S68–72.

Comments: LADA occurs in 10% of individuals older than 35 years and in 25% below that age; proved impaired beta-cell function at diagnosis of diabetes, insulin is the treatment of choice.

Fourlanos S, Dotta F, Greenbaum CJ, et al. Latent autoimmune diabetes in adults (LADA) should be less latent. *Diabetologia*, 2005; Vol. 48: pp. 2206–12.

Comments: Majority of patients become insulin-dependent within 6 years of diagnosis.

Owen KR, Stride A, Ellard S, et al. Etiological investigation of diabetes in young adults presenting with apparent type 2 diabetes. *Diabetes Care*, 2003; Vol. 26: pp. 2088–93.

Comments: LADA subjects can be identified by presence of pancreatic ß-cell antibodies, of which most useful is GAD. Have a different disease profile from type 2 diabetes, being lean and insulin sensitive with a more rapid progression to insulin treatment.

Hosszúfalusi N, Vatay A, Rajczy K, et al. Similar genetic features and different islet cell autoantibody pattern of latent autoimmune diabetes in adults (LADA) compared with adult-onset type 1 diabetes with rapid progression. *Diabetes Care*, 2003; Vol. 26: pp. 452–7.

Comments: Compares clinical parameters, C-peptide levels, pattern of islet cell-specific autoantibodies, and prevalence of predisposing genotypes in subjects with LADA and those with adult-onset type 1 diabetes with rapid progression.

Maruyama T, Shimada A, Kanatsuka A, et al. Multicenter prevention trial of slowly progressive type 1 diabetes with small dose of insulin (the Tokyo study): preliminary report. *Ann NY Acad Sci*, 2003; Vol. 1005: pp. 362–9.

Comments: Small doses of insulin effectively prevent beta-cell failure in slowly progressive type 1 diabetes. Recommend avoiding SU treatment, instead administering insulin to NIDDM patients with high GADA titer.

Schranz DB, Bekris L, Landin-Olsson M, et al. Newly diagnosed latent autoimmune diabetes in adults (LADA) is associated with low level glutamate decarboxylase (GAD65) and IA-2 autoantibodies. Diabetes Incidence Study in Sweden (DISS). *Horm Metab Res*, 2000; Vol. 32: pp. 133–8.

Comments: Young adult new-onset LADA patients have low-level GAD65Ab and IA-2Ab. The low-level autoantibodies may signify a less aggressive beta-cell autoimmunity, possibly explaining why these patients are often classified with type 2 or non-insulin-dependent diabetes.

Isomaa B, Almgren P, Henricsson M, et al. Chronic complications in patients with slowly progressing autoimmune type 1 diabetes (LADA). *Diabetes Care,* 1999; Vol. 22: pp.1347–53.

Comments: LADA patients had lower BMI, waist-to-hip ratio, fasting C-peptide concentrations, and less hypertension than the type 2 diabetic patients. Glycemic control is a stronger risk factor for retinopathy and cardiovascular disease in LADA patients than in patients with type 2 diabetes.

Turner R, Stratton I, Horton V, et al. UKPDS 25: autoantibodies to islet-cell cytoplasm and glutamic acid decarboxylase for prediction of insulin requirement in type 2 diabetes. UK Prospective Diabetes Study Group. *Lancet,* 1997; Vol. 350: pp. 1288–93.

Comments: Among young adults with type 2 diabetes, phenotype of those with ICA or GAD antibodies was similar to that of classic juvenile-onset insulin-dependent diabetes, and either phenotype or antibodies predicted insulin requirement. In older adults, phenotype was closer to that of patients without antibodies and only the presence of antibodies predicted an increased likelihood of insulin requirement.

Zimmet PZ, Tuomi T, Mackay IR, et al. Latent autoimmune diabetes mellitus in adults (LADA): the role of antibodies to glutamic acid decarboxylase in diagnosis and prediction of insulin dependency. *Diabet Med,* 1994; Vol. 11: pp. 299–303.

Comments: One of the earliest papers describing the role that testing for GAD antibodies has on detecting LADA at earliest possible stage.

ELDERLY AND DIABETES

Ana Emiliano, MD, and Rita Rastogi Kalyani, MD, MHS

DEFINITION

- Type 2 diabetes mellitus (T2DM) in older adults is a major public health problem.
- Normal aging is associated with impaired insulin sensitivity (Roder; Defronzo; Elahi) possibly due to a lower density of the glucose carrier GLUT4 in the muscle, which could contribute to insulin resistance (Houmard).
- Biological changes associated with aging may also contribute to impaired insulin sensitivity; changes include increased abdominal fat mass, decreased physical activity, mitochondrial dysfunction, hormonal changes, increased oxidative stress, and inflammation (Goulet).
- Presence of comorbidities, cognitive dysfunction, and functional disabilities affects the management of diabetes, especially in the elderly.

EPIDEMIOLOGY

- One third of adults ≥65 years has diabetes (Cowie), almost half undiagnosed. Prevalence may be even higher in nursing home residents.
- An additional 40% of elderly individuals have prediabetes (Cowie).
- T2DM prevalence in the elderly is expected to increase as individuals live longer and also due to the increasing obesity prevalence.
- Morbidity and mortality associated with diabetes complications are higher in elderly individuals (Bethel).
- Elderly-onset diabetes may be associated with a lower burden of complications such as retinopathy compared to diabetes onset in middle age (Selvin).

MANAGEMENT

- Hypoglycemia in the elderly is associated with an increased risk for cardiovascular events and is also linked to an increased dementia risk (Whitmer).
- Depression and dementia are more common in older adults with diabetes and are associated with difficulties with self-management, leading to poor glycemic control.
- Decreased muscle strength, lower muscle quality, and accelerated loss of muscle mass, especially in the lower extremities, have all been documented in older persons with diabetes (Park).
- Older adults with diabetes are 2–3 times more likely to have functional disabilities, including difficulties walking a quarter mile, lifting heavy objects, doing house work, or participating in leisure activities, compared to their counterparts (Kalyani).

DIAGNOSIS

- Though some authors have suggested that diagnostic criteria for diabetes be modified in the elderly to account for the increase in glucose intolerance associated with aging, current guidelines include same criteria as used in younger individuals (see Diagnosis and Classification of Diabetes, p. 5)

SIGNS AND SYMPTOMS

- Uncontrolled hyperglycemia in elderly individuals can manifest with polyuria, polydipsia, weight loss, and blurry vision similar to younger individuals. Symptoms, however, are not always present, increasing the risk of severe hyperglycemia.
- Hyperglycemia may more easily precipitate dehydration in the elderly, to the point of severe hyperglycemia.
- Visual decline, including blindness secondary to longstanding retinopathy, can occur and impair physical function.
- Microalbuminuria conversion to overt chronic kidney disease may occur more often in older adults with diabetes.
- Foot problems are more common due to longstanding vascular and neurologic disease. Diabetic neuropathy prevalence in the elderly as high as 40% (Young). Elderly patients with diabetes are frequently unable to inspect their own feet because of physical and cognitive disabilities increasing risk for development of foot problems.
- Falls are more common in elderly patients with diabetes due to peripheral and autonomic neuropathy, hypoglycemia, functional disabilities, impaired vision, and polypharmacy.
- Elderly women with diabetes experience urinary incontinence more frequently than women without diabetes (Jackson).

CLINICAL TREATMENT

Lifestyle Interventions

- Weight loss recommended for older adults who are overweight or obese. Debilitated nursing home residents may not be good candidates for weight loss (Wedick).
- In general, exercise beneficial even later in life as tolerated, to prevent progression to diabetes and improve survival (Mozaffarian).
- Consumption of lower glycemic index foods may be recommended (Mozaffarian).
- Smoking cessation.

Pharmacological Treatment

- Metformin may be preferred for overweight, elderly patients if no other contraindications (e.g., creatinine clearance <60 ml/min, serum creatinine >1.5 mg/dl, or congestive heart failure).

- Sulfonylureas are more likely to cause hypoglycemia in the elderly than in younger individuals. Glipizide and glimepiride are preferred over glyburide or chlorpropamide given their lower likelihood of causing hypoglycemia.
- Thiazolidinediones can be used but absolutely contraindicated in elderly patients with class III or IV heart failure.
- Alpha-glucosidase inhibitors (acarbose and miglitol) are probably safe in older adults, in spite of the limited experience.
- Dipeptidyl peptidase IV (DPP-IV) inhibitors may be attractive agents in more debilitated individuals because they are weight-neutral. Limited experience in the elderly.
- GLP-1 based therapies have the limitation of being injectable and may not be preferred in elderly patients with functional disabilities. Not a good option for frail, underweight individuals as it causes weight loss.
- The amylin analogue pramlintide may not be a good option in the elderly due to the considerable risk of hypoglycemia and the multiple daily injections required.
- Most patients with T2DM eventually require insulin. Before instituting insulin, visual acuity, manual dexterity, cognitive function, caregiver status should be evaluated.
- Long-acting, once-daily insulin regimens may be the easier and safest choice in capable individuals.

Goals of Treatment

- Healthy older adults with T2DM and a life expectancy of >5 years should have goal A1c <7% (ADA guidelines).
- Elderly individuals with multiple comorbidities, functional disabilities and/or limited expected life expectancy may benefit from less stringent A1c goals (i.e., <8%), although more rigorous studies are needed (Brown).
- Patients need to be routinely evaluated for their ability to recognize and treat hypoglycemia, which could be potentially dangerous and may limit benefits of intensive glycemic control.
- Hypoglycemia is a serious complication of diabetes treatment, especially in the elderly, and should be minimized.
- Hypoglycemia risk associated with renal impairment, coadministration of insulin sensitizers or insulin, exercise, skipped meals, caloric restriction, recent hospitalization, polypharmacy, therapy with salicylates, sulfonamides, fibric acid derivatives, and warfarin (Neumiller).

Follow-up

- Changes in hepatic and renal function in elderly patients should always be considered and medications adjusted accordingly.
- The insulin requirement of elderly patients approaching end-stage renal disease often declines due to impaired renal function and delayed renal metabolism of insulin; hypoglycemia may ensue, and insulin doses should be adjusted accordingly.
- Changes in functional status may also affect goals of treatment.

Expert Opinion

- Older adults are more likely to have abnormal glucose status, likely due to biological changes associated with aging that result in impaired insulin sensitivity.
- Less stringent hemoglobin A1c targets may be more appropriate for debilitated individuals with multiple comorbidities and limited life expectancy.
- Clinical treatment should to be tailored for the individual needs of the patient.

MANAGEMENT

REFERENCES

Kalyani RR, Saudek CD, Brancati FL, et al. Association of diabetes, comorbidities, and A1c with functional disability in older adults: results from the National Health and Nutrition Examination Survey (NHANES), 1999–2006. *Diabetes Care*, 2010; Vol. 33: pp. 1055–60.

Comments: Diabetes was associated with 2–3 times increased odds of disability across many different functional groups (p < 0.05).

American Diabetes Association. Standards of medical care in diabetes—2011. *Diabetes Care*, 2011; Vol. 34 Suppl 1: pp. S11–61.

Comments: Consensus guidelines on the management of diabetes by the American Diabetes Association.

Goulet ED, Hassaine A, Dionne IJ, et al. Frailty in the elderly is associated with insulin resistance of glucose metabolism in the postabsorptive state only in the presence of increased abdominal fat. *Exp Gerontol*, 2009; Vol. 44: pp. 740–4.

Comments: This study found that age, abdominal fat mass, and muscle mass index were significantly correlated with insulin sensitivity.

Cowie CC, Rust KF, Ford ES, et al. Full accounting of diabetes and pre-diabetes in the U.S. population in 1988–1994 and 2005–2006. *Diabetes Care*, 2009; Vol. 32: pp. 287–94.

Comments: This national representative study found that one-third of the elderly population had diabetes and three-quarters had diabetes or prediabetes.

Whitmer RA, Karter AJ, Yaffe K, et al. Hypoglycemic episodes and risk of dementia in older patients with type 2 diabetes mellitus. *JAMA*, 2009; Vol. 301: pp. 1565–72.

Comments: This study examined dementia risk in relation to the frequency of severe hypoglycemic episodes, defined as episodes that required a hospital visit/admission. Patients with a single episode had a hazard ratio for dementia of 1.26 (CI 1.10–1.49).

Mozaffarian D, Kamineni A, Carnethon M, et al. Lifestyle risk factors and new-onset diabetes mellitus in older adults: the cardiovascular health study. *Arch Intern Med*, 2009; Vol. 169: pp. 798–807.

Comments: Prospective study examining the incidence of diabetes among 4883 elderly men and women during a 10-year period. A low-risk lifestyle was associated with a significantly reduced incidence of new-onset diabetes.

Neumiller JJ, Setter SM. Pharmacologic management of the older patient with type 2 diabetes mellitus. *Am J Geriatr Pharmacother*, 2009; Vol. 7: pp. 324–42.

Comments: Comprehensive review of the use of pharmacologic agents to treat older adults with T2DM, with an emphasis on prevention of hypoglycemia and drug interactions.

Bethel MA, Sloan FA, Belsky D, et al. Longitudinal incidence and prevalence of adverse outcomes of diabetes mellitus in elderly patients. *Arch Intern Med*, 2007; Vol. 167: pp. 921–7.

Comments: Longitudinal analysis examining mortality and morbidity rates in 33,772 elderly patients newly diagnosed with diabetes compared to 25,563 elderly controls, followed from 1991–2004. The group with diabetes had an excess mortality of 9.2%.

Park SW, Goodpaster BH, Strotmeyer ES, et al. Accelerated loss of skeletal muscle strength in older adults with type 2 diabetes: the health, aging, and body composition study. *Diabetes Care*, 2007; Vol. 30: pp. 1507–12.

Comments: This study found that patients with T2DM had a 13.5% loss in knee extensor strength compared to a 9% loss in individuals without diabetes (p = 0.001). In addition, patients with type 2 diabetes also lost greater amounts of lean leg mass (p < 0.05).

Selvin E, Coresh J, Brancati FL. The burden and treatment of diabetes in elderly individuals in the US. *Diabetes Care*, 2006; Vol. 29: pp. 2415–9.

Comments: Elderly patients with middle age onset diabetes had a much greater burden of microvascular disease compared to elderly onset diabetes.

Jackson SL, Scholes D, Boyko EJ, et al. Urinary incontinence and diabetes in postmenopausal women. *Diabetes Care*, 2005; Vol. 28: pp. 1730–8.

Comments: In this study, women with diabetes reported more severe urinary incontinence, which correlated significantly with diabetes duration, peripheral neuropathy, and retinopathy.

Brown AF, Mangione CM, Saliba D, et al. Guidelines for improving the care of the older person with diabetes mellitus. *J Am Geriatr Soc*, 2003; Vol. 51: pp. S265–80.

Comments: Review article containing evidence-based recommendations to guide clinicians caring for elderly person with diabetes.

Wedick NM, Barrett-Connor E, Knoke JD, et al. The relationship between weight loss and all-cause mortality in older men and women with and without diabetes mellitus: the Rancho Bernardo study. *J Am Geriatr Soc*, 2002; Vol. 50: pp. 1810–5.

Comments: 1801 elderly men and women, with and without diabetes, were followed for 12 years. Weight loss of 10 pounds was associated with an increased hazard ratio for all-cause mortality in nondiabetic men (HR = 1.38; 95% CI 1.06–1.80) and women (HR = 1.76; 95% CI 1.33–2.34) and diabetic men (HR = 3.66; 95% CI 2.15–6.24) and women (HR = 1.65; 95% CI 0.70–3.87) after adjusting for age, smoking, and sedentary life style.

Elahi D, Muller DC, et al. Glucose tolerance, glucose utilization and insulin secretion in aging. *Novartis Found Symp*, 2002; Vol. 242: pp. 222–42, discussion 242-6.

Comments: Review article exploring basic, epidemiological, and clinical data on the development of glucose intolerance and insulin resistance with aging.

Roder ME, Schwartz RS, Prigeon RL, et al. Reduced pancreatic B cell compensation to the insulin resistance of aging: impact on proinsulin and insulin levels. *J Clin Endocrinol Metab*, 2000; Vol. 85: pp. 2275–80.

Comments: In this study, 26 older subjects (mean age 67 years) and 22 younger subjects (mean age 22 years) had their insulin sensitivity and beta-cell function assessed. The older subjects had a 50% reduction in insulin sensitivity and beta-cell function.

Houmard JA, Weidner MD, Dolan PL, et al. Skeletal muscle GLUT4 protein concentration and aging in humans. *Diabetes*, 1995; Vol. 44: pp. 555–60.

Comments: In this study, GLUT4 protein levels were lower in older individuals, irrespective of sex (men r = −0.28, women r = −0.51). GLUT4 levels were positively correlated with insulin sensitivity (r = 0.42).

Young MJ, Boulton AJ, MacLeod AF, et al. A multicentre study of the prevalence of diabetic peripheral neuropathy in the United Kingdom hospital clinic population. *Diabetologia*, 1993; Vol. 36: pp. 150–4.

Comments: A cross-sectional study of 6487 individuals with diabetes in 118 centers in the UK, ages ranging from 18–90 years. The prevalence of peripheral neuropathy in T2DM increased significantly with age, going from 5% in the 20–29 age group to 44.2% in the 70–79 age group.

DeFronzo RA. Glucose intolerance and aging. *Diabetes Care*, 1982; Vol. 4: pp. 493–501.

Comments: This article reviews the factors involved in the progressive decline of glucose tolerance seen with aging, primarily related to the intrinsic development of tissue unresponsiveness to insulin.

MANAGEMENT

STEROID-INDUCED DIABETES

Rachel Derr, MD, PhD

Definition

- Glucocorticoids (GC) such as prednisone, dexamethasone, and cortisone, are potent antiinflammatory and immunosuppressive agents, thus effective for treating a wide spectrum of diseases.
- Hyperglycemia, primarily resulting from impaired glucose transport into muscles, is a common adverse effect (Pagano).

- GC-induced hyperglycemia: diabetes-range hyperglycemia in subjects who have normal glucose tolerance when not taking GC.

EPIDEMIOLOGY

- Glucocorticoids are prescribed for roughly 10% of the inpatients at tertiary care hospitals and 3% of the outpatient population >60 years old (Donihi; Choi).
- Prevalence of glucocorticoid-induced hyperglycemia is approximately 54%–64% among inpatients at tertiary-care hospitals without a history of diabetes treated with high-dose glucocorticoids (at least 40 mg of prednisone per day for at least 2 days) (Donihi).
- Five-fold increased risk of hyperglycemia in critically ill patients in ICUs when glucocorticoids are used.
- Risk of requiring a new diabetes medication was increased 2-fold among outpatients and 4-fold among inpatients with COPD when glucocorticoids were prescribed compared to when they were not (Gurwitz; Niewoehner).
- Glucocorticoid dose is positively associated with degree of hyperglycemia and need for glucose-lowering medications (Gurwitz).

DIAGNOSIS

- No formal criteria for diagnosing steroid-induced diabetes, but it may be considered diabetes recognized for the first time in the setting of glucocorticoid (GC) use.
- Diagnostic criteria for diabetes are unchanged.
- Hyperglycemia in preexisting diabetes is usually severely worsened by GC use in any form.

SIGNS AND SYMPTOMS

- Expected signs and symptoms of hyperglycemia: worsening of polyuria, polydipsia, polyphagia, fatigue.
- Infections may be more prevalent due to combination of hyperglycemia and immunosuppression.
- Other signs and symptoms may be related to chronic exogenous steroid exposure such as buffalo hump, thin skin, easy bruisability, proximal muscle weakness, or edema.

CLINICAL TREATMENT

Possible Benefits of Treatment

- For hospitalized patients, improve hyperglycemia-related symptoms and decrease hospital length of stay.
- Reduce infections: Rates of neutropenic infections during bone marrow transplant were higher in patients with higher mean glucose during the preneutropenic period, especially in the subset who received GC while neutropenic (Derr).
- Some evidence suggests improved mortality in cancer patients: In glioblastoma multiforme patients (many receiving GC to reduce brain edema), mortality was 57% higher in patients with the highest quartile of mean glucose compared to the lowest (Derr).

Management Strategies

- If GC-induced hyperglycemia is mild, metformin and thiazolidinediones may be effective by reducing insulin resistance.
- For moderate or severe hyperglycemia and in the hospital setting, insulin is preferred because it acts immediately, allows for more flexible dosing, and is more effective.
- Some experts recommend prescribing higher ratio of nutritional insulin to basal insulin since hyperglycemia due to GC is worse postprandially (Clement).

FOLLOW-UP

- Insulin requirements will change dramatically as GC doses are adjusted, or as effects wear off following injection. Close follow-up is required.
- Anticipate the need for lower insulin doses when GC doses are weaned to avoid hypoglycemia.
- When GC doses are discontinued, glucose-lowering medications are usually no longer needed in patients with baseline normal glucose tolerance.
- Symptoms of hypoglycemia that persist after discontinuation of glucose-lowering medications should prompt evaluation for secondary adrenal insufficiency (AI). To prevent secondary AI, GC weaning should be gradual.
- Little data on risk of progression to overt diabetes among patients with previous history of GC-induced diabetes; presumably it is a risk factor for later diabetes.

EXPERT OPINION

- The effect of glucocorticoids (GC), particularly at high doses, on glucose tolerance can be dramatic and may cause symptoms or even hyperosmolar nonketotic states, as well as negatively impact outcomes in hospitalized patients.
- Warn people with diabetes who are about to receive GC (orally or by joint injection, for example) of the anticipated hyperglycemic effect.
- For inpatients on GC, monitor glucose at least daily; for outpatients with diabetes, increase monitoring while on GC.
- Symptoms of hypoglycemia that persist after discontinuation of glucose-lowering medications should prompt evaluation for secondary adrenal insufficiency (AI). To prevent secondary AI, GC weaning should be gradual.

REFERENCES

Derr RL, Ye X, Islas MU, et al. Association between hyperglycemia and survival in patients with newly diagnosed glioblastoma. *J Clin Oncol*, 2009; Vol. 27: pp. 1082–6.

   Comments: In patients with newly diagnosed glioblastoma, hyperglycemia was associated with shorter survival, after controlling for glucocorticoid dose and other confounders.

Derr RL, Hsiao VC, Saudek CD. Antecedent hyperglycemia is associated with an increased risk of neutropenic infections during bone marrow transplantation. *Diabetes Care*, 2008; Vol. 31: pp. 1972–7.

   Comments: In a bone marrow transplant population highly susceptible to infection, mean antecedent glycemia was associated with later infection risk, particularly in patients who received glucocorticoids while neutropenic.

Donihi AC, Raval D, Saul M, et al. Prevalence and predictors of corticosteroid-related hyperglycemia in hospitalized patients. *Endocr Pract*, 2006; Vol. 12: pp. 358–62.

   Comments: Using a pharmacy database at a tertiary academic hospital, evaluates prevalence of and risk factors for hyperglycemia in patients receiving high-dose glucocorticoids.

Choi HK, Seeger JD. Glucocorticoid use and serum lipid levels in US adults: the Third National Health and Nutrition Examination Survey. *Arthritis Rheum*, 2005; Vol. 53: pp. 528–35.

   Comments: Reports prevalence of glucocorticoid use in The Third National Health and Nutrition Examination Survey (1988–1994), determined from household interview regarding prescription medication use.

Clement S, Braithwaite SS, Magee MF, et al. Management of diabetes and hyperglycemia in hospitals. *Diabetes Care*, 2004; Vol. 27: pp. 553–91.

   Comments: Reviews and evaluates the evidence relating to the management of hyperglycemia in hospitals, including management in special circumstances such as glucocorticoid use.

MANAGEMENT

Niewoehner DE, Erbland ML, Deupree RH, et al. Effect of systemic glucocorticoids on exacerbations of chronic obstructive pulmonary disease. Department of Veterans Affairs Cooperative Study Group. *NEJM*, 1999; Vol. 340: pp. 1941–7.

Comments: Randomized controlled trial (RCT) that found that systemic glucocorticoids moderately improve outcomes in COPD, but hyperglycemia warranting treatment is the most frequent complication.

Gurwitz JH, Bohn RL, Glynn RJ, et al. Glucocorticoids and the risk for initiation of hypoglycemic therapy. *Arch Intern Med*, 1994; Vol. 154: pp. 97–101.

Comments: Using a Medicaid database, quantifies the risk of developing hyperglycemia requiring hypoglycemic therapy after oral glucocorticoid use.

Pagano G, Cavallo-Perin P, Cassader M, et al. An in vivo and in vitro study of the mechanism of prednisone-induced insulin resistance in healthy subjects. *J Clin Invest*, 1983; Vol. 72: pp. 1814–20.

Comments: Landmark basic science study, which found that prednisone induces insulin resistance due to depressed peripheral glucose utilization from impaired glucose transport.

Type 1 Diabetes

TYPE 1 DIABETES: RISK FACTORS

Gregory O. Clark, MD

DEFINITION

- Type 1 diabetes (T1DM) develops due to an environmental trigger in persons who are genetically susceptible.
- Genetic risk factors (see below) that determine susceptibility reflect genetic associations with disease.
- Environmental risk factors associated with susceptibility to T1DM are identified through epidemiologic study.

EPIDEMIOLOGY

- T1DM incidence is increasing 3%–4% per year worldwide, suggesting an environmental influence on disease (DIAMOND Project).
- Incidence is increasing fastest in children under 5 years old, with new cases expected to double between 2005–2020 (Patterson).
- Peak age of onset is around puberty, 10–14 years old.
- 50% of incident cases are in adults.
- Worldwide incidence of T1DM differs by >100 fold, highest in Finland and Sardinia (Italy) and lowest in China and Venezuela (Borchers).
- Generally, rates are highest in European Caucasian populations (>20 cases/year/100,000), especially in Northern Europeans and their descendants in North America, Australia, and New Zealand. Kuwait also has high rates of T1DM.
- T1DM incidence is low in Asia (<1 case/year/100,000 individuals).
- See Epidemiology of Type 1 Diabetes (p. 7).

DIAGNOSIS

- Assessment of T1DM risk via genetic testing or environmental factors is not used clinically at this time, since there are no known preventions.
- For research purposes high-risk individuals (1st-degree relatives), may be risk stratified according to genotype and presence of circulating autoantibodies (islet cell cytoplasmic autoantibodies [ICA], insulin autoantibodies, glutamic acid decarboxylase [GAD65] autoantibodies, and insulinoma-associated-2 [IA-2] autoantibodies). These antibodies are markers for early stage autoimmunity. The goal of the research is to better predict and prevent complete autoimmune destruction of beta-cell mass.
- Risk of disease development if a first-degree relative has T1DM is 5%.
- Concordance rates in identical twins is 40%–60%, suggesting that genetic risk is modulated significantly by other, presumably environmental, factors.

CLINICAL TREATMENT

Genetic Risk Factors

- There is, of course, no treatment for genetic risk factors.
- Genes for the human leukocyte antigens (HLAs) class II, which are involved in immune regulation, confer the strongest association with T1DM.

MANAGEMENT

- Specific HLA-DR and HLA-DQ haplotypes provide both susceptibility toward, and protection from, the disease.
- HLA DR3/DR4 heterozygosity confers susceptibility to T1DM, but is present in up to 2% of newborns and 30% of children who develop T1DM. Absolute risk of T1DM with this genotype is 1 in 20 (Eisenbarth).
- Other genes (non-HLA) associated with T1DM: CTLA4 (cytotoxic T-lymphocyte-associated protein 4), IFIH1 (interferon induced with helicase C domain 1), ITPR3 (inositol 1,4,5-triphosphate receptor 3), IL-2 receptor, PTPN22 (protein tyrosine phosphatase, nonreceptor type 22).
- More than 40 genetic loci have been associated with the development of T1DM (Barrett).

Environmental Risk Factors Implicated

- No environmental factors have been unequivocally linked to T1DM. Evidence for the following varies.
- Viruses (Enteroviruses, Coxsackie, Congenital rubella) may trigger the autoimmune process due to molecular mimicry (viral proteins similar to beta-cell proteins).
- The "hygiene hypothesis" suggests that a lack of childhood infections might contribute to increasing incidence of autoimmunity and allergy.
- Early infant diet: early exposure to cow's milk may lead to immune response to bovine insulin (human insulin is similar and a known important autoantigen in T1DM), gluten or other cereal-derived proteins.
- Toxins: nitrosamines.
- Geography: increasing incidence with distance from equator.
- Vitamin D deficiency: this may relate to higher incidence in more northern latitudes where there is less UV exposure.
- Obesity/weight gain: this may initiate the process due to beta-cell apoptosis exposing beta-cell antigens or accelerate the process via increased beta-cell demand due to insulin resistance, known as the "accelerator hypothesis" (Wilkin).
- High socioeconomic status.

Expert Opinion

- It is difficult to distinguish between genetic and environmental risk factors. On the island of Sardinia, for example, residents share similar genetic profile and environmental exposure but not all develop T1DM. Migrant studies help to distinguish risk factors and suggest both genetics and environment are important to the geo-epidemiology of T1DM.
- Neonatal diabetes: must assess for mutation of Kir6.2 (sulfonylurea receptor) as this accounts for half of neonatal diabetes and can be treated with high-dose oral sulfonylurea alone.

References

Borchers AT, Uibo R, Gershwin ME. The geoepidemiology of type 1 diabetes. *Autoimmun Rev*, 2010; Vol. 9: pp. A355–65.
  Comments: Detailed review of evidence related to both genetic and environmental risks of T1DM and how they interplay.

Patterson CC, Dahlquist GG, Gyürüs E, et al. Incidence trends for childhood type 1 diabetes in Europe during 1989–2003 and predicted new cases 2005–20: a multicentre prospective registration study. *Lancet*, 2009; Vol. 373: pp. 2027–33.
  Comments: Alarming results indicating a rapid increase in the incidence of T1DM in young children.

Barrett JC, Clayton DG, Concannon P, et al. Genome-wide association study and meta-analysis find that over 40 loci affect risk of type 1 diabetes. *Nat Genet,* 2009; Vol. 41: pp. 703–7.

Comments: Landmark study of genes associated with T1DM.

Eisenbarth GS. Update in type 1 diabetes. *J Clin Endocrinol Metab,* 2007; Vol. 92: pp. 2403–7.

Comments: Concise overview of the genetics of T1DM and emerging science and technology that might improve outcomes.

DIAMOND Project Group. Incidence and trends of childhood type 1 diabetes worldwide: 1990–1999. *Diabet Med,* 2006; Vol. 23: pp. 857–66.

Comments: Demonstrates worldwide increases in the incidence of T1DM.

Wilkin TJ. The accelerator hypothesis: weight gain as the missing link between Type I and Type II diabetes. *Diabetologia,* 2001; Vol. 44: pp. 914–22.

Comments: Implicates weight gain and obesity in the increasing incidence of T1DM.

TYPE 1 DIABETES: INSULIN TREATMENT

Gregory O. Clark, MD

MANAGEMENT

DEFINITION
- Type 1 diabetes mellitus (T1DM) is an autoimmune disease.
- Destruction of insulin-producing beta cells renders patients insulin deficient.
- Exogenous insulin must be used to treat T1DM (DeWitt).

EPIDEMIOLOGY
- Refer to Epidemiology of Type 1 Diabetes, p. 7.

DIAGNOSIS
- Criteria for diabetes do not change depending on the classification of the diabetes.
- Presence of circulating autoantibodies characterize T1DM: islet cell cytoplasmic autoantibodies (ICA), insulin autoantibodies, glutamic acid decarboxylase (GAD65) autoantibodies, and insulinoma-associated-2 (IA-2) autoantibodies (see Insulin Antibodies, p. 585).
- Ketoacidosis indicates insulin deficiency and usually signifies T1DM but can also occur in T2DM (Umpierrez).
- Adults with new onset T1DM (i.e., LADA) may present without ketoacidosis owing to a slower autoimmune process and can be misdiagnosed as T2DM.

SIGNS AND SYMPTOMS
- Signs of uncontrolled hyperglycemia are the same regardless of type of diabetes: polyuria, polydipsia, polyphagia, weight loss, blurred vision.
- Children with new-onset T1DM often present with diabetic ketoacidosis and require inpatient hospitalization.
- Sometimes, especially with adult-onset T1DM, hyperglycemia will be mild enough as to be asymptomatic.
- Other autoimmune conditions may be present (e.g., hypothyroidism).

CLINICAL TREATMENT
Initiating Insulin Therapy in T1DM
- Insulin therapy is indicated for everyone with diagnosed T1DM.
- Even in people whose glucose levels are near-normal ("honeymoon" or LADA), if T1DM is diagnosed (usually by positive antibodies), the current evidence recommends

starting insulin immediately, both anticipating diminished beta-cell function and to preserve some function.

- Given the anticipated lability of T1DM, generally start both long-acting and short-/fast-acting insulin.
- A clinical decision should be made as to which exact regimen to follow, and how intensive insulin treatment.
- Total daily dose (TDD) of insulin in units = weight (kg) × 0.5 (for obese patients, TDD = weight [kg] × 0.7). This is only an estimation of TDD, the dose should be further adjusted in 10%–20% increments based on individual response.
- Rapid-acting insulin can be delivered continuously via insulin pump for basal component (Walsh), without the need for long-acting insulin.

Intensive Insulin Therapy

- Preferred therapy as per results of the DCCT to reduce complications (DCCT Research Group).
- Requires 4+ shots per day.
- Carbohydrate counting allows a flexible lifestyle with regard to timing and size of meals; meals can even be skipped, although not recommended.
- Insulin dose is flexible, encouraging the patient to learn to safely adjust insulin doses.
- Frequent testing of blood glucose guides therapy (Hirsch; Bode): test at least before meals (goal: blood glucose 70–120 mg/dl), occasionally also 2 hours after meals (goal: blood glucose 140–180 mg/dl), at bedtime (goal: blood glucose 100–140 mg/dl), with symptoms of hyperglycemia or hypoglycemia and occasionally overnight.
- Prefer insulin analogs to reduce hypoglycemia and more closely mimic normal physiology (Hirsch).
- Prefer ~50% of TDD as basal insulin and ~50% as bolus insulin.
- Long-acting analogs provide constant, "basal" insulin activity—theoretically no peak in activity. Activity lasts up to 24 hours, although some people do better with split-dose long-acting insulin.
- Rapid-acting analogs are absorbed into systemic circulation faster than regular insulin. Activity peaks after 1–2 hours and dissipates at 3–5 hours.

Conventional Insulin Regimen

- Used when patients lack the resources or motivation to adhere to intensive therapy.
- Requires 2 or 3 shots per day.
- Insulin dose is fixed.
- Diet and exercise must be adjusted to compensate for fixed insulin dose.
- NPH insulin has a broad peak in activity at 4–10 hours. Activity can last 10–16 hours and is variable.
- Regular insulin peaks after 2–4 hours. Activity dissipates at 5–8 hours.
- Risk of hypoglycemia increased compared to intensive insulin therapy, especially when NPH insulin is peaking.
- AM insulin dose: 2/3 as NPH, 1/3 as regular. NPH and regular insulin can be mixed in the same syringe, or use premixed 70/30 insulin. Breakfast and lunch portions should be matched to this insulin dose. Hyperglycemia at lunch should lead to a smaller lunch. Delayed lunch often causes hypoglycemia.
- PM insulin dose: 2/3 as NPH, 1/3 as regular or use premixed 70/30 insulin. Dinner and bedtime snack portions should match this insulin dose. Early morning hypoglycemia

may result from NPH peak. Move NPH dose to before bed (3 injections/day) to reduce overnight hypoglycemia.

Basal Insulin (Long-Acting)

- Suppresses hepatic glucose and ketone production and lipolysis between meals.
- Goal to keep glucose constant in the absence of meals, exercise, or bolus insulin.
- Adjust to target fasting blood glucose 70–120 mg/dl.
- Glargine (Lantus): given once daily, usually at bedtime, cannot be mixed in the same syringe as other insulin (pH incompatibility).
- Detemir (Levemir): often given twice daily, cannot be mixed in syringe with other insulin.
- NPH insulin: given twice daily for T1DM as described previously.

Bolus Insulin (Short- or Rapid-Acting)

- Bolus dose is chosen based on nutritional and correctional component.
- Nutritional component covers meal to be consumed (i.e., insulin-to-carbohydrate ratio). A useful way to calculate I:C ratio is I:C = 500/TDD. Example: if TDD = 50 units, then use a unit of insulin for every 10 grams (500/50 = 10) of carbohydrate.
- Correctional component corrects hyperglycemia. Useful calculation is correctional factor (CF) = 1800/TDD. Example: if TDD = 30 units, then use a unit to reduce blood glucose by 60 mg/dl (1800/30 = 60) to target blood glucose (usually 120 mg/dl). Some use 1500 to calculate CF.
- Use fast-acting insulins—lispro, aspart, glulisine—equivalently.
- Regular insulin can also be used but requires administration at least 30 minutes prior to meal.

Follow-Up

- Continued communication and intensive adjustment of insulin doses in the weeks following insulin initiation is important.
- Check A1c at each visit.
- Most insulin dose adjustments should be in 10%–20% increments depending on the degree of glucose abnormality.

Expert Opinion

- Avoid insulin stacking: refers to administering additional insulin when postprandial glucose is increased and before preceding premeal insulin has acted, leading to hypoglycemia.
- Avoid hypoglycemia from exercise: patients often eat and take insulin before exercise thinking it will prevent hypoglycemia (*not true*). Exercise increases insulin sensitivity, so to prevent low blood glucose, exercise before meals and eat more or take less insulin than usual (up to 50%) depending on intensity and duration of exercise.
- Minimize lifestyle variability to minimize blood glucose variance: T1DM is characterized by high glucose variance. Encourage patients to keep meals and insulin doses small and regular to minimize glucose variability.
- Maintain realistic expectations: even the most well-controlled patients with T1DM can spend hours per day with glucoses >200 mg/dl. The goal of therapy is to maximize time spent with normoglycemia.
- Daily burden of disease management is high; consider psychological and social aspects in management plan.
- Patients often benefit from seeing healthcare providers every 3 months, adjusted according to status of the patient, including visits to educators, nutritionists, and physicians.

MANAGEMENT

REFERENCES

Hirsch IB, Bode BW, Childs BP, et al. Self-Monitoring of Blood Glucose (SMBG) in insulin-and non-insulin-using adults with diabetes: consensus recommendations for improving SMBG accuracy, utilization, and research. *Diabetes Technol Ther,* 2008; Vol. 10: pp. 419–39.

    Comments: Details the rationale for frequent self-monitoring of blood glucose to help guide therapy.

Hirsch IB. Insulin analogues. *NEJM,* 2005; Vol. 352: pp. 174–83.

    Comments: A nice review of the utility of the newer insulin analogs compared to the older, less expensive forms of insulin.

DeWitt DE, Hirsch IB. Outpatient insulin therapy in type 1 and type 2 diabetes mellitus: scientific review. *JAMA,* 2003; Vol. 289: pp. 2254–64.

    Comments: The most detailed review of scientific literature related to the use of insulin in the management of both type 1 and type 2 diabetes.

Walsh, J., Roberts, R. *Pumping Insulin: Everything You Need for Success with an Insulin Pump,* 3rd edition. San Diego: Torrey Pines Press; 2000.

    Comments: A thorough guide for both patient and physician that covers all aspects of insulin pump therapy.

Umpierrez GE, Casals MM, Gebhart SP, et al. Diabetic ketoacidosis in obese African Americans. *Diabetes,* 1995; Vol. 44: pp. 790–5.

    Comments: A characterization of 35 African Americans with type 2 diabetes admitted to Grady Memorial Hospital with ketoacidosis.

DCCT Research Group. The effect of intensive treatment of diabetes on the development and progression of long-term complications in insulin-dependent diabetes mellitus. The Diabetes Control and Complications Trial Research Group. *NEJM,* 1993; Vol. 329: pp. 977–86.

    Comments: Landmark trial showing that intensive insulin therapy, compared to conventional insulin therapy, can be used to reduce HbA1c and prevent and slow the progression of diabetes microvascular complications.

INSULIN PUMP MANAGEMENT

Christopher D. Saudek, MD

DEFINITION

- Insulin pumps (technically called continuous subcutaneous insulin infusion, CSII) deliver insulin at programmed rates, from a pump worn externally through a small catheter tip inserted into the skin. Most current brands worn on a belt, with a catheter and insertion site that is changed about every 3 days; one brand is worn directly on the skin and discarded after 3 days.
- May be linked to a glucose monitor, displaying real-time blood glucose results, but insulin delivery is *not* driven by the blood glucose result; fully closed loop delivery system does not currently exist. Insulin delivery rates and amounts are determined by the patient.
- CSII is an option for treating type 1 diabetes or unstable, insulin-requiring type 2 diabetes.
- Only use rapid-acting (e.g., aspart, lispro, or glulisine) or regular insulin.

EPIDEMIOLOGY

- Available since the 1980s, over 400,000 insulin pumps sold per year.
- Use varies widely from country to country: in the US, up to 20% of people with type 1 diabetes use a pump; in many other countries less than 1% do.
- Reports are inconsistent about whether CSII improves glycemic control, although severe hypoglycemia seems to be less frequent (Pickup).

- Incidence of ketoacidosis more common with CSII because if delivery stops, insulin delivery also immediately stops (Hanas).
- CSII is not necessarily reimbursed by Medicare in the US for people with type 2 diabetes. Medicare requires that a C-peptide assay show lack of endogenous insulin production.

CLINICAL TREATMENT

Initiation of Insulin Pump

- Patient selection is essential: best success if patient understands their diabetes well, self-monitors blood glucose multiple times daily, counts carbohydrates, is uncontrolled or subject to severe hypoglycemia on multiple dose insulin regimens, has a variable and demanding lifestyle, is comfortable with technology, and wants to use the pump.
- Prior to choosing pump therapy, a diabetes educator should review carbohydrate counting, and demonstrate pump use to potential patient.
- Insulin delivery is divided into basal rates and bolus doses. Calculate starting doses based on previous total daily insulin requirements.
- Basal rate, programmed to deliver a sequence of preprogrammed hourly rates, which repeat every 24 hours, should deliver about half the total daily dose. Example: If total daily dose (TDD) was 48 units/day, basal rate will deliver about 24 U/day, or 1.0 U/hour; bolus doses will deliver about 24 U/day total. Be conservative: start with total basal rate about 80% of patient's dose of long-acting insulin.
- Generally 2–4 different basal rates are optimal. Example: Rate 1 starting at midnight; Rate 2 increased about 30%–50% at dawn hours; Rate 3 during the day; and Rate 4 may or may not be different in the evenings.
- Bolus doses are chosen and delivered shortly before a meal is ingested, and sometimes to correct high glucose between meals.
- Typical bolus doses are (1) "nutritional" plus (2) "correctional." Nutritional is based on carbohydrate content of the meal to be ingested (example: 1 unit insulin per 15 grams carbohydrate). Correctional dose designed to bring glucose back to a target level (example: 1 unit per 30 mg/dl above a target glucose level of 120 mg/dl). These doses are only illustrations; individualize doses to each patient.
- To estimate carbohydrate ratio for patient who was not previously carbohydrate counting, use "500" (or 450) rule: 500/TDD = grams of carbohydrate covered by 1 unit of insulin. Individualize for each patient based on history. Example: if TDD 50, 500/50 = 10. Bolus 1 U per 10 g carb.
- To estimate correctional bolus, use "1800" rule for rapid-acting insulin (or 1500 for regular insulin): 1800/total daily insulin dose = mg/dl that 1 unit of insulin will lower blood glucose. Individualize for each patient based on history. Example: if TDD 45, 1800/45 = 40. Bolus 1 U per 40 mg/dl glucose above target glucose level.
- Review emergency procedures, particularly for when pump insulin delivery is interrupted for any reason (i.e., catheter malfunction), including restarting multiple dose insulin injections; patient should have long-acting insulin available if needed for emergencies.

Specialized Insulin Pump Options

- **Bolus dose calculator:** different pumps call this by different names, but it calculates amount of bolus insulin needed using preprogrammed carbohydrate ratios, insulin sensitivity factors, and target glucose levels. Patient enters grams of carbohydrate

MANAGEMENT

to be consumed and premeal blood glucose level. Insulin on board subtracted from calculated bolus dose. Pump suggests dose but patient still needs to input dose.

- **Insulin on board:** prevents overcompensating with bolus insulin by calculating time from last bolus and, based on duration of insulin effect, amount of insulin still "on board." This can be subtracted from insulin dose needed for current meal to obtain amount of additional bolus insulin to inject.
- **Square wave bolus:** slow infusion of insulin over time as opposed to standard bolus, which delivers "spike" of insulin. May be appropriate to cover high-fat or high-protein meals with delayed absorption, or in patients with slower digestion (e.g., gastroparesis).
- **Daily totals:** calculates total bolus and basal insulin dosage delivered per day.
- **Temporary basal rates:** programmed and activated by patient in situations where insulin needs may be higher or lower than usual (e.g., physical activity, illness, or menses).

FOLLOW-UP

- Must have knowledgeable healthcare professionals available, with close patient contact when initiating insulin pump therapy.
- Common follow-up issues include emergency management of discontinued insulin delivery, sick days, unusual exercise, tape allergies, and frequency of changing the insertion set.
- Some patients take "pump vacations" (e.g., for cosmetic reasons), returning to conventional insulin injections for short periods of time, although such intermittent use is not recommended.
- Discuss what to do during exercise (e.g., take pump off if <30 minutes of activity, reduce basal rate, and/or take snack beforehand).

EXPERT OPINION

- Patients must be willing and eager to use a pump; do not force a pump on an unwilling patient.
- Patients need to know that the pump is "open loop," not delivering insulin automatically but requiring input from the patient.
- Discourage unrealistic expectations; pumps may confer significant benefits, but require patients to be involved.
- Many people find insulin pump use valuable in controlling wide glucose fluctuations and more flexible than multiple daily insulin injections. Often improves both quality of life and A1c for many patients.
- Disadvantages of pump therapy include the need to be attached to pump at all times and expense. Be sure of insurance coverage before ordering a pump.
- Too many basal rates (for instance 6–10 per day) are not valuable, and suggest that the patient is using different basal rates to cover meals, rather than choosing the correct bolus dose for a meal.
- Giving bolus doses after eating a meal is not recommended.
- Also, frequently giving correctional doses between meals is not recommended, and suggests that the premeal bolus dose is too little.
- In general, bolus doses at bedtime are not recommended, but if given to cover a snack, consider more conservative dosing.
- Do not count on an insulin pump to correct poor glycemic control due to poor self-care, or to reverse established long-term diabetic complications.

REFERENCES

Hanas R, Lindgren F, Lindblad B. A 2-yr national population study of pediatric ketoacidosis in Sweden: predisposing conditions and insulin pump use. *Pediatr Diabetes,* 2009; Vol. 10: pp. 33–7.
Comments: A database review found more ketoacidosis in children using CSII.

Hirsch IB. Clinical review: realistic expectations and practical use of continuous glucose monitoring for the endocrinologist. *J Clin Endocrinol Metab,* 2009; Vol. 94: pp. 2232–8.
Comments: An excellent expert review of clinical use of CSII.

Olinder AL, Kernell A, Smide B. Missed bolus doses: devastating for metabolic control in CSII-treated adolescents with type 1 diabetes. *Pediatr Diabetes,* 2009; Vol. 10: pp. 142–8.
Comments: Emphasizes the need to use bolus doses for successful use of CSII.

Churchill JN, Ruppe RL, Smaldone A. Use of continuous insulin infusion pumps in young children with type 1 diabetes: a systematic review. *J Pediatr Health Care,* 2009; Vol. 23: pp. 173–9.
Comments: A review of CSII use in children.

Bailon RM, Partlow BJ, Miller-Cage V, et al. Continuous subcutaneous insulin infusion (insulin pump) therapy can be safely used in the hospital in select patients. *Endocr Pract,* 2009; Vol. 15: pp. 24–9.
Comments: A review of CSII use in hospitalized patients.

Noschese ML, DiNardo MM, Donihi AC, et al. Patient outcomes after implementation of a protocol for inpatient insulin pump therapy. *Endocr Pract,* 2009; Vol. 15: pp. 415–24.
Comments: A description of CSII use in hospitalized patients providing a protocol for use.

Bolli GB, Kerr D, Thomas R, et al. Comparison of a multiple daily insulin injection regimen (basal once-daily glargine plus mealtime lispro) and continuous subcutaneous insulin infusion (lispro) in type 1 diabetes: a randomized open parallel multicenter study. *Diabetes Care,* 2009; Vol. 32: pp. 1170–6.
Comments: A clinical trial comparing CSII to multiple-dose insulin using glargine insulin, found no advantage to CSII.

Noschese ML, DiNardo MM, Donihi AC, et al. Patient outcomes after implementation of a protocol for inpatient insulin pump therapy. *Endocr Pract,* 2009; Vol. 15: pp. 415–24.
Comments: A description of CSII use in hospitalized patients providing a protocol for use.

Pickup JC, Renard E. Long-acting insulin analogs versus insulin pump therapy for the treatment of type 1 and type 2 diabetes. *Diabetes Care,* 2008; Vol. 31 Suppl 2: pp. S140–5.
Comments: A comparison of CSII with multiple dose insulin, finding that there was less severe hypoglycemia on CSII in comparison with NPH insulin, though no difference when compared to use of long-acting analog insulins.

Davidson PC, Hebblewhite HR, Steed RD, et al. Analysis of guidelines for basal-bolus insulin dosing: basal insulin, correction factor, and carbohydrate-to-insulin ratio. *Endocr Pract,* 2008; Vol. 14: pp. 1095–101.
Comments: Useful review of general guidelines for using CSII.

Jeandidier N, Riveline JP, Tubiana-Rufi N, et al. Treatment of diabetes mellitus using an external insulin pump in clinical practice. *Diabetes Metab,* 2008; Vol. 34: pp. 425–v38.
Comments: Useful review of guidelines for clinical use of CSII.

Zisser H, Robinson L, Bevier W, et al. Bolus calculator: a review of four "smart" insulin pumps. *Diabetes Technol Ther,* 2008; Vol. 10: pp. 441–4.
Comments: Reviews bolus dose calculations.

Cope JU, Morrison AE, Samuels-Reid J. Adolescent use of insulin and patient-controlled analgesia pump technology: a 10-year Food and Drug Administration retrospective study of adverse events. *Pediatrics,* 2008; Vol. 121: pp. e1133–8.
Comments: A recent FDA review of reported complications of insulin pump use; the review was uncontrolled and reached over-alarming conclusions.

MANAGEMENT

Weinzimer SA, Steil GM, Swan KL, et al. Fully automated closed-loop insulin delivery versus semiautomated hybrid control in pediatric patients with type 1 diabetes using an artificial pancreas. *Diabetes Care*, 2008; Vol. 31: pp. 934–9.

Comments: Research into the future use of a "closed loop" insulin pump, with automatic insulin delivery based on continuous glucose monitoring.

Lee SW, Cao M, Sajid S, et al. The dual-wave bolus feature in continuous subcutaneous insulin infusion pumps controls prolonged post-prandial hyperglycaemia better than standard bolus in type 1 diabetes. *Diabetes Nutr Metab*, 2004; Vol. 17: pp. 211–6.

Comments: Review of how to calculate basal rates.

Pickup J, Keen H. Continuous subcutaneous insulin infusion at 25 years: evidence base for the expanding use of insulin pump therapy in type 1 diabetes. *Diabetes Care*, 2002; Vol. 25: pp. 593–8.

Comments: Not recent, but a meta-analysis of articles evaluating outcomes of CSII use over 25 years. Generally, a benefit in reducing hypoglycemia, but variable effect on lowering HbA1c.

PANCREATIC AND ISLET TRANSPLANTATION

Gregory O. Clark, MD

DEFINITION

- **Pancreas transplant** (PTx) refers to allotransplantation (human to human) of the whole pancreas, including islets of Langerhans, acinar tissue, pancreatic ducts, and blood vessels.
- **Pancreas transplant alone** (PTA) refers to pancreas transplantation without a transplanted kidney.
- **Simultaneous pancreas and kidney transplant** (SPK) involves transplanting both a pancreas and a kidney simultaneously.
- **Pancreas after kidney** (PAK) refers to PTx in a recipient who has already received a kidney transplant.
- **Islet autotransplantation** is separation of islets from a person's own pancreas and retransplantation of those islets into the same person.
- **Islet allotransplantation** is separation of islets from a donor pancreas (1%–2% of pancreas mass), transplanted by infusion via the portal vein into a recipient.

EPIDEMIOLOGY

- About 1200 pancreas transplants are performed per year, and 900 of these are SPK transplants.
- From 1999–2009, 37 registered sites have reported 631 islet allograft recipients and 501 autograft recipients to the Collaborative Islet Transplant Registry (CITR).
- United Network for Organ Sharing (UNOS) administers the organ procurement and sharing network in the US. It is a nonprofit, scientific, and educational organization, with current data on epidemiologic aspects of transplantation.

CLINICAL TREATMENT

Pancreas Transplantation

- Indications for PTx: in conjunction with a kidney transplantation for end-stage renal disease (ESRD) due to type 1 diabetes (T1DM).
- More controversial indications include life-threatening hypoglycemia unawareness, type 2 diabetes with (ESRD), or rapidly progressing complications.

- Benefits of a successful PTx: improved quality of life, insulin independence, normal glucose metabolism, cessation of hypoglycemia, regression of atherosclerosis in ~40% of cases.
- Risks: surgical procedure (cardiac morbidity, postoperative infection, anastomotic leak with enteric drainage of pancreatic exocrine secretions), lifelong immunosuppression (renal toxicity, increased risk of infection and malignancy), acute rejection rate of 4%–15%, chronic rejection of 33%–50% after 10 years (White).
- SPK transplant is most successful for both graft survival and recipient, especially when done early, prior to dialysis. Graft survival after 3 years is 85% (White).
- PAK transplant allows a living related kidney donation followed by cadaveric pancreas transplant, reducing the wait time for a kidney compared to SPK. Graft survival after 3 years is 78% (White).
- PTA is more controversial, only indication being hypoglycemia unawareness. Fewer PTAs now done due to concerns that mortality was increased from PTA versus patients waitlisted and treated medically (Venstrum). 30% of PTA recipients require kidney transplantation after 10 years due to toxic effects of immunosuppressants.

Islet Allotransplantation

- Only done in the context of well-defined research studies; not yet standard clinical care.
- Minimally invasive, avoiding risks of major surgery, although risk of immunosuppression remains.
- Islets digested from the pancreas and lodged in the liver are more susceptible to cell death; as such, results are inferior to whole organ transplantation.
- Usually requires more than a single procedure to achieve insulin independence (islets from 2 or more cadaveric donors).
- Recent success used an immunosuppressive regimen free of steroids with 1-year insulin independence rates increased from previously reported rates of 10% to 90% with the Edmonton protocol (Shapiro).
- Most patients require insulin injections again within 5 years, but even minimal remaining beta-cell function still improves metabolic control and can keep patients free of severe hypoglycemic episodes (Ryan).

Islet Autotransplantation

- Currently only performed in specialized clinical centers but reimbursed by Centers for Medicare and Medicaid Services (CMS).
- Utility is to attempt preservation of insulin secretion in person having total pancreatectomy.
- Indication is therefore total pancreatectomy (e.g., for chronic pancreatitis pain).
- Does not require immunosuppression as there is no alloimmunity to transplanted self-tissue nor autoimmunity as in type 1 diabetes.
- Prolonged islet function and insulin independence rates are superior to islet allotransplantation despite a lower beta-cell mass (Sutherland).

EXPERT OPINION

- Appropriate patients should be referred to specialized centers skilled in PTx or research in islet transplantation.
- Prior to considering transplantation therapy for hypoglycemia unawareness, we make every attempt to optimize medical therapy including consideration of continuous glucose monitoring technology.

MANAGEMENT

- Since the average patient with T1DM has one severe episode of hypoglycemia requiring assistance per year, this does not necessarily constitute an indication for PTx.
- Consider PTx for T2DM only when patient is functionally without endogenous insulin (i.e., requires insulin therapy and has very unstable blood glucose).
- Overall, we consider the potential benefit of PTx to exceed the risk when ESRD requires kidney transplantation and therefore immunosuppression.

REFERENCES

White SA, Shaw JA, Sutherland DE. Pancreas transplantation. *Lancet*, 2009; Vol. 373: pp. 1808–17.
    Comments: An excellent overview of the indications, categories, and outcomes of pancreas transplantation.

Mineo D, Pileggi A, Alejandro R, et al. Point: steady progress and current challenges in clinical islet transplantation. *Diabetes Care*, 2009; Vol. 32: pp. 1563–9.
    Comments: Review that highlights the success and progress in the field of islet transplantation that warrants broader clinical application.

Khan MH, Harlan DM. Counterpoint: clinical islet transplantation: not ready for prime time. *Diabetes Care*, 2009; Vol. 32: pp. 1570–4.
    Comments: Review that highlights remaining limitations of islet transplantation and argues for continued careful research.

Sutherland DE, Gruessner AC, Carlson AM, et al. Islet autotransplant outcomes after total pancreatectomy: a contrast to islet allograft outcomes. *Transplantation*, 2008; Vol. 86: pp. 1799–802.
    Comments: Report of one leading center's experience with islet autotransplant, comparing to islet allograft outcomes.

Ryan EA, Paty BW, Senior PA, et al. Five-year follow-up after clinical islet transplantation. *Diabetes*, 2005; Vol. 54: pp. 2060–9.
    Comments: Disappointing follow-up study from the Edmonton Protocol reporting only ~10% insulin-independence at 5 years, although ~80% retain some beneficial beta-cell function.

Venstrom JM, McBride MA, Rother KI, et al. Survival after pancreas transplantation in patients with diabetes and preserved kidney function. *JAMA*, 2003; Vol. 290: pp. 2817–23.
    Comments: Study that brings into question the utility of pancreas transplant alone in patients with preserved renal function.

Shapiro AM, Lakey JR, Ryan EA, et al. Islet transplantation in seven patients with type 1 diabetes mellitus using a glucocorticoid-free immunosuppressive regimen. *NEJM*, 2000; Vol. 343: pp. 230–8.
    Comments: Landmark study that propelled the field of islet transplantation by reporting insulin-independence for an average of 1 year after islet transplantation in patients treated with an immunosuppressive regimen free of steroids (referred to as the Edmonton Protocol).

Type 2 Diabetes

TYPE 2 DIABETES: ENVIRONMENTAL RISK FACTORS AND SCREENING

Ari Eckman, MD, and Rita Rastogi Kalyani, MD, MHS

DEFINITION
- Includes risk factors other than genetic determinants (usually associated with positive family history) for type 2 diabetes (T2DM).
- Often used to screen for T2DM.

EPIDEMIOLOGY
- American Diabetes Association (ADA) recommends diabetes screening for (1) asymptomatic persons <45 years old of age who are overweight (BMI ≥25 kg/m²) with any one additional high-risk factor (see diagnosis section here) for type 2 diabetes; or (2) persons ≥45 years of age (particularly with BMI ≥25 kg/m²) every 3 years or more regularly depending on risk status (ADA Standards of Medical Care).
- In retrospective study of over 46,000 patients ≥20 years without diabetes seen at a large academic physician practice, 66% met ADA criteria for diabetes screening; of these, 11% were <45 years with risk factors (Sheehy).
- 86% of those eligible for screening had one or more glucose tests performed; 5% of those tested were diagnosed with diabetes.
- Prevalence of high-risk factors: age ≥45 years (55%); overweight (52%); hypercholesterolemia (50%); hypertension (26%); vascular disease (6%); high-risk ethnic group (4%); prediabetes (0.4%); polycystic ovarian disease (0.4%).
- High-risk factors associated with greatest yield of new diabetes diagnoses: prediabetes (16%); polycystic ovarian disease (13%); and vascular disease (10%).
- The US Preventive Services Task Force (USPSTF) has recommended diabetes screening for patients with hypertension and hyperlipidemia since 2000; however, in the most recent 2008 update, screening only advised for asymptomatic adults with sustained blood pressure >135/80 mmHg (USPSTF guidelines).
- Only 26% met USPSTF 2008 criteria for diabetes screening in the same study (Sheehy).

DIAGNOSIS
- **ADA high-risk factors:** physical inactivity (exercising <3 times a week); high-risk ethnicity (e.g., African American, Latin American, Native American, Asian American, or Pacific Islander); women who delivered a baby >9 lbs (4kg) or had diagnosed gestational DM; hypertension; high-density lipoprotein cholesterol (HDL-C) <35 mg/dl (0.90 mmol/L) and/or triglycerides >250 mg/dl (2.82 mmol/L); women with polycystic ovarian syndrome; previously identified impaired fasting glucose or impaired glucose tolerance; clinical conditions associated with insulin resistance (e.g., severe obesity and acanthosis nigricans); history of cardiovascular disease. First-degree relative with T2DM (i.e., genetic risk factor) is also a criterion (ADA Standards of Medical Care).
- **Abdominal obesity:** waist circumference >40 inches (102 cm) in males, >35 inches (88 cm) in females, or increased waist-to-hip circumference ratio that is >0.95 in

MANAGEMENT

Caucasian men and >0.80 in Caucasian women confers higher risk; cut-offs may vary by ethnicity (Chan).
- **Other risk factors:** older age (Cowie), parity (Nicholson), low (versus moderate) alcohol use (Koppes), cigarette smoking (Willi); also (transiently) stopping smoking (Yeh), stress or depression (Golden), low socioeconomic status particularly among Latin Americans and African Americans (Aviel-Curiel; Schootman), diet (i.e., high-fat, low-fiber, Western diet) (Shai), low magnesium intake (Larsson), soda consumption (Nettleton).
- **Chronic environmental exposures:** inorganic arsenic in drinking water (Navas-Acien), organophosphate and chlorinated pesticides (Montgomery), bisphenol A (a monomer used to make hard, polycarbonate plastics), and some epoxy resins (Lang).
- **Urbanization trends:** in Pacific Island of Nauru, Pima Indians took on a more Western lifestyle leading to more obesity, and diabetes incidence went from nearly 0% to about 50% (Zimmet). In India, Asian Indians living in rural communities had diabetes prevalence of 2%, increasing to 10% after moving to an urban environment (Ramachandran).

CLINICAL TREATMENT
Modifiable Risk Factor Management for Prevention of Diabetes
- Weight loss (~5%–10%) (Knowler).
- Increase physical activity (>30 minutes at least 3–5 days/week) (Knowler).
- Decrease triglycerides and increase HDL with lifestyle modification or medication if needed.
- Treat hypertension with lifestyle modification or medication if needed.
- Cardiovascular disease prevention.
- Eliminate soft drinks and sugary foods from diet.
- High-fiber diet.
- Smoking cessation, though may transiently increase risk of T2DM (Yeh).
- Stress management.

EXPERT OPINION
- Modifiable risk factors, including obesity and physical inactivity, are the strongest environmental risk factors for developing T2DM.
- T2DM can be effectively prevented by lifestyle changes in high-risk persons (~60% risk reduction) as demonstrated in the Diabetes Prevention Program.
- Individuals from high-risk ethnic groups who also have other diabetes risk factors may be particularly vulnerable.
- Diabetes screening programs can identify individuals with high-risk factors.
- Early risk factor identification and modification is essential for prevention of diabetes.

BASIS FOR RECOMMENDATIONS
American Diabetes Association. Standards of medical care in diabetes—2011. *Diabetes Care*, 2011; Vol. 34 Suppl 1: pp. S11–61.

    Comments: American Diabetes Association consensus statement describing risk factors for diabetes and criteria for screening in asymptomatic individuals.

OTHER REFERENCES
Yeh HC, Duncan BB, Schmidt MI, et al. Smoking, smoking cessation, and risk for type 2 diabetes mellitus: a cohort study. *Ann Intern Med*, 2010; Vol. 152: pp. 10–7.

    Comments: Analyzing a cohort study, smoking predicted T2DM but cessation of smoking also caused a transient increase in T2DM incidence.

Sheehy AM, Flood GE, Tuan WJ, et al. Analysis of guidelines for screening diabetes mellitus in an ambulatory population. *Mayo Clin Proc*, 2010; Vol. 85: pp. 27–35.

Comments: Retrospective analysis of 46,991 patients without diabetes >20 years seen at Midwestern academic physician practice between years 2005–2007, investigating case-finding ability of current guidelines to screen for diabetes and prevalence of high-risk factors.

Cowie CC, Rust KF, Ford ES, et al. Full accounting of diabetes and pre-diabetes in the U.S. population in 1988–1994 and 2005–2006. *Diabetes Care*, 2009; Vol. 32: pp. 287–94.

Comments: Prevalence of diabetes and prediabetes in the United States using data from the National Health and Nutrition Examination Surveys, stratified by age, gender, and ethnicity.

Nettleton JA, Lutsey PL, Wang Y, et al. Diet soda intake and risk of incident metabolic syndrome and type 2 diabetes in the Multi-Ethnic Study of Atherosclerosis (MESA). *Diabetes Care*, 2009; Vol. 32: pp. 688–94.

Comments: Observational study that reported a 67% greater risk of incident diabetes in adults who consumed diet soda at least daily.

Navas-Acien A, Silbergeld EK, Pastor-Barriuso R, et al. Arsenic exposure and prevalence of type 2 diabetes in US adults. *JAMA*, 2008; Vol. 300: pp. 814–22.

Comments: After adjustment for biomarkers of seafood intake, total urine arsenic was associated with increased prevalence of type 2 diabetes.

Lang IA, Galloway TS, Scarlett A, et al. Association of urinary bisphenol A concentration with medical disorders and laboratory abnormalities in adults. *JAMA*, 2008; Vol. 300: pp. 1303–10.

Comments: Higher bisphenol A concentrations were associated with diabetes.

Montgomery MP, Kamel F, Saldana TM, et al. Incident diabetes and pesticide exposure among licensed pesticide applicators: Agricultural Health Study, 1993–2003. *Am J Epidemiol*, 2008; Vol. 167: pp. 1235–46.

Comments: Long-term exposure from handling certain pesticides, in particular, organochlorine and organophosphate insecticides, may be associated with increased risk of diabetes.

U.S. Preventive Services Task Force. Screening for type 2 diabetes mellitus in adults: U.S. Preventive Services Task Force recommendation statement. *Ann Intern Med*, 2008; Vol. 148: pp. 846–54.

Comments: Most recent USPSTF recommendations for diabetes screening in adults.

Avila-Curiel A, Shamah-Levy T, Galindo-Gómez C, et al. Diabetes mellitus within low socioeconomic strata in Mexico City: a relevant problem. *Rev Invest Clin*, 2007; Vol. 59: pp. 246–55.

Comments: Diabetes is highly prevalent among adults older than 30 years, mainly on the lower socioeconomic stratum in Mexico City.

Larsson SC, Wolk A. Magnesium intake and risk of type 2 diabetes: a meta-analysis. *J Intern Med*, 2007; Vol. 262: pp. 208–14.

Comments: Study suggests that increased consumption of magnesium-rich foods such as whole grains, beans, nuts, and green leafy vegetables may reduce the risk of type 2 diabetes.

Schootman M, Andresen EM, Wolinsky FD, et al. The effect of adverse housing and neighborhood conditions on the development of diabetes mellitus among middle-aged African Americans. *Am J Epidemiol*, 2007; Vol. 166: pp. 379–87.

Comments: Poor housing conditions appear to be an independent contributor to the risk of incident diabetes in urban, middle-aged African Americans.

Willi C, Bodenmann P, Ghali WA, et al. Active smoking and the risk of type 2 diabetes: a systematic review and meta-analysis. *JAMA*, 2007; Vol. 298: pp. 2654–64.

Comments: Active smoking is associated with an increased risk of type 2 diabetes.

Golden SH A review of the evidence for a neuroendocrine link between stress, depression and diabetes mellitus. *Curr Diabetes Rev*, 2007; Vol. 3: pp. 252–9.

Comments: Reviews the evidence supporting an association between stress and diabetes.

MANAGEMENT

Shai I, Jiang R, Manson JE, et al. Ethnicity, obesity, and risk of type 2 diabetes in women: a 20-year follow-up study. *Diabetes Care,* 2006; Vol. 29: pp. 1585–90.

   Comments: A diet high in cereal fiber and polyunsaturated fat and low in trans fat and glycemic load appears to have a stronger inverse association with diabetes risk among the minorities than among whites.

Nicholson WK, Asao K, Brancati F, et al. Parity and risk of type 2 diabetes: the Atherosclerosis Risk in Communities Study. *Diabetes Care,* 2006; Vol. 29: pp. 2349–54.

   Comments: Increasing parity (particularly 5 or more live births) associated with 27% increased risk for diabetes after adjustment for confounders.

Koppes LL, Dekker JM, Hendriks HF, et al. Moderate alcohol consumption lowers the risk of type 2 diabetes: a meta-analysis of prospective observational studies. *Diabetes Care,* 2005; Vol. 28: pp. 719–25.

   Comments: Moderate alcohol consumption (6–48 g/day) associated with an approximately 30% reduced risk of diabetes compared with alcohol <6 g/day in meta-analysis of 15 prospective, observational studies.

Knowler WC, Barrett-Connor E, Fowler SE, et al. Reduction in the incidence of type 2 diabetes with lifestyle intervention or metformin. *NEJM,* 2002; Vol. 346: pp. 393–403.

   Comments: Results of the Diabetes Prevention Program, demonstrating that the lifestyle intervention reduced the incidence of T2DM by 58% and metformin by 31%, as compared with placebo.

Zimmet P, Alberti KG, Shaw J. Global and societal implications of the diabetes epidemic. *Nature,* 2001; Vol. 414: pp. 782–7.

   Comments: In conjunction with genetic susceptibility, especially in certain ethnic groups, type 2 diabetes is brought on by environmental and behavioral factors such as a sedentary lifestyle, overly rich nutrition, and obesity.

Ramachandran A, Snehalatha C, Latha E, et al. Rising prevalence of NIDDM in an urban population in India. *Diabetologia,* 1997; Vol. 40: pp. 232–7.

   Comments: Increasing trend in the prevalence of type 2 diabetes in urban Indians.

Chan JM, Rimm EB, Colditz GA, et al. Obesity, fat distribution, and weight gain as risk factors for clinical diabetes in men. *Diabetes Care,* 1994; Vol. 17: pp. 961–9.

   Comments: Waist circumference was positively associated with the risk of diabetes among the top 20% of the cohort.

TYPE 2 DIABETES: GENETIC RISK FACTORS

Nisa M. Maruthur, MD, MHS

DEFINITION

- Factors that determine genetic susceptibility to type 2 diabetes.
- Single nucleotide polymorphisms (SNPs) refer to differences between individuals in a single nucleotide of a given gene's DNA sequence and are the main source of genetic variation studied for risk of diabetes to date.

EPIDEMIOLOGY

- Children of a parent with type 2 diabetes have a 40% lifetime risk of developing type 2 diabetes.
- At least 24 single nucleotide polymorphisms (including SNPs in the *TCF7L2*, *FTO*, and *PPARG* genes) are associated with type 2 diabetes, odds ratios range from 1.1 to 1.4 (see Table 2-8).
- Risk variants discovered to date likely only account for 5%–10% of the heritability of type 2 diabetes.

TABLE 2-7. SELECTED GENE LOCI FOR MARKERS ASSOCIATED WITH TYPE 2 DIABETES

Gene	Putative Function*	Proportion with Risk Allele**	Odds Ratio for Diabetes*
PPARG	adipocyte transcription factor	0.87	1.19
CDKAL1	glucose toxicity sensor in islets	0.32	1.12
SLC30A8	islet zinc transporter important for insulin storage	0.69	1.12
CDKN2A/B	islet cyclin-dependent kinase inhibitor and tumor suppressor	0.83	1.20
TCF7L2	transcription factor that regulates insulin gene	0.31	1.37
FTO	associated with BMI	0.4	1.17

* Adapted from Florez JC, Jablonski KA, Bayley N, et al. TCF7L2 polymorphisms and progression to diabetes in the Diabetes Prevention Program. *NEJM*, 2006; Vol. 355: pp. 241–50.
** Adapted from Perry JR, Frayling TM. New gene variants alter type 2 diabetes risk predominantly through reduced beta-cell function. *Curr Opin Clin Nutr Metab Care*, 2008; Vol. 11(4:) pp. 371–7.

DIAGNOSIS
- Assessment of genetic risk through family history.
- Assessment of SNPs not clinically useful in determining diabetes risk over more traditional clinical factors such as body mass index and family history.
- Test for individual SNPs are not used clinically at this time, but patients can order commercially available general genetic testing through websites like www.23andme.com, www.deCODEme.com, and www.navigenics.com.

CLINICAL TREATMENT
- No clear therapeutic gene-medication interactions at this time to guide diabetes treatment.

EXPERT OPINION
- Of variants discovered to date, variation in the *TCF7L2* gene is most consistently associated with increased risk of diabetes, and also with the largest effect.
- Use of currently known genetic risk variants does not increase the ability to predict diabetes at this time over other clinical risk factors.
- Many other single nucleotide polymorphisms (genetic variants) with small effects likely exist.

MANAGEMENT

- Other types of genetic variation (e.g., rare variants, copy number variants, and epigenetic changes) will likely explain more of the genetic susceptibility to diabetes.
- Multiple genes may affect the risk of diabetes through pathways not directly related to insulin secretion, such as eating behavior or activity level.
- Pharmacogenomics (interactions between pharmacologic agents and genes) will likely play a role in therapeutic decisions in many diseases including diabetes within the next decade.

REFERENCES

Stolerman ES, Florez JC. Genomics of type 2 diabetes mellitus: implications for the clinician. *Nat Rev Endocrinol,* 2009; Vol. 5: pp. 429–36.

Comments: Unstructured review of clinical implications of diabetes genomics.

Meigs JB, Shrader P, Sullivan LM, et al. Genotype score in addition to common risk factors for prediction of type 2 diabetes. *NEJM,* 2008; Vol. 359: pp. 2208–19.

Comments: Framingham Offspring Study participants; limited utility of genotype score over clinical factors in predicting diabetes.

Lyssenko V, Jonsson A, Almgren P, et al. Clinical risk factors, DNA variants, and the development of type 2 diabetes. *NEJM,* 2008; Vol. 359: pp. 2220–32.

Comments: Illustrates limited value of genetic information of diabetes prediction over clinical factors in European subjects.

Perry JR, Frayling TM. New gene variants alter type 2 diabetes risk predominantly through reduced beta-cell function. *Curr Opin Clin Nutr Metab Care,* 2008; Vol. 11: pp. 371–7.

Comments: Unstructured review of genetics of type 2 diabetes focused on effect of risk variants on insulin secretion.

Sladek R, Rocheleau G, Rung J, et al. A genome-wide association study identifies novel risk loci for type 2 diabetes. *Nature,* 2007; Vol. 445: pp. 881–5.

Comments: Major genome-wide association study identifying SNPs associated with type 2 diabetes.

Florez JC, Jablonski KA, Bayley N, et al. TCF7L2 polymorphisms and progression to diabetes in the Diabetes Prevention Program. *NEJM,* 2006; Vol. 355: pp. 241–50.

Comments: Diabetes Prevention Program: Confirmation that common variants in TCF7L2 are associated with type 2 diabetes risk.

Groop LC, Tuomi T. Non-insulin-dependent diabetes mellitus—a collision between thrifty genes and an affluent society. *Ann Med,* 1997; Vol. 29: pp. 37–53.

Comments: Early review of genetic basis of diabetes incorporating thrifty gene hypothesis.

TYPE 2 DIABETES: SEQUENCING THERAPIES

Christopher D. Saudek, MD

DEFINITION

- Treatment of hyperglycemia in diabetes should be progressively intensified as necessary to control blood glucose to target ranges.
- This requires, first, establishing goals, especially for hemoglobin A1c and avoidance of unacceptable hypoglycemia.
- It then requires adjusting therapy to reach those targets.

EPIDEMIOLOGY

- The risk of microvascular complications of diabetes (retinopathy, nephropathy, neuropathy) is closely related to control of blood glucose.
- Microvascular complications are a major cause of morbidity and mortality.

- Most people with diabetes do not have optimal glycemic control (average US A1c >7%), indicating the need to advance therapy more quickly.
- Prevention of macrovascular complications (cardiovascular disease) is more closely linked to control of traditional risk factors (blood pressure, lipids, smoking), which should be aggressively managed in people with diabetes, and glycemic control is also important.

Clinical Treatment

- There is no one agreed–upon sequence of treatments, although dietary modification and increased physical activity are always the basis of good care and more effective than medication in prevention of diabetes (Knowler).
- Recent guidelines suggest lifestyle therapy in addition to medication upon diagnosis, given difficulty of many patients to achieve optimal glycemic control on lifestyle therapy alone (Nathan).
- Metformin: generally first-line oral agent in treating type 2 diabetes, unless contraindicated or not tolerated. Initially 500 mg two to three times daily (often started as once daily for 2–4 weeks to reduce gastrointestinal side effects then titrated quickly).
- Maximize metformin dose (unless GI side effects limit tolerated dose).
- Current ADA and American Academy of Clinical Endocrinology (AACE) guidelines provide multiple options for additional therapy after metformin initiation.
- Add a second oral agent if glycemic control is inadequate; consider a sulfonylurea, with metformin or as a combination pill. Sulfonylureas can cause hypoglycemia and modest weight gain.
- Options for adding second or third oral drug include use of a thiazolidinedione (with additional benefits on lipids), metaglinide (for postprandial hyperglycemia), DPP-IV inhibitor (less likely to cause hypoglycemia), or early use of insulin (if A1c >8%). Review side effects and contraindications prior to initiation of additional medications for each patient.
- In specific circumstances, consider an injectable incretin analog such as exenatide (often causes weight loss), an alpha glucosidase inhibitor (e.g., for gastroparesis), or bariatric surgery (for severe obesity). Review side effects and contraindications prior to initiating additional medications.
- Always start insulin immediately in new-onset type 1 diabetes (T1DM).
- Consider initiation of insulin therapy in type 2 diabetes (T2DM) if patient already on 2–3 oral agents and still not optimally controlled.
- Intensify insulin therapy early in T1DM or uncontrolled T2DM if glycemic targets are not met or patterns of hyper- or hypoglycemia are identified.

Follow-up

- Changing treatment regimen requires follow-up more frequently than usual, depending on the circumstance.
- Consider dietary patterns and physical activity level when determining treatment regimen.

Expert Opinion

- Glycemic objective is to control hemoglobin A1c to target and avoid unacceptable hypoglycemia.
- The most common error in blood glucose management is advancing treatment regimen too slowly, allowing prolonged poor glycemic control.

MANAGEMENT

- Beware of "clinical inertia": the tendency of clinicians not to change a medical regimen even when it is not working (Bolen).
- When initiating insulin, continue oral agents to take advantage of endogenous insulin secretion, until insulin regimen is intensified and replaces endogenous insulin.
- T2DM often requires multiple oral agents and/or relatively high-dose insulin therapy.
- T1DM usually requires multiple doses of long- and short-acting insulin, usually in lower doses than for T2DM.
- Wide differences exist among clinicians' exact sequencing of oral agents; evidence favoring one sequence over others is virtually nonexistent, especially after initiation of metformin.

BASIS FOR RECOMMENDATIONS

Nathan DM, Buse JB, Davidson MB, et al. Medical management of hyperglycemia in type 2 diabetes: a consensus algorithm for the initiation and adjustment of therapy: a consensus statement of the American Diabetes Association and the European Association for the Study of Diabetes. *Diabetes Care,* 2009; Vol. 32: pp. 193–203.
   Comments: A consensus committee's recommendation on sequencing of treatment of type 2 diabetes. Quite nonspecific after initiation of metformin.

OTHER REFERENCES

American Diabetes Association. Standards of medical care in diabetes—2011. *Diabetes Care,* 2011; Vol. 34 Suppl 1: pp. S11–61.
   Comments: The annually published Standards of Medical Care published by the American Diabetes Association.

Bolen SD, Bricker E, Samuels TA, et al. Factors associated with intensification of oral diabetes medications in primary care provider-patient dyads: a cohort study. *Diabetes Care,* 2009; Vol. 32: pp. 25–31.
   Comments: An interesting study of factors that contribute to "clinical inertia," the tendency not to adjust treatment even when it is not working.

Rodbard HW, Blonde L, Braithwaite SS, et al. American Association of Clinical Endocrinologists' medical guidelines for clinical practice for the management of diabetes mellitus. *Endocr Pract,* 2007; Vol. 13 Suppl 1: pp. 1–68.
   Comments: AACE clinical guidelines for managing diabetes, describing in detail the available medications available, important characteristics, and a general statement of choices for sequencing.

Jellinger PS, Davidson JA, Blonde L, et al. Road maps to achieve glycemic control in type 2 diabetes mellitus: ACE/AACE Diabetes Road Map Task Force. *Endocr Pract,* 2007; Vol. 13: pp. 260–8.
   Comments: AACE statement of recommended sequencing on treatments.

Mooradian AD, Bernbaum M, Albert SG Narrative review: a rational approach to starting insulin therapy. *Ann Intern Med,* 2006; Vol. 145: pp. 125–34.
   Comments: A useful review of available insulins and a practical consideration of how to start and then intensify insulin regimens.

Heine RJ, Van Gaal LF, Johns D, et al. Exenatide versus insulin glargine in patients with suboptimally controlled type 2 diabetes: a randomized trial. *Ann Intern Med,* 2005; Vol. 143: pp. 559–69.
   Comments: Open label comparison of exenatide (an incretin mimetic) vs insulin glargine in type 2 diabetics who had failed oral agents. Exenatide had similar glycemic efficacy, but more weight reduction, and higher incidence of gastrointestinal side effects.

Klein S, Sheard NF, Pi-Sunyer X, et al. Weight management through lifestyle modification for the prevention and management of type 2 diabetes: rationale and strategies: a statement of the American Diabetes Association, the North American Association for the Study of Obesity, and the American Society for Clinical Nutrition. *Diabetes Care,* 2004; Vol. 27: pp. 2067–73.
   Comments: An expert committee statement of the rationale and approaches to weight control.

Yki-Järvinen H. Thiazolidinediones. *NEJM,* 2004; Vol. 351: pp. 1106–18.

    Comments: An important review of the mechanisms of action, side effects, and clinical use of thiazolidinediones.

Miller CK, Edwards L, Kissling G, et al. Nutrition education improves metabolic outcomes among older adults with diabetes mellitus: results from a randomized controlled trial. *Prev Med,* 2002; Vol. 34: pp. 252–9.

    Comments: A relatively small randomized trial in which patients were given nutrition education or not. Those educated in a sound nutrition plan showed better glycemic control.

Knowler WC, Barrett-Connor E, Fowler SE, et al. Reduction in the incidence of type 2 diabetes with lifestyle intervention or metformin. *NEJM,* 2002; Vol. 346: pp. 393–403.

    Comments: The Diabetes Prevention Program demonstrated that Intensive Lifestyle reduced incidence of diabetes by 58%, metformin by 31% in subjects with impaired glucose tolerance.

TYPE 2 DIABETES: INSULIN TREATMENT

Sherita Hill Golden, MD, MHS

MANAGEMENT

DEFINITION

- Insulin is the oldest and most effective therapy for treating hyperglycemia.
- Insulin can decrease the hemoglobin A1c (HbA1c) to any level, and there is no maximum dose of insulin beyond which glucose cannot be lowered although too aggressive lowering of HbA1c may be potentially harmful (Gerstein).
- Modern insulins are manufactured by yeast or bacteria, using recombinant DNA techniques.
- Amino acid sequences of insulin are either identical to that of human insulin, or are modified to have altered pharmacokinetic properties (analogs).

EPIDEMIOLOGY

- Data from the United Kingdom Prospective Diabetes Study (UKPDS) in individuals with type 2 diabetes showed that beta-cell function declines over time; therefore, most patients will eventually need insulin.

SIGNS AND SYMPTOMS

- Indications for initiating insulin therapy in type 2 diabetes include (1) failure to achieve glycemic targets on maximum doses of oral agents, (2) severe hyperglycemia at diagnosis (see below), or (3) contraindications to oral therapies that necessitate use of insulin as initial therapy.
- Indications for immediate insulin therapy due to severe hyperglycemia: fasting blood glucose (FBG) >250 mg/dl; random glucose >300 mg/dl; hemoglobin A1c >10%; and/or symptoms of polyuria, polydipsia, and weight loss.
- Insulin therapy should be started at any point in the treatment of type 2 diabetes when the above criteria are met or if patients have a persistently elevated A1c (≥8%) on maximal doses of oral therapy.

CLINICAL TREATMENT

- Start with single injection of bedtime intermediate-acting insulin (NPH—Neutral Protamine Hegedorn, "isophane") or bedtime or morning long-acting insulin (glargine, detirmir). Initial dose is 10 units or 0.2 units per kilogram. This is the initial basal insulin.
- Fasting self-monitored glucose (FBG) should be checked daily and the initial insulin dose increased by 2 units every 3 days until FBG is consistently in the target range (70–130 mg/dl). Use larger dose increments, such as 4 units every 3 days, if the FBG is >180 mg/dl or if patient is likely very insulin resistant (e.g., obese).

- If nocturnal hypoglycemia occurs or the FBG is <70 mg/dl, reduce bedtime insulin by 4 units or 10% (whichever is greater).
- Reassess HbA1c 2–3 months after initiating basal insulin therapy. If HbA1c is <7%, continue current therapy.
- If HbA1c is ≥7% and FBG is in the target range of 70–130 mg/dl, check blood sugar before lunch, dinner, and at bedtime to find which sugars are elevated. This guides initiation of second insulin injection.
- Add a second insulin injection as follows: (1) if prelunch BG is elevated, add a rapid-acting insulin at breakfast (i.e., lispro, aspart, glulisine); (2) if predinner BG is elevated, add NPH insulin at breakfast or a rapid-acting insulin at lunch; and (3) if prebedtime BG is elevated, add a rapid-acting insulin at dinner. When adding additional injections, start with about 4 units and adjust by 2 units every 3 days until the premeal blood sugars are within the target range (70–130 mg/dl). This rapid-acting insulin is the nutritional insulin. Alternatively, for motivated patients, carbohdyrate counting (see p. 94) can be used to calculate the amount of nutritional insulin needed.
- The average total daily dose of insulin in type 2 diabetes is ≥1 unit/kg/day due to insulin resistance (compared to a total daily dose of 0.5 units/kg/day in patients with type 1 diabetes).
- In well-educated, motivated patients, correctional, or sliding scale rapid-acting insulin, based on self-monitored blood glucose before the meal, can be added to the nutritional insulin. Examples of low, medium, and high dose correctional scales are provided in Figure 2-4, p. 71.
- Can continue oral antidiabetic agents with basal insulin; however, if glycemic targets are not reached and nutritional insulin is added, discontinue sulfonylureas, although insulin sensitizers can be continued.
- Using insulin sensitizers with insulin may reduce the total daily insulin requirement and help prevent weight gain.

FOLLOW-UP
- Patients need ongoing reassessment after the second insulin injection is added; HbA1c should be reassessed 3 months after adding the second insulin injection.
- If HbA1c not <7%, premeal blood sugars should be rechecked and depending upon which one is out of range (based on the algorithm outlined previously), add additional injections. Note that International Diabetes Federation recommends A1c goal <6.5%.
- If HbA1c remains elevated despite multiple daily injections, check blood sugars 2-hour postprandially and adjust preprandial rapid-acting insulin until postprandial readings are <180 mg/dl.
- An experienced healthcare professional should teach insulin injection technique.

EXPERT OPINION
- Higher HbA1c levels at diagnosis (i.e., >10%) indicates severe insulin deficiency and usually require immediate initiation of insulin therapy.
- A common error in treating type 2 diabetes is to initiate insulin too late, allowing poor glycemic control to continue too long.
- The ideal insulin regimen for patients without remaining endogenous insulin production inclues basal, bolus, and correctional components.

BASIS FOR RECOMMENDATIONS

Nathan DM, Buse JB, Davidson MB, et al. Medical management of hyperglycemia in type 2 diabetes: a consensus algorithm for the initiation and adjustment of therapy: a consensus statement of the American Diabetes Association and the European Association for the Study of Diabetes. *Diabetes Care,* 2009; Vol. 32: pp. 193–203.

Comments: This is a summary of the most up-to-date guidelines from the American Diabetes Association regarding medical management of hyperglycemia in patients with type 2 diabetes. It contains an insulin initiation and titration algorithm for patients with type 2 diabetes.

Rodbard HW, Jellinger PS, Davidson JA, et al. Statement by an American Association of Clinical Endocrinologists/American College of Endocrinology consensus panel on type 2 diabetes mellitus: an algorithm for glycemic control. *Endocr Pract,* 2009; Vol. 15: pp. 540–59.

Comments: This is a summary of the most up-to-date guidelines from the American Association of Clinical Endocrinologists.

OTHER REFERENCES

Action to Control Cardiovascular Risk in Diabetes Study Group, Gerstein HC, Miller ME, et al. Effects of intensive glucose lowering in type 2 diabetes. *N Engl J Med,* 2008; Vol. 358: pp. 2545–59.

Comments: The ACCORD study demonstrated an increased risk of mortality with too intensive glucose lowering (A1c <6.0%) versus an HbA1c target of 7–7.9%.

Turner RC, Cull CA, Frighi V, et al. Glycemic control with diet, sulfonylurea, metformin, or insulin in patients with type 2 diabetes mellitus: progressive requirement for multiple therapies (UKPDS 49). UK Prospective Diabetes Study (UKPDS) Group. *JAMA,* 1999; Vol. 281: pp. 2005–12.

Comments: This UKPDS study describes the progression of type 2 diabetes such that patients ultimately require insulin.

Groop LC Sulfonylureas in NIDDM. *Diabetes Care,* 1992; Vol. 15: pp. 737–54.

Comments: This study had data showing that there is a progressive decline in beta-cell function over time in patients with type 2 diabetes (4%–5% declined in function/year).

MANAGEMENT

SECTION 3
COMPLICATIONS AND COMORBIDITIES

Cardiovascular Disease, Obesity, and Risk Factors

CARDIOVASCULAR DISEASE SCREENING AND MANAGEMENT

Sheldon H. Gottlieb, MD

DEFINITION

- Cardiovascular disease (CVD) encompasses coronary heart disease (CHD) including asymptomatic disease or manifestations of angina, myocardial infarction, or sudden death due to underlying coronary artery disease; congestive heart failure (CHF); valvular heart disease; and cerebrovascular disease (stroke).
- Coronary artery disease (CAD) includes disease of the coronary arteries: epicardial coronary arteries, branching arteries, and subendocardial vessels.
- Even in the absence of known CVD, the American Diabetes Association (ADA), the American Heart Association (AHA), and the American College of Cardiology (ACC) identify diabetes as a high-risk condition for macrovascular disease.

EPIDEMIOLOGY

- CVD is a major cause of death worldwide (Yusuf).
- Risk for CVD begins to increase at age 40 and increases greatly above age 70; age is the strongest risk factor for CVD (Vasan; Wald).
- Other CVD risk factors include family history, male gender, abnormal lipids, smoking, hypertension, diabetes, abdominal obesity, psychosocial factors, consumption level of fruits, vegetables, and alcohol (lack of moderate consumption), and lack of regular physical activity (Yusuf).
- Definitions of poor, intermediate and ideal cardiovascular health and NHANES 2005-2006 prevalence estimates for AHA 2020 goals are given in Lloyd-Jones Table 3. See also *http://circ.ahajournals.org/cgi/content/full/106/25/3143*.
- Up to 80% of individuals with type 2 diabetes will develop CVD (AHA/ADA consensus statement).
- Diabetes is a major risk factor for CVD (Yusuf). Individuals with diabetes have a 2–4 times higher prevalence of CVD compared to the general population (Redberg).
- Prevalence of subclinical CVD detected using coronary CT in asymptomatic persons with coronary risk factors but no known CVD was significantly higher in persons with diabetes versus no diabetes (i.e., coronary plaques found in 91% vs 68% of individuals, respectively) (Iwaskaki).
- Diabetes traditionally considered a CVD risk factor equivalent (i.e., patients with diabetes and no history of previous MI have a similar risk [~20%] of a major cardiovascular event in the next 7 years as persons with a history of previous myocardial infarction but no diabetes) (Haffner).
- CVD is the primary cause of death in persons with diabetes, and mortality from acute myocardial infarction (MI) is much higher in persons with diabetes compared to their counterparts (Grundy).

DIAGNOSIS

- **Clinical suspicion:** those at highest risk of future CVD events are those with previous history of CHD, CHF, or stroke.
- **History:** family history of early onset CVD (<55 years in men, <65 years in women) is an important risk factor and strongest when present in both a parent and sibling (Nasir). Drawing family pedigree for diabetes and heart disease is important during initial assessment. See *http://www.americanheart.org/downloadable/heart/1170790567218Family%20Tree%20Flyer%20b-w_2007.pdf.*
- **Labs:** measure nonfasting total cholesterol and HDL-cholesterol and their ratio. Ratio of >3:1 is associated with progression of carotid intimal thickness (Emerging Risk Factors Collaboration). High-sensitivity C-reactive protein (CRP) test may be helpful in persons with intermediate CVD risk (Pearson).
- **Electrocardiogram (ECG):** on a standard resting ECG, look for left atrial enlargement, left ventricular hypertrophy (LVH), long corrected QT interval, atrial fibrillation, frequent premature atrial contraction (PAC) or premature ventricular contraction (PVC), or absence of respiratory variability in heart rate (Pop-Busui).
- **Stress testing:** graded exercise treadmill stress test preferred where possible. If uninterpretable resting ECG (i.e., left bundle branch block or major ST-T abnormalities), do stress imaging. Pharmacological stress imaging for persons who cannot undergo leg exercise. Persons with diabetes are at intermediate risk at baseline and imaging studies should be used if available. Both echocardiography and nuclear stress imaging have high negative predictive value for left main or extensive triple vessel disease (Metz).
- **Imaging:** echocardiography for LVH, left ventricle (LV) size and function, and carotid ultrasound for intimal thickness are useful.
- **Coronary CT:** can be a useful imaging test to establish coronary risk for those at intermediate risk (this will include all persons with diabetes above age 45) (Hecht). Coronary artery calcium (CAC) scores directly measure coronary artery disease burden. A significant number of persons with diabetes, at intermediate to high risk based on risk factor scoring alone may have CAC scores that reclassify them as low risk (Hecht) or high risk (Hadamitzky). CAC use in diabetes may be clinically useful and cost effective (Hecht). Radiation dose is 2 mSv, about the same as background radiation over 8 months.
- **Vascular studies:** see Peripheral Vascular Disease, p. 208.
- **Chest X-ray:** calcification of the aortic knob is often seen in patients with diabetes and is a marker for duration of diabetes, and likelihood of multivessel coronary artery disease. A cardiothoracic ratio of >0.5 is a marker for cardiac enlargement and heart failure.
- **Genomic Testing:** genes for type 2 diabetes and coronary heart disease are beginning to be identified, but no recommendations currently exist for their routine use in diagnostic evaluation.

SIGNS AND SYMPTOMS

- **Symptoms:** any complaint of chest discomfort (from midabdomen to jaw) with exertion, any limitation in walking or decreased exercise tolerance, snoring or sleep disturbance, increasing fatigue in persons middle aged and older. Description of chest

COMPLICATIONS AND COMORBIDITIES

discomfort may vary depending on age, gender, education, ethnicity, and duration of diabetes.

- **Caveat:** patients with diabetes and CVD are often asymptomatic, especially women.
- **Signs on physical examination:** blood pressure (BP) >130/80, resting heart rate (HR) >80 bpm, respiratory rate >15, arcus corneus, poor dentition, periodontal disease, stiff blood vessels on exam, increased pulse pressure (>50 mmHg), carotid bruit or murmur of aortic stenosis, a loud S4 or any S3 gallop, any signs of neuropathy, decreased ankle or knee jerks, decreased pedal pulses, any ulcerations or severe calluses on the feet.
- Tests of cognition, such as the mini-mental exam, should be part of the initial evaluation for patients with diabetes and CVD who are at risk of cognitive decline over time.
- Erectile dysfunction in younger men is associated with an increased likelihood of CAD (Miner).

CLINICAL TREATMENT

CVD Risk Calculators

- **Risk calculator:** computerized risk model, based on clinical data or clinical plus laboratory and imaging data.
- **QRISK risk calculator** (available at *http://www.QRISK.org*) is very effective when calculated with the patient at a workstation, the graphics are useful, and it calculates a "relative risk" over a 10-year span and a "heart age." This risk calculator will identify patients at intermediate risk for coronary heart disease. However, all persons with diabetes above age 45–55 are at intermediate risk. The coronary calcium score will reclassify a significant portion of these patients into a lower or higher risk category.
- **The Framingham Heart Study risk calculator** may underestimate CVD risks for people with diabetes since the study included relatively few persons with diabetes (available at *http://hin.nhlbi.nih.gov/atpiii/calculator.asp?usertype=prof*).
- Other risk calculators specifically for use in diabetes include **UKPDS** (*http://www.dtu.ox.ac.uk/riskengine/index.php*), **ARIC study** (*http://www.aricnews.net/riskcalc/html/RC1.html*), and the **ADA's Diabetes PhD** (*http://www.diabetes.org/living-with-diabetes/complications/diabetes-phd/*).

Preventive Treatment

- **Optimize risk factors:** smoking cessation; BP: <130/80, with recent studies suggesting that too aggressive lowering of BP (i.e., systolic <120 mHg) is not desirable. lipids: ratio of total cholesterol to HDL-cholesterol <3:1, LDL <100 mg/dl (target for persons with known CVD is probably <70 mg/dl), triglycerides <150 mg/dl (for persons with known disease, target probably <100 mg/dl); A1c <7.0% (benefits for reducing risk of CVD below this level are uncertain and too aggressive lowering (i.e., A1c <6%) may be associated with harm) (Yudkin; Pfeffer; Cushman; Gerstein)
- **Diabetes:** the only glucose-lowering medications that have shown net cardiovascular benefit in long-term studies of patients with type 2 diabetes are metformin and acarbose. Both drugs have pleiotropic effects. Recent studies suggest the importance of glycemic control in CVD prevention (Selvin; Hanefeld; Zhou).
- **Hypertension:** treatment of BP is essential; angiotensin-converting enzyme inhibitors often first choice for persons with diabetes. Combinations of drugs used at half recommended doses may be most effective with fewest side effects (Laws).

- Carvedilol may be particularly effective for BP lowering in African American persons with diabetes.
- Diuretics also good for BP control; the negative effect on glycemic control is minimal when used at one half dose, such as chlorthalidone 12.5 mg daily.
- **Dyslipidemia:** persons taking statins often complain of myalgias without CK elevations. Effective lipid control may often be obtained using potent and long-lasting statins such as rosuvastatin 5 to 20 mg every day.
- Given that diabetes is a high-risk condition for CVD, the NHLBI Adult Treatment Panel III (ATP III) lists diabetes as a "CVD risk equivalent" when determining LDL goals.
- **Weight loss:** bariatric surgery may have an important place in the treatment of type 2 diabetes and prevention of CVD but patients must have capacity for full understanding of the risks and potential benefits of the procedure, that include improvement in hypertriglyceridemia, low levels of HDL, hypertension, and hyperuricemia (Sjöström).
- **Lifestyle modification (diet and exercise):** see the sections on diet (p. 100) and physical activity and exercise (p. 103).
- **Aspirin therapy:** indicated in all persons with history of CVD and in persons with diabetes who have >10% risk of CVD over the next 10 years and no increased risk of bleeding (see Routine Preventive Care for more details, p. 61).

FOLLOW-UP
- Risk for patients without known CVD depends on age and risk factors. If Framingham risk or other risk scores show >10% ten-year risk, patients should be reassessed every 4–5 years (Hecht; Warburton). Frequency of reassessment for patients with known CVD is individualized and depends on risk factors, symptoms, and age.
- A position statement by the ADA/AHA/ACC has been recently published that incorporates findings from several large clinical trials of aggressive glycemic control and risk of developing cardiovascular disease, including the ACCORD, ADVANCE, and VA diabetes trials (Skyler).
- Goals of treatment for CVD are detailed in the American Diabetes Association Standards of Medical Care 2010 and the AHA/ADA consensus statement on primary prevention of CVD in persons with diabetes.
- Comprehensive list of guidelines for treatment of CVD and diabetes from US Dept. of Health and Human Services, Agency for Healthcare Research and Quality (*http://www. guideline.gov/search/search.aspx?term=diabetes+cardiovascular*).

EXPERT OPINION
- Most patients with diabetes have some degree of subclinical CVD; prevalence increases with duration of disease. Preventive screening for CVD may be appropriate, especially in those with other CVD risk factors.
- Diabetes has been called a CVD "risk equivalent," but use of the term may be contentious given considerable variability in risk for CVD (Grundy).
- Once a person has diabetes, he or she is at intermediate risk for having CVD. Smoking, family history of early cardiac disease, abdominal obesity, low HDL, erectile dysfunction in young men, and ankle brachial index <0.9 all point to increased risk.
- Risk of cardiovascular mortality rises with age in an exponential fashion.
- Approximately 15% of persons with diabetes may be reclassified as "low risk" based on coronary calcium score of 0 (Hecht).

COMPLICATIONS AND COMORBIDITIES

- We prefer use of a stress test for CVD risk stratification in symptomatic individuals, and in asymptomatic individuals at high risk for CVD prior to recommending an exercise program.
- Absence of symptoms does not exclude presence of CVD in persons with diabetes; many will be asymptomatic.
- Optimize modifiable risk factors for CVD including smoking cessation, hypertension, dyslipidemia, and encourage weight loss.
- Example of an effective medication list for most patients with type 2 diabetes and CVD: lisinopril (ACE inhibitors), carvedilol (beta-blockers), chlorthalidone (diuretics), aspirin, statin, metformin, and other diabetes medication.
- The goal for patients with diabetes and CVD is self-management supplemented by appropriate education and feedback and team management or case management as needed.

BASIS FOR RECOMMENDATIONS

American Diabetes Association. Standards of medical care in diabetes—2011. *Diabetes Care*, 2011; Vol. 34 Suppl 1: pp. S11–61.

  Comments: Summary of American Diabetes Association recommendations for routine preventive care that offers specific authoritative recommendations and is evaluated and updated yearly.

Skyler JS, Bergenstal R, Bonow RO, et al. Intensive glycemic control and the prevention of cardiovascular events: implications of the ACCORD, ADVANCE, and VA diabetes trials: a position statement of the American Diabetes Association and a scientific statement of the American College of Cardiology Foundation and the American Heart Association. *Diabetes Care*, 2009; Vol. 32: pp. 187–92.

  Comments: Joint statement ADA, AHA, ACC incorporating findings from ACCORD, ADVANCE, and VA-Diabetes studies.

Buse JB, Ginsberg HN, Bakris GL, et al. Primary prevention of cardiovascular diseases in people with diabetes mellitus: a scientific statement from the American Heart Association and the American Diabetes Association. *Diabetes Care*, 2007; Vol. 30: pp. 162–72.

  Comments: Joint statement by AHA and ADA on recommendations for primary prevention of CVD.

Grundy SM, Benjamin IJ, Burke GL, et al. Diabetes and cardiovascular disease: a statement for healthcare professionals from the American Heart Association. *Circulation*, 1999; Vol. 100: pp. 1134–46.

  Comments: The first description by the American Diabetes Association and the American Heart Association of diabetes as a CVD equivalent.

OTHER REFERENCES

Miner MM. Erectile dysfunction: a harbinger or consequence: does its detection lead to a "window of curability?". *J Androl*, 2011; Vol. 32: pp. 125–34.

  Comments: Review of data linking erectile dysfunction to risk for CAD, especially in young men.

Berger JS, Jordan CO, Lloyd-Jones D, et al. Screening for cardiovascular risk in asymptomatic patients. *J Am Coll Cardiol*, 2010; Vol. 55: pp. 1169–77.

  Comments: Recent and thorough discussion of screening to determine CV risk.

Hadamitzky M, Hein F, Meyer T, et al. Prognostic value of coronary computed tomographic angiography in diabetic patients without known coronary artery disease. *Diabetes Care*, 2010; Vol. 33: pp. 1358–63.

  Comments: Coronary artery calcium scoring identified diabetic patients at particularly high risk of major coronary events.

The ACCORD Study Group. Effects of combination lipid therapy in type 2 diabetes mellitus. *NEJM*, 2010; Vol. 362: pp. 1563–74.

  Comments: In type 2 diabetic patients, adding a fibrate to a statin did not improve CV outcomes.

Hecht HS. A zero coronary artery calcium score: priceless. *J Am Coll Cardiol*, 2010; Vol. 55: pp. 1118–20.

Comments: Impact of coronary calcium screening in persons with diabetes: a significant number will have a low CAC score and be reclassified as "low risk" for CVD.

Collins F. Has the revolution arrived? *Nature*, 2010; Vol. 464: pp. 674–5.

Comments: Genes for type 2 diabetes and coronary heart disease have been identified. Personalized genomic analysis will soon be an important tool in cardiovascular medicine.

Pop-Busui R. Cardiac autonomic neuropathy in diabetes: a clinical perspective. *Diabetes Care*, 2010; Vol. 33: pp. 434–41.

Comments: Excellent review of important and often ignored aspect of diabetes and heart disease.

Artinian NT, Fletcher GF, Mozaffarian D, et al. Interventions to promote physical activity and dietary lifestyle changes for cardiovascular risk factor reduction in adults: a scientific statement from the American Heart Association. *Circulation*, 2010; Vol. 122: pp. 406–41.

Comments: Recent review of nonpharmacologic treatment of CVD.

Pfeffer MA. ACCORD(ing) to a trialist. *Circulation*, 2010; Vol. 122: pp. 841–3.

Comments: A masterful introduction to the ACCORD trial.

Lloyd-Jones DM, Hong Y, Labarthe D, et al. Defining and setting national goals for cardiovascular health promotion and disease reduction: the American Heart Association's strategic Impact Goal through 2020 and beyond. *Circulation*, 2010; Vol. 121: pp. 586–613.

Comments: The statement from the American Heart Association regarding prevention and treatment of CVD. Section on behavioral medicine pp. 424–426 should be read by all medical practitioners.

ACCORD Study Group, Cushman WC, Evans GW, et al. Effects of intensive blood-pressure control in type 2 diabetes mellitus. *NEJM*, 2010; Vol. 362: pp. 1575–85.

Comments: A summary of the results of the ACCORD study on blood pressure.

Pencina MJ, D'Agostino RB, Larson MG, et al. Predicting the 30-year risk of cardiovascular disease: the Framingham Heart Study. *Circulation*, 2009; Vol. 119: pp. 3078–84.

Comments: Extends Framingham risk data to 30 years.

Petersson U, Ostgren CJ, Brudin L, et al. A consultation-based method is equal to SCORE and an extensive laboratory-based method in predicting risk of future cardiovascular disease. *Eur J Cardiovasc Prev Rehabil*, 2009; Vol. 16: pp. 536–40.

Comments: Clinical variables: age, sex, history of diabetes or hypertension, smoking, family history of CVD, measured hypertension, and waist/height ratio predicted 17-year history of major vascular events as well as models that included laboratory variables. The most effective estimation of CVD risk is obtained by the history and physical examination.

Shaw LJ, Min JK, Budoff M, et al. Induced cardiovascular procedural costs and resource consumption patterns after coronary artery calcium screening: results from the EISNER (Early Identification of Subclinical Atherosclerosis by Noninvasive Imaging Research) study. *J Am Coll Cardiol*, 2009; Vol. 54: pp. 1258–67.

Comments: Use of testing was appropriate in a large cohort after CAC screening.

Vasan RS, Kannel WB. Strategies for cardiovascular risk assessment and prevention over the life course: progress amid imperfections. *Circulation*, 2009; Vol. 120: pp. 360–3.

Comments: Summary of the Framingham risk assessment and advice regarding population, primary, and secondary prevention of coronary heart disease.

Emerging Risk Factors Collaboration, Di Angelantonio E, Sarwar N, et al. Major lipids, apolipoproteins, and risk of vascular disease. *JAMA*, 2009; Vol. 302: pp. 1993–2000.

Comments: Measuring nonfasting total cholesterol and HDL cholesterol without regard to triglycerides may be most practical way to evaluate and treat CV risk.

Lloyd-Jones D, Adams R, Carnethon M, et al. Heart disease and stroke statistics—2009 update: a report from the American Heart Association Statistics Committee and Stroke Statistics Subcommittee. *Circulation*, 2009; Vol. 119: pp. e21–181.

Comments: Annual statistical update of heart disease and stroke from the American Heart Association.

COMPLICATIONS AND COMORBIDITIES

Action to Control Cardiovascular Risk in Diabetes Study Group, Gerstein HC, Miller ME, et al. Effects of intensive glucose lowering in type 2 diabetes. *NEJM*, 2008; Vol. 358: pp. 2545–59.

Comments: A summary of the results of the ACCORD study on glucose lowering.

Gaede P, Lund-Andersen H, Parving HH, et al. Effect of a multifactorial intervention on mortality in type 2 diabetes. *NEJM*, 2008; Vol. 358: pp. 580–91.

Comments: The Steno-2 study demonstrated that a multifactorial intervention including multiple drug interventions and behavioral modification effectively reduced death from any cause and development of microvascular complications.

Waldstein SR, Rice SC, Thayer JF, et al. Pulse pressure and pulse wave velocity are related to cognitive decline in the Baltimore Longitudinal Study of Aging. *Hypertension*, 2008; Vol. 51: pp. 99–104.

Comments: Data suggest that treatment of risk factors for vascular stiffness may delay cognitive decline.

Stamler J. Population-wide adverse dietary patterns: a pivotal cause of epidemic coronary heart disease/cardiovascular disease. *J Am Diet Assoc*, 2008; Vol. 108: pp. 228–32.

Comments: Superb summary and analysis of data supporting title of his article. Important references.

Iwasaki K, Matsumoto T, Aono H, et al. Prevalence of subclinical atherosclerosis in asymptomatic diabetic patients by 64-slice computed tomography. *Coron Artery Dis*, 2008; Vol. 19: pp. 195–201.

Comments: This study used coronary CT to demonstrate that asymptomatic persons with diabetes and no known history of CVD had a much higher risk of coronary plaques and significant coronary stenosis compared to persons without diabetes.

Metz LD, Beattie M, Hom R, et al. The prognostic value of normal exercise myocardial perfusion imaging and exercise echocardiography: a meta-analysis. *J Am Coll Cardiol*, 2007; Vol. 49: pp. 227–37.

Comments: Distillation of extensive literature on use of two most commonly used types of exercise stress testing.

Grundy SM. Diabetes and coronary risk equivalency: what does it mean? *Diabetes Care*, 2006; Vol. 29: pp. 457–60.

Comments: Good discussion on whether the use of "coronary risk equivalent" is applicable for diabetes.

Law MR, Wald NJ, Morris JK. The performance of blood pressure and other cardiovascular risk factors as screening tests for ischaemic heart disease and stroke. *J Med Screen*, 2004; Vol. 11: pp. 3–7.

Comments: This paper is a classic and should be read carefully by all who provide medical care for persons with diabetes and especially by administrators and policy makers.

Gale EA. The Hawthorne studies—a fable for our times? *QJM*, 2004; Vol. 97: pp. 439–49.

Comments: Classic history of classic study that showed that close relationship and frequent review of process may improve outcomes. Should be read by all medical practitioners.

Selvin E, Marinopoulos S, Berkenblit G, et al. Meta-analysis: glycosylated hemoglobin and cardiovascular disease in diabetes mellitus. *Ann Intern Med*, 2004; Vol. 141: pp. 421–31.

Comments: This meta-analysis demonstrated that in pooled analysis, persons with type 2 diabetes had an 18% significantly higher risk of CVD with each 1% increase in HbA1c. In type 1 diabetes, the risk of CVD was 15% higher for each 1% increase in HbA1c but the results were not statistically significant.

Hanefeld M, Cagatay M, Petrowitsch T, et al. Acarbose reduces the risk for myocardial infarction in type 2 diabetic patients: meta-analysis of seven long-term studies. *Eur Heart J*, 2004; Vol. 25: pp. 10–6.

Comments: Meta-analysis of acarbose trials.

Sjöström L, Lindroos AK, Peltonen M, et al. Lifestyle, diabetes, and cardiovascular risk factors 10 years after bariatric surgery. *NEJM*, 2004; Vol. 351: pp. 2683–93.

Comments: In a large controlled trial of gastric bypass surgery in Sweden, cardiovascular risk factors were reduced in the bypass patients.

Yusuf S, Hawken S, Ounpuu S, et al. Effect of potentially modifiable risk factors associated with myocardial infarction in 52 countries (the INTERHEART study): case-control study. *Lancet*, 2004; Vol. 364: pp. 937–52.

Comments: The INTERHEART study reported that "Abnormal lipids, smoking, hypertension, diabetes, abdominal obesity, psychosocial factors, level of consumption of fruits, vegetables, and alcohol (lack of moderate consumption), and lack of regular physical activity account for most of the risk of myocardial infarction worldwide in both sexes and at all ages in all regions."

Pearson TA, Mensah GA, Alexander RW, et al. Markers of inflammation and cardiovascular disease: application to clinical and public health practice: a statement for healthcare professionals from the Centers for Disease Control and Prevention and the American Heart Association. *Circulation*, 2003; Vol. 107: pp. 499–511.
Comments: AHA/CDC guidelines on using hs-CRP to stratify CVD risk in practice.

Warburton RN. What do we gain from the sixth coronary heart disease drug? *BMJ*, 2003; Vol. 327: pp. 1237–8.
Comments: Editorial that reviews cost-effectiveness of drug therapy for prevention of CVD. Excellent introduction to the literature.

Redberg RF, Greenland P, Fuster V, et al. Prevention Conference VI: Diabetes and Cardiovascular Disease: Writing Group III: risk assessment in persons with diabetes. *Circulation*, 2002; Vol. 105: pp. e144–52.
Comments: Describes the increased risk of CVD in persons with diabetes.

Paffenbarger RS, Blair SN, Lee IM. A history of physical activity, cardiovascular health and longevity: the scientific contributions of Jeremy N Morris, DSc, DPH, FRCP. *Int J Epidemiol*, 2001; Vol. 30: pp. 1184–92.
Comments: Masterful review of exercise and CVD.

Zhou G, Myers R, Li Y, et al. Role of AMP-activated protein kinase in mechanism of metformin action. *J Clin Invest*, 2001; Vol. 108: pp. 1167–74.
Comments: Study of mechanism of metformin cardiovascular protection and pleiotropic effects.

Wald NJ, Hackshaw AK, Frost CD. When can a risk factor be used as a worthwhile screening test? *BMJ*, 1999; Vol. 319: pp. 1562–5.
Comments: Demonstration of when a risk factor may be useful as a screening test. Classic reference.

Haffner SM, Lehto S, Rmaa T, et al. Mortality from coronary heart disease in subjects with type 2 diabetes and in nondiabetic subjects with and without prior myocardial infarction. *NEJM*, 1998; Vol. 339: pp. 229–34.
Comments: This Finnish study demonstrated that persons with diabetes and no previous MI had as high a risk of incident MI over 7 years as persons without diabetes and history of previous MI.

Peabody FW. Landmark article March 19, 1927: the care of the patient. By Francis W. Peabody. *JAMA*, 1984; Vol. 252: pp. 813–8.
Comments: Classic essential article, written by Peabody as he was dying.

US Dept. of Health and Human Services, Centers for Medicare and Medicaid Services. http://www.cms.gov/CardiovasDiseaseScreening/. Accessed October 5, 2010.
Comments: CMS web site reviews cholesterol screening benefit for Medicare beneficiaries, who must have no signs or symptoms of CVD and must be fasting for 12 hours. There is no copay or deductible and the test may be ordered every 5 years.

COMPLICATIONS AND COMORBIDITIES

DYSLIPIDEMIA

Simeon Margolis, MD, PhD

DEFINITION

- Elevated blood levels of lipids (cholesterol and triglycerides) and/or abnormalities in the blood concentrations of lipoproteins including: increased low-density lipoprotein cholesterol (LDL-C), decreased high-density lipoprotein cholesterol (HDL-C), and increased lipoprotein(a) [Lp(a)].
- Normal fasting triglyceride levels are <150 mg/dl. Triglycerides >500 mg/dl are considered very high.

- Desirable levels of LDL-C in patients with diabetes are <100 mg/dL and probably <70 mg/dl.
- HDL-C levels are considered too low when <40 mg/dl in men and <50 mg/dl in women.
- Non-HDL cholesterol = total cholesterol – HDL-C.
- Normal levels of Lp(a) vary with the laboratory methods used to measure them.

EPIDEMIOLOGY

- Diabetic dyslipidemia: most common lipid abnormality is elevated triglycerides. Almost equally common is low levels of HDL-C (Howard).
- On average LDL-C and Lp(a) levels are no higher in individuals with diabetes compared to those without diabetes.
- Diabetic dyslipidemia is associated with greater amounts of atherogenic, small dense LDL-C.
- Severe insulin deficiency can be associated with very high triglycerides and the risk of acute pancreatitis.
- Cardiovascular disease, the most common cause of death in diabetes, is already present in about half of patients with type 2 diabetes at the time of diagnosis and is the most important long-term sequela of untreated diabetic dyslipidemia (Haffner).

DIAGNOSIS

- Obtain a fasting lipid panel (cholesterol, triglycerides, and HDL-C) at time of diagnosis and at least annually if normal during follow-up (see Lipids, p. 589).
- Small dense LDL-C can be determined by measuring apolipoprotein B or by NMR spectroscopy, measuring lipoprotein subfractions.
- In patients with hypertriglyceridemia, presence of chylomicrons can be detected by observing a lipid layer on top of plasma after overnight refrigeration.
- In patients with triglycerides over 1000 mg/dl, serum amylase and lipase may be normal with attacks of acute pancreatitis.

SIGNS AND SYMPTOMS

- No signs or symptoms are associated with modestly elevated triglycerides or with abnormal levels or LDL-C, HDL-C, or Lp(a).
- Tendon xanthomas and xanthelasma palpebra may indicate familial hypercholesterolemia, but about 50% of people with xanthelasmas have normal cholesterol levels.
- Yellow appearance of palmar creases in dysbetalipoproteinemia.
- Eruptive xanthomas (maculopapular with white "head" containing triglyceride), tuberous xanthomas around the elbows and knees, and lipemia retinalis in severe hypertriglyceridemia.
- Extremely high triglycerides may cause pancreatitis, with severe abdominal pain, nausea and vomiting.

CLINICAL TREATMENT

- **Aim:** Prevention of cardiovascular disease (Colhoun). A second goal is to prevent acute pancreatitis.
- Always begin with lifestyle measures to manage dyslipidemias. To lower LDL-C: diet containing <35% total fat calories, <7% saturated fat, <200 mg cholesterol per day.
- Weight loss and glycemic control most effective in lowering triglycerides.

- Exercise can lower triglycerides and raise HDL-C, but relatively ineffective in lowering LDL-C.
- Statins are most effective drugs to lower LDL-C and are usually starting drug for diabetic dyslipidemia (see Statins and Combination Pills, p. 415).
- Fibrates, Lovaza (omega-3-acid ethyl esters), and over-the-counter fish oil capsules are most effective treatments for very high triglycerides (see Fibric Acid Derivatives, p. 405).
- Niacin preparations are most effective drugs to raise HDL-C and generally do not significantly worsen glycemic control (Grundy) (see Niacin, p. 409).
- Pioglitazone is more effective than rosiglitazone in lowering triglycerides, raising HDL-C, and lowering LDL-C (Goldberg) (see Thiazolidinediones, p. 451).
- The bile acid sequestrant, colesevelam, improves glycemic control, lowers LDL-C by about 15%, and decreases small dense LDL (Fonseca).
- If triglycerides remain >200 mg/dl during statin treatment, consider adding a fibrate or niacin.
- Expected benefit from different lipid-lowering therapies are shown in Table 3-1.

TABLE 3-1. EXPECTED BENEFIT FROM DIFFERENT LIPID-LOWERING THERAPIES

Medication	Total and LDL Cholesterol	TG	HDL	Comments
Statins	down 25% to 50%	down 10% to 20%	up 6% to 10%	Statins are not drugs of choice if triglycerides are >500 mg/dl.
Niacin	down 10% to 25%	down 15% to 25%	up 15% to 30%	Most effective drugs to raise HDL.
Fibrates	down 10%	down 30% to 50%	up 6% to 8%	May raise LDL cholesterol when initial triglycerides >500 mg/dl.
Bile Acid Sequestrants	down 15% to 25%	0 or increased	up 6% to 8%	Should not be used in patients with elevated triglyceride levels (>200–300 mg/dl). Can raise triglycerides even more.
Ezetimibe	down 10% to 20%	0	0	Effective at lowering total and LDL cholesterol, usually used with a statin.

Courtesy of Simeon Margolis.

COMPLICATIONS AND COMORBIDITIES

FOLLOW-UP

- If lifestyle measures do not achieve targets after 4–6 weeks, add a cholesterol-lowering drug (Brunzell).
- Do lipid panel and liver enzymes 4–6 weeks after starting drug to determine its effectiveness.
- After 4–6 weeks, if LDL-C targets are not achieved and liver enzymes are normal, raise statin dose or add ezetimibe (see p. 402).
- Targets of statin treatment: LDL-C <100 mg/dl or total cholesterol/HDL-C <2.0.
- After the initial dose, further doubling of statin dose produces ~6% reduction (from baseline) in LDL-C.
- If a fibrate is added to lower triglycerides, choose fibric acid rather than gemfibrozil for lower risk of myositis. Target is non-HDL cholesterol <100 mg/dl.
- Second line therapy for hypertriglyceridemia is niacin for modestly elevated triglycerides, and either over-the-counter fish oil capsules or the prescription drug Lovaza for triglycerides >500 mg/dl (see Omega-3 Fatty Acids [Fish Oils], p. 412).
- Many experts recommend adding Niaspan if HDL-C remains <40 mg/dl in men or <50 mg/dl in women (Grundy).
- Measure CK if any complaints of muscle pain or weakness (need not measure at baseline). Stop statins and/or reduce statin dose if troublesome muscle symptoms occur to see if muscle symptoms go away. Stop statin if CK is ≥1000 mg/dl. If symptoms disappear within 2 weeks and CK was less than 1000, can restart same statin at a lower dose or choose a different statin. Use statin cautiously if CK was ≥1000 mg/dl.
- Stop statin if liver enzymes 3 times or more higher than upper limits of normal.
- Ask about muscle pain and weakness at every patient visit.

EXPERT OPINION

- Must increase statin dose or add another drug if follow-up results do not meet target.
- Initiate a statin cautiously in patients at higher risk of myositis (i.e., those on drugs like gemfibrozil, antifungal agents, or cyclosporin).
- Even modest weight loss (5% to 19% of body weight) in people who are either mildly overweight or more obese can dramatically reduce triglycerides.
- To determine effect of weight loss on triglycerides, wait until weight has stabilized; triglyceride levels may be falsely low during periods of weight loss.

BASIS FOR RECOMMENDATIONS

Brunzell JD, Davidson M, Furberg CD, et al. Lipoprotein management in patients with cardiometabolic risk: consensus statement from the American Diabetes Association and the American College of Cardiology Foundation. *Diabetes Care,* 2008; Vol. 31: pp. 811–22.

Comments: Consensus statement from ADA and American College of Cardiology regarding lipoprotein management in patients with cardiometabolic risk.

OTHER REFERENCES

Colhoun HM, Betteridge DJ, Durrington PN, et al. Effects of atorvastatin on kidney outcomes and cardiovascular disease in patients with diabetes: an analysis from the Collaborative Atorvastatin Diabetes Study (CARDS). *Am J Kidney Dis,* 2009; Vol. 54: pp. 810–9.

Comments: 2838 patients with type 2 diabetes and no prior history of cardiovascular disease were assigned to either 10 mg atorvastatin or placebo. During a median follow-up of 3.9 years, the treated group had about a 40% reduction in major cardiovascular events whether they had renal impairment or not.

Neeli H, Gadi R, Rader DJ. Managing diabetic dyslipidemia: beyond statin therapy. *Curr Diab Rep*, 2009; Vol. 9: pp. 11–7.

Comments: In the management of diabetic dyslipidemia, consideration should be given to lowering triglycerides and raising HDL-C in addition to lowering LDL-C with statins.

Mora S. Advanced lipoprotein testing and subfractionation are not (yet) ready for routine clinical use. *Circulation*, 2009; Vol. 119: pp. 2396–404.

Comments: It is not necessary to measure apoproteins or obtain particle number and size to determine risk of cardiovascular disease.

American Diabetes Association, Bantle JP, Wylie-Rosett J, et al. Nutrition recommendations and interventions for diabetes: a position statement of the American Diabetes Association. *Diabetes Care*, 2008; Vol. 31 Suppl 1: pp. S61–78.

Comments: ADA recommendations for nutritional management of diabetes.

Fonseca VA, Rosenstock J, Wang AC, et al. Colesevelam HCl improves glycemic control and reduces LDL cholesterol in patients with inadequately controlled type 2 diabetes on sulfonylurea-based therapy. *Diabetes Care*, 2008; Vol. 31: pp. 1479–84.

Comments: Colesevelam improves glycemic control and lowers LDL-C by about 15%.

El Harchaoui K, van der Steeg WA, Stroes ES, et al. Value of low-density lipoprotein particle number and size as predictors of coronary artery disease in apparently healthy men and women: the EPIC-Norfolk Prospective Population Study. *J Am Coll Cardiol*, 2007; Vol. 49: pp. 547–53.

Comments: LDL-C particle number and size are better predictors of cardiovascular disease risk than other measures of blood lipids and lipoproteins.

Goldberg RB, Kendall DM, Deeg MA, et al. A comparison of lipid and glycemic effects of pioglitazone and rosiglitazone in patients with type 2 diabetes and dyslipidemia. *Diabetes Care*, 2005; Vol. 28: pp. 1547–54.

Comments: Triglycerides fell significantly with pioglitazone but rose slightly with rosiglitazone. Pioglitazone also raised HDL-C more than rosiglitazone and was associated with a smaller rise in LDL-C.

Keech A, Simes RJ, Barter P, et al. Effects of long-term fenofibrate therapy on cardiovascular events in 9795 people with type 2 diabetes mellitus (the FIELD study): randomised controlled trial. *Lancet*, 2005; Vol. 366: pp. 1849–61.

Comments: The FIELD study randomized 9795 participants with type 2 diabetes to either fenofibrate or placebo for 5 years. Less than a third of the subjects had known cardiovascular disease. The effects on cardiovascular disease are difficult to interpret, but no dramatic benefits were observed.

Rubins HB, Robins SJ, Collins D, et al. Diabetes, plasma insulin, and cardiovascular disease: subgroup analysis from the Department of Veterans Affairs high-density lipoprotein intervention trial (VA-HIT). *Arch Intern Med*, 2002; Vol. 162: pp. 2597–604.

Comments: In the VA-HIT trial, gemfibrozil significantly reduced major cardiovascular events in men who had type 2 diabetes or insulin resistance and known coronary heart disease.

Grundy SM, Vega GL, McGovern ME, et al. Efficacy, safety, and tolerability of once-daily niacin for the treatment of dyslipidemia associated with type 2 diabetes: results of the assessment of diabetes control and evaluation of the efficacy of niaspan trial. *Arch Intern Med*, 2002; Vol. 162: pp. 1568–76.

Comments: Niacin (Niaspan) can be used to treat diabetic dyslipidemia with minimal adverse effects on glycemic control.

Huang ES, Meigs JB, Singer DE. The effect of interventions to prevent cardiovascular disease in patients with type 2 diabetes mellitus. *Am J Med*, 2001; Vol. 111: pp. 633–42.

Comments: This meta-analysis of 7 randomized trials in patients with type 2 diabetes found substantial cardiovascular benefits from lowering cholesterol levels.

Lemieux I, Lamarche B, Couillard C, et al. Total cholesterol/HDL cholesterol ratio vs LDL cholesterol/HDL cholesterol ratio as indices of ischemic heart disease risk in men: the Quebec Cardiovascular Study. *Arch Intern Med*, 2001; Vol. 161: pp. 2685–92.

Comments: Total cholesterol/HDL-C is a better predictor of cardiovascular risk than LDL-C/HDL-C.

Haffner SM, Lehto S, Rönnemaa T, et al. Mortality from coronary heart disease in subjects with type 2 diabetes and in nondiabetic subjects with and without prior myocardial infarction. *NEJM*, 1998; Vol. 339: pp. 229–34.

Comments: Individuals with diabetes but without a prior myocardial infarction have as high a risk of myocardial infarction as individuals without diabetes but with previous myocardial infarction.

Howard BV. Lipoprotein metabolism in diabetes mellitus. *J Lipid Res*, 1987; Vol. 28: pp. 613–28.

Comments: A detailed description of the lipid abnormalities in diabetes and their underlying causes.

HEART FAILURE

Sheldon H. Gottlieb, MD

DEFINITION

- **Heart failure (HF):** the heart, when functioning at a normal filling pressure, is unable to pump enough blood to meet the needs of the body, leading to maladaptive responses including volume overload (congestion), shortness of breath and fatigue, and an increased risk of sudden death.
- **Congestive heart failure (CHF)** is a less-preferred term for HF, in which symptoms and signs of congestion predominate. Most patients with HF do not have clinical signs of congestion (although BNP/ProBNP levels may be elevated, see Signs and Symptoms section) (Arnold 2006).
- **Systolic (HF):** when ejection fraction (EF) <45%.
- **Diastolic HF:** also called HF with preserved EF, when the HF occurs with EF ≥45%.
- **Chronic HF:** usually treated as an outpatient.
- **Acute decompensated HF:** a medical emergency usually requiring hospitalization.
- **Advanced HF:** when symptoms that limit normal daily activities persist despite appropriate treatment.

EPIDEMIOLOGY

- Incidence and prevalence of HF increase exponentially with age; at age 60, prevalence about 1%; by age 80, about 10%. Persons >age 40 have 20% lifetime risk of HF.
- HF is the most frequent reason for hospital admission and readmission in patients older than 65 years; most HF patients have >5 comorbid problems.
- Treatment of HF consumes 1%–3% of the total healthcare budget in developed countries.
- Annual hospitalization rates in US about 200 per 10,000 population, expected to increase; patients with chronic HF hospitalized 1 or 2 times per year on average, even with excellent care.
- 5-year mortality for HF higher than for breast or colon cancer.
- Diabetes increases risk of developing HF 3–5 fold. Women affected more than men.
- Hypertension and coronary heart disease, often in association with diabetes or metabolic syndrome, are most common etiologies of HF in developed countries. Rheumatic heart disease and cardiomyopathy due to infection (Chaga's disease in South America), HIV, or malnutrition with vitamin deficiency (beriberi) are frequent causes in developing countries.
- Strong association of smoking with HF.

DIAGNOSIS

- HF is a clinical syndrome, not a disease. Need to establish the underlying cause of HF; this may require repeated investigations.

- History of shortness of breath/fatigue and signs of congestion suggest but do not necessarily make diagnosis of HF.
- Diagnostic tests: ECG (arrhythmia, LVH, ischemia), chest X-ray (heart size and shape, cardiothoracic ratio >.5, pulmonary congestion), echocardiogram (regional and overall cardiac function, cardiomyopathy, valvular heart disease, pericardial disease, tumors), and blood tests for natriuretic peptides, BNP, and ProBNP.
- BNP and ProBNP have a very high negative predictive value: normal values rule out diagnosis of HF. High values still require clinical correlation (see below); do not differentiate between HF due to systolic or diastolic dysfunction. Normal values and cut points for HF diagnosis depend on age and renal function (Arnold 2007).
- Troponin I frequently elevated in acute decompensated HF even without coronary heart disease, due to subendocardial ischemia caused by markedly elevated left ventricular end diastolic pressure.
- Association of hemoglobin A1c with mortality in HF may be U-shaped, with lowest mortality among those with fair glycemic control (A1c = 7.1%–7.8 %) (Aguilar).
- Cardiac catheterization should be done for heart failure thought to be due to CAD or when etiology is not determined by noninvasive testing.
- Clinical suspicion guides screening for less common causes of HF: hemochromatosis, sarcoidosis, amyloidosis, HIV infection, thyroid disease (hyper- or hypo-), pheochromocytoma, rheumatological diseases, nutritional deficiencies (e.g., thiamine), sleep apnea (Arnold 2006).

SIGNS AND SYMPTOMS

- Common presenting symptoms are dyspnea, orthopnea, paroxysmal nocturnal dyspnea, fatigue, weakness, exercise intolerance, dependent edema, cough, weight gain, abdominal distension ("belly bloat"), nocturia, cool extremities. Less common presentations include cognitive impairment, altered mentation or delirium, nausea, abdominal discomfort, oliguria, anorexia, cyanosis (Arnold 2006). Nocturnal cough typically precedes decompensated HF by 7–14 days.
- Boston criteria: see Table 3-2.

TABLE 3-2. BOSTON CRITERIA FOR CONGESTIVE HEART FAILURE

Criterion	Point Value*
Category I: History	
Rest dyspnea	4
Orthopnea	4
Paroxysmal nocturnal dyspnea	3
Dyspnea on walking on level	2
Dyspnea on climbing	1

(Continued)

COMPLICATIONS AND COMORBIDITIES

TABLE 3-2. *(CONT.)*

Criterion	Point Value*
Category II: Physical examination	
Heart rate abnormality (if 91–110 beats/min, 1 point; if >110 beats/min, 2 points)	1–2
Jugular-venous pressure elevation (if >6 cm H_2O, 2 points; if >6 cm H_2O plus hepatomegaly or edema, 3 points)	2–3
Lung crackles (if basilar, 1 point; if more than basilar, 2 points)	1–2
Wheezing	3
Third heart sound	3
Category III: Chest radiography	
Alveolar pulmonary edema	4
Interstitial pulmonary edema	3
Bilateral pleural effusions	3
Cardiothoracic ratio >0.50 (posteroanterior projection)	3
Upper zone flow redistribution	2

*No more than 4 points were allowed from each of three categories, and hence the composite score, the sum of the subtotal from each category, had a maximum possible of 12 points. The diagnosis of heart failure was classified definite for a score of 8–12 points, possible for a score of 4 to 7 points, and unlikely for a score of 4 points or less.
Source: Marantz PR, Tobin JN, Wassertheil-Smoller S, et al. The relationship between left ventricular systolic function and congestive heart failure diagnosed by clinical criteria. *Circulation*, 1998; Vol. 77: pp. 607–12.

- Patients with compensated HF frequently have no signs of congestion ("warm-dry patients" when cardiac output at rest is normal; "cold-dry patients" when cardiac output at rest is low) (Nohria).
- BNP/ProBNP levels are useful when diagnosis uncertain, especially in setting of advanced pulmonary disease, and for prognosis when levels are followed serially (Doust).
- Functional capacity classes: (1) very active, (2) moderately active, (3) sedentary, (4) very sedentary or bed rest. Refer to Veterans Specific Activity Questionnaire (Myers). New York Heart Association Classification: (1) no symptoms; (2) symptoms with ordinary activity; (3) symptoms with less than ordinary activity—may require assistance to bathe and dress; (4) symptoms at rest.
- Delirium is frequently seen in elderly patients with acutely decompensated chronic HF; when HF becomes compensated, elderly often are found to have cognitive impairment.

- Older patients often present with acute decompensated HF due to pneumonia, sepsis, myocardial infarction, or acute arrhythmias such as atrial fibrillation. Valvular heart disease, most frequently aortic stenosis, is a frequent cause of HF in elderly patients who also have coronary heart disease and diabetes.
- Clinical course of chronic HF: often a slow and clinically imperceptible progression with episodes of acute decompensation. Patients with HF die suddenly or from end-stage HF with organ failure, in about equal proportions.
- Frail elderly patients frequently have delirium with decompensated HF and cognitive impairment when HF is compensated (Arnold 2007).

Clinical Treatment

Treatment

- Treat symptoms due to congestion, then find and treat precipitating causes and underlying causes of HF.
- **Acute decompensated HF** treated with diuretics, oxygen, sitting position; morphine IV is often useful to relieve agitation due to dyspnea.
- Acute decompensated HF in the elderly often due to infection; in younger patients, often due to hypertension or ischemia. Suspect sepsis in elderly patients presenting with HF.
- **Chronic HF:** Dietary sodium and fluid restriction is usually recommended, but there is limited evidence. "Moderate" dietary sodium restriction (2g/day) is reasonable. Fluid restriction (1500 ml/day) perhaps in patients with hyponatremia (sodium < 135 mmol/l); hyponatremia itself is a cardinal sign of advanced heart failure and most heart failure patients have both excess fluid and sodium that is not relieved by fluid restriction. Diet: high fiber, whole grains, fruits and vegetable, polyunsaturated fats, protein, low saturated fat, seasonings other than table salt, and moderate alcohol use (Mediterranean diet) is recommended.
- **Systolic HF** is treated with diuretics, angiotensin converting enzyme (ACE) inhibitors or angiotensin receptor blockers (ARBs), beta-blockers, aldosterone blockers, digitalis, and statins when ischemic heart disease is present. Control heart rate and blood pressure; diuretics, beta-blockers, and ACE/ARBs are the cornerstone of treatment.
- **Diastolic HF** often seen in obese patients and those with type 2 diabetes, frequently with sleep apnea. Treatment: diuretics for control of congestion, treat blood pressure, heart rate, lipids and hyperglycemia.
- Strongly evidence-based treatment is available for systolic HF; less evidence to guide treatment of diastolic HF—diuretics and renin-angiotensin blockers improve symptoms (Arnold 2006, see Figure 3-1 and Table 3-3).
- Insulin causes sodium retention and may cause volume overload and decompensated HF in patients with type 2 diabetes, especially when insulin is started at relatively high doses. Patients with HF started on insulin should follow a sodium controlled diet. A1c goals 7%–8%.
- Metformin often discontinued with HF out of concern for lactic acidosis; but evidence is scant. One prospective trial (Roberts) found reduced mortality in diabetic patients treated with metformin. FDA has removed the Black Box Warning for metformin in HF. Therefore, if normal renal function (GFR >60 ml/min), metformin may safely be continued.
- Thiazolidinediones are associated with HF with a hazard ratio of about 2:1 (Home); do not use in patients with a history of HF.

COMPLICATIONS AND COMORBIDITIES

FIGURE 3-1. ALGORITHM FOR TREATMENT OF HF

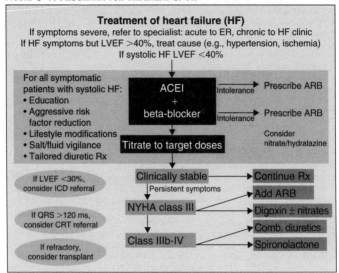

Source: Arnold JM, Liu P, Demers C, et al. Canadian Cardiovascular Society consensus conference recommendations on heart failure 2006: diagnosis and management. *Can J Cardiol*, 2006; Vol. 22(1): 23–45. Reprinted with permission from Pulsus Group, Inc.

TABLE 3-3. EVIDENCE-BASED DRUGS AND ORAL DOSES AS SHOWN IN LARGE CLINICAL TRIALS

Drug	Start Dose	Target Dose
ACE inhibitor		
Captopril	6.25 mg–12.5 mg tid	25 mg–50 mg tid
Enalapril	1.25 mg–2.5 mg bid	10 mg bid
Ramipril	1.25 mg–2.5 mg bid	5 mg bid*
Lisinopril	2.5 mg–5 mg qd	20 mg–35 mg qd
Beta-blocker		
Carvedilol	3.125 mg bid	25 mg bid

Drug	Start Dose	Target Dose
Bisoprolol	1.25 mg qd	10 mg qd
Metoprolol CR/XL+	12.5 mg–25 mg qd	200 mg qd
ARB		
Candesartan	4 mg qd	32 mg qd
Valsartan	40 mg bid	160 mg bid
Aldosterone antagonist		
Spironolactone	12.5 mg qd	50 mg qd
Eplerenone†	25 mg qd	50 mg qd
Vasodilator		
Isosorbide dinitrate	20 mg tid	40 mg tid
Hydralazine	37.5 mg tid	75 mg tid

*The Healing and Early Afterload Raducing Therapy (HEART) trial showed that 10 mg once a day (qd) was effective for attenuating left ventricular remodeling.

†Not available in Canada.

ACE, Angiotensin-converting enzyme; ARB, Angiotensin receptor blocker; bid, Twice a day; qd, Once daily; CR/XL, Controlled release/extended release; tid, 3 times a day
Source: Arnold JM, Liu P, Demers C, et al. Canadian Cardiovascular Society consensus conference recommendations on heart failure 2006: diagnosis and management. *Can J Cardiol,* 2006; Vol. 22(1): 23–45. Reprinted with permission from Pulsus Group Inc.

- HF due to valvular heart disease usually requires surgical repair or replacement of the valve. Timing requires clinical experience and consultation with a cardiologist.
- Pacemaker resynchronization useful for some patients with systolic dysfunction HF and left bundle branch block or wide QRS complexes. Recent studies provide evidence of better outcome with resynchronization pacemaker therapy for moderate HF.
- Patients who smoke cigarettes should be strongly advised to stop smoking.
- Heavy alcohol use associated with poor outcomes in HF. Moderate alcohol use (1 drink/day in women, 1–2 drinks/day in men) associated in most studies with decreased risk and improved outcomes in HF.

FOLLOW-UP

- Acute decompensated HF is a medical emergency requiring hospitalization.
- Chronic HF requires frequent outpatient follow-up; optimally, a team that includes physician, nurse, nutritionist, certified diabetes educator (CDE) and pharmacist.
- Important to determine and maintain the patient's "dry weight" (weight at which signs of congestion have resolved but BP control and renal function are not impaired).

COMPLICATIONS AND COMORBIDITIES

- Observe jugular venous pressure at every visit: patient lying supine at 45 degrees, jugular venous pressure should be just at the clavicle, or about 12–15 cm vertically from the sternal angle.
- Specific treatment goals, for patients with systolic HF: sodium 135–145 mmol/l, potassium 4.5 mmol/l, HR 55–70 bpm at rest, BP <140/90, ideally 110/70 or as tolerated by symptoms of orthostasis, weight at "dry weight", hematocrit >34%.

EXPERT OPINION

- Patients with diabetes and HF require frequent follow-up. If possible, care should not be fragmented between cardiology, endocrinology, and internal medicine. "Team Care" has repeatedly been shown to be effective for patients with HF. They may require monthly office visits if there are any concerns regarding progression of symptoms.
- Examine elderly patients who complain of feeling unwell for signs of HF and measure BNP/ProBNP.
- Maintaining the patients at their "dry weight" is essential. The patients must know their "dry weight" and must weigh themselves daily.
- Many guidelines, including Arnold 2006 recommend A1c goal of <7%, but the ideal A1c for patients with diabetes and HF may be slightly above 7% (Aguilar).
- Flu shots and pneumonia vaccination must be kept current.
- Treatment for advanced HF is essentially palliative care. End-of-life issues must be discussed with the patient and his or her family or significant others.

BASIS FOR RECOMMENDATIONS

Hunt SA, Abraham WT, Chin MH, et al. 2009 focused update incorporated into the ACC/AHA 2005 Guidelines for the Diagnosis and Management of Heart Failure in Adults: a report of the American College of Cardiology Foundation/American Heart Association Task Force on Practice Guidelines Developed in Collaboration With the International Society for Heart and Lung Transplantation. *J Am Coll Cardiol*, 2009; Vol. 53: pp. e1–e90.

Comments: Authoritative review. Lengthy, not easy to read.

Howlett JG, McKelvie RS, Arnold JM, et al. Canadian Cardiovascular Society Consensus Conference guidelines on heart failure, update 2009: diagnosis and management of right-sided heart failure, myocarditis, device therapy and recent important clinical trials. *Can J Cardiol*, 2009; Vol. 25: pp. 85–105.

Comments: Part 3 of the Canadian Cardiovascular Society review of HF. All 3 are beautifully written, concise guides to the science and art of treating patients who have HF.

Arnold JM, Howlett JG, Dorian P, et al. Canadian Cardiovascular Society Consensus Conference recommendations on heart failure update 2007: prevention, management during intercurrent illness or acute decompensation, and use of biomarkers. *Can J Cardiol*, 2007; Vol. 23: pp. 21–45.

Comments: Concise and beautifully written, many clinical pearls; detailed advice regarding when and how to use biomarkers to diagnose and treat HF. Review of use of metformin in HF is outstanding. They recommend an A1c goal of <7 for patients with diabetes and heart failure. See Expert Opinion section above for criticism of this goal.

Arnold JM, Liu P, Demers C, et al. Canadian Cardiovascular Society consensus conference recommendations on heart failure 2006: diagnosis and management. *Can J Cardiol*, 2006; Vol. 22: pp. 23–45.

Comments: Concise and beautifully written; the tables and figures are all well prepared and contain clinical pearls.

OTHER REFERENCES

Home PD, Pocock SJ, Beck-Nielsen H, et al. Rosiglitazone evaluated for cardiovascular outcomes in oral agent combination therapy for type 2 diabetes (RECORD): a multicentre, randomised, open-label trial. *Lancet*, 2009; Vol. 373: pp. 2125–35.

Comments: Thiazolidinediones must be used with great caution, if at all, in patients with HF. See also Arnold 2007.

Aguilar D, Bozkurt B, Ramasubbu K, et al. Relationship of hemoglobin A1C and mortality in heart failure patients with diabetes. *J Am Coll Cardiol*, 2009; Vol. 54: pp. 422–8.

Comments: Demonstration of "U-shaped curve" of A1c levels in HF.

Noyes K, Corona E, Veazie P, Dick AW, Zhao H, Moss AJ. Examination of the effect of implantable cardioverter-defibrillators on health-related quality of life: based on results from the Multicenter Automatic Defibrillator Trial-II. *Am J Cardiovasc Drugs*, 2009; Vol. 9(6): pp. 393–400.

Comments: Important review of use of device therapy in HF.

Roberts F, Ryan GJ. The safety of metformin in heart failure. *Ann Pharmacother*, 2007; Vol. 41: pp. 642–6.

Comments: Important review.

Doust JA, Pietrzak E, Dobson A, et al. How well does B-type natriuretic peptide predict death and cardiac events in patients with heart failure: systematic review. *BMJ*, 2005; Vol. 330: p. 625.

Comments: Biomarkers have become essential tools in the diagnosis and management of HF.

Nohria A, Tsang SW, Fang JC, et al. Clinical assessment identifies hemodynamic profiles that predict outcomes in patients admitted with heart failure. *J Am Coll Cardiol*, 2003; Vol. 41: pp. 1797–804.

Comments: Study of utility of clinical assessment of 4 different profiles of perfusion-congestion in HF patients.

Davis RC, Hobbs FD, Lip GY. ABC of heart failure. History and epidemiology. *BMJ*, 2000; Vol. 320: pp. 39–42.

Comments: First of a 10-part series on HF in the *British Medical Journal*. The presentation is outstanding; still a very useful series of articles.

Myers J, Do D, Herbert W, et al. A nomogram to predict exercise capacity from a specific activity questionnaire and clinical data. *Am J Cardiol*, 1994; Vol. 73: pp. 591–6.

Comments: The Veterans Specific Activity Scale quickly and accurately estimates exercise capacity.

Marantz PR, Tobin JN, Wassertheil-Smoller S, et al. The relationship between left ventricular systolic function and congestive heart failure diagnosed by clinical criteria. *Circulation*, 1988; Vol. 77: pp. 607–12.

Comments: Presentation of the "Boston Criteria" for diagnosis of heart failure.

HYPERTENSION

Nisa M. Maruthur, MD, MHS

DEFINITION

- Systolic blood pressure ≥130 mmHg or diastolic blood ≥80 mmHg on 2 separate days in individuals with diabetes.

EPIDEMIOLOGY

- Hypertension present in 20%–60% of those with diabetes.
- **Type 1 diabetes:** Hypertension often the result of diabetic nephropathy and may occur later.
- **Type 2 diabetes:** Hypertension is a common comorbid condition, often occurring before diabetes is diagnosed.
- Hypertension associated with both macrovascular (e.g., coronary heart disease and stroke) and microvascular (diabetic retinopathy and nephropathy) complications and death (UKPDS 36).
- Blood pressure lowering reduces complications of diabetes: macrovascular and microvascular complications and death (UKPDS 38, ADVANCE).

DIAGNOSIS

- Systolic blood pressure >130 mmHg or diastolic blood pressure >80 mmHg in seated position on 2 separate days; note this cutoff is lower than that for nondiabetes (>140/90 mmHg).

- Laboratory screening for urinalysis, CBC, electrolytes, fasting lipid profile, electrocardiogram.
- Evaluation for secondary causes of hypertension if blood pressure resistant to three or more antihypertensive agents, worsening control in previously well-controlled patient, severe hypertension (>180/110 mmHg), significant hypertensive target organ damage, onset in adults <20 years or >50 years of age, lack of family history, findings on exam or laboratory results that suggest secondary cause.
- Secondary causes of hypertension include renal artery stenosis, renal parenchymal disease, coarctation of aorta, drugs (e.g., estrogen), diet (e.g., high salt), hyperaldosteronism, pheochromocytoma, Cushing's syndrome, obstructive sleep apnea, erythropoieitin side effect, other endocrine disorders (e.g., hyperthyroidism).

SIGNS AND SYMPTOMS

- Symptoms not usually present but can include headache, chest pain, and shortness of breath.
- Signs of chronic end-organ damage include atherosclerotic vascular disease, left ventricular hypertrophy, diastolic dysfunction, chronic kidney disease, diabetic retinopathy.
- Patients with hypertensive crises may present with stroke or myocardial infarction.
- Secondary hypertension: abdominal bruit, elevated BUN/creatinine, delayed femoral pulses, presence of electrolyte abnormalities (i.e., hypokalemia, hypernatremia), paroxysmal hypertension and tachycardia, hirsutism, snoring, and daytime somnolence.

CLINICAL TREATMENT

- Systolic blood pressure 130–139 mmHg or diastolic blood pressure 80–89 mmHg: lifestyle (diet and physical activity) modification for up to 3 months and then proceed with pharmacologic therapy if blood pressure remains elevated.
- Systolic blood pressure ≥140 mmHg or diastolic blood pressure ≥90 mmHg: lifestyle modification AND pharmacologic therapy.
- Diet change to reduce blood pressure includes sodium reduction to <2.4 grams/day (JNC7).
- Dietary Approaches to Stop Hypertension (DASH) dietary pattern (high in fruits, vegetables and low-fat dairy, low in total and saturated fat), and moderation of alcohol consumption (1–2 drinks/day for men and 1 drink/day for women).
- Physical activity (aerobic and resistance training) of moderate intensity or greater for at least 150 minutes per week.
- ACE inhibitor or angiotensin receptor blocker (ARB) as initial pharmacologic therapy.
- Thiazide diuretic (if GFR ≥30 ml/min per 1.73 m²) or loop diuretic (if GFR <30 ml/min per 1.73 m²) as additional therapy to achieve goal blood pressure <130/80 mmHg.
- Add other agents (beta-blockers, calcium channel blockers, etc.) as needed to achieve blood pressure <130/80 mmHg.
- Initiate two agents for confirmed blood pressure ≥150/90 mmHg (JNC7).
- The ADVANCE Trial suggests that blood pressure lowering with a fixed combination of an ACE inhibitor and diuretic (perindopril + indapamide) may be beneficial in reducing vascular events regardless of initial hypertension status.
- Treatment of secondary causes where indicated.

FOLLOW-UP

- Home blood pressure monitoring.
- Measure blood pressure at each diabetes visit.
- Monitor potassium and GFR regularly on ACE inhibitors, ARBs, and diuretics especially with initiation of an agent or with dose change.

EXPERT OPINION

- Blood pressure control is more important than actual pharmacologic agent.
- Hypertension treatment arguably more important than glycemic control to decrease cardiovascular morbidity and mortality among patients with diabetes.

BASIS FOR RECOMMENDATIONS

American Diabetes Association. Standards of medical care in diabetes—2011. *Diabetes Care,* 2011; Vol. 34 Suppl 1: pp. S11–61.

   Comments: American Diabetes Association recommendations for diabetes care including the management of hypertension in patients with diabetes.

Chobanian AV, Bakris GL, Black HR, et al. The seventh report of the Joint National Committee on Prevention, Detection, Evaluation, and Treatment of High Blood Pressure: the JNC 7 report. *JAMA,* 2003; Vol. 289: pp. 2560–72.

   Comments: Widely accepted guideline for the treatment of hypertension with mention of special cases including diabetic hypertension; also describes use of DASH dietary pattern for reduction of hypertension.

Arauz-Pacheco C, Parrott MA, Raskin P. The treatment of hypertension in adult patients with diabetes. *Diabetes Care,* 2002; Vol. 25: pp. 134–47.

   Comments: American Diabetes association technical review of the management of hypertension in patients with diabetes.

OTHER REFERENCES

US Dept of Health and Human Services. The seventh report of the Joint National Committee on Prevention, Detection, Evaluation, and Treatment of High Blood Pressure. *NIH Publication No. 04-5230*; August 2004.

   Comments: Comprehensive report on the epidemiology, diagnosis, and management of hypertension.

Marwick TH, Hordern MD, Miller T, et al. Exercise training for type 2 diabetes mellitus: impact on cardiovascular risk: a scientific statement from the American Heart Association. *Circulation,* 2009; Vol. 119: pp. 3244–62.

   Comments: American Heart Association scientific statement to describe exercise recommendations for patients with diabetes in the context of cardiovascular disease and its risk factors.

Preis SR, Pencina MJ, Hwang SJ, et al. Trends in cardiovascular disease risk factors in individuals with and without diabetes mellitus in the Framingham Heart Study. *Circulation,* 2009; Vol. 120: pp. 212–20.

   Comments: Estimates trends in cardiovascular disease risk factors, including mean blood pressure, in the Framingham Heart Study.

Patel A, ADVANCE Collaborative Group, MacMahon S, et al. Effects of a fixed combination of perindopril and indapamide on macrovascular and microvascular outcomes in patients with type 2 diabetes mellitus (the ADVANCE trial): a randomised controlled trial. *Lancet,* 2007; Vol. 370: pp. 829–40.

   Comments: Results of the blood pressure-lowering regimen (perindopril + indapamide vs placebo) of the ADVANCE trial, a factorial trial, evaluating the effects of blood pressure-lowering and glycemic control on vascular disease in diabetes.

American Heart Association Nutrition Committee, Lichtenstein AH, Appel LJ, et al. Diet and lifestyle recommendations revision 2006: a scientific statement from the American Heart Association Nutrition Committee. *Circulation,* 2006; Vol. 114: pp. 82–96.

   Comments: American Heart Association dietary recommendations based on DASH diet.

Adler AI, Stratton IM, Neil HA, et al. Association of systolic blood pressure with macrovascular and microvascular complications of type 2 diabetes (UKPDS 36): prospective observational study. *BMJ,* 2000; Vol. 321: pp. 412–9.

Comments: UK Prospective Diabetes Study Group 36: Observational study of association between hypertension and macro- and microvascular complications and death.

[No authors listed]. Tight blood pressure control and risk of macrovascular and microvascular complications in type 2 diabetes: UKPDS 38. UK Prospective Diabetes Study Group. *BMJ,* 1998; Vol. 317: pp. 703–13.

Comments: Randomized trial (UK Prospective Diabetes Study Group 38) showing benefit of tight blood pressure control over less tight control on diabetes complications.

Appel LJ, Moore TJ, Obarzanek E, et al. A clinical trial of the effects of dietary patterns on blood pressure. DASH Collaborative Research Group. *NEJM,* 1997; Vol. 336: pp. 1117–24.

Comments: Original research article showing the blood pressure-lowering effect of the Dietary Approaches to Stop Hypertension (DASH) dietary pattern.

METABOLIC SYNDROME

Mary Huizinga, MD, MPH

DEFINITION
- Metabolic syndrome (MS) is the presence of multiple risk factors that tend to occur together and increase risk for cardiovascular disease and/or diabetes.
- Exact criteria listed under Diagnosis.
- Also called "syndrome X" or "insulin resistance syndrome."

EPIDEMIOLOGY
- Prevalence increasing, mirroring the obesity epidemic.
- Ranges from 35%–40% of the US population (Alberti; Alexander).
- Increasing age and Hispanic ethnicity are associated with increased risk of metabolic syndrome (Ford). Among African Americans, women are at an increased risk compared to men but not in Caucasians (Ford).
- No single causative factor known, but insulin resistance, physical inactivity, age, and diet may all contribute to risk.
- In patients with diabetes over the age of 50, 86% have metabolic syndrome (Alexander).
- The risk of developing diabetes is increased five-fold in those with metabolic syndrome compared to persons without metabolic syndrome (Grundy).
- HDL, blood pressure, and diabetes appear to be the most significant components of metabolic syndrome for predicting prevalent coronary heart diseases (CHD) (Alexander). In addition, these individual components have a stronger association with CHD than the syndrome (Konstantinou).
- Persons over age 50 years with metabolic syndrome but without diabetes had a CHD prevalence of 14%; those with both metabolic syndrome and diabetes had a CHD prevalence of 19%. Persons with diabetes but without metabolic syndrome had a CHD prevalence of 7.5% (Alexander).

DIAGNOSIS
- The International Diabetes Federation (IDF) and American Heart Association (AHA)/ National Heart, Lung, and Blood Institute (NHLBI) have recently agreed on the following

definition; however, the definition of elevated waist circumference varies by population and organization (Alberti). Three of the following five components must be present:

1. Elevated fasting triglycerides: ≥150 mg/dl (1.7 mmol/L) or on drug therapy
2. Low HDL: <50 mg/dl (1.3 mmol/l) in women and <40 mg/dl (1.03 mmol/L) in men or on drug therapy
3. Elevated fasting plasma glucose: ≥100 mg/dl or on drug therapy
4. Elevated blood pressure: ≥130 mmHg systolic or ≥85 mmHg diastolic or on antihypertensive drug therapy
5. Elevated waist circumference: population and organization specific definitions (see Table 3-4).

- Elevated prothrombotic markers (e.g., plasminogen activator inhibitor-1) associated with metabolic syndrome (MS) (Appel).

SIGNS AND SYMPTOMS

- Central obesity.
- Insulin resistance: acanthosis nigricans.
- Hyperglycemia: polyuria, polydipsia, fatigue, blurry vision.
- Hypertriglyceridemia: eruptive xanthomas, lipemia retinalils.
- Uncontrolled hypertension: dull headaches, dizziness.
- Other conditions associated with insulin resistance (e.g., sleep apnea).

CLINICAL TREATMENT

- Primary goal is to prevent atherosclerotic disease so general measures for cardiovascular disease prevention and management, such as smoking cessation, are indicated.
- Lifestyle changes: diet and exercise may have independent effects beyond weight loss, such as on hyperglycemia, hypertension, and hypertriglyceridemia, so patients should be encouraged to achieve a 7%–10% weight loss over 6–12 months (Alberti; Grundy).
- Medication therapy aimed at reducing individual components of MS, such as hypertension, dyslipidemia, and hyperglycemia
- Medication therapy may also be aimed at reducing cardiovascular risk factors that are not a part of MS, such as elevated LDL cholesterol.
- Framingham risk scoring should be used to better estimate 10-year atherosclerotic disease risk and may guide the use of medication therapy (available at *http://hp2010. nhlbihin.net/atpiii/CALCULATOR.asp?usertype=prof*).
- Preventive aspirin therapy may be considered in those at moderately high risk.

FOLLOW-UP

- Monitor patients with MS annually for the development of diabetes.
- Follow patients with diabetes and one or more components of MS for development of other components.
- Further diagnostic testing for atherosclerotic disease should be considered in patients with symptoms concerning for CHD (e.g., dyspnea on exertion, chest pain).

EXPERT OPINION

- Individuals with both diabetes and metabolic syndrome have a higher risk for cardiovascular disease than individuals with diabetes or metabolic syndrome alone.
- The majority of persons with diabetes have metabolic syndrome.
- Most risk factors included in MS are modifiable and amenable to lifestyle changes, which is considered primary therapy.

COMPLICATIONS AND COMORBIDITIES

TABLE 3-4. CURRENTLY RECOMMENDED WAIST CIRCUMFERENCE THRESHOLDS FOR ABDOMINAL OBESITY BY ORGANIZATION

Population	Organization (Reference)	Men	Women
Europid	IDF	≥94 cm	≥80 cm
Caucasian	WHO	≥94 cm (increased risk)	≥80 cm (increased risk)
		≥102 cm (still increased risk)	≥88 cm (still higher risk)
United States	AHA/NHLBI (ATP III)*	≥102 cm	≥88 cm
Canada	Health Canada	≥102 cm	≥88 cm
Europe	European Cardiovascular Societies	≥102 cm	≥88 cm
Asian (including Japanese)	IDF	≥90 cm	≥80 cm
Asian	WHO	≥90 cm	≥80 cm
Japanese	Japanese Obesity Society	≥85 cm	≥90 cm
China	Cooperative Task Force	≥85 cm	≥80 cm
Middle East, Mediterranean	IDF	≥94 cm	≥80 cm
Sub-Saharan African	IDF	≥94 cm	≥80 cm
Ethnic Central and South American	IDF	≥90 cm	≥80 cm

*Recent AHA/NHLBI guidlines for metabolic syndrome recognize an increased risk for CVD and diabetes at waist-circumference thresholds of ≥94 cm in men and ≥80 cm in women and identify these as optional cut points for individuals or populations with increased insulin resistance. IDF: International Diabetes Federation, WHO: World Health Organization.

Source: Alberti KG, Eckel RH, Grundy SM, et al. Harmonizing the metabolic syndrome: a joint interim statement of the International Diabetes Federation Task Force on Epidemiology and Prevention; National Heart, Lung, and Blood Institute; American Heart Association; World Heart Federation; International Atherosclerosis Society; and International Association for the Study of Obesity. *Circulation*, 2009; Vol. 120(16): p. 1640 (Table 2). Reprinted with permission of The American Heart Association.

- Medication therapy for MS factors should be considered if patient is at high risk or lifestyle therapy has failed.
- Effective management of MS components can significantly reduce future cardiovascular risk.

BASIS FOR RECOMMENDATIONS

Alberti KG, Eckel RH, Grundy SM, et al. Harmonizing the metabolic syndrome: a joint interim statement of the International Diabetes Federation Task Force on Epidemiology and Prevention; National Heart, Lung, and Blood Institute; American Heart Association; World Heart Federation; International Atherosclerosis Society; and International Association for the Study of Obesity. *Circulation*, 2009; Vol. 120: pp. 1640–5.

Comments: This article describes the latest criteria (2009) for defining the metabolic syndrome. It is a joint statement by the International Diabetes Federation and the American Heart Association/NHLBI.

Grundy SM, Cleeman JI, Daniels SR, et al. Diagnosis and management of the metabolic syndrome: an American Heart Association/National Heart, Lung, and Blood Institute Scientific Statement. *Circulation*, 2005; Vol. 112: pp. 2735–52.

Comments: Statement by the AHA/NHLBI for guidelines issued in 2005.

OTHER REFERENCES

Ogbera AO. Prevalence and gender distribution of the metabolic syndrome. *Diabetol Metab Syndr*, 2010; Vol. 2: p. 1.

Comments: Describes the prevalence of metabolic syndrome in patients with diabetes by age and gender.

Konstantinou DM, Chatzizisis YS, Louridas GE, et al. Metabolic syndrome and angiographic coronary artery disease prevalence in association with the Framingham risk score. *Metab Syndr Relat Disord*, 2010; Vol. 8: pp. 201–8.

Comments: Describes the utility of MS for predicting angiographically significant CAD.

Gardner M, Palmer J, Manrique C, et al. Utility of aspirin therapy in patients with the cardiometabolic syndrome and diabetes. *J Cardiometab Syndr*, 2009; Vol. 4: pp. 96–101.

Comments: This is a review of the mixed literature about aspirin use for the primary prevention of cardiac disease in patients with diabetes and metabolic syndrome.

Grundy SM, Cleeman JI, Daniels SR, et al. Diagnosis and management of the metabolic syndrome: an American Heart Association/National Heart, Lung, and Blood Institute Scientific Statement. *Circulation*, 2005; Vol. 112: pp. 2735–52.

Comments: Statement by the AHA/NHLBI for guidelines issued in 2005.

Appel SJ, Harrell JS, Davenport ML. Central obesity, the metabolic syndrome, and plasminogen activator inhibitor-1 in young adults. *J Am Acad Nurse Pract*, 2005; Vol. 17: pp. 535–41.

Comments: PAI-1 is associated with impaired fibrinolysis and was found to be correlated with waist circumference and metabolic syndrome in this study.

Alexander CM, Landsman PB, Teutsch SM, et al. NCEP-defined metabolic syndrome, diabetes, and prevalence of coronary heart disease among NHANES III participants age 50 years and older. *Diabetes*, 2003; Vol. 52: pp. 1210–4.

Comments: NHANES III study describing epidemiological features of metabolic syndrome using older NCEP metabolic syndrome definition. Limited to persons aged 50 years and older.

Ford ES, Giles WH, Dietz WH. Prevalence of the metabolic syndrome among US adults: findings from the third National Health and Nutrition Examination Survey. *JAMA*, 2002; Vol. 287: pp. 356–9.

Comments: Epidemiological description of metabolic syndrome from NHANES III (1988–1994).

Knowler WC, Barrett-Connor E, Fowler SE, et al. Reduction in the incidence of type 2 diabetes with lifestyle intervention or metformin. *NEJB*, 2002; Vol. 346: pp. 393–403.

Comments: Diabetes Prevention Program—a randomized controlled trial showing that ~7% weight loss significantly reduced the incidence of diabetes in persons with elevated fasting glucose.

COMPLICATIONS AND COMORBIDITIES

OBESITY

Jeanne M. Clark, MD, MPH

DEFINITION

- Excess adipose tissue that affects health.
- Defined clinically as a body mass index (BMI) of ≥30 kg/m² by the World Health Organization (WHO).
- Subdivided into Class 1 (BMI 30–34.9 kg/m²), Class 2 (BMI 35–39.9 kg/m²), and Class 3 (BMI >40 kg/m²). Overweight is BMI 25–29.9 kg/m².
- Visceral adiposity is excess adipose tissue inside the abdominal cavity.
- Visceral adiposity defined clinically as a waist circumference >35 inches (88 cm) for women, or >40 inches (102 cm) for men (WHO).

EPIDEMIOLOGY

- 2007–2008 age-adjusted prevalence of obesity overall: 33.8%; 32.2% in men and 35.5% in women. Overweight and obesity combined (BMI ≥25 kg/m²) prevalence estimate 68% overall; 72% in men and 64% in women (Flegal).
- Nearly 6% of US adults are extremely obese (Class 3).
- Non-hispanic black women have highest prevalence of obesity (49.6%).
- Past 10 years: No significant trends in obesity among women, but significant linear increase for men, apparently leveling off in most recent years (Flegal).
- Prevalence of overweight (BMI > 25 kg/m²) and obesity (BMI > 30 kg/m²) was 80% and 49%, respectively, in US adults with diabetes from 1999–2006. Prevalence of diabetes higher with increasing weight classes, from 8% (normal weight) to 43% (class 3) (Nguyen).
- WHO consultation team found a high risk of type 2 diabetes (T2DM) and cardiovascular disease among some Asian populations at BMIs lower than the existing WHO cutoff for overweight (>25 kg/m²). However, the cutoff for observed risk varies from 22–25 kg/m², but not uniformly. In other Asian populations, for high risk it varies from 26–31 kg/m². Thus, WHO cutoff points were not redefined by ethnicity (WHO Expert Consultation).
- Other organizations, such as the International Diabetes Federation, provide ethnicity-specific cutoffs for central obesity according to waist circumference (IDF Consensus Statement).

CLINICAL TREATMENT

Lifestyle Modification

- Includes combination of reduced calorie diet, physical activity, and behavioral techniques (NIH Practical Guide).
- Can result in weight loss of 5%–10% of initial body weight within 6 months.
- Reduced calorie diet: 500–1000 calories below a eucaloric diet. Eucaloric dietary requirements can be estimated fairly easily (IOM report).
- Rough guides to weight maintenance (eucaloric) requirement: Weight in pounds × 12; or weight (pounds) times 10 + 25% for low activity, 50% for moderate activity, 75% for high level of activity.
- Average weight-reducing diet for men: 1200–1600 kcals/day.
- Average weight-reducing diet for women: 1000–1200 kcals/day.

- Type of diet (low fat vs low carbohydrate vs balanced) is not as important as adherence and perseverance (see Nutrition: Overview in Diabetes, p. 89), and Nutrition for Type 2 Diabetes, p. 97).
- Moderate physical activity, like brisk walking, reduces abdominal fat and contributes modestly to weight loss.
- Behavioral techniques, such as self-monitoring, stimulus control, and meal planning, can enhance adherence and improve weight loss.
- Self-monitoring (i.e., keeping track of diet, physical activity and weight) is the most effective behavioral technique.

Medications for Weight Loss
- Medication may be indicated in patients with a BMI >30 kg/m² or 27–29.9 kg/m² with comorbid conditions (Snow).
- One medication currently FDA approved for long-term (>2 years) use: orlistat (Xenical) (see p. 539).
- Orlistat (120 mg) is a pancreatic lipase inhibitor and is given 30 minutes before each full meal.
- Orlistat produces weight loss of about 2.5–3.0 kg (6–6.5 lbs) at 1 year.
- Side effects of orlistat: diarrhea, loose fatty stool, cramping.
- Sibutramine taken off the market in October 2010 due to cardiovascular risk concerns.
- Other medications, such as phentermine and diethylpropion, are approved for short-term use (<3 months) and can produce weight loss of 3.0–3.5 kg (6.5–7.5 lbs).
- Many over-the-counter agents have been banned by the FDA and, thus, in general, should not be recommended.

Bariatric Surgery
- Bariatric surgery can be considered for patients with a BMI >40 kg/m² or >30–35 kg/m² with comorbidities (Snow) (see Bariatric Surgery, p. 84).
- Surgical procedures include: Roux-en-Y gastric bypass, gastric banding (including adjustable), biliopancreatic diversion (with or without duodenal switch), and sleeve gastrectomy.
- Many insurers require a period (typically 6 months) of medically supervised weight loss prior to surgery.
- Surgery results in weight losses of 20–40 kg (44–88 lbs), which is sustained up to 15 years.
- Weight loss is greatest with the malabsorptive procedures (biliopancreatic diversion and Roux-en-Y gastric bypass) and less with the restrictive procedures (banding, sleeve).
- Perioperative mortality is about 1%, and is lowest when done by surgeons who perform many each year.
- All other adverse events, including postoperative infections, internal (e.g., splenic) injuries, hernias, need for reoperation, etc., occur in about 20%.
- Bariatric surgery is the only obesity treatment that has been shown to reduce mortality long term (Sjostrom).

Weight-Loss Maintenance
- **With lifestyle:** continued self-monitoring and 60 minutes/day of moderate physical activity helps sustain weight loss (Wing).
- **With medication:** continued use of orlistat effective at maintaining weight loss.
- **With surgery:** on average patients maintain substantial weight loss for up to 15 years after surgery if they are compliant with diet and exercise.

COMPLICATIONS AND COMORBIDITIES

FOLLOW-UP

- Lifestyle modification: more frequent follow-up (up to weekly) is associated with greater weight loss.
- Patients consuming <800–1000 kcals/day should be monitored for electrolyte imbalances periodically.
- Medication: after medication is stopped, weight is typically regained, thus long-term treatment should be considered and discussed up front (Snow).
- If there is no weight loss after 3 months, it should be discontinued.
- Orlistat: Patients should take a multivitamin at bedtime to prevent deficiency of fat-soluble vitamins; psyllium can be used to prevent/treat diarrhea.
- Bariatric surgery: Patients need to be monitored for protein malnutrition (albumin, prealbumin), as well as electrolyte (sodium, potassium, phosphorus), vitamin (A, B_{12}, D_{12}, E, K, folic acid, thiamine) and mineral (calcium, iron, magnesium) deficiencies, and replaced as needed (Mechanik).

EXPERT OPINION

- Modest weight loss can prevent type 2 diabetes (T2DM) in those at high risk (Knowler).
- Substantial weight loss can reduce or eliminate the need for medications in some people with T2DM.
- "Resolution" of T2DM can occur within 3 months after gastric bypass surgery in many people; therefore, a diabetes management strategy should be outlined preoperatively (Mechanick).
- Maintenance of reduced body weight is, in virtually every study, far harder than losing weight initially. Successful bariatric surgery may be the exception.

BASIS FOR RECOMMENDATIONS

Snow V, Barry P, Fitterman N, et al. Pharmacologic and surgical management of obesity in primary care: a clinical practice guideline from the American College of Physicians. *Ann Intern Med*, 2005; Vol. 142: pp. 525–31.
  Comments: This article summarizes the guidelines of the American College of Physicians on the use of pharmacologic and surgical treatments for obesity.

NIH/NHLBI. *The Practical Guide: Identification, Evaluation and Treatment of Overweight and Obesity in Adults*, 2000; NIH Publication Number 00-4084. *http://www.nhlbi.nih.gov/guidelines/obesity/prctgd_c.pdf* (accessed 3/1/2011).
  Comments: This guide, available online, reviews the diagnosis and treatment of overweight and obesity.

OTHER REFERENCES

Nguyen NT, Nguyen XM, Lane J, et al. Relationship between obesity and diabetes in a US adult population: findings from the National Health and Nutrition Examination Survey, 1999–2006. *Obes Surg*, 2011; Vol. 21: 351–5.
  Comments: Describes prevalence of overweight and obesity among nationally representative sample of US adults (NHANES).

Flegal KM, Carroll MD, Ogden CL, et al. Prevalence and trends in obesity among US adults, 1999–2008. *JAMA*, 2010; Vol. 303: pp. 235–41.
  Comments: Reports obesity trends in the United States from 1999–2008 using data from the National Health and Nutrition Examination Surveys (NHANES).

Mechanick JI, Kushner RF, Sugerman HJ, et al. American Association of Clinical Endocrinologists, The Obesity Society, and American Society for Metabolic and Bariatric Surgery medical guidelines for clinical practice for the perioperative nutritional, metabolic, and nonsurgical support of the bariatric surgery patient. *Obesity* (Silver Spring), 2009; Vol. 17 Suppl 1: pp. S1–70, v.

Comments: These guidelines outline perioperative and postoperative medical care for bariatric surgery patients including management of diabetes and monitoring for nutritional deficiencies.

Segal JB, Clark JM, Shore AD, et al. Prompt reduction in use of medications for comorbid conditions after bariatric surgery. *Obes Surg*, 2009; Vol. 19: pp. 1646–56.

Comments: This analysis of medical claims data in over 6000 people who underwent bariatric surgery demonstrated that by 12 months, medication use for diabetes had decreased by 76%, compared to 59% for hyperlipidemia, and 51% for hypertension. Use of thyroid replacement and antidepressant medications decreased by less than 10%.

Svetkey LP, Stevens VJ, Brantley PJ, et al. Comparison of strategies for sustaining weight loss: the weight loss maintenance randomized controlled trial. *JAMA*, 2008; Vol. 299: pp. 1139–48.

Comments: This trial demonstrates the difficulty in getting activated patients to maintain weight. After a mean weight loss of 8.5 kg in the first 6 months, participants in the trial regained more than half the weight (4.0–5.5 kg) by 2.5 years later, but regain was less in a group getting continued personal contact.

Sjöström L, Narbro K, Sjöström CD, et al. Effects of bariatric surgery on mortality in Swedish obese subjects. *NEJM*, 2007; Vol. 357: pp. 741–52.

Comments: The Swedish Obesity Study demonstrated that subjects undergoing bariatric surgery had a 25% lower mortality than a morbidly obese comparison group after up to 15 years of follow-up. The reduced mortality was mainly due to a reduction in deaths from cardiovascular disease and cancer.

Institute of Medicine (IOM) Food and Nutrition Board. *Dietary reference intakes for energy, carbohydrate, fiber, fat, fatty acids, cholesterol, protein, and amino acids (macronutrients)*. Washington, DC: National Academy Press; 2005.

Comments: This report details the recommended energy intake for adults and references the use of the Harris-Benedict Equation. There is an easy-to-use calculator on the Mayo Clinic Website: *http://www.mayoclinic.com/health/calorie-calculator/NU00598* (accessed 3/2/2011).

Li Z, Maglione M, Tu W, et al. Meta-analysis: pharmacologic treatment of obesity. *Ann Intern Med*, 2005; Vol. 142: pp. 532–46.

Comments: This meta-analysis found that on average at 12 months, orlistat use resulted in a weight loss of 2.9 kg and sibutramine 4.5 kg. After 6 months, phentermine reduced weight by 3.6 kg and diethylpropion 3.0 kg. Side effects can be significant and differ by medication.

Maggard MA, Shugarman LR, Suttorp M, et al. Meta-analysis: surgical treatment of obesity. *Ann Intern Med*, 2005; Vol. 142: pp. 547–59.

Comments: This meta-analysis found that bariatric surgery resulted in 20–30 kg weight loss, which can be sustained over 10 years. Overall mortality was 1% with about 20% of patients having a less serious adverse event.

WHO Expert Consultation Appropriate body-mass index for Asian populations and its implications for policy and intervention strategies. *Lancet*, 2004; Vol. 363: pp. 157–63.

Comments: A WHO consultation concluded that though risk for type 2 diabetes and cardiovascular disease may be higher at lower BMI cutoffs in Asian populations (i.e., 22–25 kg/m^2), the cutoff for high risk varied between 26–31 kg/m^2. No formal attempts were made to redefine cutoff points by ethnicity.

Knowler WC, Barrett-Connor E, Fowler SE, et al. Reduction in the incidence of type 2 diabetes with lifestyle intervention or metformin. *NEJM*, 2002; Vol. 346: pp. 393–403.

Comments: This randomized trial demonstrated that an average weight loss reduced the risk of diabetes development in an at-risk population by 58%, whereas metformin reduced the risk by 31% compared to placebo.

Wing RR, Hill JO. Successful weight loss maintenance. *Annu Rev Nutr*, 2001; Vol. 21: pp. 323–41.

Comments: Data from the National Weight Control Registry indicated that people who have successfully lost weight and maintained it over several years (average weight loss of 30 kg for an average of 5.5 years) have similar habits including eating a diet low in fat, frequent self-monitoring of body weight and food intake, and high levels of regular physical activity. Weight-loss maintenance may get easier over time. Once these successful maintainers have maintained a weight loss for 2–5 years, the chances of longer-term success greatly increase.

COMPLICATIONS AND COMORBIDITIES

International Diabetes Federation. The IDF consensus worldwide definition of the metabolic syndrome. *http://www.idf.org/webdata/docs/MetSyndrome_FINAL.pdf*.

Comments: International Diabetes Federation consensus statement on definition of metabolic syndrome, which provides ethnicity-specific definitions of central obesity using different cutoffs for waist circumference.

PERIPHERAL VASCULAR DISEASE

Sheldon H. Gottlieb, MD

DEFINITION
- Peripheral vascular disease (PVD) includes disorders of the blood vessels (arteries and veins) outside the heart and brain. Persons with diabetes are especially at risk for ischemia in arteries of the legs and feet, termed lower extremity peripheral artery disease (PAD).
- Claudication is defined as limb pain with activity. It is due to muscle ischemia caused by arterial insufficiency.
- Critical leg ischemia (CLI) is defined as rest pain, ulcerations, or gangrene, with expectation of threatened limb loss within 6 months.
- "Diabetic foot syndrome" includes the combined effect of vascular and neuropathic (foot ulcer) injuries that lead to lower-extremity amputations (Bild).
- Major cause of PAD is atherosclerosis but many conditions, including venous insufficiency, mimic symptoms of PAD—these are called "pseudoclaudication"; see differential diagnosis below.

EPIDEMIOLOGY
- Exponential increase in prevalence of PAD with age in the general population, up to 60% in 85 years and older in white Europeans, little data in other populations (Bennett 2009, *QJM*).
- In <50 years old, PAD almost always due to diabetes plus another risk factor for atherosclerosis (smoking, lipids, hypertension).
- Prevalence of PAD among all persons with diabetes is 20%–30% but much higher among persons with diabetes who are smokers (Marso).
- Risk ratio for diabetes and PAD is 15:1 (i.e., persons with diabetes are 15 times more likely to develop PAD than persons without diabetes) (Bild). (In comparison, risk ratio for smoking and lung cancer is about 10:1.)
- Poor-fitting footwear is thought to be major cause of amputation in PAD (Hennis).
- Mortality of persons with PAD is high, and after any lower extremity amputation, mortality is very high, up to 80% in 5 years (Hambleton).

DIAGNOSIS
- **History:** suspect in persons age <70 years with risk factors of smoking or diabetes, or age >70 years, and symptoms of reduced physical functioning.
- **Differential diagnosis (DDX):** includes mechanical causes of nerve root irritation, arthritic and inflammatory causes, aneurysm, or Baker's cyst causing leg pain, and chronic compartment syndromes. See Table 3-6 for DDX and diagnostic clues.
- **Ankle brachial index (ABI):** key test, done on all persons with PAD to assess severity and to establish a baseline. ABI <0.9 is 95% sensitive for detecting PAD and nearly 100% specific for excluding healthy persons. ABI <0.5 associated with very poor 5-year

survival. See Grenon for instructions on how to perform ABI, and Marso for diagnostic algorithm.

- ABI may be normal at rest due to collateral flow; exercise ABI also an important test (Grenon; Marso). ABI >1.0 in diabetes often due to calcified noncompressible leg vessels.
- When CLI is present, the location and severity of vascular lesions must be determined, as well as hemodynamic requirements for successful revascularization and assessment of risk of endovascular and surgical repair.
- **Duplex ultrasound:** determines location and severity of obstruction.
- **Contrast angiography:** used when revascularization is contemplated, with caution considering renal status.

SIGNS AND SYMPTOMS

- Classification of PAD signs and symptoms include: Fontaine's Stages and Rutherford's Categories (see Table 3-5), ranging from asymptomatic to ulceration or gangrene.
- Claudication is intermittent and reproducibly associated with activity such as walking. Quantitate by distance or time (how many feet or blocks before pain?). Claudication has low sensitivity but high specificity for PAD (Marso).
- Differentiate ischemic, neuropathic, and venous leg and foot ulcers: ischemic ulcers are intensely painful; neuropathic ulcers are painless and located at pressure points of the feet or ankle; venous ulcers are mildly painful. See Table 3-6.

CLINICAL TREATMENT

- CLI is a medical/surgical emergency; urgent evaluation and revascularization may be necessary to avoid high likelihood of amputation within 6 months (Hirsch).

TABLE 3-5. DIAGNOSTIC CATEGORIES OF PAD

Fontaine		Rutherford		
Stage	Clinical	Grade	Category	Clinical
I	Asymptomatic	0	0	Asymptomatic
IIa	Mild—claudication	I	1	Mild claudication
IIb	Moderate–severe claudication	I	2	Moderate claudication
—	—	I	3	Severe claudication
III	Ischemic rest pain	II	4	Ischemic rest pain
IV	Ulceration or gangrene	III	5	Minor tissue loss
—	—	IV	6	Ulceration or gangrene

Source: Bennett PC, Silverman SH, Gill PS, et al. Peripheral arterial disease and Virchow's triad. *Thromb Haemost,* 2009; Vol. 101: pp. 1032–1040. Reprinted with permission of Schattauer GmbH and Professor Lip.

COMPLICATIONS AND COMORBIDITIES

TABLE 3-6. DIFFERENTIAL DIAGNOSIS OF INTERMITTENT CLAUDICATION

Condition	Location of Pain or Discomfort	Characteristic Discomfort	Onset Relative to Exercise	Effect of Rest	Effect of Body Position	Other Characteristics
Intermittent claudication	Buttock, thigh, or calf muscles, and rarely the foot	Cramping, aching, fatigue, weakness, or frank pain	After same degree of exercise	Quickly relieved	None	Reproducible
Nerve root compression (e.g., herniated disc)	Radiates down leg, usually posteriorly	Sharp, lancinating pain	Soon, if not immediately after onset	Not quickly relieved (also often present at rest)	Relief may be aided by adjusting back position	History of back problems
Spinal stenosis	Hip, thigh, buttocks (follows dermatome)	Motor weakness more prominent than pain	After walking or standing for variable lengths of time	Relieved by stopping only if position changed	Relief by lumbar spine flexion (sitting or stooping forward)	Frequent history of back problems, provoked by intraabdominal pressure
Arthritic, inflammatory processes	Foot, arch	Aching pain	After variable degree of exercise	Not quickly relieved (and may be present at rest)	May be relieved by not bearing weight	Variable, may relate to activity level
Hip arthritis	Hip, thigh, buttocks	Aching discomfort, usually localized to hip and gluteal region	After variable degree of exercise	Not quickly relieved (and may be present at rest)	More comfortable sitting, weight taken off legs	Variable, may relate to activity level, weather changes

Symptomatic Baker's cyst	Behind knee, down calf	Swelling, soreness, tenderness	With exercise	Present at rest	None	Not intermittent
Venous claudication	Entire leg, but usually worse in thigh and groin	Tight, bursting pain	After walking	Subsides slowly	Relief by speeded elevation	History of iliofemoral deep vein thrombosis, signs of venous congestions, edema
Chronic compartment syndrome	Calf muscles	Tight, bursting pain	After much exercise (e.g., jogging)	Subsides very slowly	Relief by speeded elevation	Typically occurs in heavily muscled athletes

Source: Norgren L, Hiatt WR, Dormandy JA, et al. Inter-Society Consensus for the Management of Peripheral Arterial Disease (TASC II). *Eur J Vasc Endovasc Surg,* 2007; Vol. 33 Suppl 1: pp. S1–S70. Reprinted with permission from Rightslink.

COMPLICATIONS AND COMORBIDITIES

- Smoking cessation essential for all persons with PAD.
- Proper foot care, including appropriate footwear and podiatric care is essential (Hirsch).
- Supervised exercise treatment, 30–45 minutes, 3 times a week for minimum of 12 weeks recommended and can be more effective than drug therapies (Hirsch).
- Blood pressure treatment goals are <130/80 mmHg in people with diabetes. Beta-blockers are not contraindicated in PAD (Hirsch).
- Treat with statins for goal LDL <70 mg/dl (Hirsch; McDermott). Beneficial effect of statins to improve function may be independent of lipid lowering (McDermott).
- Use antiplatelet and other antithrombotic drugs for severe PAD and known cardiovascular disease (Sobel). Aspirin 75–325 mg daily is recommended for patients with PAD to reduce both cardiac and stroke morbidity and mortality. Clopidogrel may be used in aspirin-intolerant patients. Primary benefit of these drugs may be to reduce incidence of stroke (McDermott).
- The evidence for benefit of glucose control in management of PAD is scant.
- Cilostazol recommended only for patients with disabling symptoms of claudication who are not candidates for revascularization (Sobel). Pentoxifylline is not effective (Marso).
- Surgical treatment indicated if symptoms of PAD are disabling, unresponsive to smoking cessation, exercise, and medications (Hirsch).

FOLLOW-UP

- Work with the patient to achieve goals of smoking cessation, titrate medications for blood pressure and lipids, improve ability to walk, and avoid CLI and lower extremity amputation.
- Specific recommendations for frequency of follow-up are individualized.

EXPERT OPINION

- For most patients with diabetes, examination of the feet will yield useful information and is an essential part of the physical examination.
- Patients with diabetes must be taught how to inspect their feet.
- Any patient with diabetes and history of cigarette smoking likely has PAD. Symptoms should be assessed during routine visits.

BASIS FOR RECOMMENDATIONS

Berger JS, Krantz MJ, Kittelson JM, et al. Aspirin for the prevention of cardiovascular events in patients with peripheral artery disease: a meta-analysis of randomized trials. *JAMA*, 2009; Vol. 301: pp. 1909–19.
  Comments: Aspirin reduced nonfatal strokes but not cardiovascular events. Despite meta-analysis, statistical power remains lacking.

Momsen AH, Jensen MB, Norager CB, et al. Drug therapy for improving walking distance in intermittent claudication: a systematic review and meta-analysis of robust randomised controlled studies. *Eur J Vasc Endovasc Surg*, 2009; Vol. 38: pp. 463–74.
  Comments: Excellent review of drug therapy for PAD symptoms.

Sobel M, Verhaeghe R, American College of Chest Physicians, et al. Antithrombotic therapy for peripheral artery occlusive disease: American College of Chest Physicians Evidence-Based Clinical Practice Guidelines (8th Edition). *Chest*, 2008; Vol. 133: pp. 815S–843S.
  Comments: Evidence-based clinical practice guideline from the American College of Chest Physicians.

Hirsch AT, Haskal ZJ, Hertzer NR, et al. ACC/AHA 2005 Practice Guidelines for the management of patients with peripheral arterial disease (lower extremity, renal, mesenteric, and abdominal aortic): a collaborative report. *Circulation*, 2006; Vol. 113: pp. e463–654.
  Comments: Complete online textbook of PAD.

OTHER REFERENCES

Grenon SM, Gagnon J, Hsiang Y. Video in clinical medicine. Ankle-brachial index for assessment of peripheral arterial disease. *NEJM*, 2009; Vol. 361: p. e40.
  Comments: Outstanding and unique teaching guide.

Bennett PC, Silverman S, Gill PS, et al. Ethnicity and peripheral artery disease. *QJM*, 2009; Vol. 102: pp. 3–16.
  Comments: Review of PAD among non-white European populations.

Bennett PC, Silverman SH, Gill PS, et al. Peripheral arterial disease and Virchow's triad. *Thromb Haemost*, 2009; Vol. 101: pp. 1032–40.
  Comments: Historical review including development of Fontaine and Rutherford classifications of claudication. Highly recommended.

Hambleton IR, Jonnalagadda R, Davis CR, et al. All-cause mortality after diabetes-related amputation in Barbados: a prospective case-control study. *Diabetes Care*, 2009; Vol. 32: pp. 306–7.
  Comments: This case-control study highlights the grave prognosis after a diabetes-related amputation.

Ankle Brachial Index Collaboration, Fowkes FG, Murray GD, et al. Ankle brachial index combined with Framingham Risk Score to predict cardiovascular events and mortality: a meta-analysis. *JAMA*, 2008; Vol. 300: pp. 197–208.
  Comments: ABI improves Framingham Risk Score prediction of cardiovascular events.

Pearce L, Ghosh J, Counsell A, et al. Cilostazol and peripheral arterial disease. *Expert Opin Pharmacother*, 2008; Vol. 9: pp. 2683–90.
  Comments: Review of the role of cilostazol in the management of PAD.

Marso SP, Hiatt WR. Peripheral arterial disease in patients with diabetes. *J Am Coll Cardiol*, 2006; Vol. 47: pp. 921–9.
  Comments: Review of PAD in major cardiology journal.

Hennis AJ, Fraser HS, Jonnalagadda R, et al. Explanations for the high risk of diabetes-related amputation in a Caribbean population of black African descent and potential for prevention. *Diabetes Care*, 2004; Vol. 27: pp. 2636–41.
  Comments: Ethnography of diabetes-related amputation.

McDermott MM, Guralnik JM, Greenland P, et al. Statin use and leg functioning in patients with and without lower-extremity peripheral arterial disease. *Circulation*, 2003; Vol. 107: pp. 757–61.
  Comments: Statins but not aspirin, ACE inhibitors, vasodilators, or beta-blockers improved function in PVD. Non-randomized but well-conducted study, highly cited.

Bild DE, Selby JV, Sinnock P, et al. Lower-extremity amputation in people with diabetes. Epidemiology and prevention. *Diabetes Care*, 1989; Vol. 12: pp. 24–31.
  Comments: Important reference, documents the evidence linking diabetes with PVD and lower-extremity amputation.

COMPLICATIONS AND COMORBIDITIES

Endocrine Diseases

ACROMEGALY

Nestoras Mathioudakis, MD, and Douglas Ball, MD

DEFINITION

- A clinical syndrome resulting from excessive secretion of growth hormone (GH).
- GH excess prior to closure of the epiphyseal plates results in gigantism; after epiphyseal plate closure, the result is acromegaly.
- Somatic and metabolic effects of chronic GH hypersecretion are predominantly mediated by high levels of insulin-like growth factor-1 (IGF-1).
- Acromegaly is an uncommon secondary cause of diabetes.
- Excess GH (1) stimulates gluconeogenesis and lipolysis, causing hyperglycemia and elevated free fatty acid levels; (2) leads to both hepatic and peripheral insulin resistance, with compensatory hyperinsulinemia. Conversely, IGF-1 increases insulin sensitivity. However, in acromegaly, increased IGF-1 levels are unable to overcome the insulin-resistant state caused by GH excess.

EPIDEMIOLOGY

- Prevalence 40–130 per million inhabitants, although may be as high as 100–1000 per million (Chanson).
- Almost always due to a GH-secreting pituitary adenoma.
- Very rare causes include excess secretion of growth hormone-releasing hormone (GHRH) by hypothalamic tumors, ectopic GHRH secretion by neuroendocrine or nonendocrine tumors (i.e., carcinoid tumors, small cell lung cancer).
- May occur as part of a genetic syndrome, including McCune-Albright syndrome, multiple endocrine neoplasia type 1 (MEN-1) syndrome, or the Carney complex. McCune-Albright syndrome is characterized by polyostotic fibrous dysplasia, cafe-au-lait spots, precocious puberty, and endocrine hyperactivity (thyrotoxicosis, gigantism, and Cushing's disease). MEN-1 results in primary endocrine hyperactivity of the pituitary, parathyroids, and pancreas. Carney complex results in myxomas, lentigenes, endocrine hyperactivity, and schwannomas (Keil).
- Slow progression of signs and symptoms and insidious course of disease often lead to delayed diagnosis; mean age at diagnosis is 40.
- Mortality rates nearly 2 times higher than general population, due to cardiovascular, cerebrovascular, or respiratory disease; increased risk of colonic neoplasia and possibly other tumors as well. Mortality risk reduced by therapy, almost to normal in patients deemed surgically cured (Melmed).
- 19%–56% of acromegalics have overt diabetes and 16%–46% have impaired glucose tolerance (Colao).
- Higher GH levels, older age, and longer disease duration predict development of symptomatic diabetes. Family history of diabetes and concomitant hypertension may increase risk (Colao).
- Diabetic ketoacidosis (DKA) rare feature of acromegaly. Severe diabetic retinopathy also a rare complication (Colao).

DIAGNOSIS

- Best single test for diagnosis is IGF-1, elevated in almost all patients with acromegaly.
- IGF-1 levels decrease with age and therefore an apparently "normal" value for an elderly patient may actually be high.
- GH measured in patients with equivocal IGF-1 levels, or when further biochemical confirmation required in patients with high IGF-1 levels.
- GH harder to interpret because secretion pulsatile and diurnal; affected by factors such as exercise, stress, sleep, and fasting. Since GH levels vary widely during the day, best not to obtain random measurements (Bonert).
- Uncontrolled diabetes can elevate serum GH levels, as can liver disease and malnutrition.
- Most specific confirmatory test to establish diagnosis is oral glucose tolerance test (OGTT). Serum GH should fall to <1 ng/ml within 2 hours of 75 g glucose ingestion. Postglucose values >2 ng/ml found in >85% of patients with acromegaly. With more highly sensitive immunoradiometric or immunochemiluminescent assays, a serum GH level >0.3 ng/ml after OGTT establishes diagnosis.
- Once GH hypersecretion confirmed, obtain MRI of the pituitary gland to look for adenoma. Most patients have a macroadenoma (tumor >1 cm) at time of diagnosis.

SIGNS AND SYMPTOMS

- Due to local tumor effects and/or systemic effects of elevated IGF-1 levels.
- **Signs:** visual field deficits (commonly bitemporal hemianopia), cranial nerve (3, 4, 5, 6) palsies, nystagmus, papilledema, acral enlargement (thickening of soft tissues of hands and feet), prognathism, widely spaced teeth, hypertrophy of frontal bones, jaw malocclusion, arthritis, proximal myopathy, oily skin, skin tags, hypertrichosis, colon polyps, hypertension, left ventricular hypertrophy, cardiomyopathy, macroglossia, goiter, visceromegaly (salivary glands, liver, spleen, kidney, prostate), acanthosis nigricans, hypercalciuria and renal calculi, hypertriglyceridemia, impaired glucose tolerance and diabetes, weight gain.
- **Symptoms:** headache, visual disturbances (loss of visual acuity, double vision), arthralgias, acroparesthesias, carpal tunnel syndrome, fatigue, heat intolerance, hyperhidrosis, sleep disturbances, obstructive and central sleep apnea, menstrual irregularities, galactorrhea, decreased libido, impotence.
- Changes in ring, glove, or shoe size suggesting acral enlargement.
- Other lab findings: hyperphosphatemia and hypercalciuria due to direct effects of GH or IGF-1 in the kidney.
- Serum insulin increased in 70% of patients.
- Imaging studies: plain films of skull show thickened calvarium, enlarged frontal and maxillary sinuses, and thickened jaw. Hand radiographs show increased soft tissue, increased width of intraarticular cartilage, "arrowhead tufting" of distal phalanges, cystic changes of carpal bones.

CLINICAL TREATMENT

Surgery

- Mainstay of treatment of GH-secreting pituitary adenomas is transsphenoidal surgery. Cure rate for microadenomas as high as 80% with experienced neurosurgeon; cure rate for macroadenomas <50%.
- Most patients with macroadenomas require adjuvant therapy (medical vs radiotherapy). Radiation therapy generally reserved as a third-line treatment because of risk of hypopituitarism.

COMPLICATIONS AND COMORBIDITIES

- Recent data show that presurgical treatment with somatostatin analogues may improve the chance of surgical cure in patients with macroadenomas (Carlsen).

Medical

- Somatostatin analogues (SSAs) (below) inhibit somatotroph cell proliferation and GH secretion. Efficacy as primary treatment: 50%–70% effective at achieving biochemical control and 50% effective at reducing tumor size. Efficacy as secondary treatment (i.e., following surgery): 20%.
- SSAs include octreotide, octreotide LAR (long-acting release), and Lanreotide Autogel (long-acting depot formulation). Octreotide administered by sub-Q injection, usually 100–250 mcg 3 times daily. Octreotide LAR administered as IM injection monthly, usually starting at 20 mg and increasing by 10-mg increments to clinical and biochemical response. Lanreotide Autogel administered by sub-Q injection monthly, with typical starting dose of 90 mg.
- Pegvisomant is a competitive inhibitor at the GH receptor level that prevents the action of native GH. Efficacy: 80%–90% effective at controlling acromegalic symptoms, but does not reduce tumor size or GH levels.
- Dopamine agonists (i.e., cabergoline, bromocriptine) may also be considered.

Diabetes Management

- Impaired glucose tolerance and diabetes generally improve following treatment of underlying disease.
- Conflicting data regarding effects of SSAs on glucose homeostasis. SSAs may reduce insulin resistance, but also impair insulin secretion. Neither SSA or surgery was associated with deterioration of glucose tolerance in one study (Colao); BMI appears to be the major predictor of worsening glycemic control.
- Reduced fasting glucose levels and hemoglobin A1c are reported following treatment with pegvisomant (Barkan).
- Management of diabetes in acromegaly is similar to general management of type 2 diabetes.
- Oral secretagogues and/or insulin sensitizers theoretically offer the greatest potential for glycemic control based on the pathophysiology of diabetes in acromegaly.
- Insulin should be started if oral agents are unsuccessful at controlling glucose.

FOLLOW-UP

- Monitor IGF-1 levels every 6 months. If not normal, maximally titrate medications. Consider combined treatment (SSA + dopamine agonist).
- Obtain MRI 3–4 months postoperatively, then every 3–6 months after starting medical therapy. If surgically cured, MRI surveillance frequency may be reduced to every 2–3 yrs. If disease not fully controlled, MRI should be performed every 6–12 months.
- Perform hormonal testing after surgery or radiation to assess anterior and posterior pituitary function (hypopituitarism/diabetes insipidus). Pituitary deficiencies can develop 10 or more years after radiation therapy.

EXPERT OPINION

- Acromegaly is a rare cause of diabetes characterized by a state of insulin resistance.
- Glycemic control is best achieved by treatment of underlying state of GH excess.
- Treatments for acromegaly (i.e., SSAs) may have potentially detrimental effects on glycemia, although the literature is conflicting.
- If diabetes persists after treatment, hyperglycemia should be managed according to standard guidelines for type 2 diabetes.

BASIS FOR RECOMMENDATIONS

Melmed S, Colao A, Barkan A, et al. Guidelines for acromegaly management: an update. *J Clin Endocrinol Metab,* 2009; Vol. 94: pp. 1509–17.

> **Comments:** This is an updated review of current management practices and guidelines.

Chanson P, Salenave S, Kamenicky P, et al. Pituitary tumours: acromegaly. *Best Pract Res Clin Endocrinol Metab,* 2009; Vol. 23: pp. 555–74.

> **Comments:** Detailed descriptions of clinical manifestations of acromegaly.

OTHER REFERENCES

Resmini E, Minuto F, Colao A, et al. Secondary diabetes associated with principal endocrinopathies: the impact of new treatment modalities. *Acta Diabetol,* 2009; Vol. 46: pp. 85–95.

> **Comments:** Good review of diabetes in various endocrine conditions.

Aghi M, Blevins LS. Recent advances in the treatment of acromegaly. *Curr Opin Endocrinol Diabetes Obes,* 2009; Vol. 16: pp. 304–7.

> **Comments:** Excellent review of the treatment modalities for acromegaly, particularly with respect to recurrent tumors.

Colao A, Auriemma RS, Galdiero M, et al. Impact of somatostatin analogs versus surgery on glucose metabolism in acromegaly: results of a 5-year observational, open, prospective study. *J Clin Endocrinol Metab,* 2009; Vol. 94: pp. 528–37.

> **Comments:** One of very few studies looking directly at direct effects of SSAs on glucose metabolism.

Bonert V. Diagnostic challenges in acromegaly: a case-based review. *Best Pract Res Clin Endocrinol Metab,* 2009; Vol. 23 Suppl 1: pp. S23–30.

> **Comments:** A case-based illustration of the diagnostic challenges of acromegaly, with emphasis on the laboratory evaluation.

Keil MF, Stratakis CA. Pituitary tumors in childhood: update of diagnosis, treatment and molecular genetics. *Expert Rev Neurother,* 2008; Vol. 8: pp. 563–74.

> **Comments:** A good review of the familial pituitary tumor syndromes.

Carlsen SM, Lund-Johansen M, Schreiner T, et al. Preoperative octreotide treatment in newly diagnosed acromegalic patients with macroadenomas increases cure short-term postoperative rates: a prospective, randomized trial. *J Clin Endocrinol Metab,* 2008; Vol. 93: pp. 2984–90.

> **Comments:** A recent study showing improved surgical cure rate with adjuvant medical therapy.

Barkan AL, Burman P, Clemmons DR, et al. Glucose homeostasis and safety in patients with acromegaly converted from long-acting octreotide to pegvisomant. *J Clin Endocrinol Metab,* 2005; Vol. 90: pp. 5684–91.

> **Comments:** This study showed improved glucose homeostasis in acromegalic patients transitioned from octreotide to pegvisomant.

CUSHING'S SYNDROME

Amin Sabet, MD

DEFINITION

- Hormonal disorder caused by prolonged exposure to high levels of glucocorticoids.
- May be due to exogenous glucocorticoids (more common) or endogenous hypercortisolemia.
- Cushing's syndrome due to an adrenocorticotropic hormone (ACTH)-secreting pituitary adenoma is referred to as Cushing's disease.
- Excess glucocorticoids, endogenous or exogenous, exert a powerful hyperglycemic effect by stimulating gluconeogenesis and inhibiting peripheral glucose utilization (insulin resistance).

EPIDEMIOLOGY

- Overt Cushing's incidence in general population: 2.4 cases per 1 million persons per year with standardized mortality ratio of 3.8 for affected persons in Spain (Etxabe).
- Occult Cushing's prevalence in diabetes: 2%–5% of overweight or obese, poorly controlled type 2 diabetes patients (Catargi).
- Approximately 25% of overweight, type 2 diabetes patients have impaired morning cortisol suppression after a low-dose overnight dexamethasone suppression test but do not necessarily have Cushing's (Catargi).
- Most common hormonal abnormality in patients with adrenal incidentaloma.

DIAGNOSIS

- Detailed history to assess for any use of exogenous glucocorticoids (oral, topical, injection, inhaled).
- CYP3A4 inhibitors (especially ritonavir) inhibit glucocorticoid clearance causing Cushing's with concurrent inhaled and injection steroid use.
- Screening: late night salivary cortisol × 2, 24-hour urine free cortisol (UFC) × 2, low-dose dexamethasone suppression test (after 1 mg dexamethasone at 11 PM, normal 8 AM cortisol <1.8 mcg/dl).
- At least two clearly abnormal (e.g., UFC >3 times upper limit of normal) tests using different test methods needed to establish diagnosis.
- False positive dexamethasone suppression test seen with increased cortisol binding globulin (e.g., estrogen-containing OCPs).
- After diagnosis of hypercortisolism, serum ACTH <5 pg/ml (1.1 pmol/L) suggests ACTH-independent disease and next step is CT or MRI adrenal imaging.
- Low or suppressed ACTH suggests ACTH-independent: usually adrenal adenoma, adrenal carcinoma, or bilateral adrenal hyperplasia.
- Normal or elevated ACTH suggests ACTH-dependent; usually due to pituitary ACTH-secreting tumor (Cushing's disease), less commonly ectopic ACTH-secreting tumor (e.g., bronchial carcinoid tumor)
- Pituitary versus ectopic ACTH: MRI pituitary (>6 mm less likely incidentaloma), high-dose 8-mg dexamethasone test (pituitary tumors more likely to suppress), corticotropin-releasing hormone (CRH) stimulation (pituitary tumors more likely to stimulate), presence of hypokalemia (more likely with ectopic), degree of ACTH elevation (may be greater with ectopic), age (ectopic less likely in young patients), inferior petrosal sinus sampling (most direct test). Detection of ectopic ACTH-secreting tumors may involve CT, MRI, PET, or octreotide scintigraphy.
- Pseudo-Cushing's: patients with marked obesity, glucose intolerance, severe depression, or alcoholism may have nonspecific manifestations of Cushing's and mildly elevated cortisol (1–3 times upper limit of normal).

SIGNS AND SYMPTOMS

- Common: centripetal obesity, facial plethora, hyperglycemia, hypertension, mood lability, easy bruisability, oligo-/amenorrhea, hirsutism/acne (ACTH-dependent).
- More specific: broad (>1 cm) purple striae, proximal muscle weakness.
- Other: bone loss, fracture, kidney stones, polydipsia, polyuria.
- Ectopic ACTH: more severe hypertension, hypokalemia, hyperpigmentation.
- Adrenal carcinoma: virilization (temporal balding, clitoromegaly, deepening voice) seen in Cushing's due to cosecretion of androgens.

- Pseudo-Cushing's: unlikely to have skin (bruising, thinning) or muscle (proximal weakness, atrophy) manifestations.

CLINICAL THERAPY

- Exogenous Cushing's: discontinue glucocorticoid therapy if possible.
- Cushing's disease: first-line: transphenoidal pituitary surgery; second-line: pituitary irradiation; definitive/third-line: bilateral total adrenalectomy requiring lifelong glucocorticoid and mineralocorticoid replacement therapy and monitoring for Nelson's syndrome (rapid enlargement of residual pituitary adenoma).
- Ectopic ACTH: surgical excision of tumor if possible. Unresectable tumors treated with adrenal enzyme inhibitor (e.g., ketoconazole, metyrapone), medical adrenalectomy (mitotane), or bilateral surgical adrenalectomy.
- ACTH-independent adrenal adenomas: unilateral adrenalectomy generally curative.
- ACTH-independent bilateral adrenal hyperplasia: most cases treated with bilateral adrenalectomy.
- Adrenal carcinoma: surgery and mitotane for resectable disease; mitotane and chemotherapy for advanced, unresectable disease; adrenal enzyme inhibitors for persistent hypercortisolemia.
- Pseudo-Cushing's: treat primary disease (i.e., depression, diabetes).
- Hyperglycemia management in Cushing's syndrome likely similar to exogenous steroid-induced hyperglycemia (see p. 149).

FOLLOW-UP

- Physiologic glucocorticoid replacement until recovery of endogenous adrenal function, which may take many months.
- Follow cortisol levels, not ACTH, for evidence of cure.
- Late relapse common after apparent surgical cure of Cushing's disease. Long-term periodic assessment of the hypothalamic-pituitary-adrenal axis required.
- Hyperglycemia, hypertension, and osteoporosis improve but often partially persist after effective therapy for Cushing's.

EXPERT OPINION

- Although testing for Cushing's not recommended in all patients with diabetes, screening is recommended for those with specific findings (myopathy, thin skin, bruising) or accumulation of new features over time.
- Pseudo-Cushing's more common than Cushing's syndrome in diabetes and requires no specific treatment except for usual diabetes management.
- Incidental pituitary and adrenal tumors are common in the general population. Imaging studies should only be performed in patients after confirming hypercortisolism.
- Late-night salivary cortisol testing is a widely available, easy-to-perform, sensitive, and specific screening test for Cushing's syndrome.
- 24-hour urine free cortisol or 1 mg overnight dexamethasone suppression are reasonable alternative screening tests that may be more widely available in the primary care setting.
- In patients with clinically suspected Cushing's and equivocal screening test results, repeat testing after several months is advisable.

COMPLICATIONS AND COMORBIDITIES

BASIS FOR RECOMMENDATIONS

Nieman LK, Biller BM, Findling JW, et al. The diagnosis of Cushing's syndrome: an Endocrine Society Clinical Practice Guideline. *J Clin Endocrinol Metab*, 2008; Vol. 93: pp. 1526–40.
   Comments: Most recent Endocrine Society consensus guidelines on diagnosis of Cushing's syndrome.

OTHER REFERENCES

Carroll T, Raff H, Findling JW. Late-night salivary cortisol measurement in the diagnosis of Cushing's syndrome. *Nat Clin Pract Endocrinol Metab*, 2008; Vol. 4: pp. 344–50.

Comments: Late night salivary cortisol testing has 92%–100% sensitivity and 93%–100% specificity for Cushing's syndrome.

Prevedello DM, Pouratian N, Sherman J, et al. Management of Cushing's disease: outcome in patients with micro-adenoma detected on pituitary magnetic resonance imaging. *J Neurosurg*, 2008; Vol. 109: pp. 751–9.

Comments: 13% of Cushing's disease patients in postoperative remission relapsed after average of 50 months.

Swearingen B, Katznelson L, Miller K, et al. Diagnostic errors after inferior petrosal sinus sampling. *J Clin Endocrinol Metab*, 2004; Vol. 89: pp. 3752–63.

Comments: Reported 90% sensitivity, 67% specificity, 99% positive predictive value (PPV), and 20% negative predictive value (NPV) using inferior petrosal sinus sampling after CRH for diagnosis of Cushing's disease.

Catargi B, Rigalleau V, Poussin A, et al. Occult Cushing's syndrome in type-2 diabetes. *J Clin Endocrinol Metab*, 2003; Vol. 88: pp. 5808–13.

Comments: Occult Cushing's syndrome seen in up to 5.5% of overweight or obese, type 2 diabetic patients.

Etxabe J, Vazquez JA. Morbidity and mortality in Cushing's disease: an epidemiological approach. *Clin Endocrinol (Oxf)*, 1994; Vol. 40: pp. 479–84.

Comments: Established Cushing's incidence of 2.4 cases per million people per year with standardized mortality ratio of 3.8 for affected persons.

Oldfield EH, Doppman JL, Nieman LK, et al. Petrosal sinus sampling with and without corticotropin-releasing hormone for the differential diagnosis of Cushing's syndrome. *NEJM*, 1991; Vol. 325: pp. 897–905.

Comments: Reported 100% sensitivity and 100% specificity using inferior petrosal sinus sampling after CRH for diagnosis of Cushing's disease.

GLUCAGONOMA

Nestoras Mathioudakis, MD, and Douglas Ball, MD

DEFINITION

- A rare tumor originating from the alpha cells of the pancreas that results in hypersecretion of glucagon.
- Mild diabetes mellitus is a classic presenting feature of glucagonoma.
- Hyperglycemia results from the glycogenolytic and gluconeogenic effects of glucagon and low insulin-to-glucagon ratio.

EPIDEMIOLOGY

- Prevalence of glucagonoma: 13.5 per 20 million people (Echenique-Elizondo).
- Glucagonomas are exceedingly rare, ~7% of all pancreatic endocrine tumors (Kindmark).
- Males and females equally affected.
- Most tumors (80%) occur sporadically, while remainder associated with multiple endocrine neoplasia type 1 (MEN-1) syndrome (pituitary, pancreatic islet cell tumors, or parathyroid tumors).
- Typical age at presentation is 40–50 years.
- Most glucagonomas (75%) malignant and have metastasized by the time of diagnosis.
- Prevalence of diabetes mellitus in glucagonoma: 38%–94% (Chastain).
- Generally, the diabetes is mild to moderate. Mean HbA1c reported at 9.8% in one series (Wermers).

DIAGNOSIS

- Necrolytic migratory erythema (NME) (described below): pathognomonic skin rash associated with glucagonoma, and generally the only clue to make the diagnosis. Skin biopsy diagnostic of NME: superficial necrolysis at edge of lesion with separation of outer epidermal layers and perivascular infiltration with lymphocytes and histiocytes (Chastain). Also seen in other disorders.
- If considered, measure glucagon. Glucagon levels >500 pg/ml strongly suggestive, and levels >1000 virtually diagnostic.
- Moderately elevated glucagon levels seen in hypoglycemia, fasting, sepsis, renal or hepatic failure, or acute pancreatitis. Modest elevations in glucagon seen with other pancreatic neuroendocrine tumors (Zollinger-Ellison syndrome, insulinoma, carcinoid).
- Less specific findings: normochromic, normocytic anemia; hypoaminoacidemia (due to amino acid oxidation and gluconeogenesis from amino acid substrates).
- If patient has classic clinical findings and/or elevated glucagon levels, then image for pancreatic mass. Abdominal CT scan with IV contrast preferred initial imaging study to localize pancreatic tumor. Unlike insulinomas, glucagonomas generally large at the time of diagnosis and more readily localizable.
- Endoscopic ultrasound (EUS) to detect tumors that are too small to be visualized by CT. Tumors as small as 2–3 mm can be seen on EUS.
- Fine needle biopsy using EUS confirms the diagnosis. Histopathology demonstrates an islet-cell tumor with positive glucagon staining by immunohistochemistry.
- Although octreotide scan has high sensitivity for glucagonomas, not usually necessary since most glucagonomas very large at presentation and easily detected by CT.
- Liver lesions suggestive of metastasis should be biopsied under CT guidance.

SIGNS AND SYMPTOMS

- 4Ds: dermatitis, diabetes, deep vein thrombosis, depression.
- **Symptoms:** weight loss, polyuria, polydypsia, abdominal pain, diarrhea, constipation, low mood.
- **Signs:** angular cheilitis, glossitis, stomatitis, blepharitis, hair thinning, dystrophic nails, anemia, ataxia, optic atrophy, proximal muscle weakness, dementia, depression.
- NME rash: erythematous papules or plaques, usually beginning in groin and perineum, then extending to buttocks, extremities, and face. Lesions enlarge and coalesce over 1–2 weeks, leaving behind blistering lesions with central clearing and psoriatic-like scaling. Lesions are often painful and pruritic.
- Related to venous thrombosis: pain, swelling, tenderness, redness/discolored skin in affected extremity, visible surface veins.
- Dilated cardiomyopathy (rare).

CLINICAL TREATMENT

Surgical Therapy

- Depends on the extent of disease at the time of diagnosis. Most common metastases: liver, regional lymph nodes, bone, adrenals, kidney, and lung. If tumor localized to pancreas at time of diagnosis, resection (simple enucleation, focal resection, Whipple) can be curative, but only successful in 30% of patients (Morgan).
- If metastatic disease with positive octreotide scan and hyperglucagonemia, options include surgical resection of liver metastases, hepatic artery chemoembolization, radiofrequency or cryoablation, and liver transplantation.

COMPLICATIONS AND COMORBIDITIES

Medical Therapy

- Somatostatin analogues (i.e., octreotide) highly effective at controlling symptoms. Typical starting dose of octreotide: 50 mcg subcutaneously 3 times daily, increasing dose gradually to control symptoms (diarrhea, NME, neurologic symptoms), then transition to a long-acting depot formulation (Sandostatin LAR).
- For extrahepatic metastases, systemic chemotherapy (streptozosin, doxorubicin) may be considered, although response rate is low (Chastain).
- Interferon alpha (IFNa) may have biochemical, radiographic, or clinical efficacy in a minority of patients (Kindmark). Use is limited by uncertain efficacy data and poor side effect profile.
- Nutritional support often needed perioperatively for associated malnutrition related to chronic hypercatabolic state. Total parental nutrition, enteral feeding, or supplements may be offered. NME may respond to infusions of amino and fatty acids.
- Radiation therapy may give symptomatic palliation to patients who are not surgical candidates.
- Diabetes usually mild and easily controlled by diet, oral agents, or insulin. Since beta-cell function preserved, insulin secretion normal, and diabetic ketoacidosis rare.
- Glycemic control for diabetes best achieved by treatment of underlying disease (i.e., tumor resection).
- In patients with metastatic disease who cannot be cured, treat hyperglycemia as standard type 2 diabetes.

FOLLOW-UP

- Yearly measurement of glucagon levels and other gastrointestinal hormones (i.e., gastrin) indefinitely, as this will allow early detection of any recurrence and detection of secondary endocrine disorders, such as Zollinger-Ellison syndrome, that may develop many years later.
- Evaluate patients regularly for development of other endocrine tumors in the setting of MEN syndrome.
- Monitor for typical complications of diabetes (retinopathy, proteinuria, neuropathy) and treat to usual lipid and blood pressure targets.

EXPERT OPINION

- Glucagonoma is an extremely rare cause of diabetes; the diagnosis requires a high level of suspicion.
- A patient with diabetes, weight loss, and the typical rash of NME should raise suspicion for this condition.
- Diabetes generally mild, but common among patients with glucagonoma.
- Glycemic control best achieved with treatment of underlying state of glucagon excess but, if not successful, can be treated with diet, oral agents, or (rarely) insulin.

BASIS FOR RECOMMENDATIONS

Kindmark H, Sundin A, Granberg D, et al. Endocrine pancreatic tumors with glucagon hypersecretion: a retrospective study of 23 cases during 20 years. *Med Oncol*, 2007; Vol. 24: pp. 330–7.

    Comments: A more recent series of glucagonoma patients showing slightly lower prevalence of diabetes in this population than previously described.

Chastain MA. The glucagonoma syndrome: a review of its features and discussion of new perspectives. *Am J Med Sci*, 2001; Vol. 321: pp. 306–20.

    Comments: An excellent clinically oriented review of the glucagonoma syndrome, with comprehensive differential diagnoses of both the NME rash and hyperglucagonemia in general.

Wermers RA, Fatourechi V, Wynne AG, et al. The glucagonoma syndrome. Clinical and pathologic features in 21 patients. *Medicine* (Baltimore), 1996; Vol. 75: pp. 53–63.

    Comments: One of a few case series of glucagonoma patients.

OTHER REFERENCES

McGevna L, Tavakkol Z. Images in clinical medicine. Necrolytic migratory erythema. *NEJM,* 2010; Vol. 362: p. e1.

    Comments: Good images of NEM.

Morgan KA, Adams DB. Solid tumors of the body and tail of the pancreas. *Surg Clin North Am,* 2010; Vol. 90: pp. 287–307.

    Comments: A good review on the surgical aspects of both endocrine and nonendocrine pancreatic tumors.

Fanelli CG, Porcellati F, Rossetti P, et al. Glucagon: the effects of its excess and deficiency on insulin action. *Nutr Metab Cardiovasc Dis,* 2006; Vol. 16 Suppl 1: pp. S28–34.

    Comments: A good review of the physiologic relationship between glucagon and insulin, and of the pathophysiology of glucagon excess in glucagonoma and other metabolic conditions.

Echenique-Elizondo M, Tuneu Valls A, Elorza Orúe JL, et al. Glucagonoma and pseudoglucagonoma syndrome. *JOP,* 2004; Vol. 5: pp. 179–85.

    Comments: A retrospective review showing a slightly higher prevalence of glucagonoma than previously reported.

van Beek AP, de Haas ER, van Vloten WA, et al. The glucagonoma syndrome and necrolytic migratory erythema: a clinical review. *Eur J Endocrinol,* 2004; Vol. 151: pp. 531–7.

    Comments: Good review of the pathophysiology of glucagonoma and the typical rash of NEM. Also includes photo images of clinical features.

Oberg K, Kvols L, Caplin M, et al. Consensus report on the use of somatostatin analogs for the management of neuroendocrine tumors of the gastroenteropancreatic system. *Ann Oncol,* 2004; Vol. 15: pp. 966–73.

    Comments: Excellent review of the mechanism of action, indications, and uses of somatostatin analogues in the management of neuroendocrine tumors. The review is not limited specifically to glucagonomas.

INSULINOMA

Ana Emiliano, MD, and Douglas Ball, MD

COMPLICATIONS AND COMORBIDITIES

DEFINITION

- A neuroendocrine tumor of the pancreas that secretes insulin autonomously.
- Unregulated insulin secretion leads to decreased hepatic glucose output and hypoglycemia (Rizza).
- A cause of endogenous hyperinsulinemic hypoglycemia.

EPIDEMIOLOGY

- Rare tumors, incidence of 4 per 1 million persons per year.
- Most commonly solitary, benign and encapsulated (approximately 87% of the time).
- May originate anywhere in the pancreas, but rarely outside the pancreas unless metastatic.
- 10% are malignant, a definition based on the presence of metastasis, found predominantly in liver and lymph nodes, sometimes bone and peritoneal tissue.
- In a 20-year cohort at the Mayo Clinic, the median age at diagnosis for all insulinomas was 50, with a range of 17–89 years (Placzkowski).
- Found in all ethnic groups.
- Sporadic in more than 90% of cases.
- Familial in 6%–10% of cases, as part of multiple endocrine neoplasia type 1 (MEN-1) or Von-Hippel Lindau syndrome (VHL).
- MEN-1 is an autosomal dominant syndrome characterized by primary hyperparathyroidism, anterior pituitary adenomas and gastroenteropancreatic neuroendocrine tumors.

Insulinomas occur in ~10% of MEN-1 patients, being the most commonly diagnosed gastroenteropancreatic neuroendocrine tumor in MEN-1, along with gastrinomas. >90% insulinomas benign, but more frequently multiple than in sporadic cases.

- VHL is an autosomal dominant syndrome including central nervous system (CNS) and retinal tumors, pheochromocytoma, islet cell tumors, and renal cell carcinoma. VHL-associated insulinomas are frequently malignant.

DIAGNOSIS

- Document Whipple's triad: neuroglycopenic symptoms with documented plasma glucose (PG) <60 mg/dl and symptom resolution with correction of hypoglycemia.
- Requires biochemical demonstration of inappropriately high plasma insulin concentrations (>3 uU/ml) during hypoglycemia (PG <60 mg/dl) (Cryer).
- In addition, an elevated plasma C-peptide level (>0.6 ng/ml), elevated plasma proinsulin level (>5 pmol/l) and a low plasma betahydroxybutyrate level (<2.7 mmol/L) occurring concomitantly with the hypoglycemia suggest endogenous hyperinsulinemia (Cryer).
- Without outpatient documentation of hyperinsulinemic hypoglycemia, a 72-hour supervised fast is recommended (See Table 3-7 for specific instructions). >97% of all patients with insulinoma develop hypoglycemia and neuroglycopenic symptoms within 48–72 hours of a supervised fast (Hirschberg).
- Exclude factitious hypoglycemia: screen urine for sulfonylureas. Measure plasma C-peptide: if suppressed in the setting of increased insulin and hypoglycemia, this suggests exogenous insulin administration.
- Other causes of hyperinsulinemic hypoglycemia: hyperinsulinism of infancy, dumping syndrome, and insulin autoimmune syndrome, among others.
- Having established clinical and biochemical confirmation of likely insulinoma, localization of the pancreatic tumor is done using ultrasound, CT, or interventional radiology.
- Transabdominal ultrasound and CT of the abdomen has a rate of detection of approximately 70% (Mathur; Boukhman).
- Endoscopic ultrasound has variable sensitivity, 40%–93%, depending on the operator (Anderson; Nikfarjam).
- Selective arterial calcium stimulation test with hepatic venous sampling (relies on calcium as secretagogue for insulin from tumor) has sensitivity of 80%–94% (Guettier; Mathur).

TABLE 3-7. 72-HOUR SUPERVISED FAST

Procedure:
1. Document patient's last meal.
2. Monitor blood glucose every hour using glucometer.
3. Collect samples every 6 hours until PG <60 mg/dl, and then every 1–2 hours.
4. Send carefully timed and stored samples for the tests listed in Table 3-8.
5. End fast when the PG <45 mg/dl with symptoms of hypoglycemia.
6. Administer glucagon 1.0 mg IV at the end of fast and measure PG 10, 20, and 30 minutes later. PG increase by >25 mg/dl or more suggests insulinoma, since insulin was inappropriately suppressing glycogenolysis during fast, reversed by glucagon.

Courtesy of Ana Emiliano and Douglas Ball.

TABLE 3-8. INTERPRETATION OF LABORATORY FINDINGS: BIOCHEMICAL TESTS/ CONFIRMATION OF INSULINOMA

Biochemical Tests	Confirmation of Insulinoma
Plasma glucose	<55 mg/dl
Insulin	>3 uU/ml*
C-peptide	>0.6 ng/ml
Pro-insulin	>5 pmol/L
Betahydroxybutyrate	<2.7 mmol/L

*when using immunochemiluminescent assay
Courtesy of Ana Emiliano and Douglas Ball.

SIGNS AND SYMPTOMS

- Most patients with insulinoma present clinically with fasting hypoglycemia (<70 mg/dl) (Service).
- About 6% of insulinomas, usually males, present with postprandial hypoglycemia (Placzkowski).
- About 20% of insulinomas present with both fasting and postprandial hypoglycemia.
- Hypoglycemia frequently manifests with neuroglycopenic as well as sympathoadrenergic symptoms.
- Metastatic disease, especially to liver, can cause severe, intractable hypoglycemia.
- Hyperphagia with weight gain can occur in patients with insulinoma (Nikfarjam).
- In estimated 20% of patients with insulinoma, symptoms are misattributed to psychiatric or neurologic disorders.

CLINICAL TREATMENT

Surgical Treatment

- Resection of the insulinoma is the treatment of choice.
- Palpation of the pancreas and intraoperative ultrasound detect insulinoma in the 83%–98% of cases.
- Distal pancreatectomy, enucleation, and pancreaticoduodenectomy most common surgical procedures (Nikfarjam).
- Tumor resection is usually curative, as most insulinomas are benign (Boukhman).
- Laparoscopic surgery is possible for small, solitary insulinomas.
- For resectable liver metastasis, surgical resection of the metastasis and the primary tumor is recommended.
- For unresectable metastatic disease of the liver, treatment options include chemoembolization, radiofrequency ablation, and cryoablation.

Medical Therapy

- Indications: (1) severe, life-threatening hypoglycemia due to unresectable metastases; (2) patient not a surgical candidate; (3) insulinoma not identified at surgery.
- Frequent carbohydrate-containing meals is the background for all medical therapy.

- Diazoxide is a first-line agent, acting by inhibiting insulin release via stimulation of alpha-adrenergic receptors. Initial dose: 150–200 mg in 2–3 divided doses, maximum dose 1200 mg daily.
- Octreotide, a somatostatin analog, inhibits insulin secretion. Unpredictable clinical response, depending on the density of somatostatin-2 receptors on the insulinoma, which is highly variable.
- Verapamil, propranolol, phenytoin, glucagon, and glucocorticoids also used to alleviate symptoms.
- See Table 3-9 for further details on symptom control and adverse effects.

TABLE 3-9. MEDICAL THERAPY FOR UNCONTROLLED HYPOGLYCEMIA

Drug	Class	Symptom Control	Adverse Effects
Diazoxide	Alpha-adrenergic agonist	50%–60% of patients	Peripheral edema, nausea, hirsutism
Octreotide	Somatostatin analog	40%–60% of patients	Bloating, abdominal cramping, malabsorption, cholelithiasis
Verapamil	Calcium channel blocker	Unknown	Constipation, peripheral edema, nausea
Propranolol	Beta-blocker	Unknown	Bradycardia, depression, may potentiate hypoglycemia
Phenytoin	Anticonvulsant	Unknown	Hypertrichosis, gingival, hypertrophy, peripheral neuropathy
Glucagon	Glucagon	Palliation	Risk of rebound hypoglycemia

Courtesy of Ana Emiliano and Douglas Ball.

FOLLOW-UP
- ~6% of patients reexperience hypoglycemia within 6 months of initial surgery. Additional localization procedures and repeat surgery are recommended.
- For patients with sporadic insulinoma, the recurrence rate was 5% at 10 years and 7% at 20 years (Service).
- Recurrence rates are higher in MEN-1: 20% at 10 and 20 years (Service).
- Recurrence within 4 years usually due to regrowth of an incompletely resected tumor.
- Prognosis favorable in benign insulinoma (Nikfarjam). With malignant insulinoma, 25%–35% 5-year survival.
- Follow-up of malignant insulinomas includes close monitoring with history and physical examination, neuroendocrine tumor markers (insulin, chromogranin A), and

imaging 3 and 6 months after initial resection, then every 6–12 months for at least 3 years postsurgery.

EXPERT OPINION

- Insulinoma should be considered in the differential for hypoglycemia, particularly in individuals who continue to have unexplained fasting hypoglycemia with high endogenous insulin levels (in contrast to hypoglycemia with high exogenous insulin use in diabetes).
- The medical workup, sometimes including a supervised fast, is the most important step in diagnosing an insulinoma.
- Establish hyperinsulinemic hypoglycemia before proceeding with localization or surgery.
- Given biochemical evidence of hyperinsulinemic hypoglycemia, preoperative localization of tumor avoids need for blind pancreatic exploration.
- Careful removal of the tumor, with the capsule, by an experienced surgeon, prevents local recurrence.
- Because insulinomas can occur throughout the pancreas, a blind partial pancreatectomy is not advisable.
- There is limited experience, and questionable survival benefit, with hepatic transplantation for unresectable liver metastasis.
- Conventional cytotoxic chemotherapy has not proved effective for malignant insulinoma. Novel therapies are under investigation, such as small molecule tyrosine kinase inhibitors and inhibitors of the mammalian target of rapamycin (mTOR).
- Depending on degree of pancreatic resection, surgery for insulinoma may rarely result in diabetes although this is unusual (see Postpancreatectomy Diabetes, p. 81).

BASIS FOR RECOMMENDATIONS

Cryer PE, Axelrod L, Grossman AB, et al. Evaluation and management of adult hypoglycemic disorders: an Endocrine Society Clinical Practice Guideline. *J Clin Endocrinol Metab,* 2009; Vol. 94: pp. 709–28.

Comments: Expert Endocrine Society consensus on the evaluation and management of hypoglycemic disorders in adults.

OTHER REFERENCES

Placzkowski KA, Vella A, Thompson GB, et al. Secular trends in the presentation and management of functioning insulinoma at the Mayo Clinic, 1987–2007. *J Clin Endocrinol Metab,* 2009; Vol. 94: pp. 1069–73.

Comments: A retrospective analysis of 237 insulinoma cases seen at the Mayo Clinic from 1987 through 2007, with an emphasis on the clinical presentation and trends in diagnostic and radiological evaluation during the 20-year period covered by the study.

Guettier JM, Kam A, Chang R, et al. Localization of insulinomas to regions of the pancreas by intraarterial calcium stimulation: the NIH experience. *J Clin Endocrinol Metab,* 2009; Vol. 94: pp. 1074–80.

Comments: Retrospective study assessing the accuracy of calcium stimulation in the preoperative localization of insulinoma in 45 patients, concluding that calcium stimulation was vastly superior to abdominal ultrasound, CT, or MRI.

Mathur A, Gorden P, Libutti SK. Insulinoma. *Surg Clin North Am,* 2009; Vol. 89: pp. 1105–21.

Comments: Comprehensive review of the clinical presentation, diagnosis, radiographic evaluation, and medical and surgical treatment of insulinoma.

Nikfarjam M, Warshaw AL, Axelrod L, et al. Improved contemporary surgical management of insulinomas: a 25-year experience at the Massachusetts General Hospital. *Ann Surg,* 2008; Vol. 247: pp. 165–72.

Comments: Retrospective review of 61 patients with sporadic and MEN-1 associated insulinoma between 1983–2007, with a description of demographics, presentation, and diagnostic workup, including an assessment of the use of endoscopic ultrasound in the preoperative evaluation.

COMPLICATIONS AND COMORBIDITIES

Hirshberg B, Livi A, Bartlett DL, et al. Forty-eight-hour fast: the diagnostic test for insulinoma. *J Clin Endocrinol Metab,* 2000; Vol. 85: pp. 3222–6.

> **Comments:** This study showed that 94.5% of 127 patients with insulinoma developed fasting hypoglycemia within 48 hours of a supervised fast, underscoring the unusual need for a complete 72-hour fast to diagnose insulinoma.

Anderson MA, Carpenter S, Thompson NW, et al. Endoscopic ultrasound is highly accurate and directs management in patients with neuroendocrine tumors of the pancreas. *Am J Gastroenterol,* 2000; Vol. 95: pp. 2271–7.

> **Comments:** A single center experience utilizing preoperative endoscopic ultrasound evaluation of 82 patients with pancreatic neuroendocrine tumors, showing that endoscopic ultrasound reached a sensitivity of approximately 93%.

Boukhman MP, Karam JH, Shaver J, et al. Insulinoma—experience from 1950 to 1995. *West J Med,* 1998; Vol. 169: pp. 98–104.

> **Comments:** Retrospective review of 67 patients with sporadic and MEN-1 associated insulinoma treated at the University of California, San Francisco from 1950–1995, looking at presentation, diagnosis, localization studies, and medical and surgical treatment.

Service FJ, McMahon MM, O'Brien PC, et al. Functioning insulinoma—incidence, recurrence, and long-term survival of patients: a 60-year study. *Mayo Clin Proc,* 1991; Vol. 66: pp. 711–9.

> **Comments:** An epidemiologic profile of insulinoma based on 224 confirmed cases seen at the Mayo Clinic from 1927 through 1986.

Demeure MJ, Klonoff DC, Karam JH, et al. Insulinomas associated with multiple endocrine neoplasia type I: the need for a different surgical approach. *Surgery,* 1991; Vol. 110: pp. 998–1004, discussion 1004-5.

> **Comments:** A retrospective analysis of seven patients with insulinoma associated with MEN-1 syndrome seen at the University of California, San Francisco and a review of 53 cases reported in the English literature.

Rizza RA, Haymond MW, Verdonk CA, et al. Pathogenesis of hypoglycemia in insulinoma patients: suppression of hepatic glucose production by insulin. *Diabetes,* 1981; Vol. 30: pp. 377–81.

> **Comments:** In patients with insulinoma, fasting hypoglycemia is due to suppression of glucose production rather than to acceleration of glucose utilization.

MALE HYPOGONADISM

See Male Hypogonadism, p. 293.

SCHMIDT'S SYNDROME

Amin Sabet, MD

DEFINITION

- Schmidt's syndrome refers to the combination of autoimmune adrenal insufficiency (Addison's disease) with autoimmune hypothyroidism and/or type 1 diabetes mellitus (T1DM), and is part of a larger syndrome known as autoimmune polyendocrine syndrome type II or polyglandular autoimmune syndrome type II (PAS II).
- The term Schmidt's syndrome is sometimes used interchangeably with PAS II.
- PAS II is a polygenic disorder that may include autoimmune thyroid disease (hypothyroidism or hyperthyroidism), T1DM, Addison's disease, primary hypogonadism, and less commonly hypoparathyroidism or hypopituitarism.
- Associated nonendocrine autoimmune conditions may be present including vitiligo, celiac disease, alopecia, pernicious anemia, myasthenia gravis, idiopathic thrombocytopenic purpura, Sjögren's syndrome, and rheumatoid arthritis.

EPIDEMIOLOGY

- Schmidt's syndrome: 1:20,000 prevalence in general population with 3:1 ratio of females to males affected (Förster).
- Peak incidence: Third–fourth decade of life.
- Familial clustering with multiple family members often affected.
- Autosomal dominant inheritance with variable penetrance likely associated with certain HLA antigens (Eisenbarth).
- Among patients with T1DM, <1% of patients have Addison's disease, whereas 2%–5% have autoimmune thyroid disease (mainly hypothyroidism) and up to 5% have celiac disease (Förster).
- Type 1 diabetes patients who developed autoimmune thyroid disease had an interval of 13.3 +/– 11.8 years between first and second endocrinopathies (Dittmar).

DIAGNOSIS

- Diagnosis of component disorders of PAS II is the same as that of the individual disorders.
- Diagnosis of T1DM and celiac disease are reviewed elsewhere (see Diagnosis and Classification of Diabetes, p. 5, and Celiac Disease and Type 1 Diabetes, p. 242).
- Diagnosis of Addison's disease (primary adrenal insufficiency due to autoimmune adrenalitis) is based on the following: (1) early morning (i.e., 7–9 AM) serum cortisol <3 mcg/dl or a serum cortisol less than 18 mcg/dl 30 or 60 minutes after a 1-mcg or 250-mcg IV bolus of cosyntropin (ACTH), respectively; (2) elevated basal serum ACTH level; (3) presence of other autoimmune disorders. Antibodies to 21-hydroxylase may aid in making the diagnosis if detectable, though abdominal CT to evaluate for other causes of adrenal insufficiency (infection, hemorrhage, metastases) is recommended.
- Diagnosis of primary hypothyroidism is based on an elevated serum TSH and low (or normal in subclinical disease) serum T4 level, whereas hyperthyroidism is diagnosed based on a low TSH with elevated (or normal in subclinical disease) serum T4 and/or T3. The presence of antithyroid antibodies (e.g., antithyroglobulin antibodies, antimicrosomal antibodies, thyroid-stimulating immunoglobulins) can be useful for diagnosis.

SIGNS AND SYMPTOMS

- In a patient with T1DM, Addison's disease may present as intermittent, severe hypoglycemia, and intermittent, severe fatigue. Decreased insulin requirements, hypotension, hyperpigmentation, and vitiligo may be present.
- Hypothyroidism may also present with fatigue, decreased insulin requirements, and hypoglycemia, whereas hyperthyroidism is associated with increased insulin requirements and hyperglycemia.
- Signs and symptoms of related autoimmune conditions (e.g., alopecia, celiac disease) may be present.

CLINICAL TREATMENT

- Treatment of the component disorders of PAS II is the same as that of the individual disorders.
- Treatment of primary hypothyroidism: physiologic thyroid hormone replacement with levothyroxine. Typical initial dose is 1.6 mcg/kg per day (lower dose in elderly and those with cardiac disease) and adjusted every 4–6 weeks according to the serum T4 and TSH.
- Chronic treatment of Addison's disease: physiologic glucocorticoid and mineralocorticoid replacement. Initial glucocorticoid regimen can be hydrocortisone

COMPLICATIONS AND COMORBIDITIES

15–25 mg per day given in 2–3 divided doses and adjusted to relieve symptoms of glucocorticoid deficiency and avoid manifestations of glucocorticoid excess. Usual initial mineralocorticoid regimen is fludrocortisone 0.1 mg/day, adjusted as needed to avoid postural hypotension and maintain normal serum potassium.

- Treatment of Addison's disease in acute illness or surgery requires increased dosing of glucocorticoid therapy according to the degree of physiologic stress.

FOLLOW-UP

- Antibody screening may help identify patients at risk for developing autoimmune gland failure. For example, GAD65 antibodies in a patient with Addison's may indicate increased risk for development of T1DM, while 21-hydroxylase antibodies in a patient with T1DM likely indicates increased risk for Addison's. However, an evidence-based approach to antibody screening is lacking.

EXPERT OPINION

- Recommend screening of people with T1DM for hypothyroidism (by measuring serum TSH) and celiac disease (by measuring tissue transglutaminase antibodies) whenever symptoms are present and/or every 1–2 years.
- In the absence of symptoms, routine screening for Addison's disease or other associated PAS II autoimmune conditions is not recommended.
- **Caution:** In a patient with coexisting hypothyroidism and Addison's disease, thyroid hormone therapy without replacement of glucocorticoids can precipitate acute adrenal insufficiency.

REFERENCES

Kahaly GJ. Polyglandular autoimmune syndromes. *Eur J Endocrinol*, 2009; Vol. 161: pp. 11–20.
  Comments: Provides review of the pathophysiology and role of genetic testing in PAS.

Owen CJ, Cheetham TD. Diagnosis and management of polyendocrinopathy syndromes. *Endocrinol Metab Clin North Am*, 2009; Vol. 38: pp. 419–36, x.
  Comments: Reviews diagnosis and management of polyendocrinopathy syndromes.

Dittmar M, Kahaly GJ. Polyglandular autoimmune syndromes: immunogenetics and long-term follow-up. *J Clin Endocrinol Metab*, 2003; Vol. 88: pp. 2983–92.
  Comments: Type 1 diabetes patients who developed autoimmune thyroid disease had an interval of 13.3 +/– 11.8 years between first and second endocrinopathies.

Förster G, Krummenauer F, Kühn I, et al. Polyglandular autoimmune syndrome type II: epidemiology and forms of manifestation. *Dtsch Med Wochenschr*, 1999; Vol. 124: pp. 1476–81.
  Comments: Reviews epidemiology of PAS II.

Eisenbarth G, Wilson P, Ward F, et al. HLA type and occurrence of disease in familial polyglandular failure. *NEJM*, 1978; Vol. 298: pp. 92–4.
  Comments: Association of HLA antigens with PAS.

SOMATOSTATINOMA

Amin Sabet, MD

DEFINITION

- Rare somatostatin-producing neuroendocrine tumors (NETs), which arise primarily in the pancreas and duodenum.

- Associated with diabetes since high somatostatin levels suppress insulin secretion (Gerich).

EPIDEMIOLOGY
- Represent 1%–2% of pancreatic islet cell tumors (He).
- Median age at diagnosis is 50 years (range 26–84 years) with equal sex distribution.
- Greater than 50% arise in pancreas, two-thirds of which are in head of pancreas.
- Most extrapancreatic somatostatinomas arise in duodenum; rarely found as primary tumors of liver, colon, or rectum.
- Most sporadic but minority can also be associated with MEN-1 syndrome.
- Duodenal somatostatinomas are associated with neurofibromatosis type 1 (NF-1)/von Recklinghausen's disease.
- Majority of somatostatinoma cases are malignant with metastases present at the time of diagnosis.
- Leads to diabetes in majority of patients with pancreatic tumors; ~10% in intestinal tumors.
- In one case series, diabetes occurred in 36% of patients with somatostatinoma (6 pancreatic, 5 duodenal) (Moayedoddin).

DIAGNOSIS
- Often discovered during evaluation of patients with abdominal pain, weight loss, or jaundice. May be discovered as an incidental finding during imaging (86% pancreatic vs 41% of extrapancreatic somatostatinomas are >2 cm) or during operation for an unrelated problem.
- If the diagnosis is suspected based on symptoms, a preoperative fasting somatostatin level ≥160 pg/ml (normal range 10–22 pg/ml) is suggestive of somatostatinoma.
- Imaging studies may be structural (endoscopic ultrasound, CT, MRI) or functional (octreotide scan).

SIGNS AND SYMPTOMS
- Most common symptoms are nonspecific: weight loss and abdominal pain.
- May present with classic triad (somatostatinoma syndrome): diabetes mellitus (decreased insulin release), cholelithiasis (decreased cholecystokinin release with decreased gallbladder contractility), and diarrhea with steatorrhea (inhibition of pancreatic enzyme and bicarbonate secretion causing decreased intestinal absorption of lipids).
- Classic triad likely occurs only in about 10% of patients, more common in pancreatic tumors.
- Duodenal somatostatinoma rarely cause this triad and may present with obstructive symptoms including pain and jaundice.
- Diabetes can range from mild glucose intolerance (more common) to ketoacidosis (Jackson).
- Rare cases of somatostatinoma presenting with hypoglycemia attributed to inhibition of glucagon and growth hormone have been reported (He).

CLINICAL TREATMENT
Surgical Therapy
- Treatment of choice is surgical resection, which is the only potentially curative therapy.
- Surgical debulking may improve symptoms in patients with metastatic disease.

Medical Therapy
- For unresectable disease, the somatostatin analog octreotide may reduce plasma somatostatin levels and improve diarrhea, hyperglycemia, and weight loss.

COMPLICATIONS AND COMORBIDITIES

- Treatment with interferon alpha may alleviate symptoms in greater than 50% of patients with pancreatic NETs although tumor response rates are low (Schöber; Bajetta).
- Palliative chemoembolization of liver metastases may provide symptomatic improvement in selected patients with metastatic pancreatic NETs.
- Results of systemic cytotoxic chemotherapy for metastatic pancreatic NETs have been disappointing, although some activity has been reported for combination streptozocin- and temozolomide-based regimens (Kouvaraki; Kulke).
- Hyperglycemia treated similar to other forms of diabetes; in addition, octreotide treatment may improve hyperglycemia.

FOLLOW-UP

- History and physical, imaging studies (CT/MRI), and fasting somatostatin level are recommended 3 and 6 months after surgical resection.
- Thereafter, clinical and biochemical surveillance are recommended every 6–12 months with imaging as clinically indicated.
- In one series of 44 patients with metastatic somatostatinoma, 5-year survival rate was 60% (Soga).
- Surgical management for pancreatic somatostatinomas (i.e., pancreatectomy) may lead to development of diabetes; glucose levels should be monitored regularly.

EXPERT OPINION

- In contrast to other causes of secondary diabetes such as acromegaly and Cushing's syndrome, which are associated with insulin resistance, somatostatinomas are associated with suppression of insulin release. This may influence choice of glucose-lowering agent for persistent hyperglycemia.
- Diabetes is usually mild and more common in pancreatic somatostatinomas.
- Pancreatectomy for pancreatic somatostatinoma may also lead to development of diabetes.

REFERENCES

He X, Wang J, Wu X, et al. Pancreatic somatostatinoma manifested as severe hypoglycemia. *J Gastrointestin Liver Dis,* 2009; Vol. 18: pp. 221–4.
   Comments: Unusual hypoglycemic presentation of somatostatinoma.

Kulke MH, Stuart K, Enzinger PC, et al. Phase II study of temozolomide and thalidomide in patients with metastatic neuroendocrine tumors. *J Clin Oncol,* 2006; Vol. 24: pp. 401–6.
   Comments: 25% objective radiologic response rate with temozolomide/thalidomide treatment of metastatic NETs.

Moayedoddin B, Booya F, Wermers RA, et al. Spectrum of malignant somatostatin-producing neuroendocrine tumors. *Endocr Pract,* 2006; Vol. 12: pp. 394–400.
   Comments: Diabetes occurred in 36% of patients with somatostatinoma (5 duodenal, 6 pancreatic) in this case series.

Kouvaraki MA, Ajani JA, Hoff P, et al. Fluorouracil, doxorubicin, and streptozocin in the treatment of patients with locally advanced and metastatic pancreatic endocrine carcinomas. *J Clin Oncol,* 2004; Vol. 22: pp. 4762–71.
   Comments: 39% objective radiologic response rate with streptozocin/5-FU/doxorubicin treatment of locally advanced and metastatic pancreatic NETs.

Soga J, Yakuwa Y. Somatostatinoma/inhibitory syndrome: a statistical evaluation of 173 reported cases as compared to other pancreatic endocrinomas. *J Exp Clin Cancer Res,* 1999; Vol. 18: pp. 13–22.
   Comments: Among 173 reported cases of somatostatinoma (83 pancreatic and 92 extrapancreatic), 5-year survival was 59.9% in patients with metastases and 100% in patients without metastases.

Angeletti S, Corleto VD, Schillaci O, et al. Use of the somatostatin analogue octreotide to localise and manage somatostatin-producing tumours. *Gut*, 1998; Vol. 42: pp. 792–4.

Comments: In 3 patients with somatostatinoma detected by octreotide scan, octreotide therapy resulted in decreased plasma somatostatinoma levels. Two patients with somatostatinoma syndrome had improved diabetes and diarrhea after treatment with octreotide.

Bajetta E, Zilembo N, Di Bartolomeo M, et al. Treatment of metastatic carcinoids and other neuroendocrine tumors with recombinant interferon-alpha-2a. A study by the Italian Trials in Medical Oncology Group. *Cancer*, 1993; Vol. 72: pp. 3099–105.

Comments: Efficacy of interferon alpha-2a in treating metastatic NETs.

Schöber C, Schmoll E, Schmoll HJ, et al. Antitumour effect and symptomatic control with interferon alpha-2b in patients with endocrine active tumours. *Eur J Cancer*, 1992; Vol. 28A: pp. 1664–6.

Comments: Efficacy of interferon alpha-2b in treating pain, diarrhea, and flushing due to progressive NETs.

Jackson JA, Raju BU, Fachnie JD, et al. Malignant somatostatinoma presenting with diabetic ketoacidosis. *Clin Endocrinol* (Oxford), 1987; Vol. 26: pp. 609–21.

Comments: Report of malignant somatostatinoma associated with ketoacidosis.

Gerich JE. Somatostatin and diabetes. *Am J Med*, 1981; Vol. 70: pp. 619–26.

Comments: Describes pathophysiology of somatostatin in reducing growth hormone, insulin, and glucagon release and role in diabetes development.

COMPLICATIONS AND COMORBIDITIES

Female Disorders

MENOPAUSAL EFFECTS ON GLYCEMIA

Melissa Yates, MD, and Wanda K. Nicholson, MD, MPH, MBA

DEFINITION
- Menopause: the cessation of menses for 12 consecutive months (Carr).
- Surgical menopause: begins the day that both ovaries are surgically removed in a previously menstruating patient.

EPIDEMIOLOGY
- Diabetes is the most common disease in the postmenopausal period (Wedisinghe).
- Increased type 2 diabetes will cause increased prevalence of postmenopausal women with diabetes. Estimated 20% of women >65 years will also have diabetes (Shih).
- Metabolic changes with menopause may contribute to development of diabetes: increased central body fat, increased LDL, and decreased HDL, and increased insulin resistance (Shih).
- Increased insulin resistance with relatively stable pancreatic insulin secretion after menopause may increase risk of developing type 2 diabetes (Wedisinghe).
- Endogenous sex hormones including higher bioavailable testosterone, higher estradiol, and lower SHBG are associated with incident diabetes in postmenopausal women and may be partially explained by higher adiposity and insulin resistance (Kalyani).
- 60% increased risk of metabolic syndrome in postmenopausal women (Carr).
- Women with type 1 diabetes have a greater incidence of premature menopause with a mean of 41.6 years, versus 51 years in women without diabetes (Dorman).
- Postmenopausal women with type 1 diabetes have a RR of 12.25 for hip fracture while type 2 diabetes have a relative risk of 1.70, compared to postmenopausal women without diabetes (Nicodemus).

SIGNS AND SYMPTOMS
- Women with diabetes may have more menopausal hot flushes and vaginal dryness than women without diabetes.
- During the perimenopause, there may be an increase in glycemic swings because of the changing endogenous sex hormone levels (Shih).

CLINICAL TREATMENT
- Due to increased risk of cardiovascular disease (CVD) after menopause, encourage control of CVD risk factors postmenopausally (Carr).
- Weight gain has stronger influence on risk of diabetes than menopause itself (Carr).
- Hormone replacement therapy (HRT) may be beneficial in symptomatic women <60 years with diabetes and without known CVD. Recommend lowest effective dose in this select group of women (Wedisinghe).
- Exogenous HRT may be associated with either favorable or unfavorable effects on glycemia depending on dose and route of treatment (Lindheim; Cagnacci).
- Due to increased risk of endometrial cancer in women with diabetes, couple estrogen therapy with progesterone therapy if uterus intact (Wedisinghe).

- For symptomatic vaginal dryness, recommend daily Replens and consideration of local estrogen therapy such as Vagifem or Estring, which have a low systemic absorption of estrogen.
- With CVD or other risk factors, would recommend nonhormonal treatments such as venlafaxine, gabapentin, or clonidine for hot flushes and vitamin D, calcium, and bisphosphonates for osteoporosis (Wedisinghe).

FOLLOW-UP

- Consider DEXA bone density screening in postmenopausal women with diabetes due to increased risk of osteoporosis.

EXPERT OPINION

- Any vaginal bleeding after starting HRT or in the postmenopausal period should be fully evaluated by a gynecologist.

REFERENCES

Wedisinghe L, Perera M. Diabetes and the menopause. *Maturitas*, 2009; Vol. 63: pp. 200–3.
  Comments: Review of the management of menopausal symptoms in the setting of diabetes.

Hadjidakis DI, Androulakis II, Mylonakis AM, et al. Diabetes in postmenopause: different influence on bone mass according to age and disease duration. *Exp Clin Endocrinol Diabetes*, 2009; Vol. 117: pp. 199–204.
  Comments: Prospective, cohort study evaluating the influence of type 2 DM on bone metabolism.

Shih J, Abrahamson M. Treatment of type 2 diabetes: an update. *Menopause Manage*, 2009; July/August: pp. 20–26.
  Comments: Review of pharmacologic management of type 2 DM in the setting of menopause.

Kalyani RR, Franco M, Dobs AS, et al. The association of endogenous sex hormones, adiposity, and insulin resistance with incident diabetes in postmenopausal women. *J Clin Endocrinol Metab*, 2009; Vol. 94: pp. 4127–35.
  Comments: Prospective study reporting that higher bioavailable testosterone, higher estradiol and lower SHBG were associated with incident diabetes in postmenopausal women, partially explained by higher adiposity and insulin resistance.

Kernohan AF, Sattar N, Hilditch T, et al. Effects of low-dose continuous combined hormone replacement therapy on glucose homeostasis and markers of cardiovascular risk in women with type 2 diabetes. *Clin Endocrinol* (Oxford), 2007; Vol. 66: pp. 27–34.
  Comments: Prospective, randomized, double-blind, placebo-controlled trial comparing markers for glucose homeostasis and cardiac risk in women with type 2 diabetes who took low-dose HRT.

Salpeter SR, Walsh JM, Ormiston TM, et al. Meta-analysis: effect of hormone-replacement therapy on components of the metabolic syndrome in postmenopausal women. *Diabetes Obes Metab*, 2006; Vol. 8: pp. 538–54.
  Comments: A meta-analysis of 107 trials regarding the effect of HRT on the metabolic syndrome.

Howard BV, Hsia J, Ouyang P, et al. Postmenopausal hormone therapy is associated with atherosclerosis progression in women with abnormal glucose tolerance. *Circulation*, 2004; Vol. 110: pp. 201–6.
  Comments: Women with abnormal glucose tolerance were noted to have increased levels of C-reactive protein and fibrinogen as well as atherosclerotic progression after 2.8 years of postmenopausal hormone therapy.

Margolis KL, Bonds DE, Rodabough RJ, et al. Effect of estrogen plus progestin on the incidence of diabetes in postmenopausal women: results from the Women's Health Initiative Hormone Trial. *Diabetologia*, 2004; Vol. 47: pp. 1175–87.
  Comments: An evaluation of the data generated from the Women's Health Initiative in regard to the effect of HRT on incidence of diabetes and its effect on insulin resistance.

Kanaya AM, Herrington D, Vittinghoff E, et al. Glycemic effects of postmenopausal hormone therapy: the Heart and Estrogen/Progestin Replacement Study. A randomized, double-blind, placebo-controlled trial. *Ann Intern Med*, 2003; Vol. 138: pp. 1–9.
  Comments: Prospective, randomized, double-blind, placebo-controlled trial comparing combined HRT use versus placebo in women with known coronary heart disease; women were followed for an average of 4.1 years.

COMPLICATIONS AND COMORBIDITIES

Carr MC. The emergence of the metabolic syndrome with menopause. *J Clin Endocrinol Metab,* 2003; Vol. 88: pp. 2404–11.

   Comments: Review of the role that estrogen deficiency plays in development of the metabolic syndrome in postmenopausal women and how these changes may contribute to overall CVD risk.

Dorman JS, Steenkiste AR, Foley TP, et al. Menopause in type 1 diabetic women: is it premature? *Diabetes,* 2001; Vol. 50: pp. 1857–62.

   Comments: Comparison of women with type 1 DM, their sisters, and control subjects, which determined a statistically significant younger age at menopause in women with type 1 DM resulting in a 17% decrease in reproductive years.

Nicodemus KK, Folsom AR, Iowa Women's Health Study. Type 1 and type 2 diabetes and incident hip fractures in postmenopausal women. *Diabetes Care,* 2001; Vol. 24: pp. 1192–7.

   Comments: Prospective cohort analysis of postmenopausal women to compare the incidence of hip fracture in women with and without diabetes.

Lindheim SR, Presser SC, Ditkoff EC, et al. A possible bimodal effect of estrogen on insulin sensitivity in postmenopausal women and the attenuating effect of added progestin. *Fertil Steril,* 1993; Vol. 60: pp. 664–7.

   Comments: An intervention trial examining the effect of varying doses of exogenous estrogen on insulin resistance. Moderate dose of estrogen improved insulin sensitivity but higher doses attenuated this benefit.

Cagnacci A, Soldani R, Carriero PL, et al. Effects of low doses of transdermal 17 beta-estradiol on carbohydrate metabolism in postmenopausal women. *J Clin Endocrinol Metab,* 1992; Vol. 74: pp. 1396–400.

   Comments: Clinical trial comparing effects of oral and transdermal estrogen on glucose metabolism. Transdermal estradiol had a beneficial effect on glucose metabolism by increasing hepatic insulin clearance.

MENSTRUAL CYCLE AND GLYCEMIA IN PREMENOPAUSAL WOMEN

Melissa Yates, MD, and Wanda K. Nicholson, MD, MPH, MBA

DEFINITION

- The menstrual cycle refers to the series of physiological changes that occur monthly in reproductive aged women to prepare for a possible pregnancy, heralded by the onset of menses during puberty (menarche).
- Uterine bleeding associated with abnormal menstrual cycles can be anovulatory or ovulatory.
- **Secondary amenorrhea:** absence of menses for more than 6 months (or 3 cycles) in women who were previously menstruating.
- **Oligomenorrhea:** fewer than 9 menstrual periods in 1 year or menstrual cycles >35 days.
- **Polymenorrhea:** regular menstrual cycles of <21 days.
- **Menorrhagia:** prolonged (>7 days) or excessive uterine bleeding at regular intervals.
- **Metrorrhagia:** irregular, frequent uterine bleeding of varying amounts and duration.
- **Intermenstrual:** uterine bleeding between cycles.

EPIDEMIOLOGY

- Both type 1 (T1DM) and type 2 (T2DM) are associated with menstrual cycle disturbances (Arrais).
- Secondary amenorrhea and oligomenorrhea are present in 20%–30% of people with T1DM (Arrais).

- Due to delayed menarche and premature onset of menopause, the period of fertility is shortened up to 17% in patients with T1DM (Arrais).
- T1DM adolescents with HbA1c >9% have a longer cycle duration, delayed menarche, and 5 times greater risk of oligomenorrhea, 12 times greater risk of amenorrhea (Gaete).
- T2DM associated with oligomenorrhea and polycystic ovarian syndrome.
- Menorrhagia can also be seen in both T1DM and T2DM, in anovulatory patients still producing estrogen.
- Two times greater risk of developing T2DM among women with menstrual cycles >40 days or too irregular to estimate (Solomon).

DIAGNOSIS

- Medical history for menstrual pattern, extent of recent bleeding, sexual activity, trauma, and symptoms of infection or systemic disease (e.g., hepatic or renal disease).
- Blood pressure, especially if considering oral contraceptive pills.
- Pelvic examination to identify alternative source of bleeding (i.e., rectum), lesions in vagina or cervix, uterine tenderness.
- Consider CBC, coagulation tests.
- Exclude pregnancy.
- Secondary amenorrhea with diabetes usually due to hypogonadotrophic hypogonadism (low FSH, LH, and estradiol).
- Anovulatory bleeding: exclude hyperprolactinemia, hypothyroidism, hyperthyroidism, polycystic ovarian syndrome, Cushing's syndrome, hypothalamic disorders (weight loss, eating disorders, stress, chronic illness, or excessive exercise).
- Ovulatory bleeding: exclude structural lesions, bleeding disorder (for menorrhagia or metrorrhagia).
- Intermenstrual bleeding: exclude IUD, cervical disease, or STDs such as gonorrhea or chlamydia.
- Ovulation status best determined by gynecologist.

SIGNS AND SYMPTOMS

- Blood glucose levels may increase during the luteal phase (second half) of the menstrual cycle, likely associated with higher endogenous sex hormone levels, and may require adjustment of insulin (Trout).
- Case reports of DKA at the time of menses in patients with T1DM (Ovalle).
- Abdominal pain, fever, vaginal discharge; signs and symptoms related to other endocrine etiologies or systemic diseases.

CLINICAL TREATMENT

Use of Hormonal Contraception

- With amenorrhea or oligomenorrhea, consider oral contraceptive pills (OCPs) such as Loestrin 1.5/30 in women without vasculopathy to improve cycle control.
- Progesterone only hormonal medications such as the Micronor OCP and the Mirena IUD have only minor influences on metabolic parameters and can be used in women with vascular disease (Visser).
- Limited data suggest no increased complications with IUD use in women with diabetes.

COMPLICATIONS AND COMORBIDITIES

- Hormonal treatments are not recommended in any of the following patients with diabetes: >35 years old, smokers, history of nephropathy, retinopathy, neuropathy, other vascular disease or diabetes duration >20 years (Vicente). The copper IUD may be used as an alternative in these patients.
- Patients with polycystic ovarian syndrome (PCOS) and/or oligomenorrhea should have a menstrual flow induced with Provera (10 mg × 10 days) at least every 3 months to decrease the risk of developing endometrial hyperplasia.

FOLLOW-UP

- Refer patients with polymenorrhea, menorrhagia, metrorrhaggia, and intermenstrual bleeding especially to a gynecologist for workup and evaluation.
- Try to improve glycemia in any woman with diabetes and menstrual cycle disturbances, although this may not restore menstrual regularity.
- Obtain estradiol, LH, FSH, prolactin, androstenedione, 17-hydroxyprogesterone levels, TSH, and 24-hour urine free cortisol to evaluate patients with menstrual disturbances that persist after improved glycemic control for other etiologies (la Marca).

EXPERT OPINION

- In reproductive-age women, HbA1c below 6.0% can reduce risk of fetal anomalies and spontaneous abortion in pregnancy.

REFERENCES

Gaete X, Vivanco M, Eyzaguirre FC, et al. Menstrual cycle irregularities and their relationship with HbA1c and insulin dose in adolescents with type 1 diabetes mellitus. *Fert Steril*, 2010; Vol. 94(5): pp. 1822–6.
   Comments: Prospective comparison of menstrual cycle irregularities in T1DM adoloescents and controls.

Ovalle F, Vaughan TA, Sohn JE, et al. Catamenial diabetic ketoacidosis and catamenial hyperglycemia: case report and review of the literature. *Am J Med Sci*, 2008; Vol. 335: pp. 298–303.
   Comments: 2 case reports of recurrent DKA at the time of the menstrual cycle.

Vicente L, Mendonça D, Dingle M, et al. Etonogestrel implant in women with diabetes mellitus. *Eur J Contracept Reprod Health Care*, 2008; Vol. 13: pp. 387–95.
   Comments: Evaluation of the effect of the etonogestrel implant (Implanon) on carbohydrate and lipid metabolism in diabetic women.

Trout KK, Rickels MR, Schutta MH, et al. Menstrual cycle effects on insulin sensitivity in women with type 1 diabetes: a pilot study. *Diabetes Technol Ther*, 2007; Vol. 9: pp. 176–82.
   Comments: Mean fasting glucose levels were higher in the luteal phase compared to the follicular phase, though the results were not significant; however, insulin adjustments may need to be made during the second half of the menstrual cycle.

Arrais RF, Dib SA. The hypothalamus-pituitary-ovary axis and type 1 diabetes mellitus: a mini review. *Hum Reprod*, 2006; Vol. 21: pp. 327–37.
   Comments: Review of the importance of evaluation of the HPO axis in diabetic patients with adequate glycemic control and menstrual irregularities.

Visser J, Snel M, Van Vliet HA. Hormonal versus non-hormonal contraceptives in women with diabetes mellitus type 1 and 2. *Cochrane Database Syst Rev*, 2006; CD003990.
   Comments: Review of 4 randomized controlled trials regarding the use of hormonal versus nonhormonal contraception in diabetic women.

Solomon, CG, Hu Fb, Dunaif, A, et al. Long or highly irregular menstrual cycles as a marker for risk of type 2 diabetes mellitus. *JAMA*, 2001; Vol. 286: pp. 2421–6.
   Comments: Part of the Nurses Health Study II noting a significantly increased risk of T2DM in women with a history of irregular or long menstrual cycles.

la Marca A, Morgante G, De Leo V. Evaluation of hypothalamic-pituitary-adrenal axis in amenorrhoeic women with insulin-dependent diabetes. *Hum Reprod*, 1999; Vol. 14: pp. 298–302.

Comments: Stress induced activation of the hypothalamic-pituitary-adrenal axis may lead to hypogonoadotrophic amenorrhea.

POLYCYSTIC OVARIAN SYNDROME

Amin Sabet, MD

DEFINITION

- Polycystic ovarian syndrome (PCOS) is a heterogenous disorder with major features including menstrual irregularity, androgen excess, and/or polycystic ovaries.

EPIDEMIOLOGY

- Most common endocrine disorder of premenopausal women. Estimated prevalence of 6%–7% in general population worldwide.
- Present in up to 91% of women with euestrogenic normogonadotropic ovulatory dysfunction (Broekmans).
- Up to 35% of women with PCOS have impaired glucose tolerance and 10% have type 2 diabetes by age 40 years (Ehrmann).
- Up to 41% of adult women with type 1 diabetes have PCOS using Rotterdam criteria (see Diagnosis section here), compared with 11.9% prevalence using 1990 NIH diagnostic criteria (Codner).

DIAGNOSIS

- **NIH criteria** (1990): Exclusion of other conditions that cause menstrual irregularity and androgen excess and presence of both menstrual irregularity due to oligo- or anovulation and clinical or biochemical evidence of hyperandrogenism.
- **Rotterdam criteria** (2003): Exclusion of other conditions that cause menstrual irregularity and androgen excess and presence of at least two of the following: (1) oligoovulation or anovulation; (2) clinical and/or biochemical evidence of hyperandrogenism; (3) polycystic ovaries by ultrasound (>11 follicles measuring 2–9 mm in each ovary).
- Conditions to be excluded for diagnosis of PCOS: pregnancy, congenital adrenal hyperplasia (CAH), androgen-secreting tumors, hypothyroidism, hyperprolactinemia, Cushing's syndrome.
- Lab tests: serum HCG, prolactin, TSH, LH, FSH, free testosterone, DHEA-S, 17-OH progesterone, 1 mg overnight dexamethasone suppression test (if symptoms/signs of Cushing's present).
- In PCOS, LH to FSH ratio often elevated. Androgrens including free testosterone and DHEA-S usually high.
- Nonclassic CAH is suggested by elevated AM serum 17-OH progesterone in early follicular phase and confirmed by measurement of 17-OH progesterone after ACTH stimulation.
- Women with androgen-secreting tumors typically present with amenorrhea, progressive hirsutism, virilization (deepening voice, clitoromegaly), free testosterone >150 mg/dl or DHEA-S >800 mcg/dl, and low LH.

COMPLICATIONS AND COMORBIDITIES

- Pelvic ultrasound not needed for NIH criteria.
- Consider screening for impaired glucose states including fasting blood glucose and/or oral glucose tolerance test.

SIGNS AND SYMPTOMS

- Menstrual irregularity characterized by oligomenorrhea or amenorrhea with typical onset in peripubertal period (primary amenorrhea) or after weight gain (secondary amenorrhea).
- Anovulatory infertility is frequently seen.
- Hyperandrogenism characterized by hirsutism (excessive terminal body hair in male pattern), acne, and/or male pattern hair loss.
- Chronic anovulation can lead to endometrial hyperplasia, dysfunctional uterine bleeding, and possibly endometrial cancer.
- Can occur in normal weight individuals.

CLINICAL TREATMENT

- Weight loss often improves hyperandrogenism, menstrual irregularity, and infertility.
- Hirsutism generally managed with estrogen-progestin contraceptive (OCP) medication (usually containing ethinyl estradiol in a dose of 20–35 mcg/day and a nonandrogenic progestin such as norgestimate, desogestrel, or drospirenone).
- Spironolactone (starting dose of 50 mg once or twice daily, can be increased to 100 mg twice daily) has additional benefit in hirsutism but should not be used without contraception since maternal spironolactone use may prevent normal sex characteristics in the developing male fetus.
- Metformin therapy can be used to manage metabolic derangements associated with PCOS (obesity, insulin resistance); may decrease androgen levels and improve menstrual irregularity.
- Endometrial protection may be accomplished via estrogen-progestin OCP or intermittent progestin therapy such as medroxyprogesterone acetate 10 mg daily for 7–10 days every 1–2 months.
- Clomiphene citrate is first-line drug therapy for induction of ovulation in women with PCOS, although metformin may also be effective.
- Hyperglycemia in people with PCOS and diabetes is managed no differently than in others with diabetes.

FOLLOW-UP

- Surveillance for and treatment of prevalent comorbid conditions: obesity, insulin resistance, type 2 diabetes, dyslipidemia (typically high triglycerides and low HDL), fatty liver, and sleep apnea.

EXPERT OPINION

- Given that ultrasonographic criteria of polycystic ovaries may be difficult to document and that otherwise normal women may have polycystic ovaries, we continue to use the 1990 NIH criteria to make the diagnosis of PCOS.
- Women with typical features of PCOS (onset of menstrual irregularity in peripubertal period, overweight/obesity) and mild hirsutism may not require measurement of serum androgens, whereas those with moderate to severe or progressive hirsutism, any virilization, or onset of menstrual irregularity after age 20 should be tested for testosterone and DHEA-S excess to evaluate for androgen-secreting tumor.

- In overweight or obese women with PCOS, we typically consider metformin as a first-line therapy given its favorable metabolic effects and potential efficacy as an agent to lower androgen levels and correct menstrual irregularity.
- Based on limited available data (Cheung), we consider referral for endometrial biopsy in women with PCOS and a history of fewer than 5 menstrual periods yearly.

BASIS FOR RECOMMENDATIONS

Polycystic Ovary Syndrome Writing Committee. American Association of Clinical Endocrinologists position statement on metabolic and cardiovascular consequences of polycystic ovary syndrome. *Endocr Pract*, 2005; Vol. 11: pp. 126–34.

  Comments: American Association of Clinical Endocrinologists' position statement regarding metabolic aspects of PCOS.

Rotterdam ESHRE/ASRM-sponsored PCOS Consensus Workshop Group. Revised 2003 consensus on diagnostic criteria and long-term health risks related to polycystic ovary syndrome (PCOS). *Hum Reprod*, 2004; Vol. 19: pp. 41–7.

  Comments: 2003 Rotterdam consensus on PCOS diagnostic criteria.

Zawadski, JK, Dunaif, A. Diagnostic criteria for polycystic ovary syndrome: Towards a rational approach. In Dunaif A, Givens JR, Haseltine FP, Merriam GE, (Eds.), *Polycystic Ovary Syndrome.* Oxford, UK: Blackwell Publishing; 1992: pp. 59–69.

  Comments: NIH diagnostic criteria for PCOS.

OTHER REFERENCES

Nestler JE. Metformin for the treatment of the polycystic ovary syndrome. *NEJM*, 2008; Vol. 358: pp. 47–54.

  Comments: Review of metformin therapy for PCOS.

Legro RS, Barnhart HX, Schlaff WD, et al. Clomiphene, metformin, or both for infertility in the polycystic ovary syndrome. *NEJM*, 2007; Vol. 356: pp. 551–66.

  Comments: Infertile women with PCOS treated with clomiphene had a 3-fold higher live-birth rate compared with those treated with metformin.

Broekmans FJ, Knauff EA, Valkenburg O, et al. PCOS according to the Rotterdam consensus criteria: Change in prevalence among WHO-II anovulation and association with metabolic factors. *BJOG*, 2006; Vol. 113: pp. 1210–7.

  Comments: Using Rotterdam criteria, PCOS was present in 91% of women with euestrogenic normogonadotropic ovulatory dysfunction.

Codner E, Soto N, Lopez P, et al. Diagnostic criteria for polycystic ovary syndrome and ovarian morphology in women with type 1 diabetes mellitus. *J Clin Endocrinol Metab*, 2006; Vol. 91: pp. 2250–6.

  Comments: Among adult women with type 1 diabetes, 38.1% had clinical hyperandrogenism, 23.8% had biochemical hyperandrogenism, 19% had menstrual dysfunction, and 40.5% had PCOS based on Rotterdam criteria (vs 11.9% using 1990 NIH criteria).

Ehrmann DA. Polycystic ovary syndrome. *NEJM*, 2005; Vol. 352: pp. 1223–36.

  Comments: Current review of PCOS.

Cheung AP. Ultrasound and menstrual history in predicting endometrial hyperplasia in polycystic ovary syndrome. *Obstet Gynecol*, 2001; Vol. 98: pp. 325–31.

  Comments: Among women with PCOS, intermenstrual interval <3 months and endometrial thickness >7 mm were predictors of endometrial hyperplasia.

Ehrmann DA, Barnes RB, Rosenfield RL, et al. Prevalence of impaired glucose tolerance and diabetes in women with polycystic ovary syndrome. *Diabetes Care*, 1999; Vol. 22: pp. 141–6.

  Comments: 35% and 10% prevalence of IGT and type 2 diabetes, respectively, in women with PCOS.

COMPLICATIONS AND COMORBIDITIES

Gastrointestinal Diseases

CELIAC DISEASE AND TYPE 1 DIABETES

Octavia Pickett-Blakely, MD, MHS, and Mary Huizinga, MD, MPH

DEFINITION
- Celiac disease (CD) is a gluten-sensitive enteropathy characterized by autoimmune mucosal inflammation and abnormal villous architecture leading to small bowel malabsorption.

EPIDEMIOLOGY
- The prevalence of CD in the general US population is 0.4% to 1.0% (Collin; Green; Rewers).
- The prevalence of CD in patients with type 1 diabetes ranges from 1% to 16.4% (Rewers).
- In patients with CD, the prevalence of type 1 diabetes is 5% to 10% (Rewers).
- Type 1 diabetes is diagnosed before CD in 90% of patients.
- Given the wide spectrum of disease, there is no defined time period of celiac disease presentation after diabetes diagnosis.

DIAGNOSIS
- Serology: used as a noninvasive screening test in high-risk populations, includes positive antitissue transglutaminase (tTG), antigliadin, or antiendomysial (EM) IgA (antigliadin only) or IgG antibodies (all) while on a gluten-containing diet. Antiendomysial and tissue transglutaminase antibodies and a quantitative IgA are usually tested simultaneously during initial screening.
- Gold standard: upper endoscopy with duodenal biopsy showing intraepithelial lymphocytosis, crypt hyperplasia, and villous hyperplasia that improve with a gluten-free diet.
- Genetic testing: HLA-DR2 and HLA-DR8 have high negative predictive value and are useful in asymptomatic individuals with a family history of celiac disease or autoimmune disease like type 1 diabetes. In type 1 diabetes, this is not the recommended CD screening algorithm but is an alternative.

SIGNS AND SYMPTOMS
- Classic symptoms: diarrhea and weight loss.
- Other gastrointestinal symptoms: bloating, abdominal pain.
- Generalized symptoms: fatigue, failure to thrive.
- Biochemical abnormalities: iron-deficiency anemia, abnormal transaminases, hypoalbuminemia, hypocalcemia from vitamin D deficiency.
- Osteopenia or osteoporosis.
- Infertility.
- Neuropsychiatric symptoms.
- Dermatitis herpatiformis: an itchy, prurutic eruption of red blisters (usually on the knees, elbows, or buttocks) that may later be associated with an intense burning.
- Other autoimmune conditions (e.g., hypothyroidism).

CLINICAL TREATMENT

- Gluten-free diet: eliminates wheat, rye, and barley. Common gluten free foods include fresh fish, meats, milk, cheese, fruits, and vegetables.
- A gluten-free diet in diabetics is challenging because wheat products would be encouraged due to of their low glycemic index; however, gluten-free substitutes often also have low glycemic indices.
- Gluten-free substitutes are often expensive and may be difficult to access.
- Repletion of micronutrient deficiencies (e.g., iron, vitamin D, B12, folate).
- Fertility counseling.

FOLLOW-UP

- All patients with celiac disease should be screened for osteoporosis with bone densitometry.
- Symptoms and histology generally improve within 2–4 weeks of initiation of a gluten-free diet and can completely resolve with dietary adherence.
- Patients should be screened for micronutrient deficiencies and evaluated by an experienced dietician/nutritionist.
- ADA clinical practice guidelines recommend antibody screening in type 1 diabetes with signs or symptoms (e.g., iron-deficiency anemia, hypocalcemia, fatigue, bloating) suggestive of CD; however, widespread screening in asymptomatic patients is not recommended (ADA).
- Repeat antibody screening in patients with changes in symptomatology (e.g., weight loss, failure to gain weight in children), though definite intervals of testing are undefined (ADA).

EXPERT OPINION

- Up to 2.5% of patients with celiac disease may have isolated IgA deficiency and therefore will have falsely negative tTG, endomysial, and gliadin IgA antibody tests; quantitative IgA testing is useful in these situations and often performed with initial screening.
- Patients with symptoms despite adherence to a strict gluten free-diet should have an evaluation for hidden sources of gluten, secondary diagnoses (e.g., lactose malabsorption), and complications of celiac sprue (e.g., mucosal associated T-cell lymphoma).
- Asymptomatic type 1 diabetes patients can be screened using serologic testing; however, those with persistent symptoms should undergo diagnostic testing with upper endoscopy and small bowel biopsy.
- Although celiac disease increases the risk of small intestinal adenocarcinoma and T-cell lymphoma, there are no established screening guidelines. The clonal expansion of T-cells is thought to be a gluten-independent process and thus may develop despite strict adherence to a gluten free diet (DiSabatino).
- Glycemic control may improve in patients with type 1 diabetes and celiac disease who are adherent to a gluten-free diet, although data are limited (Amin).
- There are numerous online resources for CD patients, including *http://www.celiac.org/* and *http://www.gluten.net*.

BASIS FOR RECOMMENDATIONS

American Diabetes Association. Standards of medical care in diabetes—2011. *Diabetes Care*, 2011; Vol. 34 Suppl 1: pp. S11–61.

    Comments: Provides clinical practice guidelines for screening type 1 diabetes patients for CD.

COMPLICATIONS AND COMORBIDITIES

OTHER REFERENCES

Sollid LM, Lundin KE. Diagnosis and treatment of celiac disease. *Mucosal Immunol*, 2009; Vol. 2: pp. 3–7.
  Comments: Novel targets for treatment of CD.

Di Sabatino A, Corazza GR. Celiac disease. *Lancet*, 2009; Vol. 373: pp. 1480–93.
  Comments: Review of pathogenesis of CD.

Green PH, Cellier C. Celiac disease. *NEJM*, 2007; Vol. 357: pp. 1731–43.
  Comments: Excellent general review of CD.

Rewers M. Epidemiology of celiac disease: what are the prevalence, incidence, and progression of celiac disease? *Gastroenterology*, 2005; Vol. 128: pp. S47–51.
  Comments: Review of the epidemiology of CD.

Rewers M, Liu E, Simmons J, et al. Celiac disease associated with type 1 diabetes mellitus. *Endocrinol Metab Clin North Am*, 2004; Vol. 33: pp. 197–214, xi.
  Comments: Review of the epidemiology of CD in type 1 diabetes.

Amin R, Murphy N, Edge J, et al. A longitudinal study of the effects of a gluten-free diet on glycemic control and weight gain in subjects with type 1 diabetes and celiac disease. *Diabetes Care*, 2002; Vol. 25: pp. 1117–22.
  Comments: Small, case-control study showing improved glycemic control in diabetics treated with a gluten-free diet.

GASTROPARESIS

Octavia Pickett-Blakely, MD, MHS, and Mary Huizinga, MD, MPH

DEFINITION
- Delayed gastric emptying in the absence of a mechanical gastric outlet obstruction.
- The result of hyperglycemia-associated autonomic dysfunction and vagus nerve damage.
- Absence of other etiologies of delayed gastric emptying (e.g., narcotics, previous vagotomy).

EPIDEMIOLOGY
- Diabetes is the most common known cause of gastroparesis.
- Up to 50% of patients with diabetes have objective evidence of delayed gastric emptying but may not have clinical manifestations (Kong).
- Female sex and the presence of autonomic neuropathy, retinopathy, and renal microvasculopathy are positive predictors of delayed gastric emptying in diabetes (Jones; Koçkar).

DIAGNOSIS
- Clinical history suggestive of gastroparesis (see Signs and Symptoms here).
- Objective evidence of abnormal solid phase gastric emptying by scintigraphy, retained gastric contents noted on upper endoscopy, or barium X-ray.
- Scintigraphy measures the rate of exit (in minutes) of a radioisotope-labeled solid and liquid meal ingested by the patient. Delayed gastric emptying is greater than 10% of the meal retained in the stomach 4 hours after ingestion (Camilleri).
- Liquid phase gastric emptying is often normal and, thus, is not useful in the diagnosis of diabetic gastroparesis (Tack).
- Other methods to objectively measure gastric emptying: isotope labeled breath test (not available in the US), wireless capsule endoscopy (not commonly used), antroduodenal manometry.

SIGNS AND SYMPTOMS
- Early satiety
- Abdominal pain
- Nausea
- Vomiting
- Bloating
- Postprandial fullness
- Physical examination findings suggestive of volume depletion, epigastric distension, epigastric tenderness
- Presence of autonomic neuropathy and/or other diabetes complications

CLINICAL TREATMENT

Dietary Therapy
- Small frequent meals with low fiber and fat content.
- Nutritional supplementation if dietary intake needs are not met (via oral supplements, postpyloric enteral nutrition, or parental nutrition).

Medical Therapy
- Prokinetic therapy: first-line therapy that includes Metoclopramide (p. 429), Erythromycin (p. 427), Domperidone (available in Canada and Europe; p. 424).
- Metoclopramide is most commonly used in the US, but its use is limited by neurologic side effects like tardive dyskinesia, while erythromycin use can be complicated by prolongation of the QT interval and tachyphalaxis (Haans).
- Symptomatic therapy: antiemetics and nonnarcotic analgesics (usually used in addition to prokinetics as second-line agents).

Endoscopic/Surgical Therapy
- Pyloric botulinum toxin injection has been utilized; however, large randomized trials are needed to evaluate this treatment. Its current use is in those refractory to medical therapy and the duration of effect (if effective) is variable (Haans; DeSantis).
- Gastric electrical stimulators have been shown to improve symptoms in patients refractory to medical therapy without necessarily any improvement in gastric emptying compared to placebo (Haans; Tack).
- Roux-en-Y gastric bypass reduces the symptoms of gastroparesis in patients with diabetes who are having a bariatric surgery procedure for weight loss.

FOLLOW-UP
- Patients should be followed in short, frequent intervals as an outpatient.
- Screening for micronutrient deficiencies should be performed in patients with significant weight loss and/or malnutrition.
- Patients should be followed by a nutritionist/dietician.
- Referral to a gastroenterologist is recommended in patients with symptoms suggestive of gastroparesis. Additional workup including upper endoscopy may be warranted to investigate other etiologies of symptoms.

EXPERT OPINION
- Diabetic gastroparesis is a difficult entity to diagnose and treat.
- The medical management of diabetic gastroparesis is limited by few options with debilitating side effects.
- There is poor symptom correlation with objective studies of gastric emptying, which further complicates the disease management.

COMPLICATIONS AND COMORBIDITIES

- Diabetic gastroparesis can result in erratic glycemic control as a result of unpredictable oral intake and nutrient absorption.
- Although suboptimal glycemic control has been positively associated with delayed gastric emptying and gastroparesis-related hospitalizations, there is little prospective data to suggest that euglycemia improves diabetic gastroparesis outcomes (Uppalapati).

REFERENCES

Uppalapati SS, Ramzan Z, Fisher RS, et al. Factors contributing to hospitalization for gastroparesis exacerbations. *Dig Dis Sci*, 2009; Vol. 54: pp. 2404–9.
Comments: Study investigating factors related to morbidity related to diabetic gastroparesis.

Tack J. Gastric motor and sensory function. *Curr Opin Gastroenterol*, 2009; Vol. 25: pp. 557–65.
Comments: Review article outlining the pathophysiology of gastroparesis.

Sugumar A, Singh A, Pasricha PJ. A systematic review of the efficacy of domperidone for the treatment of diabetic gastroparesis. *Clin Gastroenterol Hepatol*, 2008; Vol. 6: pp. 726–33.
Comments: Systematic review of domperidone's use in diabetic gastroparesis.

Camilleri M. Clinical practice. Diabetic gastroparesis. *NEJM*, 2007; Vol. 356: pp. 820–9.
Comments: Review article that outlines the diagnosis and treatment of diabetic gastroparesis.

Haans JJ, Masclee AA. Review article: the diagnosis and management of gastroparesis. *Aliment Pharmacol Ther*, 2007; Vol. 26 Suppl 2: pp. 37–46.
Comments: Review article outlining the diagnosis and treatment of diabetic gastroparesis.

Hasler WL. Gastroparesis: symptoms, evaluation, and treatment. *Gastroenterol Clin North Am*, 2007; Vol. 36: pp. 619–47, ix.
Comments: Review of the epidemiology, presentation, and treatment of diabetic gastroparesis.

DeSantis ER, Huang S. Botulinum toxin type A for treatment of refractory gastroparesis. *Am J Health Syst Pharm*, 2007; Vol. 64: pp. 2237–40.
Comments: Review of botulinum toxin's use in gastroparesis.

Kong MF, Horowitz M. Diabetic gastroparesis. *Diabet Med*, 2005; Vol. 22 Suppl 4: pp. 13–8.
Comments: Review of diabetic gastroparesis.

Koçkar MC, Kayahan IK, Bavbek N. Diabetic gastroparesis in association with autonomic neuropathy and micro-vasculopathy. *Acta Med Okayama*, 2002; Vol. 56: pp. 237–43.
Comments: Study investigating the correlation between gastric emptying and parameters of autonomic neuropathy and microvasculopathy in diabetics.

Jones KL, Russo A, Stevens JE, et al. Predictors of delayed gastric emptying in diabetes. *Diabetes Care*, 2001; Vol. 24: pp. 1264–9.
Comments: An observational study investigating the predictors of delayed gastric emptying in T1DM, T2DM, and normal controls.

NONALCOHOLIC FATTY LIVER DISEASE

Mariana Lazo, MD, ScM, PhD, and Jeanne M. Clark, MD, MPH

DEFINITION

- **Nonalcoholic fatty liver disease (NAFLD):** fatty infiltration of the liver, exceeding 5% of liver weight. In biopsy specimens, >5%–10% macrosteatotic hepatocytes.
- By definition, requires exclusion of alcohol as a potential cause. Acceptable levels of alcohol consumption are controversial but in general <20 grams/day (2 drinks) in men and

<10 grams/day (1 drink) in women are considered safe, and below the cutoff associated with increased risk of cirrhosis (30 grams/day in men and 20 grams/day in women).

- **Primary NAFLD:** common term for typical NAFLD associated with central obesity and/or type 2 diabetes (T2DM) or insulin resistance (IR), without another specific etiology.
- **Secondary NAFLD:** NAFLD in the absence of insulin resistance; associated with other causes such as medication use (glucocorticoids, tamoxifen, amiodarone, HAART, diltiazem), disorders of lipid metabolism (abetalipoproteinemia, lipodystrophy, Weber-Christian syndrome, Andersen's disease), total parenteral nutrition, and jejunoileal bypass surgery. Many cases of secondary NAFLD likely represent an exacerbation of often unrecognized primary NAFLD.
- **Nonalcoholic steatohepatitis (NASH):** a more severe form of NAFLD characterized by inflammation, ballooned hepatocytes, and/or fibrosis on biopsy. NAFLD can progress to cirrhosis.

EPIDEMIOLOGY

- NAFLD considered the most common chronic liver disease in the United States (Clark) and probably worldwide.
- In the general population, prevalence of NAFLD based on liver enzymes or imaging (ultrasound or MRI) ranges from 3%–30% (Lazo; Argo).
- Among people with T2DM, prevalence of NAFLD is 50%–80% (Lazo).
- Adults with T2DM are at much higher risk for cirrhosis compared to the general population, possibly due to NAFLD (Clark; Caldwell).
- Non-Hispanic whites and Hispanics at higher risk.
- Predictors of more severe disease: age >40–50 years; female sex; severe obesity; hypertension; diabetes; hypertriglyceridemia; elevated ALT, AST, GGT; AST: ALT ratio >1.

DIAGNOSIS

- All spectrums of disease can be seen even with normal liver test levels.
- The American Gastroenterological Association (AGA) Medical Position Statement recommends a progressive diagnostic approach. Step (1): Serum liver tests: AST, ALT, alkaline phosphatase, serum bilirubin, albumin levels, and prothrombin time; Step (2): Evaluate for coexisting treatable conditions (hepatitis C, autoantibodies); Step (3): An alcohol consumption evaluation by interviewing the patient and family members. If AST or ALT are abnormal, ongoing alcohol consumption <20–30 grams/day (2–3 drinks) and other causes of liver disease excluded, then Step (4): Perform imaging (ultrasonography, CT scan, or MRI).
- Currently, no imaging method distinguishes between fatty liver, steatohepatitis, and fibrosis but can help exclude biliary tract or focal liver diseases.
- To detect the presence of liver fat, sonography is more sensitive than CT scan, less expensive, and has no radiation risk. MRI primarily used in research settings to quantify the amount of fat in the liver.
- Transient elastography: based on ultrasound technology measures tissue elasticity and correlates well with liver stiffness in patients with viral hepatitis. Not validated in NAFLD patients who tend to be overweight or obese.
- Gold standard for diagnosis is liver biopsy, staging (extent of injury), and grading (degree of activity) of NAFLD. NAFLD activity score (NAS) ranging from 0 to 8 is a composite score based on findings of steatosis, inflammation, and hepatocyte injury. Fibrosis scored separately, ranging from 0 to 4: 0–2 = minimal, 3–4 = bridging fibrosis

COMPLICATIONS AND COMORBIDITIES

and cirrhosis. A higher NAS indicates greater damage. Designed for use in clinical trials of NASH.

- Limitations of liver biopsy: patient inconvenience, potential for complications, and sampling error.
- Noninvasive markers of fibrosis: proprietary fibrosis scores (Fibrospect, Hepascore, and Fibroscore) based on a combination of biochemical serum assays and routine lab tests and can reliably identify those with either minimal or advanced disease; however a substantial gray zone precludes accurate fibrosis diagnosis and staging. Currently, none have been FDA approved and their utility in NAFLD remains uncertain.
- Many patients have elevated cholesterol and triglycerides.

SIGNS AND SYMPTOMS

- Most common: asymptomatic (48%–100%), fatigue (70%), right upper quadrant pain (up to 50%).
- Palmar erythema and spider angiomas in cirrhosis.
- Clinical findings associated with metabolic syndrome commonly seen.
- Hepatomegaly and acanthosis nigricans in children.
- Lipoatrophy/lipodystrophy.

CLINICAL TREATMENT

Non-Pharmacologic

- Diet and exercise are the cornerstones of therapy. Weight loss of 5%–7% effectively improves steatosis and other histological features of NAFLD and reduces risk of progression (Harrison; Promrat).
- Avoid rapid weight loss, which can cause histological exacerbation.
- Exercise only without weight loss: Recent evidence suggests it may help. Encourage increased physical activity level even in the absence of weight loss.
- Diet composition: The effects of specific diets on NAFLD are not known. Recommend a balanced diet such as that endorsed by the American Diabetes Association or American Heart Association.

Pharmacologic (Non-FDA Approved) Therapy

- Thiazolidinediones: Pioglitazone significantly improves histological outcomes (Sanyal; Ratziu) and, because of other benefits in the treatment of T2DM, can be considered drug of choice for NAFLD in those with T2DM.
- Biguanides: Metformin usually used only in research settings. Pilot data have shown mixed results.
- Antioxidants: Pilot data suggest improvement with vitamin E (Sanyal).
- Cytoprotective agents: Large RCT of ursodeoxycholic acid showed no histologic benefit.

General Considerations

- Glycemic control: ideally A1c <7%.
- Alcohol use: limited especially if more severe disease.
- Concomitant use of medications that may promote steatohepatitis (e.g., amiodarone, tamoxifen) requires weighing risk and benefits.
- Avoid workplace exposure to hepatotoxic substances (e.g., hydrocarbon solvents).
- Patient education/immunization to prevent viral hepatitis.

FOLLOW-UP

- No conclusive recommendations for disease surveillance.
- Most commonly used endpoints: histological, liver test (enzymes), and metabolic parameters.
- Other less commonly used endpoints: serologic fibrosis markers, imaging techniques.
- Referral to a gastrointestinal specialist may be indicated for consideration of a liver biopsy and/or experimental therapies.

EXPERT OPINION

- Patients with T2DM have a higher risk of liver-related morbidity and mortality.
- Biopsy is the gold standard method to diagnose, stage, and grade NAFLD; however, it is not usually performed in the initial evaluation.
- Laboratory tests to rule out other potential causes of liver disease are the most common initial approach.
- Lifestyle changes remain a cornerstone of initial management.
- Currently, no FDA-approved medication therapy, although thiazolidinediones may be preferred in patients with both NAFLD and T2DM.

BASIS FOR RECOMMENDATIONS

American Gastroenterological Association. American Gastroenterological Association medical position statement: nonalcoholic fatty liver disease. *Gastroenterology*, 2002; Vol. 123: pp. 1702–4. Available for download at *http://www.aasld.org/practiceguidelines/Documents/Practice%20Guidelines/position_nonfattypg.pdf*.
   Comments: Summary of the Medical Position Statement.

Sanyal AJ, American Gastroenterological Association. AGA technical review on nonalcoholic fatty liver disease. *Gastroenterology*, 2002; Vol. 123: pp. 1705–25.
   Comments: Most comprehensive and recent official review of nonalcoholic fatty liver disease.

OTHER REFERENCES

Promrat K, Kleiner DE, Niemeier HM, et al. Randomized controlled trial testing the effects of weight loss on nonalcoholic steatohepatitis. *Hepatology*, 2010; Vol. 51: pp. 121–9.
   Comments: Small RCT of lifestyle intervention on Biopsy proven NASH showing significant effect of ≥7% weight loss on liver histology: steatosis, inflammation, ballooning, and NAS score.

Sanyal AJ., et al. A randomized controlled trial of pioglitazone or vitamin E for nonalcoholic steatohepatitis (PIVENS) [Abstract]. *Hepatology*, 2009; Vol. 50 (Suppl): p. LB4 .
   Comments: 24-month RCT of pioglitazone in biopsy proven NASH showing a significant effect on liver histology: Steatosis, inflammation, ballooning (borderline P = 0.08).

Ratziu V, Zelber-Sagi S. Pharmacologic therapy of non-alcoholic steatohepatitis. *Clin Liver Dis*, 2009; Vol. 13: pp. 667–88.
   Comments: Excellent narrative review of treatment of NAFLD.

Argo CK, Caldwell SH. Epidemiology and natural history of non-alcoholic steatohepatitis. *Clin Liver Dis*, 2009; Vol. 13: pp. 511–31.
   Comments: Excellent narrative review of the Natural History of NAFLD.

Ratziu V, Giral P, Jacqueminet S, et al. Rosiglitazone for nonalcoholic steatohepatitis: one-year results of the randomized placebo-controlled Fatty Liver Improvement with Rosiglitazone Therapy (FLIRT) Trial. *Gastroenterology*, 2008; Vol. 135: pp. 100–10.
   Comments: 12-month randomized controlled trial (RCT) of rosiglitazone in NASH showing a significant effect on liver transaminases, insulin resistance, and steatosis.

Lazo M, Clark JM. The epidemiology of nonalcoholic fatty liver disease: a global perspective. *Semin Liver Dis*, 2008; Vol. 28: pp. 339–50.
   Comments: Comprehensive narrative review of the epidemiology of NAFLD.

COMPLICATIONS AND COMORBIDITIES

Harrison SA, Day CP. Benefits of lifestyle modification in NAFLD. *Gut,* 2007; Vol. 56: pp. 1760–9.
  Comments: Excellent review of the mechanism and experimental studies of lifestyle effects in NAFLD.

Harrison SA, Torgerson S, Hayashi PH. The natural history of nonalcoholic fatty liver disease: a clinical histopathological study. *Am J Gastroenterol,* 2003; Vol. 98: pp. 2042–7.
  Comments: Paper that provided key data of the progression of NAFLD.

Marchesini G, Bugianesi E, Forlani G, et al. Nonalcoholic fatty liver, steatohepatitis, and the metabolic syndrome. *Hepatology,* 2003; Vol. 37: pp. 917–23.
  Comments: This paper, along with others, has provided substantial evidence of the link between insulin resistance and NAFLD.

Mofrad P, Contos MJ, Haque M, et al. Clinical and histologic spectrum of nonalcoholic fatty liver disease associated with normal ALT values. *Hepatology,* 2003; Vol. 37: pp. 1286–92.
  Comments: Paper that showed the limitation of liver enzymes, especially ALT as a surrogate marker of liver injury.

Neuschwander-Tetri BA, Caldwell SH. Nonalcoholic steatohepatitis: summary of an AASLD Single Topic Conference. *Hepatology,* 2003; Vol. 37: pp. 1202–19.
  Comments: Expert review of NAFLD. A good summary of its pathophysiology, epidemiology, and treatment, as well as current gaps in the literature.

Clark JM, Brancati FL, Diehl AM. The prevalence and etiology of elevated aminotransferase levels in the United States. *Am J Gastroenterol,* 2003; Vol. 98: pp. 960–7.
  Comments: Paper that showed for the first time the high prevalence of presumed NAFLD in the general population.

Clark JM, Diehl AM. Nonalcoholic fatty liver disease: an underrecognized cause of cryptogenic cirrhosis. *JAMA,* 2003; Vol. 289: pp. 3000–4.
  Comments: One of the first studies suggesting that most cases of cryptogenic cirrhosis could be related to NAFLD.

Brunt EM, Janney CG, Di Bisceglie AM, et al. Nonalcoholic steatohepatitis: a proposal for grading and staging the histological lesions. *Am J Gastroenterol,* 1999; Vol. 94: pp. 2467–74.
  Comments: Provides a widely accepted scoring system for grading and staging histologically NAFLD.

Matteoni CA, Younossi ZM, Gramlich T, et al. Nonalcoholic fatty liver disease: a spectrum of clinical and pathological severity. *Gastroenterology,* 1999; Vol. 116: pp. 1413–9.
  Comments: Another paper that provided key data of the progression of NAFLD.

Caldwell SH, Oelsner DH, Iezzoni JC, et al. Cryptogenic cirrhosis: clinical characterization and risk factors for underlying disease. *Hepatology,* 1999; Vol. 29: pp. 664–9.
  Comments: One of the first studies suggesting that most cases of cryptogenic cirrhosis could be related to NAFLD.

PANCREATIC CANCER

See Pancreatic Cancer, p. 258.

PANCREATITIS

Reza Alavi, MD, MHS, MBA, and Jeanne M. Clark, MD, MPH

DEFINITION
- Refers to inflammation of the pancreas.
- Common etiologies of acute pancreatitis include gallstones, alcohol, hypercalcemia, drugs, infections, and trauma.

EPIDEMIOLOGY

- The annual incidence of acute pancreatitis ranges from 4.9 to 35 per 100,000 population. People with type 2 diabetes have almost a three-fold greater risk of acute pancreatitis compared to those without diabetes (Vege).
- Drug-induced pancreatitis is generally uncommon with diabetes medications (Balani).
- Extreme hypertriglyceridemia, >1000 mg/dl (chylomicronemia), can cause chronic pancreatitis.
- Other etiologies include cystic fibrosis, autoimmune disorders, pancreatic anomalies (e.g., pancreas divisum).
- During acute pancreatitis, 50% of patients have glucose intolerance, but few require insulin administration (Gorelick).
- In chronic pancreatitis, up to 50% have reported overt diabetes (Wakasugi), and up to 70% when pancreatic calcification is present (Gorelick).
- Overall, mortality in hospitalized patients with acute pancreatitis is ~10% (range 2%–22%).
- Mortality rates unaffected by diabetes status (Cavallini).

DIAGNOSIS

- Serum amylase rises within 6–12 hours of onset, usually to >3 times the upper limit of normal (more sensitive test).
- Serum lipase is a more specific test.
- Serial measurements do NOT predict prognosis or alter management.
- White blood cell count is usually elevated even in the absence of infection.
- Always check serum electrolytes, especially calcium.
- Consider toxicology screen, lipid profile, blood cultures to evaluate for secondary etiologies.
- Pancreas-dedicated CT scan with oral and IV contrast is the most important imaging test, looking for pancreatic necrosis.
- Abdominal plain films help to exclude other causes of abdominal pain such as obstruction and bowel perforation.
- Abdominal ultrasound can show a diffusely enlarged and hypoechoic pancreas, and can also detect gallstones in the gallbladder.

SIGNS AND SYMPTOMS

- Upper abdominal pain
- Nausea and vomiting
- Fever and tachycardia
- Abdominal distention, epigastric tenderness and guarding
- Shallow respirations due to diaphragmatic irritation
- Vasodilatory shock in severe acute pancreatitis without sepsis

CLINICAL TREATMENT

- ICU monitoring for severe pancreatitis, including pancreatic necrosis, organ failure, or pleural effusion at admission; high severity of disease score (i.e., APACHE-II).
- Fluid resuscitation with 250–300 cc/hr of isotonic saline for 24–48 hours if the cardiac status permits (Tenner).
- Correction of electrolyte and metabolic abnormalities.
- Supplemental oxygen to keep pulse oxygen levels above 95%.

- Pain management: Meperidine usually favored over morphine because morphine increases sphincter of Oddi pressure, but no clinical evidence that morphine actually aggravates or causes pancreatitis or cholecystitis.
- Nutritional support if likely to remain fasting for >7 days. Nasojejunal tube feeding (using an elemental or semi-elemental formula) is preferred to parenteral nutrition.
- Prophylactic antibiotics to prevent pancreatic infection is NOT routinely recommended (Banks), although imipenem/meropenem may help if >30% pancreatic necrosis (Villatoro).
- ERCP indicated for the clearance of bile duct stones in severe pancreatitis or cholangitis, if poor candidate for cholecystectomy, or postcholecystectomy in those with persistent biliary obstruction.
- Surgical treatment may be required in patients with intractable pain from chronic pancreatitis.

FOLLOW-UP
- After necrotizing pancreatitis, high prevalence of IGT due to both loss of beta-cell function and insulin resistance.
- Perform cholecystectomy after recovery in patients with gallstone pancreatitis, within 7 days after recovery in mild pancreatitis, and 3–4 weeks after in severe necrotizing pancreatitis.
- Exocrine pancreatic insufficiency can be common in chronic pancreatitis with both type 1 and type 2 diabetes.
- Exocrine pancreatic insufficiency is treated with low-fat diet and administration of exogenous pancreatic enzymes.

EXPERT OPINION
- Glucose intolerance occurs frequently in chronic pancreatitis, but overt diabetes usually occurs late in the course of disease.
- Diabetes is more common with chronic calcifying disease, particularly early calcifications.
- Diabetes in patients with chronic pancreatitis usually requires insulin treatment and has increased risk of hypoglycemia (presumably due to both alpha- and beta-cell damage).
- Although preliminary reports suggesting exenatide, sitagliptin, and sitagliptin/metformin increase the risk of drug-induced pancreatitis, the data are inconclusive at this point (Drucker).

REFERENCES
Drucker DJ, Sherman SI, Gorelick FS, et al. Incretin-based therapies for the treatment of type 2 diabetes: evaluation of the risks and benefits. *Diabetes Care,* 2010; Vol. 33: pp. 428–33.
> Comments: Excellent recent review of incretin-based therapies and rare adverse events including acute pancreatitis.

Balani AR, Grendell JH. Drug-induced pancreatitis: incidence, management and prevention. *Drug Saf,* 2008; Vol. 31: pp. 823–37.
> Comments: Drug-induced pancreatitis.

Vege SS, Yadav D, Chari ST. Pancreatitis. In Talley NJ, Locke GR, Saito YA (Eds.), *GI Epidemiology,* 1st edition. Malden, MA: Blackwell Publishing; 2007: pp. 221–225.
> Comments: Epidemiology of pancreatitis.

Forsmark CE, Baillie J, AGA Institute Clinical Practice and Economics Committee, et al. AGA Institute technical review on acute pancreatitis. *Gastroenterology,* 2007; Vol. 132: pp. 2022–44.
Comments: AGA guidelines.

Banks PA, Freeman ML, Practice Parameters Committee of the American College of Gastroenterology. Practice guidelines in acute pancreatitis. *Am J Gastroenterol,* 2006; Vol. 101: pp. 2379–400.
Comments: Detailed practice guidelines.

Villatoro E, Bassi C, Larvin M. Antibiotic therapy for prophylaxis against infection of pancreatic necrosis in acute pancreatitis. *Cochrane Database Syst Rev,* 2006; CD002941.
Comments: Antibiotic therapy for severe pancreatitis.

Cavallini G, Frulloni L, Bassi C, et al. Prospective multicentre survey on acute pancreatitis in Italy (ProInf-AISP): results on 1005 patients. *Dig Liver Dis,* 2004; Vol. 36: pp. 205–11.
Comments: Italian epidemiological study of incidence, hospitalization, and mortality rates.

Tenner S. Initial management of acute pancreatitis: critical issues during the first 72 hours. *Am J Gastroenterol,* 2004; Vol. 99: pp. 2489–94.
Comments: Initial management.

Malka D, Hammel P, Sauvanet A, et al. Risk factors for diabetes mellitus in chronic pancreatitis. *Gastroenterology,* 2000; Vol. 119: pp. 1324–32.
Comments: The risk of diabetes mellitus is not influenced by elective pancreatic surgical procedures other than distal pancreatectomy in patients with chronic pancreatitis.

Dervenis C, Johnson CD, Bassi C, et al. Diagnosis, objective assessment of severity, and management of acute pancreatitis. Santorini consensus conference. *Int J Pancreatol,* 1999; Vol. 25: pp. 195–210.
Comments: Diagnosis using plasma concentrations of pancreatic enzymes is reliable.

Wakasugi H, Funakoshi A, Iguchi H. Clinical assessment of pancreatic diabetes caused by chronic pancreatitis. *J Gastroenterol,* 1998; Vol. 33: pp. 254–9.
Comments: Among 154 patients with chronic pancreatitis, 50% had diabetes.

Gorelick FS. Diabetes mellitus and the exocrine pancreas. *Yale J Biol Med,* 1984; Vol. 56: pp. 271–5.
Comments: Review of epidemiology and pathophysiology of diabetes associated with pancreatitis.

POSTPANCREATECTOMY DIABETES

See Postpancreatectomy Diabetes, p. 81.

Hematologic Diseases/Malignancy

ANEMIA (DIABETES)

See Anemia, p. 579.

CANCER AND DIABETES

Hsin-Chieh Yeh, PhD, and Frederick L. Brancati, MD, MHS

DEFINITION
- Cancer or malignant neoplasm refers to uncontrolled cell growth, invasion into adjacent tissues, and spread to other locations in the body via lymph or blood (i.e., metastases).
- Benign tumors do not invade or metastasize.

EPIDEMIOLOGY

Incident Cancer
- Diabetes associated with increased risk of non-Hodgkin lymphoma (Chao) and cancer of breast (Larsson, 2007), colorectum (Larsson, 2005), endometrium (Friberg), liver (El-Serag), and pancreas (Huxley).
- Negatively associated with risk of prostate cancer (Kasper).
- Hypotheses about possible link between diabetes and cancer include:
  1. Insulin is known to stimulate cell proliferation (Giovannucci).
  2. Hyperglycemia promotes tumor growth (Saydah; Rinaldi).
  3. Shared risk factors such as obesity (Giovannucci), diet, physical inactivity (Roberts), hepatitis C (White), and NAFLD (Clark).

Diabetes and Cancer Death
- Diabetes associated with increased risk of death from colon and pancreatic cancers in both men and women; increased risk of death from liver and bladder cancers in men; and increased risk of death from breast cancer in women (Coughlin).
- Also reported positive associations with death from: esophagus, liver, and colon/rectum cancers in men; and liver and cervix cancers in women (Jee).

Diabetes in Cancer Patients
- Meta-analyses showed diabetes associated with an increased mortality in patients with any cancer (HR = 1.44), cancers of the endometrium (HR = 1.76), breast (HR = 1.61), colorectum (HR = 1.32), and prostate (Barone; Snyder).
- Meta-analysis showed diabetes associated with increased odds of postoperative mortality across all cancer types (HR = 1.5) (Barone).
- Hyperglycemia associated with shorter duration of complete remission in patients with acute lymphocytic leukemia (Weiser).
- Hyperglycemia associated with shorter survival in patients with newly diagnosed glioblastoma (Derr).

Diabetes and Prostate Cancer
- Negatively associated with risk of prostate cancer (Kasper).
- Androgen deprivation therapy causes changes in body composition, alterations in lipid profiles, and decreased insulin sensitivity in men (Faris).

- Androgen deprivation therapy significantly increases risk for diabetes mellitus in men (Alibhai).

Obesity and Cancer

- A meta-analysis (Renehan) showed BMI strongly associated with:
  - esophageal adenocarcinoma (RR 1.52), thyroid (RR 1.33), colon (RR 1.24), and renal (RR 1.24) cancers (all p <0.001)
  - endometrial (RR 1.59), gallbladder (RR 1.59), esophageal (RR 1.51), and renal (RR 1.34) cancers in women (all p <0.05)
  - weaker positive associations with cancer and malignant melanoma in men
- Patients with gastric bypass surgery had a lower risk of cancer mortality compared to severely obese patients (Adams).

CLINICAL TREATMENT

Diabetes Treatment and Cancer Risk

- Recent studies suggest metformin (Currie; Bodmer) and thiazolidinediones (Blanquicett) may decrease the risk of cancer but further studies are ongoing.
- Cumulative insulin use possibly associated with increased cancer mortality rates (Bowker), while specific insulins have not been definitively linked to increased cancer risk (Currie).

EXPERT OPINION

- The above risks are statistical associations that are subject to a number of confounders and cannot be considered to prove causality.
- Therefore, in the person with diabetes, more vigilant use of established screening approaches, such as for colon cancer, may be indicated; but generally not indicated to scare patients by emphasizing statistical associations.
- As for treatment, again, use caution in drawing clinical conclusions about using either metformin or insulin based on possible associations with cancer.

BASIS FOR RECOMMENDATIONS

Giavannucci E, Harlan DM, Archer MC, et al. Diabetes and cancer: a consensus report. *CA Cancer J Clin,* 2010; Vol. 60: pp. 207–21.

Comment: A consensus report from the American Diabetes Association and American Cancer Society that reviews the current state of knowledge regarding the association of diabetes and cancer, including possible biological mechanisms.

OTHER REFERENCES

Barone BB, Yeh HC, Snyder CF, et al. Postoperative mortality in cancer patients with preexisting diabetes: systematic review and meta-analysis. *Diabetes Care,* 2010; Vol. 33: pp. 931–9.

Comments: The landmark systematic review reports that compared with their nondiabetic counterparts, cancer patients with preexisting diabetes are approximately 50% more likely to die after surgery.

Snyder CF, Stein KB, Barone BB, et al. Does pre-existing diabetes affect prostate cancer prognosis? A systematic review. *Prostate Cancer Prostatic Dis,* 2010; Vol. 13: pp. 58–64.

Comments: Reports pre-existing diabetes is associated with increased long-term, overall mortality, receiving radiation therapy, complication rates, recurrence, and treatment failure.

Faris JE, Smith MR Metabolic sequelae associated with androgen deprivation therapy for prostate cancer. *Curr Opin Endocrinol Diabetes Obes,* 2010; Vol. 17: pp. 240–6.

Comments: Concludes androgen deprivation therapy is associated with diabetes mellitus, and linked to cardiovascular morbidity.

COMPLICATIONS AND COMORBIDITIES

Bodmer M, Meier C, Krähenbühl S, et al. Long-term metformin use is associated with decreased risk of breast cancer. *Diabetes Care,* 2010; Vol. 33: 1935-5548; pp. 1304–8.

Comments: Evaluates whether use of oral hypoglycemic agents is associated with an altered breast cancer risk in women.

Derr RL, Ye X, Islas MU, et al. Association between hyperglycemia and survival in patients with newly diagnosed glioblastoma. *J Clin Oncol,* 2009; Vol. 27: pp. 1082–6.

Comments: Reports hyperglycemia is associated with shorter survival, after controlling for glucocorticoid dose and other confounders.

Alibhai SM, Duong-Hua M, Sutradhar R, et al. Impact of androgen deprivation therapy on cardiovascular disease and diabetes. *J Clin Oncol,* 2009; Vol. 27: pp. 3452–8.

Comments: Continuous androgen deprivation therapy use for at least 6 months in older men is associated with an increased risk of diabetes and fragility fracture.

Currie CJ, Poole CD, Gale EA The influence of glucose-lowering therapies on cancer risk in type 2 diabetes. *Diabetologia,* 2009; Vol. 52: pp. 1766–77.

Comments: Examines the risk of development of solid tumors in relation to treatment with oral agents, human insulin, and insulin analogues.

Chao C, Page JH. Type 2 diabetes mellitus and risk of non-Hodgkin lymphoma: a systematic review and meta-analysis. *Am J Epidemiol,* 2008; Vol. 168: pp. 471–80.

Comments: Type 2 diabetes mellitus is associated with altered immune function and chronic inflammation, which are also implicated in the pathogenesis of non-Hodgkin lymphoma. This study summarizes findings from the current literature on the association between history of type 2 diabetes mellitus and risk of non-Hodgkin lymphoma.

Rinaldi S, Rohrmann S, Jenab M, et al. Glycosylated hemoglobin and risk of colorectal cancer in men and women, the European prospective investigation into cancer and nutrition. *Cancer Epidemiol Biomarkers Prev,* 2008; Vol. 17: pp. 3108–15.

Comments: The results of this study suggest a mild implication of hyperglycemia in colorectal cancer, which seems more important in women than in men, and more for cancer of the rectum than of the colon.

White DL, Ratziu V, El-Serag HB. Hepatitis C infection and risk of diabetes: a systematic review and meta-analysis. *J Hepatol,* 2008; Vol. 49: pp. 831-44.

Comments: Reports excess diabetes risk with HCV infection in comparison to non-infected controls. The excess risk observed in comparison to HBV-infected controls suggests a potential direct viral role in promoting diabetes risk.

Renehan AG, Tyson M, Egger M, et al. Body-mass index and incidence of cancer: a systematic review and meta-analysis of prospective observational studies. *Lancet,* 2008; Vol. 371: pp. 569–78.

Comments: This comprehensive paper reports that an increased BMI is associated with increased risk of common and less common malignancies.

Blanquicett C, Roman J, Hart CM. Thiazolidinediones as anti-cancer agents. *Cancer Ther,* 2008; Vol. 6: pp. 25–34.

Comments: Discusses studies employing TZDs as anti-cancer therapies for the most common types of cancers including lung, breast, and colon, and explores the principal PPAR-gamma-dependent and -independent mechanisms by which TZDs exert their anti-tumor effects.

Larsson SC, Mantzoros CS, Wolk A. Diabetes mellitus and risk of breast cancer: a meta-analysis. *Int J Cancer,* 2007; Vol. 121: pp. 856–62.

Comments: This study assesses the evidence regarding the association between diabetes and risk of breast cancer. Analysis of all 20 studies showed that women with diabetes had a statistically significant increased risk of breast cancer.

Friberg E, Orsini N, Mantzoros CS, et al. Diabetes mellitus and risk of endometrial cancer: a meta-analysis. *Diabetologia*, 2007; Vol. 50: pp. 1365–74.

Comments: Provides a quantitative assessment of the association between diabetes and risk of endometrial cancer, including both case-control studies and cohort studies.

Adams TD, Gress RE, Smith SC, et al. Long-term mortality after gastric bypass surgery. *NEJM*, 2007; Vol. 357: pp. 753–61.

Comments: Concludes that long-term total mortality after gastric bypass surgery is significantly reduced, particularly deaths from diabetes, heart disease, and cancer.

El-Serag HB, Hampel H, Javadi F. The association between diabetes and hepatocellular carcinoma: a systematic review of epidemiologic evidence. *Clin Gastroenterol Hepatol*, 2006; Vol. 4: pp. 369–80.

Comments: A systematic review and a meta-analysis to estimate the magnitude and determinants of association between diabetes and hepatocellular carcinoma.

Kasper JS, Giovannucci E. A meta-analysis of diabetes mellitus and the risk of prostate cancer. *Cancer Epidemiol Biomarkers Prev*, 2006; Vol. 15: pp. 2056–62.

Comments: This study suggests an inverse relationship between diabetes and prostate cancer.

Clark JM. The epidemiology of nonalcoholic fatty liver disease in adults. *J Clin Gastroenterol*, 2006; Vol. 40 Suppl 1: pp. S5–10.

Comments: This article reviews the prevalence of NAFLD and the factors associated with this disorder, and with the more advanced stages of NAFLD, including nonalcoholic steatohepatitis (NASH) and fibrosis.

Bowker SL, Majumdar SR, Veugelers P, et al. Increased cancer-related mortality for patients with type 2 diabetes who use sulfonylureas or insulin. *Diabetes Care*, 2006; Vol. 29: pp. 254–8.

Comments: Explores the association between antidiabetic therapies and cancer-related mortality in patients with type 2 diabetes, suggesting that agents that increase insulin levels might promote cancer.

Larsson SC, Orsini N, Wolk A. Diabetes mellitus and risk of colorectal cancer: a meta-analysis. *J Natl Cancer Inst*, 2005; Vol. 97: pp. 1679–87.

Comments: A meta-analysis of published data on the association between diabetes and the incidence and mortality of colorectal cancer. Support a relationship between diabetes and increased risk of colon and rectal cancer in both women and men.

Huxley R, Ansary-Moghaddam A, Berrington de González A, et al. Type-II diabetes and pancreatic cancer: a meta-analysis of 36 studies. *Br J Cancer*, 2005; Vol. 92: pp. 2076–83.

Comments: Type 2 diabetes is widely considered to be associated with pancreatic cancer, but whether this represents a causal or consequential association is unclear. This article provides a meta-analysis to examine this association.

Roberts CK, Barnard RJ. Effects of exercise and diet on chronic disease. *J Appl Physiol*, 2005; Vol. 98: pp. 3–30.

Comments: The purpose of this review is to 1) discuss the effects of exercise and diet in the prevention of chronic disease, 2) highlight the effects of lifestyle modification for both preventing disease progression and reversing existing disease, and 3) suggest potential mechanisms for beneficial effects.

Jee SH, Ohrr H, Sull JW, et al. Fasting serum glucose level and cancer risk in Korean men and women. *JAMA*, 2005; Vol. 293: pp. 194–202.

Comments: Reports elevated fasting serum glucose levels and a diagnosis of diabetes are independent risk factors for several major cancers, and the risk tends to increase with an increased level of fasting serum glucose.

Weiser MA, Cabanillas ME, Konopleva M, et al. Relation between the duration of remission and hyperglycemia during induction chemotherapy for acute lymphocytic leukemia with a hyperfractionated cyclophosphamide, vincristine, doxorubicin, and dexamethasone/methotrexate-cytarabine regimen. *Cancer*, 2004; Vol. 100: pp. 1179–85.

Comments: Determines the prevalence of hyperglycemia during induction chemotherapy for acute lymphocytic leukemia.

COMPLICATIONS AND COMORBIDITIES

Saydah SH, Platz EA, Rifai N, et al. Association of markers of insulin and glucose control with subsequent colorectal cancer risk. *Cancer Epidemiol Biomarkers Prev*, 2003; Vol. 12: pp. 412–8.

Comments: This study supports the hypothesis that perturbations in insulin and glucose control may influence colorectal carcinogenesis.

PANCREATIC CANCER

Reza Alavi, MD, MHS, MBA, and Frederick L. Brancati, MD, MHS

DEFINITION

- Exocrine pancreatic cancers are most commonly adenocarcinomas of pancreatic ductal and acinar cells and their stem cells.
- Endocrine (islet-cell) pancreatic cancers are classified by the hormones that they secrete: insulin, gastrin, glucagon, somatostatin, or VIP.

EPIDEMIOLOGY

- Fourth leading cause of cancer-related death in the United States among both men and women (Jemal).
- Rare before the age of 45, but the incidence rises sharply thereafter.
- Incidence is greater in males than females (male-to-female ratio 1.3:1) and in blacks (14.8 per 100,000 in black males compared to 8.8 per 100,000 in the general population).
- Exocrine pancreatic cancers are far more common (e.g., adenocarcinoma in >95%) compared to endocrine tumors that are rare.
- Compared to their nondiabetic counterparts, adults with type 1 or type 2 diabetes are two-fold more likely to develop pancreatic cancer (Everhart).
- Abnormal glucose metabolism has also been associated with increased pancreatic cancer mortality (Gapstur).
- Approximately 1% of diabetes subjects over age 50 years will be diagnosed with pancreatic cancer within 3 years of first meeting criteria for diabetes (Chari).
- There is more evidence that diabetes leads to cancer, not the reverse (i.e, early cancer leading to diabetes due to destruction of islet cells) (Stolzenberg-Solomon).
- Other risk factors: cigarette smoking, obesity, diet, physical inactivity, alcohol, and potentially aspirin use (Schernhammer).

DIAGNOSIS

- Diagnosis and staging can often be done by imaging rather than exploratory surgery.
- Endoscopic ultrasound: 90% sensitivity, 90% specificity, and useful for staging.
- Pancreas-dedicated CT scan: 90% sensitivity, 95% specificity, and useful for staging.
- Ultrasound: 80% sensitivity, 90% specificity.
- Endoscopic retrograde cholangiopancreatography (ERCP): 90% sensitivity, 90% specificity.
- MRI scan: 90% sensitivity, 90% specificity.
- Fine needle aspirate: 90% sensitivity, 98% specificity.
- Serum markers (CA 19-9) have good sensitivity and specificity on larger tumors, but have limited role in diagnosing small, surgically resectable cancers.

SIGNS AND SYMPTOMS

- History: abdominal pain, appetite loss, jaundice, pale-colored stools, unusual belching, weight loss, and unusual bloating.

- Physical findings: abdominal mass, ascites, nontender but palpable gallbladder, left supraclavicular lymphadenopathy (Virchow's node).
- The majority of patients have unresectable disease by the time symptoms occur.
- New-onset glucose intolerance or diabetes arising in a thin older adult may raise suspicion of pancreatic cancer (Chari).
- The most common sites of distant metastases include the liver, peritoneum, lungs, and, less frequently, bone.
- Many patients with pancreatic cancer have a hypercoagulable state (Trousseau's syndrome).

CLINICAL TREATMENT

- Treatment depends on the stage of cancer, and whether the patient is a good surgical candidate (only 15%–20% candidates for pancreatectomy).
- Surgical treatments for pancreatic head tumors: standard pancreaticoduodenectomy (Whipple procedure), total pancreatectomy, regional pancreatectomy, or pylorus-preserving pancreaticoduodenectomy.
- Pancreatic tail tumors can be resected by distal subtotal pancreatectomy combined with splenectomy.
- There is no consensus regarding the optimal management (chemotherapy vs chemoradiotherapy) of patients after resection of a pancreatic adenocarcinoma.
- The optimal management of locally advanced, unresectable nonmetastatic disease is also controversial. Therapeutic options: radiation therapy (RT) alone, chemoradiotherapy, and chemotherapy alone.
- In advanced pancreatic cancer, systemic chemotherapy (gemcitabine monotherapy or 5-FU-based combination therapy) can improve disease-related symptoms and survival when compared to best supportive care alone (Yip).
- Postpancreatectomy diabetes can occur depending on type of surgery (see Postpancreatectomy Diabetes, p. 81).

FOLLOW-UP

- Regardless of the therapy chosen, median survival is approximately 8–12 months for patients with locally advanced unresectable disease, and 3–6 months for those who present with metastases.
- The focus for most pancreatic cancer patients eventually becomes palliation of symptoms.
- Palliation of jaundice is usually accomplished by the placement of an expandable metal stent.
- Duodenal obstruction can be addressed by posterior retrocolic gastrojejunostomy whenever biliary bypass is performed.
- Symptomatic gastric outlet obstruction are treated with endoscopically placed expandable metal stents.
- Pain is addressed with opioid analgesics, celiac plexus neurolysis (CPN), or radiation therapy.
- There is a particularly high incidence of thromboembolic (both venous and arterial) events, particularly in the setting of advanced disease.

EXPERT OPINION

- Although adults with prediabetes or diabetes are at higher risk for developing pancreatic cancer, there is no definitive evidence that glucose control affects risk of pancreatic cancer.

COMPLICATIONS AND COMORBIDITIES

- Patients who have both pancreatic cancer and diabetes, either before or after surgery, often have unstable glycemic control.
- While pancreatic cancer may be present in older people with new-onset diabetes, we do not routinely work up new-onset diabetes for possible cancer in the absence of other suggestive signs or symptoms.
- The utility of diagnosing pancreatic cancer in new-onset diabetes (i.e., cure rate) needs further evaluation.
- Although pancreas-dedicated CT scan with three-dimensional reconstruction is the preferred method to diagnose and stage pancreatic cancer, endoscopic ultrasound is also reasonable depending on local experience and expertise.
- Inform patients that pancreatectomy may cause diabetes, and follow blood glucose levels carefully.

REFERENCES

Jemal A, Siegel R, Ward E, et al. Cancer statistics, 2009. *CA Cancer J Clin,* 2009; Vol. 59: pp. 225–49.
   Comments: Epidemiology of pancreatic cancer.

Yip D, Karapetis C, Strickland A, et al. Chemotherapy and radiotherapy for inoperable advanced pancreatic cancer. *Cochrane Database Syst Rev,* 2006; Vol. 3: CD002093.
   Comments: Chemotherapy appears to prolong survival in people with advanced pancreatic cancer and can confer clinical benefits and improve quality of life.

Chari ST, Leibson CL, Rabe KG, et al. Probability of pancreatic cancer following diabetes: a population-based study. *Gastroenterology,* 2005; Vol. 129: pp. 504–11.
   Comments: Adults with new-onset diabetes were 8 times more likely to be diagnosed with pancreatic cancer within 3 years than the general population.

Stolzenberg-Solomon RZ, Graubard BI, Chari S, et al. Insulin, glucose, insulin resistance, and pancreatic cancer in male smokers. *JAMA,* 2005; Vol. 294: pp. 2872–8.
   Comments: Provides good evidence that the metabolic derangements related to diabetes are a cause of pancreatic cancer. The elevated risk of pancreatic cancer in people with diabetes cannot be explained solely by the cancer's effect on islet cell function during its subclinical phase.

Schernhammer ES, Kang JH, Chan AT, et al. A prospective study of aspirin use and the risk of pancreatic cancer in women. *J Natl Cancer Inst,* 2004; Vol. 96: pp. 22–8.
   Comments: >14 tab/wk of aspirin for more than 4 years increases relative risk of pancreatic cancer by 1.8-fold.

Hochwald SN, Zee S, Conlon KC, et al. Prognostic factors in pancreatic endocrine neoplasms: an analysis of 136 cases with a proposal for low-grade and intermediate-grade groups. *J Clin Oncol,* 2002; Vol. 20: pp. 2633–42.
   Comments: Prognosis of endocrine pancreatic cancer.

Gapstur SM, Gann PH, Lowe W, et al. Abnormal glucose metabolism and pancreatic cancer mortality. *JAMA,* 2000; Vol. 283: pp. 2552–8.
   Comments: Abnormal glucose metabolism increases the relative risk of pancreatic cancer death by 1.5- to 2-fold

Everhart J, Wright D. Diabetes mellitus as a risk factor for pancreatic cancer. A meta-analysis. *JAMA,* 1995; Vol. 273: pp. 1605–9.
   Comments: Diabetes increases odds of pancreatic cancer by two-fold.

Infectious Diseases

AMPUTATIONS

Lee J. Sanders, DPM

DEFINITION

- **Minor lower extremity amputation (LEA):** toe(s), ray(s), transmetatarsal, and midfoot amputation.
- **Major lower extremity amputation (LEA):** below-knee transtibial amputation (BKA) of the lower leg distal to the tibial tuberosity; above-knee amputation (AKA) of the leg through the femur (supracondylar, midthigh, or high thigh).
- **Guillotine amputation:** an open amputation for uncontrolled pedal sepsis, through a circular incision down bone, allowing for quick removal of septic focus and direct examination of muscle compartments for extension of infection.
- **Autoamputation:** dry gangrene allowed to demarcate and proceed to amputation without surgical intervention.

EPIDEMIOLOGY

- Approximately two-thirds of all LEAs occur in people with diabetes (leading cause).
- Risk factors: peripheral arterial disease, peripheral sensory neuropathy, ulceration, infection, renal disease, smoking, and prior amputation.
- Half of all LEAs occur >65 years of age.
- In 2003, rate per 1000 persons with DM = 5.0 among blacks and 3.2 among whites in US.
- Diabetic foot ulcers (DFUs) precede 85% of amputations.
- A higher percentage of distal amputations (toes, rays, and transmetatarsal) are performed in individuals with diabetes; >50% of amputations in persons with diabetes are performed at the level of the foot (40% toe, 13% transmetatarsal).

DIAGNOSIS

- Relies on accurate diagnosis of risk factors for amputation.
- Diabetes is strongly associated with femoral-popliteal and tibial (infrapopliteal) atherosclerotic disease.
- Diagnosis of peripheral vascular disease (PVD) requires a detailed assessment for absence of femoral, popliteal, and pedal pulses (see Peripheral Vascular Disease, p. 208).
- Ankle-brachial index (ABI): the ratio of the systolic blood pressure at the ankle divided by systolic blood pressure at the arm (normal ABI = 0.91–1.30; severe ischemia = ABI <0.4) (Hirsch).
- In patients with DM, ABIs may be artifactually elevated due to calcification of the arterial wall; 10% will have noncompressible vessels.
- Anatomic studies: (1) Gold standard for vascular imaging is conventional X-ray angiography but should only be performed when considering a revascularization intervention; (2) duplex ultrasound (allows direct visualization of vessels); (3) magnetic resonance angiography (MRA) (noninvasive with minimal risk); and (4) CT angiography (CTA) (Hirsch).

COMPLICATIONS AND COMORBIDITIES

- Regardless of the imaging tool used, arterial stenosis is seen as narrowing of vessels, abrupt interruption of flow, or inability to visualize a branch.
- Pulse volume recordings provide a qualitative assessment of blood flow; toe pressures >68 mmHg and transcutaneous oxygen (TcPO2) levels >30 mmHg can accurately predict healing of a transmetatarsal, midfoot, or below knee amputation.
- See Peripheral Neuropathy, p. 319, and Foot Ulcers, p. 264, for diagnosis of these important risk factors.

SIGNS AND SYMPTOMS

- **PVD:** absent pedal pulses, dependent rubor, pallor on elevation, loss of hair on dorsum of the foot, shiny scaly skin, thickening of the toenails, intermittent claudication.
- **Acute limb ischemia (ALI):** sudden decrease in limb perfusion that threatens tissue viability; 5 Ps: pain, pallor, pulseless, paresthesias, and paralysis.
- **Critical limb ischemia (CLI):** chronic ischemic rest pain in the forefoot, toes and/ or leg, ischemic ulcers, tissue necrosis, or gangrene attributable to objectively proven arterial occlusive disease.
- Moderate to severe aerobic or anaerobic infection with tissue necrosis.
- Rutherford classification of peripheral arterial disease severity used to classify degree of ischemia and salvageability of the limb (Table 3-5) (Hirsch).

CLINICAL TREATMENT

- Treatment for ALI and CLI is described in the Gangrene and Critical Limb Ischemia section (see p. 309).
- Among those with unreconstructable disease ~40% of the cases of CLI will require major amputation within 6 months of initial diagnosis (Hirsch).
- Level of amputation is determined by degree of tissue damage and infection, tissue oxygen perfusion, rehabilitation potential of the patient, and the clinical judgment of the surgeon (skin temperature, hair growth, tissue bleeding, viable muscle, and wounds without tension).
- **Goals of minor LEA:** (1) eliminate nonviable tissue, (2) provide a foot that has the best chance to heal, (3) provide a functional and cosmetically acceptable partial foot, (4) prevent major amputation of the leg.
- **Goals of major LEA:** (1) eliminate nonviable tissue, (2) provide a stump that has the best chance to heal, (3) provide a stump with best chance of long-term function.

FOLLOW-UP

- Close follow-up of patients post-major LEA is needed, because they have a 4%–30% risk of mortality at 30 days, and a 20%–37% risk of significant morbidity (MI, stroke, and infection).
- Intensive treatment of all risk factors is needed because of poor overall prognosis: patient survival in the National Surgical Quality Improvement Program (NSQIP) amputation series for BKA and AKA was 57% and 39% at 3 years (Nehler).
- Also requires intensive prevention program for surviving limb, because 15% of patients with initially successful BKA will be converted to an AKA at 2 years, likely due to more proximal atherosclerotic occlusive vascular disease, flexion contracture of the knee, and the development of nonhealing wounds on the BKA stump (Nehler).
- Another 15% of patients with initially successful BKA will suffer a major contralateral amputation.

EXPERT OPINION

- Comprehensive multidisciplinary foot care programs can reduce amputation rates by 45%–85%.
- These statistics highlight the importance of close follow-up and intensive preventive measures.
- Major LEA confers a poor overall prognosis.

BASIS FOR RECOMMENDATIONS

Hirsch AT, Haskal ZJ, Hertzer NR, et al. ACC/AHA 2005 Practice Guidelines for the management of patients with peripheral arterial disease (lower extremity, renal, mesenteric, and abdominal aortic): a collaborative report from the American Association for Vascular Surgery/Society for Vascular Surgery, Society for Cardiovascular Angiography and Interventions, Society for Vascular Medicine and Biology, Society of Interventional Radiology, and the ACC/AHA Task Force on Practice Guidelines (Writing Committee to Develop Guidelines for the Management of Patients With Peripheral Arterial Disease)—Summary of Recommendations endorsed by the American Association of Cardiovascular and Pulmonary Rehabilitation; National Heart, Lung, and Blood Institute; Society for Vascular Nursing; Trans Atlantic Inter-Society Consensus; and Vascular Disease Foundation. *Circulation*, 2006; Vol. 113: pp. e463–654.

   Comments: The ACC/AHA guidelines can be downloaded for free from the American Heart Association, *http://circ.ahajournals.org/cgi/reprint/113/11/1474.*

OTHER REFERENCES

Johannesson A, Larsson GU, Ramstrand N, et al. Incidence of lower-limb amputation in the diabetic and non-diabetic general population: a 10-year population-based cohort study of initial unilateral and contralateral amputations and reamputations. *Diabetes Care*, 2009; Vol. 32: pp. 275–80.

   Comments: In the general population aged >45 years, the incidence of vascular lower-limb amputations at or proximal to the transmetatarsal level is 8 times higher in diabetic than in nondiabetic individuals. One in four amputees may require contralateral amputation and/or reamputation. 74% of all amputations were transtibial.

Canavan RJ, Unwin NC, Kelly WF, et al. Diabetes-and nondiabetes-related lower extremity amputation incidence before and after the introduction of better organized diabetes foot care: continuous longitudinal monitoring using a standard method. *Diabetes Care*, 2008; Vol. 31: pp. 459–63.

   Comments: In the South Tees area of the UK, major diabetes-related LEA rates have fallen over a continuous 5-year period, while major nondiabetes LEA rates increased, after introduction of diabetes foot care program. The biggest improvement in LEA incidence was seen in the reduction of repeat major LEAs.

Ziegler-Graham K, MacKenzie EJ, Ephraim PL, et al. Estimating the prevalence of limb loss in the United States: 2005 to 2050. *Arch Phys Med Rehabil*, 2008; Vol. 89: pp. 422–9.

   Comments: In the year 2005, 1.6 million persons were living with loss of a limb in the United States. 42% were nonwhite and 38% (608,000) had an amputation secondary to vascular disease with a comorbid diagnosis of DM.

Eskelinen E, Eskelinen A, Albäck A, et al. Major amputation incidence decreases both in non-diabetic and in diabetic patients in Helsinki. *Scand J Surg*, 2006; Vol. 95: pp. 185–9.

   Comments: Decrease in major amputation rates among diabetic as well as nondiabetic patients attributed to increased interest in amputation prevention, with a contribution by vascular surgeons.

Jeffcoate WJ. The incidence of amputation in diabetes. *Acta Chir Belg*, 2005; Vol. 105: pp. 140–4.

   Comments: Reported incidence of amputation varies enormously between countries, races, and communities, but gives an indication of the suffering and costs caused by disease of the foot in diabetes. Quality of care of foot disease in diabetes can, and should, be best assessed in terms of survival, function/incapacity, and well-being.

Lavery LA, Armstrong DG, Wunderlich RP, et al. Diabetic foot syndrome: evaluating the prevalence and incidence of foot pathology in Mexican Americans and non-Hispanic whites from a diabetes disease management cohort. *Diabetes Care*, 2003; Vol. 26: pp. 1435–8.

   Comments: Incidence of amputation is higher in Mexican Americans compared to non-Hispanic whites, despite rates of ulceration, infection, vascular disease, and lower-extremity bypass.

COMPLICATIONS AND COMORBIDITIES

Centers for Disease Control and Prevention (CDC). Lower extremity amputation episodes among persons with diabetes—New Mexico, 2000. *MMWR*, 2003; Vol. 52: pp. 66–8.

Comments: Median age of persons was 66. Incidence was twice a high for men as for women. Overall age adjusted LEA rate was 3.4 per 1000 persons with DM.

Leggetter S, Chaturvedi N, Fuller JH, et al. Ethnicity and risk of diabetes-related lower extremity amputation: a population-based, case-control study of African Caribbeans and Europeans in the United kingdom. *Arch Intern Med*, 2002; Vol. 162: pp. 73–8.

Comments: Amputation risk in African Caribbeans is one-third that of Europeans and is explained by low smoking, neuropathy, and peripheral vascular disease rates.

Wrobel JS, Mayfield JA, Reiber GE. Geographic variation of lower-extremity major amputation in individuals with and without diabetes in the Medicare population. *Diabetes Care,* 2001; Vol. 24: pp. 860–4.

Comments: Diabetes-related amputation rates exhibit high regional variation. Adjusted rate of major amputation for individuals with diabetes was 3.83 per 1000. Diabetes amputations accounted for 53% of major amputations.

Adler AI, Boyko EJ, Ahroni JH, et al. Lower-extremity amputation in diabetes. The independent effects of peripheral vascular disease, sensory neuropathy, and foot ulcers. *Diabetes Care,* 1999; Vol. 22: pp. 1029–35.

Comments: Prospective study to identify risk factors for LEA in individuals with diabetes. Showed that peripheral sensory neuropathy, PVD, foot ulcers, former amputation, and treatment with insulin are independent risk factors for LEA in patients with diabetes.

Centers for Disease Control and Prevention (CDC). Age-Adjusted Hospital Discharge Rates for Nontraumatic Lower Extremity Amputation per 1000 Diabetic Population, by Race, United States, 1980 to 2003. *http://www .cdc.gov/diabetes/statistics/lea/diabetes_complications/fig6.htm.*

Comments: From 1980 through 2003, the adjusted rate of hospital discharge for nontraumatic lower extremity amputation per 1000 persons with diabetes was higher among blacks than among whites. In 2003, the age-adjusted LEA rate per 1000 persons with diabetes was 5.0 among blacks and 3.2 among whites.

Sanders LJ. Ray and Transmetatarsal Amputations. In Fischer JE, (Ed.), *Mastery of Surgery,* Fifth Edition. Philadelphia: Lippincott, Williams and Wilkins; 2007: pp. 2193–2207.

Comments: This well-illustrated chapter covers minor (local) amputations of the foot, indications, criteria for wound healing, surgical techniques, complications, and functional outcomes. Attention should be directed to preserving foot function, achieving a durable, cosmetically acceptable result and whenever possible preventing major amputation of the leg.

Nehler MR, Halandres P. Major Lower Extremity Amputation. In Fischer JE, (Ed.), *Mastery of Surgery,* Fifth Edition. Philadelphia: Lippincott, Williams and Wilkins; 2007: pp. 2211–2220.

Comments: Nicely illustrated chapter discusses indications, preoperative planning, determining level of amputation, surgical technique, and functional outcomes for major LEA.

FOOT ULCERS

Lee J. Sanders, DPM

DEFINITION

- Diabetic foot ulcer (DFU): a nonhealing or poorly healing partial- or full-thickness wound below the ankle in an individual with diabetes, critical in the natural history of the diabetic foot.
- Most common sites: plantar surface of foot (metatarsal heads and midfoot), and toes (dorsal interphalangeal joints or distal tip).
- Pathogenesis: DFUs frequently caused by repetitive injury to an insensate foot.

EPIDEMIOLOGY

- Ill-fitting shoes are the most frequent cause of DFUs.
- Risk factors for DFUs: peripheral neuropathy, peripheral vascular disease, foot deformities (hammertoes, clawtoes, prominent metatarsal heads, bunion, rocker-bottom foot), vibratory perception threshold (VPT) 25V or greater, past foot ulcer, visual impairment, diabetic nephropathy (especially patients on dialysis), poor glycemic control, and cigarette smoking.
- Incidence: annual population-based incidence in people with diabetes is from 1.9% to 2.2%.
- Prevalence range: from 1.8% in South Asians living in the UK to 11.8% in the US.
- Lifetime risk for DFUs estimated to be as high as 25%.
- DFUs most common precursor of amputation; 85% of amputations are preceded by an active foot ulcer.
- Ulcer related costs per episode average $13,179 (range $1,892 to $27,721) and increase with severity level (Stockl). Hospitalization is a major cost driver.

DIAGNOSIS

- Classified as neuropathic, ischemic or neuroischemic, based upon the presence or absence of ischemia in the common background of neuropathy. Several specific classifications exist and are listed here.
    - **Wagner-Meggitt classification:** foot ulcers are divided into six grades based on depth, presence, or absence of infection and gangrene. All grades except 5 can be converted to a Grade 0 foot. *Grade 0:* skin is intact; *Grade 1:* superficial ulcer; *Grade 2:* deep ulcer reaches tendon, bone, or joint capsule; *Grade 3:* deeper tissues involved with abscess, osteomyelitis, or tendinitis with extension along midfoot compartments of tendon sheaths; *Grade 4:* gangrene of toe, toes, or forefoot; surgical ablation is indicated; *Grade 5:* gangrene involves the whole foot; salvage not possible. Amputation below the knee (Wagner).
    - **University of Texas (UT) Classification:** the UT system assesses ulcer depth, the presence of wound infection and signs of ischemia. *Grade 0:* intact skin (pre- or postulcerative site that has healed); *Grade 1:* superficial wound not involving tendon, capsule, or bone; *Grade 2:* wound penetrating to tendon or capsule; *Grade 3:* wound penetrating bone or joint. Within each grade there are four stages: stage A: clean wound; stage B: nonischemic infected wounds; stage C: ischemic noninfected wounds; and stage D: ischemic infected wounds (Oyibo).
    - **The PEDIS system:** diabetic foot ulcer classification for research purposes. Evaluates five important clinical characteristics, **P**erfusion, **E**xtent/size, **D**epth/tissue loss, **I**nfection, and **S**ensation (International Working Group on the Diabetic Foot, http://www.iwgdf.org).

SIGNS AND SYMPTOMS

- Early signs of emerging DFU: mild erythema, elevated skin temperature, blister formation, and serous or serosanguinous drainage on socks or bed linen.
- Neuropathic ulcers: usually surrounded by callus, located at the tips of the toes, on the tops of the interphalangeal joints, and beneath the metatarsal heads, and painless unless infected.
- Neuroischemic ulcers: usually located on the margins of the foot, over boney prominences (first and fifth metatarsal heads). A halo of erythema often surrounds the ulcer. Often associated with pain secondary to ischemia or infection.

COMPLICATIONS AND COMORBIDITIES

CLINICAL TREATMENT

Comprehensive Foot Examination and Risk Assessment

- Early detection of foot lesions and aggressive care can reduce risk for amputation.
- Requires detailed history and careful systematic inspection of the feet in a well-lit room.
- Must include neurologic, vascular, dermatologic, and musculoskeletal assessment.
- Inspect footwear to determine correct fit (length, width, and depth), condition (state of wear, protruding seams or nails), and suitability for the individual's foot structure and function.
- Shoes should serve to accommodate foot deformities and to protect the high-risk foot from injury.
- ADA Risk Classification (Table 3-10): Risk categories 0–3, determined by the presence and combination of the following risk factors: peripheral neuropathy with loss of protectice sensation (LOPS), peripheral arterial disease (PAD), foot deformity, and history of foot ulcer or amputation.
- Treatment recommendations and follow-up are based upon the level of risk.

Medical and Surgical Treatment

- Wound debridement with scalpel to remove callus and necrotic tissue can be done in primary care setting, but preferable to refer to diabetic foot specialist.
- Wound dressings to control exudate and maintain moist environment.
- Mechanical off-loading (cornerstone of treatment for plantar ulcers): total contact cast (TCC), Scotch cast boot or removable cast walker (RCW). Once DFU is healed, evaluate for custom-molded insoles/orthotics and therapeutic footwear.
- Infection: diabetic foot infections require attention to local (foot) and systemic (metabolic) issues and coordinated management by a multidisciplinary foot care team.
- Avoid prescribing antibiotics for uninfected ulcerations, wounds lacking purulence, or any manifestations of inflammation.
- Determine the need for surgical and infectious disease consultation.
- Superficial ulcer with infection: debridement and oral antibiotics targeted at *Staphylococcus aureus* and *Streptococci* (see *Johns Hopkins ABX Guide*, Diabetic Foot Infection, p. 6).
- Infected wounds may require: incision and drainage, excision of infected necrotic tissues, local amputation, revascularization.
- Deep (limb threatening) infection: emergent surgical drainage, debridement of necrotic tissues, broad-spectrum intravenous antibiotics targeted at gram-positive and gram-negative organisms including anaerobes (see *Johns Hopkins ABX Guide*, Diabetic Foot Infection, p. 6).
- Smoking cessation.

FOOTWEAR

- Footwear is a major modifiable risk factor.
- Shoes should be "foot shaped," with roomy toe box, snugly fitting heel cup, heels low (<5 cm high), shoe lining smooth, sole sufficiently thick to prevent puncture wounds, shoe fastened with lace or strap to hold the foot back in the shoe, athletic shoes useful if sufficiently long, broad, and deep.
- Wearing socks is advisable to reduce friction.

TABLE 3-10. RISK CLASSIFICATION BASED ON THE COMPREHENSIVE FOOT EXAMINATION

Risk Category	Definition	Treatment Recommendations	Suggested Follow-up
0	No LOPS, no PAD, no deformity	• Patient education including advice on appropriate footwear.	Annually (by generalist and/or specialist)
1	LOPS ± deformity	• Consider prescriptive or accommodative footwear. • Consider prophylactic surgery if deformity cannot be safely accommodated in shoes. Continue patient education.	Every 3–6 months (by generalist or specialist)
2	PAD ± LOPS	• Consider prescriptive or accommodative footwear. • Consider vascular consultation for combined follow-up.	Every 2–3 months (by specialist)
3	History of ulcer or amputation	• Same as category 1. • Consider vascular consultation for combined follow-up if PAD present.	Every 1–2 months (by specialist)

Source: Boulton AJ, Armstrong DG, Albert SF, et al. Comprehensive foot examination and risk assessment: a report of the task force of the foot care interest group of the American Diabetes Association, with endorsement by the American Association of Clinical Endocrinologists. *Diabetes Care*, 2008; Vol. 31(8): pp. 1679–85. Reprinted with permission from The American Diabetes Association.

COMPLICATIONS AND COMORBIDITIES

- Custom-made (bespoke) shoes can accommodate moderate-to-severe foot/ankle deformities and partial foot amputations.
- In hot climates, sandals should have closed toes.
- AVOID stiff leather dress shoes, high heels, thin soles, slip-on style, and flip-flops (thongs).

EXPERT OPINION
- Most common combination of factors resulting in DFUs are peripheral neuropathy and foot deformity and trauma.
- The most predictive single risk factor for ulceration is a past history of ulceration or amputation.

- The habit of going barefoot is common in developing countries, increasing risk of DFUs.
- Patients must understand the implications of sensory loss, the importance of appropriate, properly fitted footwear, and avoidance of barefoot walking.

BASIS FOR RECOMMENDATIONS

Apelqvist J, Bakker K, van Houtum WH, et al. Practical guidelines on the management and prevention of the diabetic foot: based upon the International Consensus on the Diabetic Foot (2007), prepared by the International Working Group on the Diabetic Foot. *Diabetes Metab Res Rev*, 2008; Vol. 24 Suppl 1: pp. S181–7.

Comments: Basic principles of prevention and treatment of the diabetic foot, based upon the International Consensus on the Diabetic Foot (2007), prepared by the International Working Group on the Diabetic Foot. Five key elements of foot management: regular inspection and examination, identification of risk, education (patient, family, provider), appropriate footwear, and treatment of nonulcerative pathology.

Boulton AJ, Armstrong DG, Albert SF, et al. Comprehensive foot examination and risk assessment: a report of the task force of the foot care interest group of the American Diabetes Association, with endorsement by the American Association of Clinical Endocrinologists. *Diabetes Care*, 2008; Vol. 31: pp. 1679–85.

Comments: ADA Task Force Report, risk classification based on comprehensive foot examination. Can be downloaded from *Diabetes Care*: *http://care.diabetesjournals.org/content/31/8/1679.full.pdf+html?sid=fd69ef11-8a67-4647-9f2e-5c25ed282ef0* (accessed 3/3/2011).

Lipsky BA, Berendt AR, Deery HG, et al. Diagnosis and treatment of diabetic foot infections. *Clin Infect Dis*, 2004; Vol. 39: pp. 885–910.

Comments: Foot infections in persons with diabetes cause severe morbidities and are the most common proximate, nontraumatic cause of amputations. This guideline provides a framework for treating all diabetic patients with a suspected foot infection.

OTHER REFERENCES

Stockl K, Vanderplas A, Tafesse E, et al. Costs of lower-extremity ulcers among patients with diabetes. *Diabetes Care*, 2004; Vol. 27: pp. 2129–34.

Comments: 2253 adult patients with DM who had a lower-extremity ulcer episode during 2000 and 2001 were identified by claims data. Mean age was 68.9 years, 59% of patients were male. Total ulcer-related costs averaged $13,179 per episode and increased with severity level.

Schaper NC. Diabetic foot ulcer classification system for research purposes: a progress report on criteria for including patients in research studies. *Diabetes Metab Res Rev*, 2004; Vol. 20 Suppl 1: pp. S90–5.

Comments: International Working Group on the Diabetic Foot (IWGDF) classification system for diabetic foot ulcers, for research purposes.

Oyibo SO, Jude EB, Tarawneh I, et al. A comparison of two diabetic foot ulcer classification systems: the Wagner and the University of Texas wound classification systems. *Diabetes Care*, 2001; Vol. 24: pp. 84–8.

Comments: Increasing stage, regardless of grade, associated with increased risk of amputation and prolonged healing time. UT system's inclusion of stage makes it a better predictor of outcome.

Wagner FW. The dysvascular foot: a system for diagnosis and treatment. *Foot Ankle*, 1981; Vol. 2: pp. 64–122.

Comments: Wagner classification of diabetic foot ulcers is based on the depth of the skin lesion and the presence or absence of infection and gangrene. It is still widely used to describe the natural history of the dysvascular foot.

Bakker K, Foster A, van Houtum W, Riley P (Eds.). *Diabetes and Foot Care: Time to Act*. A joint publication of the International Diabetes Federation and the International Working Group on the Diabetic Foot. 2005. ISBN 2-930229-40-3.

Comments: This publication is the fourth of the International Diabetes Federation's Time to Act series. It is written by international experts and aims to increase awareness of diabetic foot problems worldwide, to demonstrate the benefits of preventive strategies and to convince stakeholders to engage in implementing diabetic foot care services.

Edmonds ME, Foster AVM, Sanders LJ (Eds.). *A Practical Manual of Diabetic Foot Care*, Second Edition. Oxford, UK: Blackwell Publishing; 2008. ISBN 978-1-4051-6147-3.

Comments: BMA Medical Book of the Year, 2004. Comprehensive assessment, staging, and treatment of the diabetic foot with a global perspective.

HIV-ASSOCIATED DIABETES

Todd T. Brown, MD, PhD

DEFINITION

- Human immunodeficiency virus (HIV) is a retrovirus that causes acquired immune deficiency syndrome (AIDS) by infecting helper T cells of the immune system, leading to immunosuppression and opportunistic infections. Modern antiretroviral therapy can effectively control HIV replication and has greatly improved the prognosis for HIV-infected patients.
- HIV-associated diabetes refers to diabetes occurring among individuals with HIV who may not otherwise have traditional risk factors for diabetes.

EPIDEMIOLOGY

- Insulin resistance (IR) and diabetes mellitus (DM) are common among HIV+ individuals.
- Incidence of DM is 4 times greater in HIV+ men on highly active antiretroviral therapy (HAART) compared to HIV− men (Brown).
- Complications such as kidney disease and cardiovascular disease may occur more frequently in HIV+ versus HIV− individuals (Neuhaus).
- Risk factors for IR/DM in HIV: abdominal fat accumulation (i.e., lipodystrophy), peripheral lipoatrophy, family history of DM, obesity, age, hepatitis C positivity, low CD4 nadir, black/Hispanic race.
- Certain protease inhibitors (PIs) may have a direct effect on insulin resistance. Lopinavir/ritonavir is the PI in current use most associated with IR.
- Stavudine and zidovudine are also associated with insulin resistance.
- Consider glycemic effects of other medications commonly used for HIV−related comorbidities: corticosteroids, growth hormone, megestrol acetate, immunosuppressants, atypical antipsychotics
- In HIV+ patients, DM associated with two times higher risk for coronary artery disease (Worm).

DIAGNOSIS

- DM is diagnosed using the same criteria with or without HIV.
- HbA1c underestimates glycemia in HIV+ patients on HAART by ~0.8% (Kim).
- No accepted role for clinical use of insulin levels to assess IR.

CLINICAL TREATMENT

- Balanced diet and regular exercise crucial. Recommend ADA diet.
- Lifestyle modification shown to improve metabolic parameters in HIV-infected patients.
- Aggressive risk factor modification for coronary disease: lipid control, HTN control (generally with ACE-I or ARB), smoking cessation, cocaine avoidance, aspirin therapy.

COMPLICATIONS AND COMORBIDITIES

- First-line treatment: metformin. Some consider pioglitazone first-line for HIV-infected patients with lipoatrophy, as this is associated with modest increases in subcutaneous fat.
- Metformin: reduces hepatic IR. Associated with reduced visceral fat, blood pressure, triglycerides (TG) (decreased 10%–20%) in HIV+ patients. Some studies have shown decreased limb fat with metformin; use with caution in patients with lipoatrophy. Enhanced theoretical risk of lactic acidosis with nucleoside reverse transcriptase inhibitors (NRTIs), liver disease, and congestive heart failure (CHF).
- TZDs (pioglitazone and rosiglitazone): reduce peripheral IR as peroxisome proliferator-activated receptor (PPAR) gamma agonists. Effect on lipoatrophy controversial. Pioglitzaone may be better than rosiglitazone for lipoatrophy, but no head-to-head trials. Effect present only on those not on stavudine or zidovudine. Some increase in TG with rosiglitazone but not pioglitazone. Rosiglitazone may increase cardiovascular risk. Lipid profile with rosiglitazone less favorable than pioglitazone. Maximum effect after several weeks.
- Use sulfonylureas, meglitinides, exenatide, sitagliptin, or acarbose as second-line therapies.
- No accepted role for pharmacologic interventions for those with IR or prediabetes. Metformin can be considered in overweight, young patients with prediabetes per ADA guidelines.
- Consider switching from PI to non-nucleoside reverse transcriptase inhibitor (NNRTI)-based regimen provided viral control not jeopardized.
- Consider low-dose (10–15 units) bedtime glargine, detimer, or NPH insulin in combination with oral antidiabetic agents if failing oral agents. Insulin effective for glucose control with individualized regimen.
- Note: newer PIs (atazanavir, darunavir) are not associated with insulin resistance.

FOLLOW-UP

- In routine management of HIV, check fasting glucose at baseline, prior to, 3 and 6 months after HAART initiation, then yearly if normal.
- In people with DM, self-monitor blood glucose 1–2 times per day on oral agents, 2–4+ times/day if on insulin. Monitoring may be more or less intensive depending on the stability of glycemia.
- Monitor HbA1c every 3–6 months, depending on control. Goal <7%, with caveat regarding accuracy of A1c in HIV-infected persons.
- Patients with prediabetes should be screened at 3- to 6-month intervals.
- Monitoring for complications: dilated fundoscopic exam by ophthalmology; spot urine for microalbumin; and foot exam with inspection, monofilament, and vibration testing at baseline and every 6–12 months (see Routine Preventive Care, p. 61).

EXPERT OPINION

- With effective HAART, HIV+ patients are living longer and age-related comorbidities, such as DM, are gaining importance.
- Due to effects of antiretroviral medications and/or chronic HIV infection, kidney disease and cardiovacular disease occur at higher than expected frequencies.
- Multiple risk factor modification is essential.

REFERENCES

Neuhaus J, Angus B, Kowalska JD, et al. Risk of all-cause mortality associated with nonfatal AIDS and serious non-AIDS events among adults infected with HIV. *AIDS,* 2010; Vol. 24: pp. 697–706.

Comments: A large cohort study showing the importance of non-AIDS events on mortality in HIV-infected persons.

Kim PS, Woods C, Georgoff P, et al. A1C underestimates glycemia in HIV infection. *Diabetes Care,* 2009; Vol. 32: pp. 1591–3.

Comments: Important paper demonstrating the underestimation of glycemia by A1c in HIV+ patients.

Samaras K. Prevalence and pathogenesis of diabetes mellitus in HIV-1 infection treated with combined antiretroviral therapy. *J Acquir Immune Defic Syndr,* 2009; Vol. 50: pp. 499–505.

Comments: Good review article regarding insulin resistance and DM in HIV+ patients.

Worm SW, Wit SD, Weber R, et al. Diabetes mellitus, preexisting coronary heart disease, and the risk of subsequent coronary heart disease events in patients infected with human immunodeficiency virus: the Data Collection on Adverse Events of Anti-HIV Drugs (D:A:D Study). *Circulation,* 2009; Vol. 119: pp. 805–11.

Comments: This study of 33,347 HIV-infected persons found that preexisting DM was associated with two times higher risk of heart disease.

Wohl DA, McComsey G, Tebas P, et al. Current concepts in the diagnosis and management of metabolic complications of HIV infection and its therapy. *Clin Infect Dis,* 2006; Vol. 43: pp. 645–53.

Comments: Recommendations regarding the management of metabolic abnormalities in HIV+ patients.

Brown TT, Cole SR, Li X, et al. Antiretroviral therapy and the prevalence and incidence of diabetes mellitus in the multicenter AIDS cohort study. *Arch Intern Med,* 2005; Vol. 165: pp. 1179–84.

Comments: Shows that the risk of incident DM is higher in HIV+ men on HAART compared to HIV-men.

Hadigan C, Corcoran C, Basgoz N, et al. Metformin in the treatment of HIV lipodystrophy syndrome: a randomized controlled trial. *JAMA,* 2000; Vol. 284: pp. 472–7.

Comments: Shows metformin may be effective in the treatment of central fat accumulation in HIV+ patients.

INFECTIOUS DISEASES AND DIABETES

Paul Auwaerter, MD

DEFINITION

- Diabetes is commonly associated with an increased risk of certain infections; however, good data to support this contention are often limited.
- According to Boyko and Lipsky's review of epidemiological data and risks, "probable" means data support the association, "possible" means presence or absence of the association cannot be confirmed from available information, and "doubtful" indicates that data do not support a link.
- **Probable** increased risk of infection: asymptomatic bacteriuria, lower extremity infections, increased postsurgical infections after sternotomy or total hip replacement, Group B *Streptococcal* infections and reactivation tuberculosis (TB) in American Indians.
- **Possible** increased risk of infection: genitourinary infections such as bacterial cystitis, pyelonephritis, candidal vaginitis; respiratory tract infections including pneumonia, influenza, chronic bronchitis, primary or reactivation TB, zygomycete infections (e.g., mucormycosis), malignant otitis media; Fournier's gangrene.
- **Doubtful** increased risk of infection: *S. aureus* infections, chronic sinusitis.

COMPLICATIONS AND COMORBIDITIES

- Incidence of infections associated with diabetes mellitus (DM) difficult to discern based on available data.
- Diabetes associated with three-fold higher risk of infection-related mortality in persons with history of cardiovascular disease (Bertoni).
- Diabetic ketoacidosis (DKA) and the hyperosmolar hyperglycemic state (HHS): infection is leading precipitant with pneumonia and urinary tract infections (UTIs) most common reasons.
- **Genitourinary (GU) infections:** bacteriuria 2–4 times higher in DM. Less data support increase risk of UTI or pyelonephritis, but likely higher in both women and men. In case reports of emphysematous cystitis, a majority have DM. Candidal UTI, especially *C. glabrata*, frequently cited as common in DM, but slender data support this association. Commonly believed that candidal vulvovaginitis more common in DM, but no data support this notion.
- **Lower extremity (LE) infections:** more common, including diabetic foot infection, cellulitis, and osteomyelitis. Amputation in DM 15 times greater than in non-DM.
- **Surgical site infections:** studies suggest higher rates of sternal wound infections after coronary artery bypass graft (CABG) requiring redo sternotomy and also saphenous vein graft harvest site infections. Total hip infection rates are also higher in diabetes compared to no diabetes. Although some studies looking at a broad range of surgical procedures find increased rates of infections (10.7% vs 1.8%), other studies found similar rates regardless of diabetes status.
- Most convincing data suggest that higher risk for tuberculosis occurs in American Indians with diabetes.
- **Group B *Streptococcal* infections:** case series have described DM occurring in 9.4%–45.8% of patients.
- **Respiratory:** *S. pneumoniae* leading cause of pneumonia but true for most series of community-acquired infection. Mortality for pneumonia or influenza higher in DM patients based upon several studies.
- **Zygomycoses:** (includes *Mucor, Rhizopus, Cunninghamella* and *Absidia* fungal species) case series have high rates in DM (up to 70%) and DKA is said to be a special risk factor.
- **Necrotizing fasciitis/Fournier's gangrene:** diabetes is the most common listed comorbidity in case series (approximately 10% of patients).

- **GU infections:** asymptomatic bacteruria defined as $>10^5$ organisms/ml in 2 consecutive urine specimens with or without presence of white blood cells (WBCs). Cystitis or pyelonephritis defined by symptoms and urinalysis: leukocyte esterase (+), nitrite (+), urine with >10 WBC/hpf, culture $>10^5$ organisms per ml. Emphysematous complicated UTI (cystitis or pyelonephritis) with gas seen in renal or bladder structures.
- **DKA:** leukocytosis of 10,000–15,000 mm^3 common and may not indicate infection, if $>25,000$ mm^3 or $>10\%$ bandemia consider due to infection until proven otherwise.
- **Rhinocerebral zygomycosis:** invasive sinusitis in patient usually with eschar present. Obtain sinus CT or MRI along with otolaryngology consultation. Definitive diagnosis by showing hyphae invading tissue + culture.

- **Malignant otitis externa:** high prevalence of diabetes in case reports. Etiology mostly due to *Pseudomonas aeruginosa* or *Aspergillus* species. Historically with high mortality, although now much lower with effective antibiotic therapy and imaging studies.

SIGNS AND SYMPTOMS

- **Severe, necrotizing soft tissue infections:** necrotizing fasciitis, Fournier's gangrene may present fulminantly (as in type II Group A *Streptococcal* infection) within 24 hours of onset or more slowly over 2–5 days as in mixed aerobic/anaerobic pathogens typically of type I infections. Pain may be out of proportion to physical findings. Skin discoloration, bullae, and thin/foul discharge (not pus) develop routinely without intervention.
- **Rhinocerebral zygomycosis:** sinus complaints, eschar of the palate that may invade bone and brain and yield cranial nerve palsies.
- **Malignant otitis externa:** otalgia, ear canal erythema, or eschar. May cause facial nerve paralysis with progression to involve CN IX, X, XI and XII +/– skull osteomyelitis.
- **Group B *Streptococcal* (GBS) infections:** higher risk due to diabetes seen with skin/soft tissue infections, bone/joint infections, and UTIs—often with concomitant bacteremia.
- **GU:** if patient without symptoms this is asymptomatic bacteriuria regardless of whether leukocytes are present or absent in urine.

CLINICAL TREATMENT

- **Candidal vulvovaginitis:** topical suppositories first-line therapy (e.g., OTC: clotrimazole, butoconazole, miconazole, tioconazole) or topical nystatin 100,000 U/d, use short course (1–3 d) for mild sx, >7–14 d if severe, recurrent, or abnormal host. Systemic therapy: fluconazole 150 mg PO single dose (wait 3 d for response). Boric acid 600-mg gel capsule intravaginal daily × 14 d effective especially for non-albicans species or refractory infections.
- **LE infections:** see Foot Ulcers (p. 264) and Osteomyelitis (p. 275). Cellulitis treated with agents to cover staphylococcal +/– MRSA and Gram-negative bacteria (i.e., Cephalexin 500 mg PO four times daily, Amoxicillin/Clavulanate 875 mg–1000 mg PO twice daily, or Clindamycin 300 mg PO three times daily) for 14 days.
- **Pneumonia:** guidelines for community-acquired pneumonia or hospital-acquired pneumonia do not distinguish diabetes from nondiabetes. Influenza-related mortality may be higher in DM and is considered a high-risk condition for which early antiviral treatment should be considered.
- **Rhinocerebral zygomycosis:** surgical debridement critical, performed on an emergent basis. Antifungal therapy traditionally polyene-based (liposomal amphotericin 5 mg/kg IV q24h) but posaconazole and combination therapy (caspofungin and lipid amphotericin B [amB]) reported to have role in salvage therapy or yield improved outcomes over historical cohorts treated with polyene alone. Fluconazole, voriconazole, and echinocandin monotherapy ineffective. Need to correct underlying acidosis and hyperglycemia if present.
- **Malignant otitis externa:** irrigation, aural toilet, ear wick, and topical antibiotic therapy (i.e., eardrops). Oral systemic therapy typically used in addition to topical: ciprofloxacin 500 mg PO twice-daily × 10–14 d. Refractory infection or resistant organisms may require parenteral antipseudomonal drugs guided by sensitivity data from culture. Role of surgery unclear.

COMPLICATIONS AND COMORBIDITIES

- **GU infections:** asymptomatic bacteruria = no antimicrobial treatment needed. Uncomplicated UTI treated for longer course in DM (i.e., 7–10 d), otherwise similar to non-DM (i.e., nitrofurantoin 50–100 mg PO daily, amoxicillin-clavulanate 500/125 mg PO twice daily, or trimethoprim-sulfamethotrexate DS 1 tab PO daily).
- **GBS:** treatment depends on location of infection, penicillin preferred therapy.

FOLLOW-UP

- The best studies documenting decreased wound infection rates with achieving optimal glucose control have been done in the post-CABG patient population.

EXPERT OPINION

- Diabetes is often cited as increasing the risk of infection for many conditions; however, data truly linking a diabetic condition to infectious risk are absent for most conditions.
- Hyperglycemic state appears to affect the function of neutrophils with impairment of phagocytosis, chemotaxis and migration, as well as intracellular lysis of organisms.
- Other predisposing factors may include abnormal tissue perfusion due to peripheral vascular disease and microcirculatory abnormalities.
- Peripheral neuropathy due to diabetes is clearly a risk factor for diabetic foot infection.
- Patients with abnormal bladder function due to neuropathy are at higher risk of UTI.

BASIS FOR RECOMMENDATIONS

Boyko EJ, Lipsky BA. Infection and diabetes. In Harris, MI (Ed.), *Diabetes in America*, 2nd edition. Washington, DC: National Institutes of Health, 1995; pp. 485–499.

    Comments: Authors review available literature to establish whether there is an association with infections commonly considered to be more common in the setting of diabetes. There are some surprising findings, such as insufficient evidence to strongly link rhinocerebral mucormycosis to diabetes or DKA—although this may reflect the available data rather than a true lack of an association. Some studies that support a link date to the 1970s or earlier and relevance in the modern era may be questioned. To access online: *http://diabetes.niddk. nih.gov/dm/pubs/america/index.htm.*

OTHER REFERENCES

Kitabchi AE, Umpierrez GE, Miles JM, et al. Hyperglycemic crises in adult patients with diabetes. *Diabetes Care*, 2009; Vol. 32: pp. 1335–43.

    Comments: Although infections remain the leading cause of DKA and HHS, suggested algorithms for treatment do not incorporate any formal evaluation of infection or antibiotic therapy but leave this to the clinician to sort through.

Dooley KE, Chaisson RE. Tuberculosis and diabetes mellitus: convergence of two epidemics. *Lancet Infect Dis*, 2009; Vol. 9: pp. 737–46.

    Comments: Authors suggest that the increasing rate of diabetes in both developing world and developing countries may be leading to increased rates of TB. Article is most helpful where highlighting issues in the comanagement of diabetes and TB infection.

Marchant MH, Viens NA, Cook C, et al. The impact of glycemic control and diabetes mellitus on perioperative outcomes after total joint arthroplasty. *J Bone Joint Surg Am*, 2009; Vol. 91: pp. 1621–9.

    Comments: Large retrospective review examining patients with uncontrolled DM (n = 3973) and controlled DM (n = 105,485), and no DM (n = 920,555). Those with uncontrolled DM had increased odds of UTI (adjusted OR = 1.97; 95% CI = 1.61–2.42) and wound infection (adjusted OR ratio = 2.28; 95% CI = 1.36–3.81), among other conditions. Overall mortality was higher, OR 3.23, 95% CI = 1.87–5.57.

Shine TS, Uchikado M, Crawford CC, et al. Importance of perioperative blood glucose management in cardiac surgical patients. *Asian Cardiovasc Thorac Ann*, 2007; Vol. 15: pp. 534–8.

Comments: Although data substantiating the dangers of hyperglycemia leading to complications after cardiac surgery are robust, there is less supporting the role of tight glucose control to avoiding complications. Authors review the studies looking at intensive insulin use.

Nicolle LE, Bradley S, Colgan R, et al. Infectious Diseases Society of America guidelines for the diagnosis and treatment of asymptomatic bacteriuria in adults. *Clin Infect Dis*, 2005; Vol. 40: pp. 643–54.

Comments: Asymptomatic pyuria with or without the presence of WBCs is not an indication for treatment. Screening urinalysis is not recommended for diabetic women.

Bertoni AG, Saydah S, Brancati FL. Diabetes and the risk of infection-related mortality in the U.S. *Diabetes Care*, 2001; Vol. 24: pp. 1044–9.

Comments: Longitudinal study suggested a three-fold increased risk in mortality due to infection in patients with diabetes and cardiovascular disease (CVD), but not in those lacking CVD.

Slovis CM, Mork VG, Slovis RJ, et al. Diabetic ketoacidosis and infection: leukocyte count and differential as early predictors of serious infection. *Am J Emerg Med*, 1987; Vol. 5: pp. 1–5.

Comments: Given that leukocytosis is a common feature of DKA, this emergency department study of 153 patients found that only the presence of a left shift with significant bandemia (>10%) correlated with the presence of actual infection (100% [19/19] and a specificity of 80% [98/122]).

OSTEOMYELITIS

Paul Auwaerter, MD

DEFINITION
- **Osteomyelitis (OM):** infection of the bone.
- **Acute OM:** first presentation of osteomyelitis, <2 weeks duration, no bony necrosis/ sequestrum, usually hematogenously acquired.
- **Chronic OM:** not clearly defined but may include failure of prior OM treatment, symptoms >3 weeks, presence of necrotic bone/sinus tract, or discharge.
- No widely agreed-upon definitions or guidelines for treatment of OM in setting of diabetic foot infection (DFI) (see Foot Ulcer, p. 264).
- Two general categories of OM: (1) occurring within context of DFI (most common by far) and (2) other sites.

EPIDEMIOLOGY
- OM may afflict up to 20% of patients with DFI (Berendt).
- OM due to DFI usually a consequence of neuropathy, callus formation, and/or ischemia causing an ulcer that then involves periosteum and then bone.
- Risk factors for OM/DFI: duration of diabetes mellitus >10 years, peripheral neuropathy, abnormal foot structure/maldistribution of weight over the plantar surface, peripheral vascular disease, smoking, poor diabetic control, skin/nail disease (e.g., maceration, puncture wound, tinea pedis, onychomycosis), male gender.
- Acute OM: uncommon, usually hematologic origin; in adults mostly affects the axial skeleton (discitis/vertebral osteomyelitis).
- Chronic OM: predominant bone infection in DM. Usually due to contiguous problem: ulceration > trauma > surgery.
- Microbiology: *Staphylococcal* species most common (*S. aureus* including MRSA), *Streptococcus* species (including Group A), *Enterobacteriaceae*, anaerobes. *Enterococci* often recovered, role usually uncertain. OM often polymicrobial.

COMPLICATIONS AND COMORBIDITIES

DIAGNOSIS

- Suspect when ulcer fails to heal as expected.
- **Differential:** neuroosteoarthropathy (may also coexist, frequently causes positive bone scans without infection present).
- Probing (steel probe) to bone often used. Positive test increases likelihood of OM; negative test reduces likelihood. If bone fragments observed, OM is definite.
- **Imaging:** plain radiographs are inexpensive and usually obtained. Many findings such as periosteal reaction, soft tissue swelling, irregularity of cortical bone, and demineralization are relatively nonspecific and therefore require other testing. More advanced findings such as areas of sclerosis with adjacent radiolucencies or bony destruction are very suggestive. For chronic OM, the overall sensitivity of plain films is high although the specificity is low. For acute OM, a minimum 2–3 weeks to see early changes of OM.
- MRI: preferred test to evaluate bone and soft tissues (especially small bones, for larger bones CT adequate). Occasionally, acute Charcot neuroosteoarthropathy (see Charcot Joint Disease [Diabetes Neuropathic Osteoarthropathy], p. 302) may be read as OM.
- Bone scan (Tc-99): Not recommended. Although superior to plain films, many false positives due to noninfectious causes (overlying inflammation, neuroosteopathy).
- WBC scans: expensive, less sensitive than bone scans. Use mainly when MRI unavailable.
- PET scan: role uncertain, limited studies suggest good sensitivity/specificity.
- **Lab:** ESR >70 mm/hr or elevated CRP suggestive; however, limited bone involvement (e.g., toe) may not be associated with increased ESR or CRP. ESR and CRP elevations are nonspecific, and may be elevated by other active processes (cellulitis, etc.). Blood cultures uncommonly positive.
- **Definitive diagnosis:** Bone biopsy required, given chronic nature and wide range of possible microbial etiologies. Patient should be off antibiotics for at least 48 hours, preferably longer. One or more pathogens recovered from involved bone (+compatible histopathology) makes the diagnosis. Obtain by needle biopsy through uninvolved skin or by operative approach. False negatives due to sampling error, fastidious organisms (anaerobes; or uncommonly actinomyces or mycobacterial species) or prior antibiotic therapy. False positives due to contamination from skin flora or other colonizing bacteria of the wound.
- Unfortunately, bone biopsy not widely utilized. If not obtained, important to note that wound swab often does not represent actual pathogens in bone. If wound swab performed, most clinicians can use to guide general selection of antibiotics, especially for *S. aureus* (MRSA) infection (Mackowiak).

SIGNS AND SYMPTOMS

- DFI OM: most commonly toes > metatarsal heads > calcaneum > midfoot (if Charcot neuropathic arthropathy present).
- Acute OM often accompanied by local pain and redness overlying bone + constitutional symptoms + fever.
- Chronic OM often without pain, fever, or constitutional symptoms. In DFI, consider if nonhealing ulcer, sinus tract, bone observed or probed.

CLINICAL TREATMENT

- General approach: secure accurate microbiologic diagnosis (difficult, need surgeon or invasive radiologist) and remove necrotic bone and devitalized surrounding soft tissue in chronic infection.

- Without severe, acute infection, antibiotics can typically be held pending microbiological diagnosis. If severe, empiric antibiotics should be directed against Gram positives (staph, strep), Gram negatives (coverage of *P. aeruginosa* not needed unless suspicious), and anaerobes (see below). Initial therapy may be with oral or parenteral therapy.
- **Antibiotics:** Empiric: therapy should cover *Streptococci*, *Staphylococci*, and gram-negative bacteria (GNB), also anaerobes especially if a fetid foot. Examples: vancomycin 15 mg/kg IV q12h (MRSA, strep), clindamycin 600 mg IV q8 or 450 mg PO q6–8 (strep, MSSA, some MRSA, anaerobes), piperacillin-tazobactam 3.375 g IV q 4–6h (MSSA, strep, GNB including *Pseudomonas aeruginosa*, anaerobes), ertapenem 1 g IV q24h (MSSA, strep, GNB except *P. aeruginosa*, anaerobes), ciprofloxacin 400 mg IV q8–12h or 750 mg PO twice daily (GNB including *P. aeruginosa*).
- Pathogen-directed therapy: use susceptibilities to guide, combination therapy may be required for polymicrobial infection. See Table 3-11.
- Suppressive or consolidative regimens: use susceptibilities to guide; some commonly used suggestions follow. *Staphylococcus*: (MSSA or MRSA): trimethoprim/sulfamethoxazole DS 1–2 tabs PO twice daily, minocycline or doxycycline 100 mg PO twice daily, clindamycin 300–450 mg PO 3 or 4 times daily, linezolid 600 mg PO twice daily (beware of long-term complications of anemia, thrombocytopenia, peripheral neuropathy, or optic neuritis). Some add rifampin 600 mg PO once daily. *Streptococci*, GNB, anaerobes: amoxicillin/clavulanate

TABLE 3-11. PATHOGEN-SPECIFIC THERAPIES

- **MSSA:** nafcillin or oxacillin 2 g IV q4h, cefazolin 2 g IV q8h, ceftriaxone 2 g IV q24h.

- **MRSA:** vancomycin 15 mg/kg IV q12h (goal trough level 15–20mg/dl), daptomycin 6–8 mg/kg IV q24h.

- **Staph (MSSA, MRSA), strep, anaerobes:** clindamycin 600 mg IV q6h or 900 mg IV q8h.

- **Strep species:** penicillin G 2–4 MU IV q4–6h or ampicillin 2 g IV q6h (+/– gentamicin 1.0 mg/kg IV q8h for *S. agalactiae* or enterococcal species).

- **GNB/anaerobes:** ampicillin/sulbactam 2 g IV q6h, ticarcillin/clavulanate 3.1 g IV q4–6h, piperacillin/tazobactam 3.375 g IV q4–6h, meropenem 500–1000 mg IV q8h.

- **GNB:** ciprofloxacin 400 mg IV q12h (may make early transition to oral therapy: 750 mg PO q12h) or levofloxacin 750 mg IV (then PO) once daily.

- **GNB:** ceftriaxone 2 g IV q24h or cefotaxime 2 g IV q6–8h or ceftazidime 2 g IV q8h or cefepime 2 g IV q12h.

- **GNB, MSSA, strep, anaerobes:** ertapenem 1 g IV q24h (convenient for outpatient parenteral therapy).

Courtesy of Paul Pham, PharmD, Johns Hopkins University School of Medicine.

COMPLICATIONS AND COMORBIDITIES

500 mg PO q8h, moxifloxacin 400 mg once daily. GNB: ciprofloxacin 750 mg PO twice daily or levofloxacin 500–750 mg once daily. Anaerobes: metronidazole 500 mg PO 3 times daily.

- Duration: acute OM usually treated for 4–6 wks with parenteral antibiotics. Chronic OM more variable and depends upon pathogen, degree of debridement, whether there is intent to cure, and/or prevention of relapsing infection. If curative intent, use IV or oral therapy (with good bioavailability) for 6 weeks at a minimum, often longer—12 to 24 wks; some follow ESR/CRP and treat until normalization (assuming removal of any sequestrum). If noncurative intent, may treat a "flare" for 6 weeks +/– subsequent secondary suppression.
- **Surgical:** removal of necrotic bone essential for cure of chronic osteomyelitis. Other strategies including tissue or muscle flaps or bone grafting. Whether to amputate depends on whether sufficient medical/surgical options exist or failed. Also, level of amputation should take into consideration functional result desired and likelihood of recurrent ulcer/OM (e.g., AKA or BKA better than TMA).
- **Adjunctive therapies:** consider revascularization, local delivery of antibiotics via pump to bone, or use of antibiotic-impregnated beads, hyperbaric oxygen (controversial).
- Other items deemed important to good outcomes: good glycemic control, smoking cessation, non-weight bearing (if foot involved). Consult with podiatrist, surgeon, or wound-care specialist.

Follow-up

- Failure usually due to inadequate debridement, wrong antibiotic (especially if bone biopsy not performed), host problem (e.g., vascular insufficiency, immune suppression), or noncompliance.
- Little good data to suggest that predominantly medical or surgical management of diabetic OM should be favored. Overall success rates reported range 60%–90% (Berendt; Calhoun).
- OM increases likelihood that patient may require amputation (if OM due to DFI) (see Amputations, p. 261).
- After successful treatment, dynamics of weight-bearing in the foot often altered. Podiatry involvement encouraged and footwear changes often needed.

Expert Opinion

- Superficial cultures of ulcers or sinus tracts are unreliable. They should not guide therapy if bone biopsy is possible, except if *S. aureus* is recovered.
- No antibiotic studies have shown superiority for any agent or combination.
- Antibiotics with excellent bone penetration (based on animal studies): clindamycin, fluoroquinolones, and rifampin. Poor bone penetration typical of cefazolin and other beta-lactams. Unclear if this has any impact on human clinical outcomes.
- Several staging systems for OM have been described (Waldvogel, Cierny-Mader), but these are more useful to surgeons than initial diagnostic evaluation or treatment.
- Surgical intervention for foot-salvage individualized. Strategies used include amputation, two-stage debridement with secondary closure, primary debridement to bleeding bone with grafting (muscle, skin).

Basis for Recommendations

Berendt AR, Peters EJ, Bakker K, et al. Diabetic foot osteomyelitis: a progress report on diagnosis and a systematic review of treatment. *Diabetes Metab Res Rev,* 2008; Vol. 24 Suppl 1: pp. S145–61.

> Comments: Systematic literature review highlights that there are insufficient data regarding medical versus surgical management or antibiotic choice to make firm recommendations.

Calhoun JH, Manring MM. Adult osteomyelitis. *Infect Dis Clin North Am,* 2005; Vol. 19: pp. 765–86.

   Comments: Good overall review of OM including pathogenesis, diagnosis and management—both medical and surgical.

OTHER REFERENCES

Johnston B, Conly J. Osteomyelitis management: More art than science? *Can J Infect Dis Med Microbiol,* 2007; Vol. 18: pp. 115–8.

   Comments: Authors present information from human and animal studies that support the rather thin evidence available for typically employed clinical recommendations.

Zuluaga AF, Galvis W, Saldarriaga JG, et al. Etiologic diagnosis of chronic osteomyelitis: a prospective study. *Arch Intern Med,* 2006; Vol. 166: pp. 95–100.

   Comments: When carefully performed, bone culture yield was 94%. Importantly there was only a 30% correlation of bone versus non-bone cultures, although when *S. aureus* was present this increased to 42%. This study emphasizes that non-bone cultures are not appropriate to guide therapy.

Termaat MF, Raijmakers PG, Scholten HJ, et al. The accuracy of diagnostic imaging for the assessment of chronic osteomyelitis: a systematic review and meta-analysis. *J Bone Joint Surg Am,* 2005; Vol. 87: pp. 2464–71.

   Comments: Useful meta-analysis that examined 23 chronic OM clinical studies compared to histological diagnosis. Sensitivity data included PET (96%), MRI (84%), Tc-99 bone scan (82%), WBC scan (61%), combined bone/wbc scans (78%). Specificity data included PET (91%), MRI (60%), Tc-99 bone scan (25%), wbc scan (84%), combined bone/wbc scans (84%). Overall, bone scans clearly suffer from lack of specificity. PET looks like the lead technology; however, it worked best on the axial skeleton and not peripheral skeleton. WBC scans might have the best diagnostic accuracy; however, sensitivity favors MRI imaging. PET imaging suffers from having relatively few, good studies to guide on its utility.

Mader JT, Shirtliff M, Calhoun JH. Staging and staging application in osteomyelitis. *Clin Infect Dis,* 1997; Vol. 25: pp. 1303–9.

   Comments: Authors compare two commonly employed classification systems (Waldvogel, Cierny-Mader) in OM as well as others.

Mackowiak PA, Jones SR, Smith JW. Diagnostic value of sinus-tract cultures in chronic osteomyelitis. *JAMA,* 1978; Vol. 239: pp. 2772–5.

   Comments: Often cited study showing that sinus tract cultures in chronic OM are only useful if they yield *S. aureus.* In this study, sinus tract cultures only yielded 44% of the pathogens retrieved from bone. However, there was ~90% correlation if *S. aureus* was retrieved from the sinus tract.

WOUND HEALING

Lee J. Sanders, DPM

DEFINITION

- **Wound healing:** the body's natural process of dermal or epidermal tissue regeneration. Involves a cascade of events: activation of keratinocytes, fibroblasts, macrophages, platelets, and endothelial cells. Healing consists of new epithelium, decreased area and depth of the wound, and no drainage.
- **Impaired wound healing (IWH):** lack of orderly process of healing, associated with morbidity, amputations, mortality, and healthcare costs. IWH is associated with hyperglycemia and advanced glycation end products (AGE), decreased cell and growth factor response, and endothelial dysfunction with decreased local angiogenesis.
- Poor healing has impaired angiogenesis and vasculogenesis with reduced vascular endothelial growth factor (VEGF). Bone marrow-derived endothelial progenitor cells (EPCs), essential for neovascularization, are decreased in DM. Keratinocyte

and fibroblast migration and proliferation also decreased. Matrix metaloproteinases (MMPs) also play a major role in wound healing and are in excess in wound fluid.

- The diabetic foot refers to a constellation of pathological conditions (neuropathy, ischemia, ulceration, infection—"the fetid foot," Charcot foot, and gangrene) of which the diabetic foot ulcer (DFU) is the most characteristic.

EPIDEMIOLOGY

- Failure of normal wound healing after cutaneous ulceration is the most prevalent component cause leading to amputation in 81% of cases (Pecoraro).
- Predisposing factors: (1) abnormal cellular/inflammatory pathways, (2) peripheral neuropathy, and (3) ischemia. Hyperglycemia, advanced glycation end products (AGE) as well as physiologic impairments complicate the healing process. Ability to fight infection and to mount an adequate inflammatory response is impaired.
- Factors that negatively affect wound healing: diabetes, aging, obesity, malnutrition, decreased oxygenation of wound, smoking, and impaired renal function.

DIAGNOSIS

- Identify the causes of the wound: ischemia, neuropathy, minor trauma, callus, infection, and/or foot deformities.
- Assess the need for hospitalization or outpatient treatment, and diagnostic tests (wound culture, metabolic panel, CBC with differential, radiographs and vascular studies).
- Assess wound: PEDIS-Perfusion, Extent/size, Depth/tissue loss, Infection, Sensation.
- Describe anatomic location, appearance, temperature, purulence, and odor.
- Sterile probe to evaluate depth and extent of wound. Identify undermining of the skin edges, sinus tracts, abscess, or penetration to tendon, bone, or joint. Wound depth is important to outcome.

SIGNS AND SYMPTOMS

- Uninfected wounds may be remarkably asymptomatic, due to peripheral sensory neuropathy. Neuroischemic wounds are often painful, as are moderate to severely infected wounds.
- Cellulitis >2 cm, lymphangitic streaking, deep-tissue abscess, gangrene, and involvement of muscle, tendon, joint, or bone are signs of moderate infection.
- The presence of fever, chills, tachycardia, hypotension, confusion, vomiting, leukocytosis, acidosis, severe hyperglycemia, or azotemia indicate systemic toxicity and/or metabolic instability, characteristic of severe infection.

CLINICAL TREATMENT

- **Fundamentals:** cleanse the wound (with sterile saline or wound cleanser); sharp wound debridement; appropriate wound dressing; adequate off-loading device; infection control; metabolic control; and revascularization of ischemic limbs.
- **Wound debridement:** sharp removal of callus and necrotic tissue. Maintenance debridement of chronic wounds is advised to "jump-start" the wound and keep it in a healing mode.
- **Infection control:** local (foot) and systemic (metabolic) issues; avoid antibiotics for uninfected ulcers, wounds lacking purulence or any manifestations of inflammation. Bacterial contamination and colonization of a wound does not constitute infection. For superficial ulcers, with infection target *Staphylococcus aureus* and *Streptococci* with systemic antibiotics. Wound bioburden is best treated with wound cleansing and debridement.

- **Off-loading:** Relief of mechanical stress (pressure, shear, and repetitive injury) on the foot to treat and prevent further insult, using total contact cast (TCC) (the gold standard), instant TCC (iTCC), removable cast walkers (RCWs), Scotch cast boot, crutches, and wheel chairs.
- **Dressings:** Select according to the characteristics of the wound (dry, exudative, infected, necrotic, partial or full thickness). There is no single best dressing for all wounds, and type of dressings may change throughout the process of wound healing. A physiologic moist wound environment promotes epithelialization of the wound and helps to prevent desiccation. Dressings serve as a barrier to the external environment, prevent further trauma, minimize the risk of infection, and optimize the wound milieu. See Table 3-13 for description of commonly used passive and active dressings.
- **Advanced therapies:** Topical growth factors (PDGF-BB), protease inhibitors, bioengineered skin substitutes. Cryopreserved human skin allografts and living skin equivalents serve as biologic dressings, contributing growth factors, cytokines, and collagen to the wound. See Table 3-13 for description of commonly used biological wound care products.
- **Negative pressure wound therapy (NPWT):** an open-cell foam dressing covered with an adhesive drape, connected to a vacuum pump, creating subatmospheric pressure. Most commonly used device is the Vacuum Assisted Closure (V.A.C.) (KCI, San Antonio, TX). Negative pressure wound therapy is widely applied, although the evidence base is weak.
- **Footwear and orthoses:** Before wound has healed, evaluate for appropriate footwear, orthoses, and braces.
- **Key points:** off-load high pressure areas, accommodate foot deformities (hammertoes, bunions, prominent metatarsal heads, midfoot collapse, and partial foot amputations) and brace instability of the foot/ankle. Therapeutic footwear and/or braces should be available to patients once wounds have healed and before resuming full weight bearing.

FOLLOW-UP

- Longer duration wounds are less likely to heal.
- Impaired renal function and dialysis are important predictors of long-term outcome.
- Percent change in foot ulcer area at 4 weeks' observation is a powerful predictor of healing at 12 weeks.

EXPERT OPINION

- **Note:** literature reviews provide a weak level of evidence for the clinical efficacy or superiority of different wound care products (Bergin). Silver-impregnated wound dressings and topical agents for the treatment of DFUs are expensive. Cell-derived wound care products in addition to standard care generate very high costs. However, high costs may be offset by faster healing rates and shorter treatment periods (Langer).
- Cost, duration of treatment, and potential risk of infection and amputation highlight critical role of treating poorly healing wounds.
- Chronic wounds are more likely to become infected, require hospitalization/surgery, and to incur increased costs.
- Patients with peripheral sensory neuropathy should be continually reminded of the implications of sensory loss and associated risks of recurrent ulceration, infection, and amputation.
- Multidisciplinary team management including podiatrists or wound care specialists, along with early detection and intervention, patient education, and close monitoring, is key to prevention and treatment of diabetic foot wounds.

COMPLICATIONS AND COMORBIDITIES

TABLE 3-12. PASSIVE, ACTIVE, AND BIOLOGIC WOUND CARE PRODUCTS

Category	Function	Properties	Examples	Indications and Use
Passive Dressings				
Alginates	Absorption, Packing	Conformable and absorbent. Nonwoven spun fibers derived from brown seaweed. Composed of calcium alginate, through ion exchange mechanism (Ca for Na), forms hydrophilic gel as fluid is absorbed. Absorb up to 20 times their weight.	Sorbsan, Kaltostat, Restore, CalciCare, Nu-derm, Algisite M, Seasorb. Available as sheets and rope.	Full-thickness contaminated and infected wounds. Moderate to heavy exudate. Pack loosely into wound. Requires a secondary dressing to secure. Change daily.
Foams	Absorption, Packing	Semipermeable, polyurethane foam. Nonadhesive, hydrophillic, polymeric. They hold exudate away from wound bed.	Allevyn, Lyofoam, PolyMem, Tielle, Copa	Partial- and full-thickness wounds. Minimal to heavy exudate, infected wounds. Primary dressing extends on to the periwound skin and requires a cover dressing. Change dressing every 3–7 days.
Gauze	Absorption, Packing	Woven or nonwoven. Sterile and nonsterile. Sponges, pads, ropes, strips, and rolls. Can be impregnated with petrolatum, antimicrobials, and saline.	Curity Gauze, SpongeKerlix, NuGauze Packing	Partial- and full-thickness wounds. Infected wounds. Packing large wounds. Adheres to wound tissue, nonselective debridement. Limited moisture retention. Frequent dressing changes are needed 2–3×/day.

Hydrocolloid	Absorption	Hydrophillic, occlusive dressing. Carboxymethylcellulose, pectin orgelatin. Pastes, powders, and sheets. Impermeable, waterproof barrier. Sheet hydrocolloids are adhesive.	Duoderm, Restore, Tegasorb, Comfeel	Partial- and full-thickness wounds. Conformable. Minimal to moderate exudates. Take care not to tear skin when removing dressings. Dressings react with wound drainage, leaving anodorous gel in the wound. Change every 5–7 days.
Hydrogel	Maintains moist wound milieu	Glycerin or water-based semipermeable dressings. Available as sheets, viscous gels, or granulate form. Sheets contain up to 96% water and maintain a moist wound milieu. Autolytic debridement property. Cooling and soothing effect on the wound.	Aquaflo, Curafil, Hypergel, Vigilon, Intrasite gel	Partial- and full-thickness wounds. Dry to minimal exudate. Necrotic and infected wounds. Used in combination with other dressings.
Transparent film	Protects	Thin transparent adhesive polyurethane film. Semipermeable, nonabsorptive. Provides autolytic debridement. Requires a border of dry intact skin.	Op-Site, Tegaderm, Polyskin II	Nondraining partial-thickness wounds. Traps wound fluid under dressing. Not recommended for infection. Change dressing every 3–5 days.

(Continued)

COMPLICATIONS AND COMORBIDITIES

TABLE 3-12. PASSIVE, ACTIVE, AND BIOLOGIC WOUND CARE PRODUCTS *(CONT.)*

Category	Function	Properties	Examples	Indications and Use
Active Dressings				
Elemental antimicrobials	Decreases bioburden	Semiocclusive dressings containing silver and iodine. Cadexomer iodine is nontoxic to fibroblasts at concentrations up to 0.45%. Bacteria are trapped within the cadexomer beads. Silver has bacteriostatic properties.	Silver sulfadiazine cream, Silver impregnated dressings, Cadexomer iodine	May be used to control or reduce wound bioburden. Use of elemental antimicrobials should be prudent and limited to 2–4 weeks.
Oxidized Regenerated Cellulose (ORC)/collagen	Absorbent, Renders MMPs inactive	Sterile freeze dried matrix sheet of ORC and collagen, absorbs wound exudate forms a biodegradable gel. Chemically binds to matrix metalloproteases (MMPs) rendering them inactive. Elevated protease levels in chronic wound fluid impedes wound healing by degrading newly formed granulation tissue and proteins.	Promogran (Systagenix Wound Management)	Partial- and full-thickness exudating wounds. Apply directly to the whole wound bed. For a wound with low or no exudate, hydrate with saline or Ringer's solution. Cover with either gauze, a nonadhering or a hydropolymer dressing in order to maintain a moist wound environment.
Enzyme-debriding agents	Nonsurgical enzymatic debridement	Collagenase and papain-urea. Reduce wound bioburden, debride necrotic tissue, and promote granulation tissue.	Santyl Ointment (collagenase), Accuzyme (Papain-urea)	Partial- or full-thickness necrotic wounds. For patients who are poor surgical candidates or wounds that need less aggressive debridement.

			If eschar is present, cross-hatch with scalpel blade. Cleanse wound with saline and gauze sponge, apply directly to wound once daily, cover with gauze as secondary dressing. Discontinue when granulation tissue forms.
		TheraGauze (Soluble Systems, Newport News, VA)	Partial- and full-thickness wounds. Infected and non-infected wounds. Dry to heavily exudating wounds.

Note: Fenestrate dressing for moderate to heavily exudative wounds. Requires a cover dressing, transparent film or dressing of choice. Change 2–3×/week.

To remove: if dry, first moisten with saline. Can be used as a cover dressing for skin grafts and donor sites, and for the delivery of topical antiseptic or antibiotic solutions. |
| Skin Moisture Rebalancing Technology ("SMRT" dressing) | Moisture, Regulating | Nonstick, inert breathable polymer-integrated into a nonwoven polyester/rayon substrate. Regulates moisture differentially across wound bed (release and absorption). Moisture without maceration. | |

(Continued)

TABLE 3-12. PASSIVE, ACTIVE, AND BIOLOGIC WOUND CARE PRODUCTS (CONT.)

Category	Function	Properties	Examples	Indications and Use
Cell-Derived Products for Treatment of DFUs				
Growth factors: PDGF-BB	Promote wound healing	Recombinant platelet-derived growth factor (PDGF). Chemo-attractant and mitogen for fibroblasts. Stimulates extracellular matrix and granulation tissue. **FDA BOXED WARNING:** Contraindicated in patients with neoplasms at the site of application. An increased risk of mortality secondary to malignancy remote from the site of treatment has been observed in patients treated with 3 or more tubes of REGRANEX Gel in a post-marketing retrospective cohort study. REGRANEX Gel should only be used when the benefits can be expected to outweigh the risks.	REGRANEX (beca-plermin) Gel 0.01% (Ortho-McNeil)	Indicated for treatment of DFUs that extend deep into the subcutaneous tissue and have an adequate blood supply. Wound debridement is a vital adjunct to treatment with beca-plermin. Apply once/day in measured quantity and cover with moist dressing. Change dressing in 12 hours, cleanse with saline and apply a moist saline dressing.
Bioengi-neered skin	Promote wound healing	**Apligraf:** Bilayered living human skin substitute with an allogeneic dermis and well-differentiated allogeneic epidermis.	Apligraf (Organogen-esis, Canton, MA), Dermagraft (Advanced BioHealing, La Jolla, CA)	BSSs are expensive; however increased ulcer-free time coupled with reduced risk of infection and amputation may offset initial costs.

Substitutes (BSSs)		Constructed by culturing human foreskin-derived neonatal fibroblasts in a bovine type 1 collagen matrix, and adding epidermal keratinocytes.	Apligraf is indicated for treatment of venous leg ulcers and DFUs.
		Produces cytokines and growth factors associated with normal wound healing.	Dermagraft is indicated for use in the treatment of full-thickness DFUs >6 weeks duration, which extend through the dermis, but without tendon, muscle, joint capsule, or bone exposure.
		Dermagraft: A cryopreserved human fibroblast-derived dermal substitute composed of fibroblasts, extracellular matrix, and a bioabsorbable scaffold.	Refer to manufacturer's guidelines for specific instructions.
		Manufactured from human fibroblast cells derived from newborn foreskin. Assists in restoration of the dermal bed, facilitates re-epithelialization of the wound.	
Human Skin Allografts			
Cadaveric human skin allografts	Promote wound healing	**TheraSkin:** Cryopreserved human skin allograft with both epidermis and dermis layers.	For treatment of diabetic foot ulcers (DFUs) and venous leg ulcers (VLUs) that have failed to respond to >4 weeks of conservative wound care.
		TheraSkin (Soluble Systems, Newport News, VA)	

(Continued)

COMPLICATIONS AND COMORBIDITIES

TABLE 3-12. PASSIVE, ACTIVE, AND BIOLOGIC WOUND CARE PRODUCTS (CONT.)

Category	Function	Properties	Examples	Indications and Use
		Cellular integrity has been preserved. It contains a biologically active extracellular matrix, which provides growth factors to the wound. An effective natural barrier to help control infection and assist in the promotion of granulation tissue and epithelialization. Decreases fluid and protein loss. **GammaGraft:** Gamma-irradiated human skin allograft. Epidermis and dermis are preserved but without living cells. Packaged in airtight foil and preserved in a penicillin/gentamycin solution. Can be stored at ambient temperature for up to 2 years. **GraftJacket:** An acellular dermal tissue matrix made from human donor skin, which undergoes a process that removes the epidermis and dermal cells. Serves as a framework to support cellular repopulation and vascularization. Packaged in a peel-pouch, freeze-dried and sealed in a foil bag. It is shipped at ambient temperature and then refrigerated to maximize shelf life.	GammaGraft (Promethean LifeSciences, Inc., Pittsburgh, PA) GraftJacket (Wright Medical Technology, Inc., Arlington, TN)	Ulcers should be free of infection or underlying osteomyelitis. Must have adequate blood supply, ABI 0.65 or greater. DFUs, VLUs, full-thickness ulcers, Mohs surgery sites, skin graft donor sites, partial-thickness wounds, burns. Wounds must be clean with no infection. DFUs, repair or replacement of damaged or inadequate integumental tissues. Contraindicated in infected or nonvascular surgical sites, and in patients with autoimmune or connective tissue diseases. Refer to manufacturer's guidelines for specific instructions.

Source: Sanders LJ, Frykberg RG. The Charcot Foot (Pied de Charcot). In: Bowker J, Pfeifer MA, eds. Levin and O'Neal's The Diabetic Foot. 7th ed. Philadelphia: Elsevier Inc.; 2008.

- The diabetes healthcare provider should be generally familiar with the use of different wound care products.

BASIS FOR RECOMMENDATIONS

Falanga V, Brem H, Ennis WJ, et al. Maintenance debridement in the treatment of difficult-to-heal chronic wounds. Recommendations of an expert panel. *Ostomy Wound Manage,* 2008; Vol. Suppl: pp. 2–13, quiz 14–5.

Comments: Consensus development conference on treatment of chronic wounds.

Bergin SM, Wraight P. Silver based wound dressings and topical agents for treating diabetic foot ulcers. *Cochrane Database Syst Rev,* 2006; CD005082.

Comments: Results reveal no randomized clinical trials (RCTs) or controlled clinical trials (CCTs) evaluating the effect of silver-based products on infection and healing of diabetic foot ulcers. The authors were unable to determine whether silver-based dressings and topical agents result in benefits or harms for people with diabetes-related foot ulcers.

American Diabetes Association. Consensus Development Conference on Diabetic Foot Wound Care: 7–8 April 1999, Boston, Massachusetts. *Diabetes Car,* 1999; Vol. 22: pp. 1354–60.

Comments: Consensus position statement on 6 questions: (1) What is the value of treating a diabetic foot wound? (2) What is the biology of wound healing? (3) How should diabetic foot wounds be assessed and classified? (4) What are the appropriate treatments for foot wounds? (5) How should new treatments be evaluated? and (6) How can recurrent foot wounds be prevented?

OTHER REFERENCES

Langer A, Rogowski W. Systematic review of economic evaluations of human cell-derived wound care products for the treatment of venous leg and diabetic foot ulcers. *BMC Health Serv Res,* 2009; Vol. 9: p. 115.

Comments: Cell-derived wound care products in addition to standard care generate very high costs. Economic analysis suggests that the initial high costs of these products may be offset by (1) restricted use to ulcers that are unresponsive to healing, (2) higher healing rates and shorter treatment periods, (3) fewer complications, and (4) fewer inpatient episodes. Further research is necessary to obtain better estimates of the clinical benefits.

Ghanassia E, Villon L, Thuan Dit Dieudonné JF, et al. Long-term outcome and disability of diabetic patients hospitalized for diabetic foot ulcers: a 6.5-year follow-up study. *Diabetes Care,* 2008; Vol. 31: pp. 1288–92.

Comments: 60.9% of patients had ulcer recurrence, 43.8% underwent amputation (24 minor and 15 major), and 51.7% died. The global long-term outcome of patients hospitalized for DFUs was poor. Multivariate analysis showed age and impaired renal function/albuminuria as independent predictors of wound healing failure.

Gregor S, Maegele M, Sauerland S, et al. Negative pressure wound therapy: a vacuum of evidence? *Arch Surg,* 2008; Vol. 143: pp. 189–96.

Comments: Institute for Research in Operative Medicine and Institute for Quality and Efficiency in Health Care systematic review of RCTs and non-RCTs comparing NPWT and conventional therapy for acute and chronic wounds. Main outcomes of interest were wound healing variables. Conclusion: Although there is some indication that NPWT may improve wound healing, the body of evidence is insufficient to clearly prove an additional clinical benefit. From 2003–2004, revenue for vacuum-assisted closure increased by 45% to $700 million.

Payne WG, Salas RE, Ko F, et al. Enzymatic debriding agents are safe in wounds with high bacterial bioburdens and stimulate healing. *Eplasty,* 2008; Vol. 8: p. e17.

Comments: Collagenase and papain-urea appear beneficial and safe even in wounds with high bacterial loads, and appear to significantly aid extent and rate of healing.

Brem H, Tomic-Canic M. Cellular and molecular basis of wound healing in diabetes. *J Clin Invest,* 2007; Vol. 117: pp. 1219–22.

Comments: Available online: *http://www.jci.org/articles/view/32169/pdf.*

Gallagher KA, Liu ZJ, Xiao M, et al. Diabetic impairments in NO-mediated endothelial progenitor cell mobilization and homing are reversed by hyperoxia and SDF-1 alpha. *J Clin Invest,* 2007; Vol. 117: pp. 1249–59.

Comments: This study aimed to determine mechanisms responsible for the diabetic defect in circulating and wound endothelial progenitor cells (EPCs). EPCs are essential in vasculogenesis and wound healing.

COMPLICATIONS AND COMORBIDITIES

Bryant RA, Nix, DP. *Acute and Chronic Wounds: Current Management Concepts*, Third Edition. St. Louis, MO: Mosby Elsevier; 2007. ISBN-13: 978-0-323-03074-8

Comments: Comprehensive all-inclusive resource on the management of acute and chronic wounds, with emphasis on the multidisciplinary team approach to wound management.

Armstrong DG, Lavery LA, Wu S, et al. Evaluation of removable and irremovable cast walkers in the healing of diabetic foot wounds: a randomized controlled trial. *Diabetes Care,* 2005; Vol. 28: pp. 551–4.

Comments: Intent-to-treat analysis showed that modification of a standard RCW wrapped with a cohesive bandage or plaster bandage (iTCC), to increase patient adherence to pressure off-loading, had a higher proportion of ulcers that healed than in the RCW group (82.6 vs 51.9%). Those treated with an iTCC healed significantly sooner (41.6 + 18.7 vs 58.0 + 15.2 days, p = 0.02).

Lobmann R, Schultz G, Lehnert H. Proteases and the diabetic foot syndrome: mechanisms and therapeutic implications. *Diabetes Care,* 2005; Vol. 28: pp. 461–71.

Comments: Review article: the biology of normal wound healing, pathogenesis of wound healing in chronic wounds, cytokines and growth factors, MMPs in wound healing, and clinical studies with growth factors and protease inhibitors.

Lipsky BA, Berendt AR, Deery HG, et al. Diagnosis and treatment of diabetic foot infections. *Clin Infect Dis,* 2004; Vol. 39: pp. 885–910.

Comments: IDSA Guidelines for the evaluation, classification, and treatment of diabetic foot infections. Contains suggested empirical antibiotic regimens based on clinical severity. Can be downloaded free from *http://www.journals.uchicago.edu/doi/pdf/10.1086/424846.*

Sheehan P, Jones P, Caselli A, et al. Percent change in wound area of diabetic foot ulcers over a 4-week period is a robust predictor of complete healing in a 12-week prospective trial. *Diabetes Care,* 2003; Vol. 26: pp. 1879–82.

Comments: 276 patients randomized to either a moistened gauze dressing or a collagen/oxidized regenerated cellulose dressing (Promogran). Wound area measurements were performed at baseline and after 4 weeks. The percent change in wound area at 4 weeks in those who healed was 82%, whereas in those who failed to heal the percent change in wound area was 25%.

Armstrong DG, Nguyen HC, Lavery LA, et al. Off-loading the diabetic foot wound: a randomized clinical trial. *Diabetes Care,* 2001; Vol. 24: pp. 1019–22.

Comments: The proportions of healing for patients treated with TCC, RCW, and half-shoe were 89.5%, 65.0%, and 58.3%, respectively. A significantly higher proportion of patients were healed by 12 weeks in the TCC group.

Reiber GE, Vileikyte L, Boyko EJ, et al. Causal pathways for incident lower-extremity ulcers in patients with diabetes from two settings. *Diabetes Care,* 1999; Vol. 22: pp. 157–62.

Comments: The Rothman model of causation was applied to the diabetic foot ulcer condition. The most frequent component causes for lower-extremity ulcers were a critical triad of neuropathy, minor foot trauma, and foot deformity, present in >63% of patient's causal pathways.

Pecoraro RE, Reiber GE, Burgess EM. Pathways to diabetic limb amputation. Basis for prevention. *Diabetes Care,* 1990; Vol. 13: pp. 513–21.

Comments: The authors define the causal pathways responsible for 80 consecutive initial lower-extremity amputations. Most pathways were composed of multiple causes. 46% of the amputations were attributed to ischemia, 59% to infection, 61% to neuropathy, 81% to faulty wound healing, 84% to ulceration, 55% to gangrene, and 81% to initial minor trauma.

Male Disorders

ERECTILE DYSFUNCTION

Amin Sabet, MD

DEFINITION
- Impaired ability to achieve or maintain an erection sufficient for satisfactory sexual activity.
- Multifactorial pathophysiology of erectile dysfunction (ED) in diabetes: endothelial/smooth muscle dysfunction, autonomic neuropathy, hypogonadism, psychological/interpersonal factors, antihypertensive medication side effects (e.g., diuretics, beta-blockers).

EPIDEMIOLOGY
- General population: common condition with prevalence increasing from 5.1% (prior to age 40) to 70.2% (after age 70).
- Diabetes: over age of 20 years, age-adjusted prevalence of erectile dysfunction (ED) is 38.6% in men with diabetes versus 18.4% in men without diabetes (Selvin).
- Associated conditions: neuropathy (peripheral, autonomic), retinopathy, poor glycemic control, longer duration of diabetes.
- ED is an independent predictor of CAD and adverse cardiac events in diabetes (2 times greater risk) (Gazzaruso).

DIAGNOSIS
- **History:** libido (correlates with androgen function), medication use (SSRIs, spironolactone, clonidine, thiazide diuretics, beta-blockers, ketoconazole, cimetidine), illicit drug use, onset of symptoms (rapid onset suggests psychogenic).
- **Exam:** visual fields (defects with pituitary macroadenomas causing hypogonadism), pulses (femoral, peripheral), gynecomastia (seen in hypogonadism), testes, penile plaques (Peyronie's disease).
- **Laboratory testing:** HbA1c, testosterone, prolactin, TSH (also see Male Hypogonadism, p. 293).
- **Other testing:** postage stamp and snap gauge testing have been largely replaced by devices such as the Rigi-Scan, which provide more accurate and reproducible information about nocturnal rigidity and tumescence.
- Complete lack of nocturnal/morning erections on nocturnal penile tumescence testing suggests neurologic or vascular disease.

CLINICAL TREATMENT
- Poor glycemic control is associated with ED, but evidence is insufficient to show that improved glycemic control reverses ED.
- Androgen therapy is appropriate for hypogonadal patients with ED.
- First-line: PDE5 inhibitors (see Sildenafil, p. 421, vardenafil, tadalafil).
- Second-line: Vacuum-assisted filling devices.
- Third-line: Transurethral or intracavernosal PGE1 (alprostadil).
- Fourth-line: Surgical implantation of penile prosthesis.

COMPLICATIONS AND COMORBIDITIES

- PDE5 inhibitors contraindicated in men taking nitrates; may be hazardous in setting of cardiac ischemia, heart failure, and use of CYP3A4 inhibitors (decrease drug clearance) or alpha-adrenergic antagonists (possible hypotension).
- Rare reports of nonarteritic anterior ischemic optic neuropathy in setting of PDE5 inhibitor use; causal relationship not established.

FOLLOW-UP

- Consider urology referral, especially for patients refractory to PDE5 inhibitor therapy.

EXPERT OPINION

- PDE5 inhibitors improve ED in the majority of patients with type 1 and type 2 diabetes (Rendell) and should be tried first, although may be relatively less efficacious than in men without diabetes.
- PDE5 inhibitors should not be prescribed in men taking nitrates.
- Caution is advised regarding concomitant use of PDE5 inhibitors with alpha-blockers as the combination of these two vasodilator medications may result in hypotension.
- Psychological factors contributing to ED may include depression, performance anxiety, and relationship (including marital) problems.
- Psychosexual counseling may be useful as an adjunct to pharmacologic therapy (Melnik).

REFERENCES

Gazzaruso C, Solerte SB, Pujia A, et al. Erectile dysfunction as a predictor of cardiovascular events and death in diabetic patients with angiographically proven asymptomatic coronary artery disease: a potential protective role for statins and 5-phosphodiesterase inhibitors. *J Am Coll Cardiol*, 2008; Vol. 51: pp. 2040–4.
  Comments: ED independently predicts major adverse cardiac events (HR 2.1) in diabetics with asymptomatic CAD.

Selvin E, Burnett AL, Platz EA. Prevalence and risk factors for erectile dysfunction in the US. *Am J Med*, 2007; Vol. 120: pp. 151–7.
  Comments: Overall prevalence of ED in men aged 20 and over is 18.4% in nondiabetic versus 38.6% (age-adjusted) in diabetic men.

Melnik T, Soares BG, Nasselo AG. Psychosocial interventions for erectile dysfunction. *Cochrane Database Syst Rev*, 2007; CD004825.
  Comments: In men treated with sildenafil, group psychotherapy may improve ED.

Rendell MS, Rajfer J, Wicker PA, et al. Sildenafil for treatment of erectile dysfunction in men with diabetes: a randomized controlled trial. Sildenafil Diabetes Study Group. *JAMA*, 1999; Vol. 281: pp. 421–6.
  Comments: Sildenafil improved ED in 56% of diabetic men.

Feldman HA, Goldstein I, Hatzichristou DG, et al. Impotence and its medical and psychosocial correlates: results of the Massachusetts Male Aging Study. *J Urol*, 1994; Vol. 151: pp. 54–61.
  Comments: 52% prevalence of ED in men age 40–70 (general population).

Wein AJ, Van Arsdalen KN. Drug-induced male sexual dysfunction. *Urol Clin North Am*, 1988; Vol. 15: pp. 23–31.
  Comments: Commonly used meds causing ED.

McCulloch DK, Campbell IW, Wu FC, et al. The prevalence of diabetic impotence. *Diabetologia*, 1980; Vol. 18: pp. 279–83.
  Comments: Among diabetic men, ED is common and best correlates with proliferative retinopathy and symptomatic autonomic neuropathy.

MALE HYPOGONADISM

Amin Sabet, MD

DEFINITION

- Hypogonadism in a male refers to decreased spermatogenesis and/or testosterone action.
- Classified as primary (resulting from testicular disease) or secondary (resulting from pituitary or hypothalamic disease).
- Hypogonadism may be a cause of, but is to be distinguished from, erectile dysfunction.
- Total testosterone level that is 2.5 standard deviations below the mean in young adults or less than ~300 ng/dl.
- Clinical criteria are more ambiguous.

EPIDEMIOLOGY

- In cross-sectional studies, between 20%–64% of men with diabetes have hypogonadism; higher prevalence rates in the elderly (Dhindsa; Kalyani).
- Diabetes risk factor for hypogonadism through various mechanisms including increased body weight; decreased sex hormone binding globulin (SHBG); suppression of gonadotrophin release or Leydig cell testosterone production; cytokine-mediated inhibition of testicular steroid production; and increased aromatase activity contributing to relative estrogen excess.
- Low testosterone levels independent risk factor for type 2 diabetes, even after adjusting for adiposity, possibly due to androgen receptor polymorphisms, alterations in glucose transport, or reduced antioxidant effect (Stellato; Kalyani).

DIAGNOSIS

- Diagnose hypogonadism based on decreased sperm count and/or low testosterone levels relative to age-matched reference values (i.e., <300–400 mg/dl).
- Due to diurnal testosterone fluctuations, measure testosterone at 8 AM in addition to FSH, LH.
- Total testosterone may not accurately reflect gonadal status in obese (low SHBG) and elderly patients (high SHBG); free and bioavailable testosterone levels should be checked if hypogonadism suspected.
- Free and bioavailable testosterone levels can be measured directly or calculated from total testosterone, albumin, and SHBG (online calculator available at *http://www.issam.ch/freetesto.htm*).
- In hypogonadal men, high luteinizing hormone (LH)/follicle-stimulating hormone (FSH) indicates primary hypogonadism and normal or low FSH/LH indicates secondary hypogonadism.
- Primary hypogonadism differential diagnosis: infection (i.e., mumps), trauma, chemotherapy, radiation exposure, cryptorchidism, Klinefelter syndrome.
- Secondary hypogonadism differential diagnosis: hypopituitarism, hyperprolactinemia, hypothyroidism, hemochromatosis, long-term opioid use, obesity.
- Chronic systemic illnesses such as HIV, liver disease/cirrhosis, renal failure, and diabetes may have mixed effects but are more likely to be associated with secondary hypogonadism (Kalyani).
- In primary hypogonadism, peripheral blood karyotype analysis should be performed to evaluate for Klinefelter syndrome (47 XXY).

COMPLICATIONS AND COMORBIDITIES

- In secondary hypogonadism, measure serum prolactin, thyroxine, morning cortisol, and iron saturation, and obtain pituitary MRI.

SIGNS AND SYMPTOMS

- Symptoms of postpubertal hypogonadism include sexual dysfunction, infertility, gynecomastia, reduced energy, depressed mood or diminished sense of well-being, increased irritability, difficulty concentrating, hot flushes, decreased bone density, weakness, fatigue, anemia, decreased lean body mass, and increased body fat.
- Loss of male secondary sex characteristics, such as body hair distribution and muscle mass, may take years to occur after onset of hypogonadism.
- Eunuchoid proportions (length of lower > upper body segment; arm span 5 cm or more longer than height) indicate prepubertal onset of hypogonadism.
- Small testicular size (normal ≥25 cc) on physical examination.

CLINICAL TREATMENT

- Men should have both a low serum testosterone level and symptoms classically associated with hypogonadism before testosterone replacement therapy is offered.
- Primary treatment is testosterone therapy with goal of restoring testosterone levels to normal range and symptomatic improvement.
- Testosterone treatment contraindicated in presence of active prostate cancer or breast cancer and may worsen erythrocytosis, obstructive sleep apnea, severe lower urinary tract symptoms, or severe congestive heart failure.
- Transdermal testosterone is available as gel, patch, or buccal testosterone tablet.
- Testosterone patch: inital dose is 5 mg per day but may result in application site reactions.
- Testosterone 1% gel: initial dose is 5 g (50 mg testosterone) per day and is usually preferred as first-line therapy since application site reactions are less.
- Testosterone enanthate and cypionate are administered intramuscularly. Initial dose 150–200 mg injected every 2 weeks; often preferred in children. Usually not preferred in adults since testosterone levels will have nonphysiological peaks and troughs.
- Intramuscular testosterone therapy improves obesity and glycemic control in patients with diabetes (Kapoor).

FOLLOW-UP

- Monitor symptoms 3 months after initiating testosterone therapy and regularly thereafter.
- Monitor testosterone levels 2–3 months after initating testosterone therapy and every 6 months thereafter. If given IM, levels should be checked midway between injections.
- Perform digital rectal exam (DRE) and check prostate-specific antigen (PSA) and hematocrit at baseline, 3 months after initiating testosterone therapy, and every 6–12 months thereafter.
- Obtain urology consultation if PSA >4 ng/ml, if PSA increases by >1.4 ng/ml within any 1-year period, PSA velocity >0.4 ng/ml per year for >2 years, or if abnormal findings on DRE.
- Stop therapy and assess for hypoxia and sleep apnea if hematocrit exceeds 54%.
- Consider also checking lipid panel and liver function tests.
- Measure bone mineral density after 1–2 years of testosterone therapy in hypogonadal men with osteoporosis.

EXPERT OPINION

- Diabetes more likely to be associated with secondary hypogonadism.
- Benefits of testosterone treatment may include not only improvement of hypogonadal symptoms, but also better glycemic control and reduced obesity in persons with diabetes.

- Commonly available free testosterone assay by direct radioimmunoassay (RIA) is unreliable and should not be used to diagnose hypogonadism.
- The most reliable and efficient approach we use is to start with total testosterone measurement. If this is normal, then hypogonadism can be excluded. If the total testosterone is low in a patient with obesity and/or diabetes, free testosterone is calculated from total testosterone, SHBG, and albumin (Rosner).
- Because testosterone levels fluctuate even in early morning, measurement should be repeated to confirm low levels on at least two occasions prior to making diagnosis of hypogonadism.
- Testosterone gel is preferred for treatment, avoiding the nonphysiologic peaks and troughs of testosterone injection as well as application site reactions of testosterone patch, but care must be taken to avoid skin transfer to women and children.

BASIS FOR RECOMMENDATIONS

Bhasin S, Cunningham GR, Hayes FJ, et al. Testosterone therapy in adult men with androgen deficiency syndromes: an endocrine society clinical practice guideline. *J Clin Endocrinol Metab*, 2006; Vol. 91: pp. 1995–2010.

Comments: Endocrine Society practice guideline on treatment of hypogonadism.

OTHER REFERENCES

Laughlin GA, Barrett-Connor E, Bergstrom J. Low serum testosterone and mortality in older men. *J Clin Endocrinol Metab*, 2008; Vol. 93: pp. 68–75.

Comments: Men 50 and older with testosterone levels in the lowest quartile were 40% more likely to die within 20 years than men with higher testosterone.

Selvin E, Feinleib M, Zhang L, et al. Androgens and diabetes in men: results from the Third National Health and Nutrition Examination Survey (NHANES III). *Diabetes Care*, 2007; Vol. 30: pp. 234–8.

Comments: Men with free and bioavailable testosterone in the lowest tertile were 4 times more likely to have diabetes than those with testosterone levels in the third tertile.

Rosner W, Auchus RJ, Azziz R, et al. Position statement: utility, limitations, and pitfalls in measuring testosterone: an Endocrine Society position statement. *J Clin Endocrinol Metab*, 2007; Vol. 92: pp. 405–13.

Comments: Endocrine Society position statement regarding measurement of testosterone.

Kalyani RR, Gavini S, Dobs AS. Male hypogonadism in systemic disease. *Endocrinol Metab Clin North Am*, 2007; Vol. 36: pp. 333–48.

Comments: Summary of manifestation and treatment of hypogonadism in various chronic systemic illnesses.

Kalyani RR, Dobs AS Androgen deficiency, diabetes, and the metabolic syndrome in men. *Curr Opin Endocrinol Diabetes Obes*, 2007; Vol. 14: pp. 226–34.

Comments: Describes the bidirectional association of hypogonadism and diabetes, in addition to possible mechanisms and an algorithm for evaluating suspected hypogonadism in persons with diabetes.

Kapoor D, Goodwin E, Channer KS, et al. Testosterone replacement therapy improves insulin resistance, glycaemic control, visceral adiposity and hypercholesterolaemia in hypogonadal men with type 2 diabetes. *Eur J Endocrinol*, 2006; Vol. 154: pp. 899–906.

Comments: Randomized-controlled crossover trial of intramuscular testosterone therapy versus placebo in hypogonadal men with diabetes for 3 months in random order. HOMA-IR, A1c, and fasting glucose all signficantly improved with testosterone therapy.

Mohr BA, Guay AT, O'Donnell AB, et al. Normal, bound and nonbound testosterone levels in normally ageing men: results from the Massachusetts Male Aging Study. *Clin Endocrinol* (Oxford), 2005; Vol. 62: pp. 64–73.

Comments: Suggested cutoffs for abnormally low total testosterone level as less than 8.7, 7.5, 6.8, and 5.4 nm (251, 216, 196, and 156 ng/dl) for men in their 40s, 50s, 60s, and 70s, respectively.

COMPLICATIONS AND COMORBIDITIES

Dhindsa S, Prabhakar S, Sethi M, et al. Frequent occurrence of hypogonadotropic hypogonadism in type 2 diabetes. *J Clin Endocrinol Metab*, 2004; Vol. 89: pp. 5462–8.

Comments: 33% of patient with type 2 diabetes were hypogonadal.

Stellato RK, Feldman HA, Hamdy O, et al. Testosterone, sex hormone-binding globulin, and the development of type 2 diabetes in middle-aged men: prospective results from the Massachusetts male aging study. *Diabetes Care*, 2000; Vol. 23: pp. 490–4.

Comments: Odds ratio for future diabetes of 1.58 for a 1 SD decrease in free testosterone.

Muscle, Skin, and Bone Diseases

AMPUTATIONS

See Amputations, p. 261.

BONE DISEASE

Kendall F. Moseley, MD, and Todd T. Brown, MD, PhD

DEFINITION

- Osteoporosis and osteopenia are the most important bone diseases observed in type 1 diabetes mellitus (T1DM) and type 2 diabetes mellitus (T2DM), characterized by decreased bone mass and structural deterioration of bone tissue, leading to bone fragility and increased susceptibility to fracture.
- On bone density measurements via dual energy X-ray absorptiometry (DXA): a T-score between +1.0 and −1.0 standard deviations (SD) is considered normal bone density, a score between −1.0 and −2.5 SD is osteopenia, and a score that is below −2.5 SD is osteoporosis; Z-scores are used for men <50 years and premenopausal women.
- Osteomalacia is softening of the bone resulting from impaired bone mineralization with calcium and vitamin D.
- Charcot foot is a result of bone loss in the foot or ankle causing microfractures, ligament laxity, and bony destruction, exacerbated by neuropathy and the patient's inability to perceive ongoing trauma (see Charcot Joint Disease [Diabetic Neuropathic Osteoarthropathy], p. 302).

EPIDEMIOLOGY

- According to the National Osteoporosis Foundation (NOF), low bone mass affects over 55% of persons greater than 50 years of age; in the US, greater than 10 million people have osteoporosis, while 34 million have low bone mass.
- Prevalence of osteoporosis and osteopenia varies in T1DM depending on whether individual has reached peak bone mass, duration of diabetes, and degree of glycemic control (Mastrandrea).
- Among middle-aged persons with T1DM, 30%–60% have osteopenia and 10%–30% have osteoporosis when compared to age-matched controls (Wada).
- Bone density is on average higher for persons with T2DM when compared to healthy control subjects, although this population likely more susceptible to fracture at the hip and nonvertebral sites (Vestergaard).
- Prevalence and incidence of low bone mass and fracture in T2DM varies and depends upon disease control, duration, and degree of end-organ damage (i.e., neuropathy, nephropathy, retinopathy) (Leidig-Bruckner).

DIAGNOSIS

- See definition section for specific diagnostic criteria.
- DXA is the gold standard for areal densiometry measurements (see Bone Mineral Density, p. 550).

- Volumetric quantitative CT scan and calcaneal ultrasound are alternative modalities for bone mineral density (BMD) measurement.
- Screening: No specific guidelines for osteoporosis or osteopenia in diabetes mellitus.
- Current NOF general recommendations: bone density testing in women >65 years or men >70 years if no risk factors for osteoporosis (Heinemann).
- Screening for men and women >50 years if one or more risk factors for osteoporosis or bone disease (i.e., steroid use, hyperparathyroidism, malnutrition, maternal hip fracture).
- Screening for men and women regardless of age if there is a history of fragility fracture.
- Incidental identification of low bone mass or poor bone mineralization may be diagnosed on routine X-rays.
- Low serum 25-hydroxyvitamin D level (<15 ng/ml) with concurrent elevated intact parathyroid hormone (iPTH) may herald osteomalacia.
- Elevated serum iPTH level observed in secondary hyperparathyroidism due to renal disease or vitamin D deficiency can lead to bone disease.

Signs and Symptoms

- Signs and symptoms of bone disease the same for persons with and without diabetes mellitus.
- Osteoporosis and osteopenia usually clinically silent diseases.
- Low-trauma fractures or recurrent fractures at any age in T1DM or T2DM should raise suspicion of bone disease.
- Fragility fractures resulting from low bone density are a major source of osteoporosis-induced pain and morbidity.
- Sudden onset pain, focal back pain, or spinal process tenderness to physical exam could indicate vertebral fracture.
- Severe hip pain, hip swelling, and inability to walk following a fall could indicate hip fracture.
- Severe vitamin D deficiency may manifest as bone pain and fatigue.
- Increased prevalence of celiac disease and vitamin D deficiency in T1DM; symptoms including abdominal pain, bloating, and diarrhea.
- Bowing of the legs in childhood observed with vitamin D deficiency/rickets in children.

Clinical Treatment

Diabetes and Complication Management

- Optimize glycemic control to minimize advanced glycation end product (AGE) deposition in bone (Schwartz).
- Optimize glycemic control and diet to minimize malnutrition, especially in early T1DM.
- HbA1c <7% to minimize microvascular and macrovascular complications, which can contribute to and exacerbate bone disease and fall risk (Schwartz).
- Retinopathy and neuropathy screening, prevention, and treatment for fall and fracture reduction.
- Nephropathy prevention and treatment to normalize calcium, phosphate, and vitamin D handling.
- Prevention and reduction of peripheral and microvascular disease to optimize blood supply to bone and maintain bone quality.
- Orthostatic hypotension, if untreated, may increase fall and fracture risk in persons with autonomic dysfunction.
- Minimize hypoglycemic episodes which can lead to syncope, falls, and fractures (Schwartz).

Diet and Lifestyle
- NOF dietary and lifestyle recommendations apply to general and diabetic population with bone disease.
- Calcium 1000 mg and vitamin D 400–800 IU daily in adults <50 years old; calcium 1200 mg and vitamin D 800–1000 IU daily in adults >50 years old and in those with known bone disease.
- Consider dietary supplements if inadequate intake in food sources alone or if malabsorption present.
- High-dose vitamin D repletion for vitamin D deficiency or insufficiency with ergocalciferol or cholecalciferol.
- Protein intake up to 15% of daily caloric intake.
- Maintain healthy weight (BMI 18.5–24.9 kg/m^2).
- Weight-bearing exercise and resistance exercises to strengthen bone (i.e., biomechanical forces) (Daly).
- Moderate aerobic exercise for cardiovascular health and weight maintenance.
- Home safety evaluation and hazard identification for fall prevention.
- Hip protectors of potential benefit in the elderly.

Pharmacologic Therapy
- If osteoporosis present and/or high risk for fracture, pharmacologic therapy often needed in addition to exercise, calcium, and vitamin D (see Expert Opinion on FRAX calculations); therapeutic options the same for persons with and without diabetes mellitus.
- Antiresorptive medications to inhibit osteoclast-mediated bone resorption but use limited to those without renal failure.
- Bisphosphonates most common antiresorptive medications (alendronate, risedronate, ibandronate, zoledronic acid).
- Dose recommendations: alendronate 70 mg orally weekly; risedronate 35 mg orally weekly OR 150 mg monthly; ibandronate 150 mg orally monthly; zoledronic acid 5 mg IV yearly.
- Raloxifene, an antiresorptive, and a selective estrogen receptor modifier (SERM): dose 60 mg orally daily.
- Denosumab, a monoclonal antibody against RANK ligand, recently approved in November 2010 as the newest antiresorptive medication on the market.
- Teriparitide (recombinant PTH) the only approved anabolic therapy on the market for treatment of osteoporosis; dose 20 mcg SQ daily for up to 2 years.
- Estrogen and/or hormone replacement therapy, controversial in postmenopausal osteoporosis treatment (cardiovascular complications).
- Testosterone in hypogonadal men beneficial to bone.
- When possible, avoid medications, which might have adverse effects on bone metabolism (steroids, antiepileptic medications, thiazolidinediones in those with known bone disease) (Kahn).

Other Interventions
- Physical therapy to optimize core strength and transfers, minimize falls and fracture risk.
- Vertebroplasty and fixation for vertebral pain management and spine stabilization.
- Orthopedic specialist required for Charcot foot management including limited weight bearing, total contact casting, possible surgical intervention.
- Diagnose and treat other secondary causes of bone loss (i.e., Cushing's disease, primary hyperparathyroidism, rheumatoid arthritis).

COMPLICATIONS AND COMORBIDITIES

- Typical workup of secondary causes of osteoporosis: iPTH, 24-hour urine calcium, testosterone, SPEP, UPEP, phosphate, magnesium, 25-hydroxyvitamin D (consider 1,25 hydroxyvitamin D in patients with renal disease).

FOLLOW-UP

History and Physical Exam

- Fractures, bone pain
- Fall history, syncope
- Kidney stones (hypercalciuria)
- New medications that might worsen bone loss (i.e., thiazolidinediones, steroids, antiseizure, breast or prostate cancer therapies)
- Compliance or side effects with osteoporosis medications
- Height loss, worsening kyphosis
- Point tenderness to spinal process palpation, anterior tibial pain

Biochemical Evaluation

- Diabetes management per routine.
- No definite screening guidelines for vitamin D deficiency, but consider yearly serum levels of 25-hydroxyvitamin D (see Vitamin D, p. 553).
- If progressive bone loss despite therapy, readdress other secondary causes of osteoporosis.
- Consider measurement of markers of bone resorption (N-telopeptide or C-telopeptide) if person on long-standing pharmacologic therapy with question of efficacy.
- Measure serum uric acid and calcium 2 weeks after teriparitide initiation.

Imaging

- Vertebral fracture evaluation with PA/lateral spine X-rays for new back pain, point tenderness.
- DXA yearly to every 2 years in those initiated on osteoporosis therapy.
- DXA yearly in those with low bone density being monitored for therapy initiation.
- Repeat DXA in those with previously normal bone density who have suffered a new fracture.

EXPERT OPINION

- Although T2DM associated with higher BMD on DXA than healthy age-matched population, fracture risk may be up to two-fold higher (Vestergaard).
- Mainstay of improving insulin sensitivity in T2DM is weight loss, although BMD may also decrease with body mass index.
- PPAR gamma agonists (thiazolidnediones) influence mesenchymal stem cell differentiation into adipocytes rather than osteoblasts, leading to bone loss and increased risk of fracture; prescription should be limited to those considered at low risk for bone disease (Vestergaard).
- Fracture risk assessment tool, FRAX (*http://www.shef.ac.uk/FRAX/index.htm*), aids in calculating 10-year major osteoporotic and hip fracture risk based on patient information and risk factors for bone loss; type 1 diabetes considered secondary cause of osteoporosis in this model.
- Consider and screen for syndromes with combined osteoporosis and diabetes phenotype in the appropriate patient: Klinefelter syndrome, Turner's syndrome, Cushing's syndrome, polyglandular autoimmune syndrome type II, and hereditary hemochromatosis.

REFERENCES

Adami S. Bone health in diabetes: considerations for clinical management. *Curr Med Res Opin,* 2009; Vol. 25: pp. 1057–72.
Comments: Discussion of bone fragility in T2DM despite high BMD.

Vestergaard P. Bone metabolism in type 2 diabetes and role of thiazolidinediones. *Curr Opin Endocrinol Diabetes Obes,* 2009; Vol. 16: pp. 125–31.
Comments: Discussion of PPAR gamma agonist effect on bone metabolism.

Schwartz AV, Garnero P, Hillier TA, et al. Pentosidine and increased fracture risk in older adults with type 2 diabetes. *J Clin Endocrinol Metab,* 2009; Vol. 94: pp. 2380–6.
Comments: Advanced glycation end products as a cause of poor bone quality in T2DM.

Wada S, Kamiya S, Fukawa T. Bone quality changes in diabetes. *Clin Calcium,* 2008; Vol. 18: pp. 600–5.
Comments: Mechanisms by which diabetes affects bone remodeling and structure.

Schwartz AV, Vittinghoff E, Sellmeyer DE, et al. Diabetes-related complications, glycemic control, and falls in older adults. *Diabetes Care,* 2008; Vol. 31: pp. 391–6.
Comments: Reduction of diabetic complications and hypoglycemia may reduce fall risk.

Kahn SE, Zinman B, Lachin JM, et al. Rosiglitazone-associated fractures in type 2 diabetes: an Analysis from A Diabetes Outcome Progression Trial (ADOPT). *Diabetes Care,* 2008; Vol. 31: pp. 845–51.
Comments: Increased 5-year fracture incidence in women taking rosiglitazone compared with metformin or glyburide.

Mastrandrea LD, Wactawski-Wende J, Donahue RP, et al. Young women with type 1 diabetes have lower bone mineral density that persists over time. *Diabetes Care,* 2008; Vol. 31: pp. 1729–35.
Comments: Failure to achieve peak bone density in T1DM as a cause of future bone disease and fracture.

Vestergaard P. Discrepancies in bone mineral density and fracture risk in patients with type 1 and type 2 diabetes—a meta-analysis. *Osteoporos Int,* 2007; Vol. 18: pp. 427–44.
Comments: Meta-analysis describing higher fracture rate in T1DM and T2DM despite BMD differences in both groups.

de Liefde II, van der Klift M, de Laet CE, et al. Bone mineral density and fracture risk in type-2 diabetes mellitus: the Rotterdam Study. *Osteoporos Int,* 2005; Vol. 16: pp. 1713–20.
Comments: Increased nonvertebral fracture risk in T2DM (HR 1.69) compared to healthy subjects.

Daly RM, Dunstan DW, Owen N, et al. Does high-intensity resistance training maintain bone mass during moderate weight loss in older overweight adults with type 2 diabetes? *Osteoporos Int,* 2005; Vol. 16: pp. 1703–12.
Comments: Use of resistance exercise to minimize bone loss in attempts at weight loss in T2DM.

Malluche HH, Mawad H, Monier-Faugere MC. The importance of bone health in end-stage renal disease: out of the frying pan, into the fire? *Nephrol Dial Transplant,* 2004; Vol. 19 Suppl 1: pp. i9–13.
Comments: Diabetic nephropathy with resultant renal osteodystropy.

Leidig-Bruckner G, Ziegler R. Diabetes mellitus a risk for osteoporosis? *Exp Clin Endocrinol Diabetes,* 2001; Vol. 109 Suppl 2: pp. S493–514.
Comments: Possible pathophysiology of bone disease in T1DM versus T2DM.

Heinemann DF. Osteoporosis. An overview of the National Osteoporosis Foundation clinical practice guide. *Geriatrics,* 2000; Vol. 55: pp. 31–6; quiz 39.
Comments: National Osteoporosis Foundation clinical guidelines.

Barrett-Connor E, Kritz-Silverstein D. Does hyperinsulinemia preserve bone? *Diabetes Care,* 1996; Vol. 19: pp. 1388–92.
Comments: Fasting insulin levels positively correlated with BMD, suggesting an anabolic role.

World Health Organization Collaborating Centre for Metabolic Bone Diseases, University of Sheffield, UK. FRAX calculator. Available online *http://www.shef.ac.uk/FRAX/index.htm.* (accessed 3/3/2011)
Comments: Fraction risk assessment tool.

COMPLICATIONS AND COMORBIDITIES

CHARCOT JOINT DISEASE (DIABETIC NEUROPATHIC OSTEOARTHROPATHY)

Lee J. Sanders, DPM

DEFINITION

- Diabetic neuropathic osteoarthropathy (DNOAP) also commonly known as Charcot joint disease (CJD).
- A potentially disabling complication of diabetes, that results in deformity and instability of the foot or ankle with the subsequent development of ulceration and infection that can ultimately lead to amputation.
- Acute condition: a sudden, unexpected, and often unrecognized neuropathic arthropathy, often preceded by unrecognized minor trauma; characterized by rapidly progressive localized inflammation with erythema, swelling, and elevated skin temperature; and associated with joint subluxation, dislocation, fractures, osteolysis, and foot deformity.
- Chronic condition: characterized by resolution of inflammation, exuberant ossification, increased bone density, restoration of stability, and foot deformity.

EPIDEMIOLOGY

- Diabetes is the leading cause of neuropathic osteoarthropathy of the foot and ankle.
- Prevalence of DNOAP between 0.08% and 13% of people with diabetes (Frykberg; Sanders).
- Incidence of DNOAP <1%. A prospective study of 1666 patients found incidence of Charcot arthropathy was 8.5/1000 per year (Lavery).
- In type 1 diabetes: average age at onset: 33.5 years; average duration of diabetes: 20 years.
- In type 2 diabetes: average age at onset: 57 years; average duration of diabetes: 15 years.
- DNOAP is associated with an elevated risk of major amputation and mortality (28% at 5 years) (Sohn).
- Risk factors: peripheral neuropathy (essential), age, duration of diabetes, weight, diminished bone mineral density, localized osteopenia, and history of pancreas-kidney transplant.
- Affects both sexes equally.

DIAGNOSIS

- Peripheral neuropathy is an absolute requirement for the diagnosis of DNOAP.
- Pathogenesis: multifactorial, sensorimotor neuropathy, autonomic neuropathy, minor trauma.
- Associated factors: diminished bone mineral density (BMD), proinflammatory cytokines.
- Differential diagnosis of acute DNOAP: cellulitis, acute gouty arthritis, osteomyelitis, and deep vein thrombosis.
- Differential diagnosis of chronic DNOAP: diabetes mellitus (primary cause), alcoholic neuropathy, leprosy, tabes dorsalis, syringomyelia, and congenital insensitivity to pain.
- Laboratory: normal WBC count (no evidence of infection), normal C-reactive protein, normal serum uric acid, negative duplex scan, positive bone scan (nonspecific, cannot distinguish CJD from osteomyelitis, can be false positive in absence of infection).
- Radiology: No X-ray or MRI differences between Charcot foot and osteomyelitis.
- Early radiographic examination may be negative or with subtle findings.
- Bone biopsy is recommended if the diagnosis remains equivocal.

SIGNS AND SYMPTOMS

- A rocker-bottom foot deformity with collapse of the midfoot is the hallmark of DNOAP.
- Earliest presentation may be consistent with incipient osteoarthritis.
- Acute CJD presentation: signs of an acute inflammatory process with mild to moderate pain, swelling, localized erythema, and elevated skin temperature. May have joint effusion, bone resorption, joint subluxation, dislocation, and instability.
- Three radiographic stages (Eichenholtz): development, coalescence, and reconstruction as CJD evolves from acute to chronic.
- Five anatomic patterns (Sanders and Frykberg): I: forefoot joints; II: tarsometatarsal joints; III: midtarsal and naviculocuneiform joints; IV: ankle and/or subtalar joints; V: isolated to calcaneus.
- Patterns I, II, and III often associated with ulceration; Pattern IV causes most severe structural deformity and instability, highest risk of amputation.
- Misdiagnosis and delay of treatment allows for uninterrupted mechanical stress of weight-bearing, with resultant soft tissue injury (ulcers), microfractures, fractures, dislocations, subluxation, bone resorption, disorganization and fragmentation, soft tissue edema, increased joint mobility, and deformity. Can lead to amputation.
- Evolution of the Charcot foot: see Figure 3-2 below.

CLINICAL TREATMENT

- Goals of therapy: preventing progression of foot/ankle deformity, ulceration, or reulceration.
- Quality of life goals include the ability to continue working, be independently mobile, and wear shoes.
- **Cornerstone of therapy for acute CJD:** immediate off-loading of the foot with elimination of physical stress. Brief period of bed rest with elevation of the extremity to reduce swelling, followed by cast immobilization with, optimally, serial application

FIGURE 3-2. EVOLUTION OF THE CHARCOT FOOT

Stage 0 Prodromal period	Stage 1 Development	Stage 2 Coalescence	Stage 3 Reconstruction
Swelling Local warmth Mild erythema Clinical instability Radiographic changes are absent or minimal	Debris formation at articular margins Fragmentation of subchondral bone Subluxation Dislocation Erosion of articular cartilage Bone resorption Osteolysis and osteopenia Disorganization and fragmentation of bone Soft tissue edema Increased joint mobility	Lessening of edema Absorption of fine debris Healing of fractures Fusion and coalescence of larger fragments Loss of vascularity Sclerosis of bone	Further repair and remodeling of bone Fusion & rounding of large fragments Revascularization Diminution of sclerosis Restoration of stability Increased bone density Exuberant ossification **Deformity**

Resorption of Bone   Repair

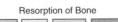

Source: Sanders LJ, Frykberg RG. The Charcot Foot (Pied de Charcot). In: Bowker J, Pfeifer MA, eds. *Levin and O'Neal's The Diabetic Foot.* 7th ed. Philadelphia: Elsevier, Inc.; 2008.

COMPLICATIONS AND COMORBIDITIES

of total contact casts (TCC) or a removable cast walker (RCW) made irremovable to facilitate compliance (Sanders).
- Prolonged non-weight-bearing and subsequent protected weight-bearing are recommended.
- **Braces and custom footwear:** with reduction of swelling, warmth and erythema and radiographic evidence of bone healing (Eichenholtz stages 2 and 3), transition to partial weight-bearing in RCW, ankle foot orthosis (AFO), Charcot Restraint Orthotic Walker (CROW), or a patella-tendon-bearing brace (PTB) and custom shoe.
- **Antiresorptive pharmacologic agents:** bisphosphonates and calcitonin affect bone remodeling cycle, but not currently approved for prevention or treatment of CJD.
- **Surgical management:** controversial. Primary indication is failed conservative treatment. Less certain indications: foot/ankle instability, deformity, chronic ulceration, and progressive joint destruction. Complication rates are high especially in feet with chronic ulceration. Lack long-term surgical outcomes studies.

Follow-up

- Average time of immobilization leading to resolution of acute CJD is 10 months (7–15 months).
- High-risk individuals require professional foot care and lifelong surveillance for the prevention, early identification, and treatment of foot complications.
- A multidisciplinary team approach to care is recommended.

Expert Opinion

- Early recognition and timely treatment will often result in more satisfactory outcomes.
- The key to treatment is prevention of deformity and ulceration by off-loading the foot/ankle and avoiding further injury until the bone and soft tissues heal.

References

Sohn MW, Lee TA, Stuck RM, et al. Mortality risk of Charcot arthropathy compared with that of diabetic foot ulcer and diabetes alone. *Diabetes Care*, 2009; Vol. 32: pp. 816–21.
Comments: Charcot arthropathy is associated with higher mortality risk than diabetes alone and with lower risk than foot ulcer.

Sanders LJ, Frykberg RG. The Charcot Foot (Pied de Charcot). In Bowker J, Pfeifer MA, (Eds.), *Levin and O'Neal's The Diabetic Foot*, Seventh Edition. Philadelphia: Elsevier Inc.; 2008: pp. 257–283.
Comments: Review of the pathogenesis, natural history, and management of the Charcot foot. Anatomic patterns of bone and joint involvement are illustrated. Emerging research is reviewed, including the putative role of antiresorptive pharmacologic agents, proinflammatory cytokines, and osteoclastogenesis and the RANKL/OPG signaling pathway.

Sanders LJ. What lessons can history teach us about the Charcot foot? *Clin Podiatr Med Surg*, 2008; Vol. 25: pp. 1–15, v.
Comments: Contemporary historical perspective on the Charcot foot. Contains original 19th century illustrations from primary source materials.

Frykberg RG, Belczyk R. Epidemiology of the Charcot foot. *Clin Podiatr Med Surg*, 2008; Vol. 25: pp. 17–28, v.
Comments: The actual incidence of CJD is likely greater than that reported. The diagnosis is delayed or missed in 25% of the cases.

Burns PR, Wukich DK. Surgical reconstruction of the Charcot rearfoot and ankle. *Clin Podiatr Med Surg*, 2008; Vol. 25: pp. 95–120, vii–viii.
Comments: Overview of surgical management of the Charcot foot, including basic surgical principles and techniques. Outcomes and scientific evidence-based medicine regarding Charcot ankle and hindfoot deformity is minimal.

Lavery LA, Armstrong DG, Wunderlich RP, et al. Diabetic foot syndrome: evaluating the prevalence and incidence of foot pathology in Mexican Americans and non-Hispanic whites from a diabetes disease management cohort. *Diabetes Care,* 2003; Vol. 26: pp. 1435–8.

    Comments: A prospective study of 1666 patients from a disease management program in Texas found the incidence of Charcot arthropathy was 8.5/1000 per year.

Hoché G, Sanders LJ. On some arthropathies apparently related to a lesion of the brain or spinal cord, by Dr. J-M Charcot, January 1868. *J Hist Neurosci,* 1992; Vol. 1: pp. 75–87.

    Comments: Translation of J-M Charcot's 1868 paper on the tabetic arthropathies. Contains 4 clinical case observations and a discussion of 2 main groups of arthropathies manifesting in the course of progressive locomotor ataxia.

Eichenholtz SN. Charcot joints. Springfield, IL: Charles C. Thomas, 1966: p. 227.

    Comments: This is Sidney Eichenholtz's classic monograph on Charcot joints, in which he describes three well-defined radiographic stages in the evolution of this condition. His classification is the most commonly accepted taxonomy of neuroarthropathy.

NIH Office of Rare Diseases and National Institute of Diabetes and Digestive and Kidney Diseases (NIDDK). Summary Report: Charcot Neuroarthropathy Workshop, September 17–18, 2008. Bethesda, MD. Report can be downloaded from the NIDDK website. *http://www3.niddk.nih.gov/fund/other/neuroarthropathy/SummaryReport.pdf* (accessed 3/3/2011).

    Comments: NIH Office of Rare Diseases and NIDDK cosponsored workshop, Charcot Neuroarthropathy Recent Progress and Future Directions.

DERMATOLOGIC MANIFESTATIONS OF DIABETES

Mary Huizinga, MD, MPH

COMPLICATIONS AND COMORBIDITIES

DEFINITION

- Dermatologic manifestations of diabetes are common and come in numerous forms (Romano).
- Skin findings may help diagnose diabetes (e.g., acanthosis nigricans) or reflect long-term complications of diabetes (e.g., necrobiosis lipoidica diabeticorum [NLD]).
- The dermatologic manifestations may be due to deposition of advanced glycosylation end products (AGEs), infectious etiologies, autoimmune conditions, or related to pharmacologic therapy for diabetes (i.e., insulin).
- Often, skin manifestations reflect other coexisting conditions such as dyslipidemia.

EPIDEMIOLOGY

- Approximately half of all patients with diabetes will have some dermatological manifestations (Chakrabarty; Romano).
- Autoimmune skin findings are more common in T1DM than T2DM (Romano).
- Infectious skin findings are most prevalent in poorly controlled diabetes (Romano).

DIAGNOSIS

- Diagnosis can often be made by examination of the skin.
- Occasionally, such as with NLD, punch biopsy, culture, or imaging is needed to confirm diagnosis.

SIGNS AND SYMPTOMS

- **Acanthosis nigricans:** hyperpigmented, velvety plaques in skin folds—most commonly the axillae and flexural areas of the posterior neck. A manifestation of insulin resistance, usually in type 2 diabetes and polycystic ovarian syndrome; asymptomatic.

Differential includes paraneoplastic syndrome, a sign of a gastrointestinal malignancy, or drug reaction (Higgins; Ahmed).

- **Diabetic dermopathy (shin spots):** groupings of macules or plaques on the lower leg, which may recede or progress; progression may involve an increase in the number of spots, enlargement of spots, and the spots may become hyperpigmented and/or depressed ("shallow"). Occurs in up to 40% of patients with diabetes, men > women, usually in the setting of other microvascular complications. May be due to slowly healing trauma (Ahmed; van Hatten).

- **Necrobiosis lipoidica diabeticorum (NLD):** begins as a violaceous patch, expanding slowly with a red border and yellow-brown central area; over time, the central area atrophies and becomes waxy with telangiectasias—ulceration occurs in 35% of cases. Rare, occurring in 0.3% of people with diabetes; typically occurs in women in third to fourth decade and may appear many years before the onset of diabetes. Unless ulceration occurs, asymptomatic and only occasionally of cosmetic concern (Ferringer; Cohen; Paron).

- **Diabetic bullae:** rapid onset of painless, tense, serous blisters on plantar surface of feet, hands, and legs; usually heal in 2–4 weeks. Occur in longstanding diabetes (Romano; Ferringer; Ahmed; van Hattem; Paron).

- **Yellow nails, palms, or soles:** common, without known pathological consequence. Unknown etiology but may be due to deposition of advanced glycosylation products or, less likely, elevated carotene (Paron; Ahmed; Ferringer).

- **Skin infections:** occur in 20%–60% of patients with diabetes. (1) *Candida: Staphylococcus* and *Streptococcus* especially common, affecting intertriginous areas (groin, under breasts, axillae), vagina (vaginitis) in women, penis (balinitis) in men. Most common with poor glycemic control. (2) *Necrotizing fasciitis:* rapidly progressive infection of skin and soft tissue, mixed bacterial origin; consider in patients with signs of cellulitis who appear septic. (3) *Malignant external otitis:* invasive infection of external auditory ear canal—most commonly, pseudomonas—may spread to surrounding structures; clinical exam reveals tenderness of pinna with purulent drainage. CT or MRI needed to determine extent of bony involvement. (4) *Erythrasma:* common skin infection of skin folds (axillae, groin, spaces between digits, intergluteal folds), usually due to *Corynebacterium.* (5) *Rhinocerebral mucormycosis:* rare but life threatening, occurs more often in the elderly, due to fungal infection with zygomycetes; presents with fever, facial cellulitis, periorbital edema, facial numbness, proptosis, and/or blindness. CT/MRI used to assess extent of involvement (Romano; Ahmed; Chakrabarty, Carfrae).

- **Scleroderma-like changes:** Prevalence ranges from 2.5%–50%; affects T1DM and T2DM, with no race or sex preference. Asymmetric nonpitting thickening and hardening of the skin or hands (sclerodactyly) and/or neck, shoulders, and back (scleredema diabeticorum or scleredema of Bushke). Often occurs with joint problems; clinical course is progressive with increasing involvement and stiffness (Cole; Sattar; Brik; Ahmed; Ferringer; Yosipovitch).

- **Reactions to insulin:** (1) *Lipoatrophy:* areas with loss of subcutaneous fat, may be as large as 5–10 cm. May have immunological basis or due to lipolytic components of insulins. Risk increases with repeated injection at same site. Insulin absorption from effective sites can be erratic. Less common with newer insulins than with beef/pork insulin. (2) *Lipohypertrophy:* areas of marked subcutaneous lipid hypertrophy, often 1–15 cm circumference, raised 3–5 cm. This is the most common skin complication of insulin therapy. Also reduced with newer insulins. Like lipoatrophy, associated with injection into same site repeatedly, and can cause erratic insulin absorption. (3) *Local allergic reactions:* erythema, pruritis, and induration. These reactions are short-lived and resolve within a few weeks. (Paron; Richardson)

- **Dyslipidemias associated with diabetes:** (1) *Hypertriglyceridemia:* if severe (>1000 mg/dl), eruptive xanthomata are showers of macular papules with white tip (triglyceride) and mildly erythematous base, most often on upper or lower extremities. Resolve with resolution of hypertriglyceridemia. (2) *Hypercholesterolemia:* xanthelasma (yellowish plaques in palpebrae of eye lids); tendon xanthomata; tuberous xanthomata (elbows, knees). (3) *Dysbetalipoproteinemia:* palmar xanthomata, an unusual dyslipidemia associated with elevated very-low-density lipoprotein (VLDL) remnants and chylomicrons; total cholesterol and triglycerides >90th percentile.

CLINICAL TREATMENT
AGE-Related

- **Acanthosis nigricans (AN):** treat insulin resistance with weight reduction, exercise, metformin, or thiazolidinediones, although little evidence that AN responds. Lactic acid cream or retinoic acid may soften lesions; Accutane will reduce lesions but they will recur when drug stopped (Higgins; van Hatten).
- **Diabetic dermopathy (shin spots):** treatment directed at the prevention of secondary infection (Chakrabarty).
- **Necrobiosis lipoidica diabeticorum:** no standard therapy—local steroid injections or topical creams are used with controversial results. In severe cases, skin grafting may be required.
- **Diabetic bullae:** usually resolves without intervention. If uncomfortable, bullae may be drained; topical antibiotics may be used to prevent secondary infection.
- **Yellow skin:** no treatment exists.

Skin Infections

- **Candida infections:** keep affected area dry, treat with topical antifungals. Oral antifungals rarely required for superficial candidiasis (Hay; Guitart).
- **Cellulitis:** elevation of affected area, maintain hydration of skin to avoid cracking; empiric antibiotic therapy should cover *Staphylococcus aureus* +/– MRSA and gram-negative bacteria.
- **Necrotizing fasciitis:** surgical evaluation and intravenous antibiotics must be delivered rapidly (Ahmed).
- **Malignant external otitis:** prolonged course of quinolones, debridement may be required (Ahmed; Carfrae).
- **Erythrasma:** erythromycin 250 mg 4 times a day for 14 days (Holdiness).
- **Rhinocerebral mucormycosis:** urgent intravenous amphotericin B and surgical debridement.
- For more details on treatment, also see Infectious Diseases and Diabetes, p. 271.

Autoimmune

- **Scleroderma-like changes:** treatments have mixed results—options include photopheresis, radiotherapy, cyclosporin, and high-dose penicillin; no effective treatment known for scleredema diabeticorum (Van Hattem; Ferringer).

COMPLICATIONS AND COMORBIDITIES

Reactions to Insulin

- **Lipoatrophy:** rotate insulin injection site or mode of delivery. Occasionally, for severe cases, consider adding glucocorticoid to insulin for injection.
- **Lipohypertrophy:** rotate injection sites. Occasionally, liposuction has been used to achieve cosmetic improvement.
- **Local allergic reactions:** usually resolves spontaneously, but addition of glucocorticoid to insulin has been used, as has desensitization or changing to insulin pump therapy.

Coexisting Conditions

- **Dyslipidemia:** treat the underlying condition.

EXPERT OPINION

- Dermatologic manifestations of diabetes are common.
- Most cutaneous manifestations are related to hyperglycemia (AGEs), autoimmune, or infectious etiologies due to pharmacologic therapy or comorbidities.
- Prognosis and treatment varies greatly depending on the type of dermatological manifestation.

REFERENCES

Chakrabarty A, Norman RA, Phillips TJ. Cutaneous manifestations of diabetes. In Norman RA (Ed.), *Diagnosis of Aging Skin Diseases.* London: Springer-Verlag; 2008; Online ISBN 978-1-84628-678-0; pp. 253–263.
  Comments: Review of skin manifestations of diabetes.

Van Hattem S, Bootsma AH, Thio HB. Skin manifestations of diabetes. *Cleve Clin J Med,* 2008; Vol. 75: pp. 772, 774, 776–7 passim.
  Comments: Review of skin manifestations of diabetes.

Carfrae MJ, Kesser BW. Malignant otitis externa. *Otolaryngol Clin North Am,* 2008; Vol. 41: pp. 537–49, viii–ix.
  Comments: Review of malignant otitis externa.

Higgins SP, Freemark M, Prose NS. Acanthosis nigricans: a practical approach to evaluation and management. *Dermatol Online J,* 2008; Vol. 14: p. 2.
  Comments: Review of management for acanthosis nigricans.

Ahmed I, Goldstein B. Diabetes mellitus. *Clin Dermatol,* 2006; Vol. 24: pp. 237–46.
  Comments: Review of skin manifestations of diabetes.

Richardson T, Kerr D Skin-related complications of insulin therapy: epidemiology and emerging management strategies. *Am J Clin Dermatol,* 2003; Vol. 4: pp. 661–7.
  Comments: Skin-related complications of insulin therapy.

Richardson T, Kerr D. Skin-related complications of insulin therapy: epidemiology and emerging management strategies. *Am J Clin Dermatol,* 2003; Vol. 4: pp. 661–7.
  Comments: Review of skin-related complications of insulin therapy.

Holdiness MR. Management of cutaneous erythrasma. *Drugs,* 2002; Vol. 62: pp. 1131–41.
  Comments: Review of treatments for erythrasma.

Ferringer T, Miller F. Cutaneous manifestations of diabetes mellitus. *Dermatol Clin,* 2002; Vol. 20: pp. 483–92.
  Comments: Review of skin manifestations of diabetes.

Paron NG, Lambert PW. Cutaneous manifestations of diabetes mellitus. *Prim Care,* 2000; Vol. 27: pp. 371–83.
  Comments: Review of cutaneous manifestations of diabetes.

Hay RJ. The management of superficial candidiasis. *J Am Acad Dermatol,* 1999; Vol. 40: pp. S35–42.
  Comments: Review of superficial candidiasis.

Romano G, Moretti G, Di Benedetto A, et al. Skin lesions in diabetes mellitus: prevalence and clinical correlations. *Diabetes Res Clin Pract,* 1998; Vol. 39: pp. 101–6.
  Comments: Prevalence of skin manifestations found in 60% of patients.

Yosipovitch G, Hodak E, Vardi P, et al. The prevalence of cutaneous manifestations in IDDM patients and their association with diabetes risk factors and microvascular complications. *Diabetes Care,* 1998; Vol. 21: pp. 506–9.
  Comments: Cross-sectional study of 238 insulin dependent patients and 122 controls; scleroderma-like changes found in 39% of patients.

Cohen O, Yaniv R, Karasik A, et al. Necrobiosis lipoidica and diabetic control revisited. *Med Hypotheses,* 1996; Vol. 46: pp. 348–50.
  Comments: Review of necrobiosis lipoidica.

Guitart J, Woodley DT. Intertrigo: a practical approach. *Compr Ther,* 1994; Vol. 20: pp. 402–9.
  Comments: Review of superficial candidiasis.

Brik R, Berant M, Vardi P. The scleroderma-like syndrome of insulin-dependent diabetes mellitus. *Diabetes Metab Rev,* 1991; Vol. 7: pp. 120–8.
  Comments: Scleroderma-like syndromes.

Sattar MA, Diab S, Sugathan TN, et al. Scleroedema diabeticorum: a minor but often unrecognized complication of diabetes mellitus. *Diabet Med,* 1988; Vol. 5: pp. 465–8.
  Comments: Cross-sectional study of 100 persons with diabetes; 14% had scleredema diabeticorum.

Cole GW, Headley J, Skowsky R. Scleredema diabeticorum: a common and distinct cutaneous manifestation of diabetes mellitus. *Diabetes Care,* 1983; Vol. 6: pp. 189–92.
  Comments: Review, case series, and prospective analysis of patients with diabetes; prevalence of scleredema in patients with diabetes was 2.5%.

FOOT ULCERS

See Foot Ulcers, p. 264.

GANGRENE AND CRITICAL LIMB ISCHEMIA

Lee J. Sanders, DPM

COMPLICATIONS AND COMORBIDITIES

DEFINITION

- Gangrene is necrosis of tissue associated with ischemia (dry gangrene) or infection (wet gangrene).
- Gas gangrene is a type of wet gangrene caused by anaerobic bacteria (*Clostridium*), especially *C. perfringens*.
- The term critical limb ischemia (CLI) should be used for all patients with chronic ischemic rest pain, ulcers, or gangrene attributable to objectively proven arterial occlusive disease; if untreated, natural history could lead to major amputation within 6 months.
- The pathophysiology of CLI is complex in the diabetic foot, influenced by the interaction of arterial insufficiency, neuropathy, ulceration, and infection; reduced perfusion, below the level required to sustain basal tissue metabolism, results in slowly progressive tissue death and amputation.

EPIDEMIOLOGY

- The incidence of CLI is approximately 500–1000 per million persons per year (Dormandy).
- Chronic CLI is most often precipitated by diffuse or multisegmental atherosclerotic arterial occlusive disease.

- Patients with CLI have the same cardiovascular risk factor profile as patients with claudication; risk factors include smoking, hypertension, diabetes, and hyperlipidemia.
- The risk of developing CLI is greater in individuals with diabetes.
- The progression of CLI to gangrene has been reported to be 40% in diabetes compared with 9% in no diabetes patients.
- Chronic CLI is associated with a 1-year mortality rate ~20%. Nearly 50% of cases require revascularization for limb salvage. 40% of patients with unreconstructable disease will require amputation within 6 months of initial diagnosis (Hirsch).
- Patients with both peripheral arterial disease (PAD) and diabetes are ~10 times more likely to require an amputation than those with PAD alone.
- In the Rochester, MN, population-based cohort study of diabetes, the incidence of new episodes of gangrene in patients with diabetes and no lower extremity arterial disease (LEAD) was reported as 4.5 per 1000 person-years of study. In patients with both diabetes and LEAD, the incidence of gangrene was 29.6 per 1000 person-years in men and 37.1 per 1000 person-years in women (Melton).
- Risk factors for gangrene include peripheral arterial disease, peripheral neuropathy, infection, trauma, and delayed wound healing.

DIAGNOSIS

- Diagnosis is made by detailed clinical history (ischemic rest pain, intermittent claudication, chronic nonhealing wound), physical examination (absence of pedal pulses, trophic skin changes, ischemic ulceration, or skin necrosis), noninvasive evaluation for PAD (ABI), vascular laboratory evaluation (segmental pressures, pulse volume recordings, preoperative transcutaneous oxygen tension [TcPO2] mapping), and anatomic studies (duplex ultrasound, magnetic resonance angiography, and contrast X-ray angiography).
- Wet gangrene "fetid foot": extensive necrosis or gangrene, malodorous. Often with mixed polymicrobial infection.
- Pathogens: mixed aerobic gram-positive cocci, including *Enterococci*, *Enterobacteriaceae*, nonfermenting gram-negative rods and obligate anaerobes.
- Severity of ischemia: Rutherford classification Grades III (minor tissue loss) and IV (ulceration or gangrene). See Table 3-5 in Peripheral Vascular Disease, p. 209.

SIGNS AND SYMPTOMS

- Gangrene usually affects the digits, and in severe cases, the forefoot.
- Mummification of the toes and autoamputation may occur in the absence of infection (dry gangrene); a line of demarcation is often present, below which temperature drops off suddenly, indicating the change in perfusion.
- In the presence of infection, the skin may feel warm and the necrotic tissue is moist and malodorous (wet gangrene).
- Moderate infection severity: systemically well, metabolically stable; one or more of the following: cellulitis >2 cm, lymphangiitic streaking, spread beneath superficial fascia, deep tissue abscess, gangrene, involvement of muscle tendon, joint, or bone.
- Severe infection severity: systemic toxicity or metabolic instability (e.g., fever, chills, tachycardia, hypotension, confusion, vomiting, leukocytosis, acidosis, severe hyperglycemia, or azotemia).
- Patients with critical arterial insufficiency present with severe pain, often in the distal part of the foot or toe; ischemic rest pain at night and severely impaired walking

capacity due to claudication; loss of hair growth on the dorsum of the foot and toes; thick dystrophic toenails; pallor of the skin on elevation of the limb and rubor on dependency.

- Arterial ulcers involve the tips of the toes, the heels, and areas of small radius of curvature (e.g., the first and fifth metatarsal heads) from shoe pressure.

CLINICAL TREATMENT

- **Aggressive risk factor interventions:** smoking cessation, glycemic control, aggressive blood pressure control (ACE inhibitors, beta-blockers, calcium channel blockers), antiplatelet therapy (ASA, clopidogrel), lipid-lowering agents (statins), as well as exercise rehabilitation and cilostazol for claudication.
- **Systemic antibiotics:** required in patients who develop cellulitis or spreading infection in ischemic ulcers or gangrene but should not delay more definitive treatment.
- **Revascularization:** ideal treatment for CLI is the elimination or bypass of occlusions in the larger arteries by percutaneous angioplasty (PTA) or stent procedures.
- Venous bypass grafts for CLI are considered the gold standard.
- **Pharmacologic therapy:** to modify the consequences of low perfusion pressure on the distal microcirculation.
- **Hyperbaric oxygen (HBO) therapy:** controversial as an adjunct to antibiotics and aggressive surgical debridement, but indications may include necrotizing fasciitis, gas gangrene, chronic refractory osteomyelitis, and infected diabetic foot ulcers.
- **Pain management:** adequate treatment of ischemic pain is mandatory in all patients with CLI and may require short-term use of narcotics.
- Topical antibiotics, growth factors, and debriding agents (enzymes) are unlikely to be successful as the sole therapy in treating patients with CLI.
- The decision regarding the most appropriate intervention should be made by a multidisciplinary team after consideration of the following issues: extent of gangrene and infection, vascular lesion morphology, comorbidities, risk of surgery for the individual patient, previous procedures (bypass or angioplasty), patient's life expectancy, rehabilitation potential, and local expertise and experience with particular surgical or endovascular procedures.
- Dry gangrene in neuroischemic feet requires vascular consultation, wound debridement, and/or amputation, or autoamputation.
- Wet gangrene in neuropathic feet requires intravenous antibiotics and surgical debridement or amputation.
- Wet gangrene in neuroischemic feet requires intravenous antibiotics and consideration of surgical debridement, and/or revascularization surgery.

FOLLOW-UP

- Diabetic patients with CLI are at very high risk for MI, stroke, and vascular death.
- Decreased peripheral perfusion leads to limb loss without appropriate revascularization.
- Timely referral of patients with CLI to a podiatrist and vascular specialist improves the chances of limb salvage.
- Prognosis for well-vascularized neuropathic patients with gangrene of the toe(s) secondary to infection or trauma is much better than for neuroischemic patients with gangrene associated with CLI.
- CLI is never completely or permanently cured because the underlying peripheral arterial disease continues to progress.

COMPLICATIONS AND COMORBIDITIES

- Clinical success after lower extremity revascularization for ischemic tissue loss is determined by intrinsic patient factors and not by method of revascularization. Diabetes patients with impaired ambulatory status and gangrene have an 85.2% probability of failure, whereas patients with ESRD, impaired ambulatory status, gangrene, and a prior vascular intervention, have a 92.8% probability of failure.

Expert Opinion

- Differentiate ischemic pain (severe, worse on leg elevation or walking, associated with signs of ischemia) from neuropathic pain (unassociated with walking, usually relatively symmetrical, associated with signs of neuropathy but not ischemia). A given patient may have both, but ischemic pain is suggestive of CLI.
- In contrast to patients with intermittent claudication, the prognosis of CLI is very poor. CLI patients are at high risk for mortality and amputation.

Basis for Recommendations

Hirsch AT, Haskal ZJ, Hertzer NR, et al. ACC/AHA 2005 guidelines for the management of patients with peripheral arterial disease (lower extremity, renal, mesenteric, and abdominal aortic): executive summary. A collaborative report from the American Association for Vascular Surgery/Society for Vascular Surgery, Society for Cardiovascular Angiography and Interventions, Society for Vascular Medicine and Biology, Society of Interventional Radiology, and the American College of Cardiology (ACC)/American Heart Association (AHA) Task Force on Practice Guidelines: writing Committee to Develop Guidelines for the Management of Patients With Peripheral Arterial Disease. *J Am Coll Cardiol*, 2006; Vol. 47: pp. 1239–312.

> Comments: The ACC/AHA guidelines address the diagnosis and management of atherosclerotic, aneurysmal, and thromboembolic peripheral arterial diseases (PADs).

Dormandy JA, Rutherford RB. Management of peripheral arterial disease (PAD). TASC Working Group. Trans Atlantic Inter-Society Consensus (TASC). *J Vasc Surg*, 2000; Vol. 31: pp. S1–S296.

> Comments: TransAtlantic Inter-Society Consensus (TASC) document on the management of peripheral arterial disease. Comprehensive monograph on the epidemiology, natural history, risk factors, evaluation, and medical and surgical management of PVD.

Other References

Taylor SM, York JW, Cull DL, et al. Clinical success using patient-oriented outcome measures after lower extremity bypass and endovascular intervention for ischemic tissue loss. *J Vasc Surg*, 2009; Vol. 50: pp. 534–41; discussion 541.

> Comments: The purpose of this study was to retrospectively examine success after lower extremity revascularization for tissue loss using patient-oriented measures and to include patients who underwent both open surgical bypass and endovascular procedures. Type of intervention was not a significant factor in either bivariate or logistic regression analysis.

Mohler E, Giri J, American College of Cardiology, et al. Management of peripheral arterial disease patients: comparing the ACC/AHA and TASC-II guidelines. *Curr Med Res Opin*, 2008; Vol. 24: pp. 2509–22.

> Comments: Findings and conclusions: Both documents agree on the need for aggressive management of patients with PAD. In spite of these recommendations, there is a general lack of adherence to the current guidelines—a critical concern considering the high morbidity and mortality associated with the disease.

Nather A, Bee CS, Huak CY, et al. Epidemiology of diabetic foot problems and predictive factors for limb loss. *J Diabetes Complications*, 2008; Vol. 22: pp. 77–82.

> Comments: Detailed prospective study of 202 patients during the period January 2005–May 2006, to evaluate the epidemiology of diabetic foot problems (DFP) and predictive factors for major lower extremity amputations. Results: 192 patients had DM2, mean age 60 years, male to female ratio of 1:1. 72.8% of patients had poor endocrine control and 42.1% had sensory neuropathy. Common DPF = gangrene (31.7%), infection (28.7%), ulcer 27.7%, cellulitis (6.4%), necrotizing fasciitis (3.5%), and Charcot osteoarthropathy (2.0%). Surgery was performed in 74.8% of patients, major amputation in 27.2% (below-knee in 20.3% and above knee in 6.9%).

Kaide CG, Khandelwal S. Hyperbaric oxygen: applications in infectious disease. *Emerg Med Clin North Am*, 2008; Vol. 26: pp. 571–95, xi.

Comments: Review article discussing the application of hyperbaric oxygen (HBO) as an adjunctive treatment of certain infectious processes.

Lipsky BA, Berendt AR, Deery HG, et al. Diagnosis and treatment of diabetic foot infections. *Clin Infect Dis*, 2004; Vol. 39: pp. 885–910.

Comments: Infectious Disease Society of America (IDSA) guidelines for the diagnosis and treatment of diabetic foot infections. Document can be downloaded from *http://www.journals.uchicago.edu/doi/abs/10.1086/424846*.

Melton LJ, Macken KM, Palumbo PJ, et al. Incidence and prevalence of clinical peripheral vascular disease in a population-based cohort of diabetic patients. *Diabetes Care*, 1981; Vol. 3: pp. 650–4.

Comments: Rochester, MN, population-based cohort of diabetic patients. In the cohort with diabetes and gangrene, survival was poor, with only 39% alive after 2 years.

Joslin, EP. The menace of diabetic gangrene. *NEJM*, 1934; Vol. 211(1): pp. 16–20.

Comments: Joslin noted that following the introduction of insulin, mortality from diabetic coma had fallen significantly from 60% to 5%. Yet, deaths from diabetic gangrene (of the foot and leg) had risen significantly. Joslin observed that gangrene increased with age and duration of diabetes. There was almost always a history of injury to the foot that could be elicited from the patient. Burns and ill-fitting shoes caused the most common injuries. Joslin firmly believed that gangrene and amputations were preventable. His remedy was a team approach to diabetes care.

MUSCULOSKELETAL DISEASES

Mary Huizinga, MD, MPH

DEFINITION

- A number of musculoskeletal disorders (MSDs) are associated with diabetes.
- Joints most often affected include shoulders, hands, and feet.
- Many of the MSDs associated with diabetes are systemic.
- Duration of diabetes is a significant risk factor for most MSDs regardless of the type of diabetes.

EPIDEMIOLOGY

- MSDs are common in diabetes. In one study, half of people with diabetes had one MSD affecting the hand, and a quarter had two MSDs (Gamstedt).
- **Carpal tunnel syndrome:** prevalence of 20% in persons with diabetes but can be as high as 75% (Gamstedt; Chaudhuri).
- **Dupuytren's contracture:** reported in up to 40% of persons with diabetes (Gamstedt; Noble).
- **Flexor tenosynovitis:** "trigger" finger described in up to 20% of persons with diabetes; related to duration of diabetes regardless of glycemic control (Gamstedt).
- **Adhesive capsulitis:** reported in 19%–29% of persons with diabetes; risk factors include increased age, longer duration of diabetes, Dupuytren's contracture, and retinopathy (Pal; Balci).
- **Calcific periarthritis:** 3 times more common in patients with diabetes than in patients without diabetes; associated with older age, longer duration of diabetes, and insulin use (Mavrikakis).

COMPLICATIONS AND COMORBIDITIES

- **Limited joint mobility:** prevalence ranges from 8%–58% depending on population; increased with longer duration of diabetes, worse glycemic control, retinopathy, nephropathy, increasing age, and cigarette smoking.
- **Diabetic sclerodactyly:** see Dermatological Manifestations of Diabetes, p. 305.
- **Stiff-person disease:** very rare disease of progressive muscle stiffness in type 1 diabetes (Helfgott).
- **Diabetic muscle infarction:** rare complication of diabetes where the muscle infarcts spontaneously (Trujillo-Santos).
- **Osteoarthritis:** can be associated with diabetes; likely due to obesity (Hochberg).
- **Rheumatoid arthritis (RA):** chronic inflammation in RA plus chronic glucocorticoid use may increase risk of type 2 diabetes in these patients; no evidence to link T1DM to RA although both may be present in polyglandular autoimmune conditions (Doran; Simard).

DIAGNOSIS

- **Carpal tunnel syndrome:** limited joint movement due to median nerve entrapment; Hoffmann-Tinel sign (tapping wrist at median nerve to elicit symptoms) and Phalen's sign (acute wrist flexion for 30–60 seconds to elicit symptoms); electrodiagnostic tests that show median nerve dysfunction (Preston).
- **Dupuytren's contracture:** joint stiffness of the hand due to fibrosis of palmar fascia and triangular puckering of skin or nodules over flexor tendons without signs of inflammation of the joints; disease course highly variable with regression in up to 10% (Gudmundsson).
- **Flexor tenosynovitis:** palpable nodule forms on the flexor tendon; thumb, third, and fourth digits are most likely to be involved and may be bilateral (Ryzewicz).
- **Adhesive capsulitis:** advanced form of "frozen shoulder" (a reversible shoulder contraction) where adhesions have formed leading to significant loss of range of motion (abduction and rotation); demonstration that limited range of motion not due to arthritis or other process (Sheridan).
- **Calcific periarthritis:** also known as calcific tendinitis, refers to deposition of calcium hydroxyapatite crystals in tendons around the shoulder joint; diagnosed by presence of calcifications in shoulder tendons on X-ray (Siegal; Mavrikakis).
- **Limited joint mobility:** limited movement of joints, especially the small joints of the hands, thought to be due to the glycosylation of collagen; "prayer sign" (unable to flatten hands together), and "table top test" (unable to flatten palm on table top) (Kapoor).
- **Stiff-person disease:** diagnoses strongly suggested by the presence of anti-GAD antibodies in type 1 diabetes; physical exam and EMG also useful (Duddy).
- **Diabetic muscle infarction:** often a diagnosis of exclusion; creatinine kinase may or may not be elevated; ultrasonography and MR imaging may be useful; muscle biopsy will reveal muscular necrosis and edema with occusional of arterioles (Trujillo-Santos).
- **Osteoarthritis:** plain radiographs show deterioration of the joint (Feydy).

SIGNS AND SYMPTOMS

- **Carpal tunnel syndrome:** pain and paraesthesia in the thumb, second, and third digits, and radial half of the fourth digit.
- **Dupuytren's contracture:** major symptom is flexor contraction of one or more digits at the metacarpophalangeal joint.
- **Flexor tenosynovitis:** pain on flexing tendon(s); in hand, with point tenderness.
- **Adhesive capsulitis:** symptoms include limited and painful range of shoulder motion.

- **Calcific periarthritis:** only a third may be symptomatic (shoulder pain).
- **Limited joint mobility:** painless decrease in motion, decreased grip strength (also seen with Dupuytren's contracture).
- **Stiff-person disease:** primarily affects spine and lower extremities and associated with autoimmune diseases (like T1DM).
- **Diabetic muscle infarction:** usually affects lower extremities but may very rarely affect upper extremities. Bilateral in one-third of cases, recurrence at same site in 50% of cases; pain, swelling, and tenderness and may be associated with a mild fever.
- **Osteoarthritis:** joint pain; most common site is knee.

CLINICAL TREATMENT
General

- **Limited joint mobility:** optimize glycemic control, discontinue smoking, physical therapy for passive stretching. Little evidence exists for drug therapy but penicillamine and aldose reductase inhibitors have been used as well as glucocorticoid injections (Kapoor).
- **Stiff-person disease:** most effective treatments are benzodiazepines and exercise (Duddy).
- **Diabetic muscle infarction:** best treatment unclear but options include (1) rest and analgesics; (2) antiplatelet agents and/or anti-inflammatories; or (3) surgical removal (Trujillo-Santos).
- **Osteoarthritis:** physical therapy, NSAIDs, glucocorticoid injections, surgery for replacement of joint (Crosby).

Hand

- **Carpal tunnel syndrome:** exclude hypothyroidism; options include splinting wrist, NSAIDs, glucocorticoid injections, and surgery (Preston).
- **Dupuytren's contracture:** for mild disease, passive stretching and lanolin massage; for more advanced disease, glucocorticoid injection of nodules and surgery to release the fascia (Trojian).
- **Flexor tenosynovitis:** glucocorticoid injection or surgery; repeat surgeries occasionally necessary (Ryzewicz).

Shoulder

- **Adhesive capsulitis:** physical therapy, glucocorticoid injection, hydroplasty (intraarticular dilation), and, as a last resort, surgery (Sheridan).
- **Calcific periarthritis:** joint aspiration, glucocorticoid injection, or surgical removal (Siegal).

Feet

- **Charcot joint (or foot):** See Charcot Joint Disease (Diabetic Neuropathic Osteoarthropathy), p. 302.

FOLLOW-UP

- Many treatments require referrals to specialists such as a rheumatologist, dermatologist, orthopedic surgeon, or physical therapist.

EXPERT OPINION

- MSDs are commonly seen in diabetes.
- Good glycemic control, regular physical activity, and the cessation of smoking may decrease the risk of some MSDs.
- Diabetes-associated MSDs should be considered in persons with diabetes who complain of joint pain or decreased movement.
- Appropriate management often involves referral to a specialist.

COMPLICATIONS AND COMORBIDITIES

REFERENCES

Siegal DS, Wu JS, Newman JS, et al. Calcific tendinitis: a pictorial review. *Can Assoc Radiol J,* 2009; Vol. 60: pp. 263–72.
  Comments: A review of calcific tendinitis with examples of radiographic findings.

Duddy ME, Baker MR. Stiff person syndrome. *Front Neurol Neurosci,* 2009; Vol. 26: pp. 147–65.
  Comments: Review of stiff-person syndrome.

Feydy A, Pluot E, Guerini H, et al. Role of imaging in spine, hand, and wrist osteoarthritis. *Rheum Dis Clin North Am,* 2009; Vol. 35: pp. 605–49.
  Comments: Review of imaging in osteoarthritis.

Crosby J. Osteoarthritis: managing without surgery. *J Fam Pract,* 2009; Vol. 58: pp. 354–61.
  Comments: Review of nonsurgical treatment of osteoarthritis.

Doran M. Rheumatoid arthritis and diabetes mellitus: evidence for an association? *J Rheumatol,* 2007; Vol. 34: pp. 460–2.
  Comments: Discussion of the links between diabetes and rheumatoid arthritis.

Simard JF, Mittleman MA. Prevalent rheumatoid arthritis and diabetes among NHANES III participants aged 60 and older. *J Rheumatol,* 2007; Vol. 34: pp. 469–73.
  Comments: NHANES III examination of the association between diabetes and rheumatoid arthritis. No significant association was found.

Trojian TH, Chu SM. Dupuytren's disease: diagnosis and treatment. *Am Fam Physician,* 2007; Vol. 76: pp. 86–9.
  Comments: Review of Dupuytren's contracture.

Ryzewicz M, Wolf JM. Trigger digits: principles, management, and complications. *J Hand Surg Am,* 2006; Vol. 31: pp. 135–46.
  Comments: Description of stenosing flexor tenosynovitis.

Sheridan MA, Hannafin JA. Upper extremity: emphasis on frozen shoulder. *Orthop Clin North Am,* 2006; Vol. 37: pp. 531–9.
  Comments: Description of adhesive capsulitis and frozen shoulder.

Lindsay JR, Kennedy L, Atkinson AB, et al. Reduced prevalence of limited joint mobility in type 1 diabetes in a UK clinic population over a 20-year period. *Diabetes Care,* 2005; Vol. 28: pp. 658–61.
  Comments: Decreased prevalence of limited joint mobility from 1981–2002 (from 43%–23%). Authors hypothesized this was due to better glycemic control.

Trujillo-Santos AJ. Diabetic muscle infarction: an underdiagnosed complication of long-standing diabetes. *Diabetes Care,* 2003; Vol. 26: pp. 211–5.
  Comments: Systematic review of case reports of diabetic muscle infarction. 166 episodes were found in the literature.

Smith LL, Burnet SP, McNeil JD. Musculoskeletal manifestations of diabetes mellitus. *Br J Sports Med,* 2003; Vol. 37: pp. 30–5.
  Comments: Review of various arthropathies seen in diabetes, including adhesive capsulitis.

Cagliero E, Apruzzese W, Perlmutter GS, et al. Musculoskeletal disorders of the hand and shoulder in patients with diabetes mellitus. *Am J Med,* 2002; Vol. 112: pp. 487–90.
  Comments: 200 diabetes and 100 nondiabetes patients enrolled and examined for hand and shoulder disorders. MSDs of hand and shoulder found in 39% of persons with diabetes and 9% of controls.

Frost D, Beischer W. Limited joint mobility in type 1 diabetic patients: associations with microangiopathy and subclinical macroangiopathy are different in men and women. *Diabetes Care,* 2001; Vol. 24: pp. 95–9.
  Comments: Limited joint movement is associated with microvascular disease in men.

Gudmundsson KG, Arngrimsson R, Jónsson T. Eighteen year follow-up study of the clinical manifestations and progression of Dupuytren's disease. *Scand J Rheumatol,* 2001; Vol. 30: pp. 31–4.
  Comments: Cohort to study progression of Dupuytren's contracture; not limited to persons with diabetes.

Helfgott SM. Stiff-man syndrome: from the bedside to the bench. *Arthritis Rheum,* 1999; Vol. 42: pp. 1312–20.
  Comments: Review of the stiff-person syndrome and its association with diabetes.

Balci N, Balci MK, Tüzüner S. Shoulder adhesive capsulitis and shoulder range of motion in type II diabetes mellitus: association with diabetic complications. *J Diabetes Complications,* 1999; Vol. 13: pp. 135–40.
  Comments: Shoulder adhesive capsulitis was found in 29%; associated with other MSDs, increasing age, duration of diabetes, retinopathy.

Preston DC, Shapiro BE. Median neuropathy. In *Electromyography and Neuromuscular Disorders: Clinical-Electrophysiologic Correlations.* Boston: Butterworth-Heinemann; 1998.
  Comments: Description of carpal tunnel syndrome.

Arkkila PE, Kantola IM, Viikari JS. Limited joint mobility in type 1 diabetic patients: correlation to other diabetic complications. *J Intern Med,* 1994; Vol. 236: pp. 215–23.
  Comments: Limited joint mobility found in 58% of persons with diabetes and 14% of controls. Limited joint mobility was associated with duration of diabetes, retinopathy, and nephropathy.

Gamstedt A, Holm-Glad J, Ohlson CG, et al. Hand abnormalities are strongly associated with the duration of diabetes mellitus. *J Intern Med,* 1993; Vol. 234: pp. 189–93.
  Comments: Cross-sectional study of 100 persons with diabetes; one hand abnormality found in 50%, more than one abnormalities found in 26%. Associated with duration of diabetes but not glycemic control.

Eadington DW, Patrick AW, Frier BM. Association between connective tissue changes and smoking habit in type 2 diabetes and in non-diabetic humans. *Diabetes Res Clin Pract,* 1991; Vol. 11: pp. 121–5.
  Comments: Cigarette smoking was associated with limited joint mobility and Dypuytren's contracture in persons with and without diabetes.

Hochberg MC. Epidemiology of osteoarthritis: current concepts and new insights. *J Rheumatol Suppl,* 1991; Vol. 27: pp. 4–6.
  Comments: Review of several studies for prevalence of osteoarthritis.

Mavrikakis ME, Drimis S, Kontoyannis DA, et al. Calcific shoulder periarthritis (tendinitis) in adult onset diabetes mellitus: a controlled study. *Ann Rheum Dis,* 1989; Vol. 48: pp. 211–4.
  Comments: Examination of calcific shoulder periarthritis (tendinitis)—32% of patients with diabetes had shoulder calcification compared to 10% of the control group.

Chaudhuri KR, Davidson AR, Morris IM. Limited joint mobility and carpal tunnel syndrome in insulin-dependent diabetes. *Br J Rheumatol,* 1989; Vol. 28: pp. 191–4.
  Comments: Carpal tunnel is present in 75% of persons with diabetes who have limited joint mobility.

Kapoor A, Sibbitt WL. Contractures in diabetes mellitus: the syndrome of limited joint mobility. *Semin Arthritis Rheum,* 1989; Vol. 18: pp. 168–80.
  Comments: Description of limited joint mobility.

Pal B, Anderson J, Dick WC, et al. Limitation of joint mobility and shoulder capsulitis in insulin- and non-insulin-dependent diabetes mellitus. *Br J Rheumatol,* 1986; Vol. 25: pp. 147–51.
  Comments: Limitation of shoulder mobility found in 49% of patients with T1DM, 52% of patients with T2DM, and 20% of controls. Those with joint limitations had longer duration of diabetes and increased prevalence of retinopathy. Shoulder capsulitis was found in 19% of persons with diabetes and 5% of controls.

Noble J, Heathcote JG, Cohen H. Diabetes mellitus in the aetiology of Dupuytren's disease. *J Bone Joint Surg Br,* 1984; Vol. 66: pp. 322–5.
  Comments: 42% of persons with diabetes had signs of Dupuytren's contracture.

COMPLICATIONS AND COMORBIDITIES

OSTEOMYELITIS

See Osteomyelitis, p. 274.

VITAMIN D

See Vitamin D, p. 553.

WOUND HEALING

See Wound Healing, p. 279.

Neurologic Diseases

PERIPHERAL NEUROPATHY

Michael Polydefkis, MD, MHS, and Donna Westervelt, CRNP, MS, CDE

DEFINITION

- Diabetic peripheral neuropathy (DPN) is the most common neuropathy in diabetes.
- DPN is a length-dependent, sensory predominant peripheral neuropathy in which symptoms begin at the distal ends of the longest peripheral nerves (i.e., those that extend to the feet).
- Neuropathy in a person with diabetes may not be due to diabetes alone (Gorson).

EPIDEMIOLOGY

- DPN prevalence varies from ~25% when assessed with questionnaires or simple examination to ~70%, when assessed using peripheral nerve tests such as autonomic function testing, nerve conduction testing, and quantitative sensory testing (Laughlin).
- Risk factors for DPN include poor glycemic control, duration of diabetes, and cardiovascular risk factors such as hypertension, elevated cholesterol, tobacco use, and hypertryglyceridemia. Height and BMI also increase risk.
- DPN can occur early in diabetes, can be a presenting symptom, and can be associated with impaired glucose tolerance (IGT).
- DPN is an established risk factor for amputation.

DIAGNOSIS

- The diagnosis of DPN is made on the basis of patient history, physical examination, and diagnostic testing (England).
- Neuropathy usually begins in the toes and feet and spreads in a caudal to rostral fashion.
- Bedside sensory examination tests include monofilament, vibratory threshold, proprioception, and pinprick tests. These assess different types of sensory nerves. Loss of sensation in the toes and feet can be detected by each of these measures though the exact sequence can vary among individual patients.
- Loss of monofilament sensation (called loss of protective sensation) is an established risk factor for diabetic foot ulceration and subsequent amputation.
- Electrophysiological changes associated with diabetic peripheral neuropathy are measured with the nerve conduction test, which assesses large, myelinated sensory nerve fibers. A reduction in conduction velocity represents demyelination of large sensory axons while a reduction in nerve amplitude represents axon loss. It is possible for patients to have DPN and show normal results to this test because the tested fibers comprise only 20% of sensory nerve fibers.
- Punch skin biopsy is a relatively noninvasive test that requires 3-mm skin punches to be taken. After histological processing, nerve fibers can be viewed. This test assesses small unmyelinated sensory nerve fibers and is a more sensitive measure of DPN than nerve conduction velocity (NCV) testing (Griffin).
- Patients with IGT-associated DPN typically have abnormal skin biopsies that gradually involve large myelinated nerve fibers.
- Other diagnostic tests include quantitative sensory testing and detailed autonomic testing.

COMPLICATIONS AND COMORBIDITIES

SIGNS AND SYMPTOMS

- Symptoms of DPN are symmetric, sensory, and follow the caudal to rostral (foot to head) pattern. They vary widely from pronounced neuropathic pain, to little or no symptoms.
- Sometimes, an absence of sensation (numbness) is the predominant symptom, while other patients experience pronounced neuropathic pain.
- The pain of DPN is often described as burning, which can be associated with electric-like shocks.
- Patients also complain of a "pins and needles" tingling that can be painful and annoying. Symptoms often made worse by prolonged standing or walking, are typically worse at night, and can be associated with allodynia that interferes with sleep.
- When symptoms reach the level of the knee in the lower extremities, symptoms in the fingers also usually begin to develop. Similarly, patients can develop symptoms over the anterior chest and abdomen when symptoms extend to the level of the elbows in the upper extremities. It would not be typical, however, to have symptoms in the hands but not feet.
- Patients can develop little or no DPN despite years of poorly controlled diabetes, while others develop signs and symptoms very early.
- DPN can be seen in impaired glucose states (i.e., IGT).

CLINICAL TREATMENT

Prevention

- The best preventative treatment for DPN is improved glycemic control. This will result in a slower rate of progression, and can also stabilize existing peripheral neuropathy.
- Improved glycemic control is unlikely to result in reversal of DPN; peripheral nerve function will not usually improve once lost, although many patients note reduced pain levels with improved glycemic control.

Regenerative Strategies

- There is no FDA-approved agent for the treatment, reversal, or stabilization of DPN although as a class, aldose reductase inhibitors (ARI) have shown promise. Agents within this class have been withdrawn in some countries due to hepatic or renal toxicity, while another is actively used in Japan. There is a large trial of an ARI compound, ranirestat, underway in the US and Europe (Oates).

Symptomatic Treatment

- Two FDA approved agents are available for treatment of DPN-associated neuropathic pain—duloxetine and pregabalin—as well as several classes of agents such as tricyclic antidepressants and opiates that have consistently demonstrated efficacy. See Treatment of Neuropathic Pain, p. 534.

FOLLOW-UP

- Follow-up of a patient with DPN requires routine, detailed examinations, as well as repeated counseling and education.
- Be aware of other causes of neuropathy that can affect people with diabetes and lead to rapid progression of neurologic disability. If rapid changes occur, consider vitamin deficiencies, toxic exposures, or autoimmune neuropathies.
- Metformin may interfere with vitamin B12 absorption, and B12 levels should be checked to rule out B12 deficiency as a cause of neuropathy (Bell).

EXPERT OPINION

- Diagnostic testing consisting of screening laboratory studies, NCV testing, and/ or punch skin biopsies are appropriate to confirm the diagnosis of DPN and rule out other causes. Other conditions such as lumbar radiculopathy, focal nerve entrapments, and intrinsic foot disorders (plantar fasciitis or arthropathies) can mimic DPN.

- Reevaluate if distinct change of symptoms: development of weakness, changes in neuropathic pain, or development of a non-length-dependent pattern.

- Focus on glycemic control as well as cardiovascular risk factors, since hypertension and elevated cholesterol also contribute to DPN (Tesfaye).

- Some studies have shown an association between statin medications and peripheral neuropathy, although there is not enough evidence to justify discontinuing use in patients with DM, given the cardiovascular benefits of statins.

- Surgical decompression of nerves has been proposed as a treatment for DPN. With proven focal demyelination due to compression, surgical decompression is clinically indicated; but it is not clear that surgical decompression of nerves improves symptoms of DPN itself.

REFERENCES

Bell DS. Metformin-induced vitamin B12 deficiency presenting as a peripheral neuropathy. *South Med J,* 2010; Vol. 103: pp. 265–7.
> **Comments:** A recent report that metformin may interfere with B12 absorption.

Laughlin RS, Dyck PJ, Melton LJ, et al. Incidence and prevalence of CIDP and the association of diabetes mellitus. *Neurology,* 2009; Vol. 73: pp. 39–45.
> **Comments:** Review of chronic inflammatory demyelinating polyneuropathy (CIDP) in diabetes.

England JD, Gronseth GS, Franklin G, et al. Practice parameter: evaluation of distal symmetric polyneuropathy: role of laboratory and genetic testing (an evidence-based review). Report of the American Academy of Neurology, American Association of Neuromuscular and Electrodiagnostic Medicine, and American Academy of Physical Medicine and Rehabilitation. *Neurology,* 2009; Vol. 72: pp. 185–92.
> **Comments:** A recent practice parameter on diagnosis of peripheral neuropathy.

Oates PJ. Aldose reductase, still a compelling target for diabetic neuropathy. *Curr Drug Targets,* 2008; Vol. 9: pp. 14–36.
> **Comments:** A pertinent review of ARI trials and their potential for success.

Gorson KC, Ropper AH. Additional causes for distal sensory polyneuropathy in diabetic patients. *J Neurol Neurosurg Psychiatry,* 2006; Vol. 77: pp. 354–8.
> **Comments:** A first-rate review of other causes of neuropathy in diabetes.

Tesfaye S, Chaturvedi N, Eaton SE, et al. Vascular risk factors and diabetic neuropathy. *NEJM,* 2005; Vol. 352: pp. 341–50.
> **Comments:** An excellent longitudinal study that demonstrates cardiovascular risk factors associated with DPN.

Griffin JW, McArthur JC, Polydefkis M. Assessment of cutaneous innervation by skin biopsies. *Curr Opin Neurol,* 2001; Vol. 14: pp. 655–9.
> **Comments:** Reviews the role of different nerve fibers in peripheral neuropathy and for skin biopsy in diagnosis.

Brownlee M. Biochemistry and molecular cell biology of diabetic complications. *Nature,* 2001; Vol. 414: pp. 813–20.
> **Comments:** A detailed review of the postulated pathogenesis of DPN with a focus on oxidative stress.

COMPLICATIONS AND COMORBIDITIES

AMYOTROPHY

Michael Polydefkis, MD, MHS

DEFINITION

- An underdiagnosed condition referred to by different names including "diabetic proximal amyotrophy," "diabetic lumbosacral plexopathy," "diabetic lumbosacral radiculoplexopathy," "ischemic mononeuropathy multiplex," "femoral-sciatic neuropathy," "femoral neuropathy," "diabetic cachexia," and "Bruns-Garland syndrome."
- Classically, a monophasic illness characterized by acute or subacute, progressive, asymmetrical lower limb muscle weakness (i.e., back, buttocks, or thigh) a few weeks after severe pain onset with variable degrees of recovery.
- Patients typically also have diabetic peripheral neuropathy (DPN).
- Differentiated from diabetic polyneuropathy by the spatial pattern of involvement, time course, and prominent motor involvement.
- Important to diagnose diabetic amyotrophy (DA) because treatment differs from DPN.

EPIDEMIOLOGY

- Epidemiology not well established, but overall prevalence estimated at ~1%; more common in T2DM than T1DM.
- Classically occurs in middle- to older-aged adults, but also described in children.
- Increasing evidence that an immune-mediated inflammatory microvasculitis, resulting in ischemic nerve damage, may be the underlying pathogenic process (Chan).
- Often associated with poor glycemic control.

DIAGNOSIS

- Diagnosis based on clinical presentation, distinction from DPN, and electrodiagnostic testing.
- Hallmark is proximal lower extremity weakness that may be asymmetric.
- **Electrodiagnostic findings:** multifocal denervation in paraspinous and leg muscles on EMG and reduced sensory and motor action potentials on nerve conduction testing.
- **Nerve biopsy:** rarely required to make the diagnosis. Pathologic findings notable for ischemic injury and microvasculitis, prompting physicians to treat DA with immunomodulating therapies when diagnosed early, although no evidence of benefit (Chan).
- **Lumbar puncture:** CSF protein often elevated.
- **MRI:** imaging of the lumbar spine and lumbosacral plexus can be helpful to exclude infiltrating disorders in subacute cases.
- Conditions that can mimic DA include ALS, mononeuropathy multiplex, limb girdle muscular dystrophy, acute radiculopathies, and other plexopathies such as carcinomatous infiltration or radiation plexitis.

SIGNS AND SYMPTOMS

- Pain is severe; even stoic patients may seek emergency care, requiring multiple agents including opiates.
- Weakness also not subtle and typically 50% of patients will be wheelchair dependent.

- Proximal leg muscles weakness (quadriceps, hip flexors, extensors) compared to distal sensation abnormalities in DPN.
- Knee reflex usually absent.
- Symptoms progress over months; mean 6.2 months in one case series (Bastron).
- However, duration may be variable, ranging from a few months to several years.
- Usually unilateral, though it can be bilateral or even involve thoracic nerves.
- Patients often have substantial concomitant weight loss that approaches 50 lbs.
- Rarely a presenting complication of diabetes.

CLINICAL TREATMENT

- Early diagnosis critical for therapeutic intervention such as steroids or intravenous immunoglobulin (IVIg).
- Immunotherapy options consist of IVIg or IV methylprednisolone (MP). MP will increase blood glucose or insulin requirement (see Steroid-Induced Diabetes, p. 149) and IVIg carries risk of acute renal failure. Patients with glomerular filtration rate (GRF) <50 ml/min should be especially well hydrated and monitored closely.
- Recovery occurs more slowly without medical treatment, although definitive evidence is lacking due to the rarity of the condition.
- Treatment is otherwise largely supportive, including pain medication and physical therapy. Hospitalization is rarely needed.
- Treat patients who become wheelchair- or bed-bound for risk of DVT.
- Patients may require subacute rehabilitation and outpatient physical therapy.

FOLLOW-UP

- Most have a good functional recovery within 12–24 months. Occasional relapses can occur.
- Little evidence that glycemic control affects prognosis, although it is anecdotally recommended.

EXPERT OPINION

- Most important to recognize and diagnose DA, and distinguish it from DPN.
- While DA is more alarming compared to DPN, the prognosis is better.
- Though patients with DA typically do improve spontaneously, we, and most neurologists, treat with IVIg or IV methylprednisolone when diagnosed early.

REFERENCES

Chan YC, Lo YL, Chan ES. Immunotherapy for diabetic amyotrophy. *Cochrane Database Syst Rev*, 2009; CD006521.
   Comments: This systemic review of the literature found only one clinical trial for DA and concluded "there is presently no evidence from RCT to support any recommendation on the use of any immunotherapy treatment in diabetic amyotrophy."

Dyck PJB, Brien P, Bosch EP, et al. The multi-centre double-blind controlled trial of IV methylprednisolone in diabetic lumbosacral radiculoplexusneuropathy. *Neurology*, 2006; Vol. 66 (5, Suppl 2): p. A191.
   Comments: This abstract reports a trend toward a beneficial effect of IV methylprednisolone in DA.

Dyck PJ, Windebank AJ. Diabetic and nondiabetic lumbosacral radiculoplexus neuropathies: new insights into pathophysiology and treatment. *Muscle Nerve*, 2002; Vol. 25: pp. 477–91.
   Comments: Describes the pathology of DA from fascicular nerve biopsies.

Barohn RJ, Sahenk Z, Warmolts JR, et al. The Bruns-Garland syndrome (diabetic amyotrophy). Revisited 100 years later. *Arch Neurol*, 1991; Vol. 48: pp. 1130–5.
   Comments: An excellent historical review of DA as well as a case series that demonstrates the heterogeneity of DA presentations.

COMPLICATIONS AND COMORBIDITIES

Bastron JA, Thomas JE. Diabetic polyradiculopathy: clinical and electromyographic findings in 105 patients. *Mayo Clin Proc,* 1981; Vol. 56: pp. 725–32.

> Comments: Includes 105 patients with diabetic amyotrophy: age of onset 36–83 years; symptoms progressed over mean of 6.2 months; 9.5% of patients had painless muscle weakness.

Casey EB, Harrison MJ. Diabetic amyotrophy: a follow-up study. *Br Med J,* 1972; Vol. 1: pp. 656–9.

> Comments: Early case reports of DA describing age of onset and other clinical features.

AUTONOMIC NEUROPATHY

Michael Polydefkis, MD, MHS, and Kathleen Burks, MSN, CRNP

DEFINITION

- Diabetic autonomic neuropathy (DAN) is a common, underappreciated complication of diabetes with significant negative impact on survival and quality of life.
- Involvement of autonomic nerves in diabetes follows a length-dependent pattern. The longest autonomic nerve—the vagus nerve—is the first affected, and provides 75% of parasympathetic tone, with a broad range of effects.
- Later, loss of sympathetic nerve function can also occur.

EPIDEMIOLOGY

- Prevalence estimates of DAN depend on the criteria used and population studied. In general, rates increase with the degree of testing performed.
- In one population-based study, visceral autonomic neuropathy, based upon symptoms, had prevalence of 5.5% (Dyck).
- In contrast, another community-based study reported prevalence of DAN, as defined by abnormal heart rate variability (HRV) tests, of 16.7% (Ziegler).
- Cardiovascular autonomic neuropathy, defined as abnormal results in more than 2 of 6 autonomic function tests, among 1171 diabetic patients across 22 European diabetic centers was 25.3% for T1DM and 34.3% for T2DM (Zeigler).
- Patients with DAN are at increased risk of cardiovascular (CV) events and death. The usual diurnal variation in myocardial infarction (MI) is reversed in DAN patients, with less frequent MI in morning, more in the evening hours.
- Patients with DAN affecting cardiovascular system (C-DAN) have a 5-fold increase of mortality rate at 5 years compared to subjects without C-DAN. (Valensi).

DIAGNOSIS

- Diagnosis of DAN is based upon the organ system affected.
- Most prominent clinical autonomic signs and symptoms in diabetes include the pupil, sweat glands, genitourinary system, gastrointestinal tract system, adrenal medullary system, and the cardiovascular system.
- **C-DAN** causes abnormal heart rate (HR) control as well as abnormal central and peripheral vascular tone. Often presents as increased resting HR due to preferential loss of vagal parasympathetic tone, but increased HR variability, with reduced cardiac ejection fraction, systolic dysfunction, and decreased diastolic filling, may be the earliest indicators of C-DAN. With progression, HR can become fixed due to loss of both sympathetic and parasympathetic function.

- Orthostatic hypotension (a fall in systolic BP >30 mmHg upon standing) is also common, attributed to loss of sympathetic innervation of splanchnic vasomotor fibers and reduced peripheral resistance.
- C-DAN diagnosis may require tilt-table, or heart rate variability testing, in an EMG and/ or cardiac clinical laboratory.
- **Sudomotor dysfunction:** anhidrosis of the extremities, sometimes accompanied by compensatory hyperhidrosis in the trunk. With progression, diffuse anhidrosis.
- Gustatory sweating—abnormal sweating over the face, head, neck, shoulders, and chest after eating—can also be seen.
- Formal diagnosis of sudomotor dysfunction: detailed assessment of sweat production either through quantitative sweat axon reflex test (sweat production in response to the iontophoresis of acetylcholine) or a thermoregulatory sweat test (assessing territories of sweat production through the application of moisture sensitive powder. Subjects lie in a controlled sauna chamber and sweat production is detected by the powder changing color when it contacts moisture).
- **Gastrointestinal diabetic autonomic symptoms (GI-DAN):** common, often reflecting upper or lower GI autonomic neuropathy.
- GI symptoms reflect both the vagal nerve (responsible for esophageal and gastric motility) and intrinsic enteric neurons. Often impossible to distinguish between the two and diagnosis relies largely on motility studies such as esophageal scintigraphy and gastric emptying studies. Pathologically, abnormalities in gastric mucosal innervation.
- Delayed gastric emptying can lead to bezoars in stomach that also interfere with nutrient delivery to the small bowel and cause unstable diabetes.
- Diabetic diarrhea is typically profuse, watery, lasting hours or days and frequently alternates with constipation (see Gastroparesis, p. 244).
- **Erectile Dysfunction (ED):** multifactorial, including neuropathy, vascular disease, metabolic control, nutrition, endocrine disorders, psychogenic factors, and medications. Parasympathetic dysfunction of the penis results in reduced relaxation of the corpus cavernosa and reduced blood flow (see Erectile Dysfunction, p. 291).
- **Neurogenic bladder:** diagnosed by a postvoid residual volume of >150 ml, and a risk factor for urinary infections (UTIs). More than two UTIs in a year suggests possible neurogenic bladder. The bladder is innervated by sympathetic, parasympathetic, and somatic nerves and the earliest signs of dysfunction in diabetes are related to impaired bladder sensation producing an elevated micturition reflex threshold (see Bladder Disorders in Diabetes, p. 384).

SIGNS AND SYMPTOMS

- Clinical symptoms of autonomic neuropathy DAN generally do not occur until long after the onset of diabetes. Subclinical autonomic dysfunction, however, can occur within a year of diagnosis in type 2 diabetes (T2DM) and within 5 years in type 1 diabetes (T1DM).
- Symptoms of DAN are based upon the organ system involved.
- **C-DAN:** symptoms typically include dizziness, weakness, fatigue, and visual blurring. Symptoms of more advanced C-DAN include postural hypotension, exercise intolerance, asymptomatic cardiac ischemia, and intraoperative cardiovascular lability. C-DAN also confers an increased risk of death due to MI.

COMPLICATIONS AND COMORBIDITIES

- **Sudomotor dysfunction:** symptoms are typically subtle, including heat intolerance and central hyperhydrosis. Lack of sweat production in the feet is believed to predispose patients to ulcer formation.
- **GI-DAN:** classified into upper and lower GI involvement. Upper GI include heartburn, dysphagia for solids, early satiety, anorexia, nausea, vomiting, epigastric discomfort, and bloating, while lower GI involvement causes alternating diarrhea and constipation.
- **ED:** See Erectile Dysfunction, p. 291.
- **Neurogenic bladder:** symptoms are variable and include hesitancy in micturition, weak stream, and dribbling. Ultimately, incomplete bladder emptying, bladder overdistension, and urine retention predispose patients to UTIs.

CLINICAL TREATMENT

- **C-DAN:** Intensive glycemic and multifactorial treatment slows C-DAN (Gaede) and there is evidence that pharmaceutical-grade alpha-lipoic acid (not available in the US) slows the progression. Discontinue medications that can produce/aggravate orthostasis. Can treat orthostasis with mineralocorticoids (such as 9-å-fluorohydrocortisone, initiated at 0.1 mg/day and increased, as needed to 0.5 mg daily) and peripherally activing sympathomimetics (such as midodrine, dose titrated from 2.5 mg to 10 mg 3 times a day). Unfortunately, symptoms generally do not respond until fluid retention and edema develop.
- **Sudomotor dysfunction:** anticholinergic agents such as trihexyphenidyl, propantheline, or scopolamine, although efficacy limited by other anticholinergic effects, such as dry mouth, urinary retention, and constipation. Glycopyrolate is successful in some patients with gustatory sweating. Intracutaneous injection of botulinum toxin type A is useful as a focal treatment.
- **GI-DAN:** 4–6 small meals per day and reduction of dietary fat content also helpful. Prokinetic agents for gastroparesis include metoclopramide, domperidone, erythromycin, and levosulpiride. The severe and intermittent nature of diabetic diarrhea makes treatment and assessment difficult and best done in a GI clinic.
- **ED:** withdrawal of offending medications coupled with psychological counseling, medical treatment, or surgery. Medical treatment includes guanine monophosphate type-5 phosphodiesterase inhibitors that enhance blood flow to the corpora cavernosae with sexual stimulation. Other therapies include the injection of vasoactive substances such as papaverine, phentolamine, and prostaglandin E1 into the corpus cavernosum; transurethral delivery of vasoactive agents; and mechanical devices, such as a vacuum erection device or constricting rings. Penile prosthetic implants available if these therapies fail or are not tolerated by the patient.
- **Neurogenic bladder:** instruct patients to palpate bladder and, if they are unable to initiate micturition when bladder is full, use Crede's maneuver to start flow of urine every 4 hours. Parasympathomimetics such as bethanechol (10 to 30 mg 3 times a day) sometimes partially helps. Extended sphincter relaxation can be achieved with an alpha 1-blocker, such as doxazosin. Clean intermittent self-catheterization may also be necessary.

FOLLOW-UP

- Regular follow-up of patients with DAN to assess symptoms and effects of the medications.

- ADA consensus statement suggests that screening for DAN should be instituted at diagnosis for T2DM and 5 years after diagnosis for T1DM. Screening typically consists of a history and an examination for signs of autonomic dysfunction focusing on HR variability, including expiration-to-inspiration ratio and in response to Valsalva and standing.
- Repeat screening annually; if positive, appropriate diagnostic tests and symptomatic treatments should be instituted.

EXPERT OPINION

- Autonomic symptoms that produce disability or that affect QOL do occur.
- Systematic, annual review of autonomic symptoms is critical to diagnosis.
- Treatment is generally best reserved for specialized clinics.

REFERENCES

Pop-Busui R, Low PA, Waberski BH, et al. Effects of prior intensive insulin therapy on cardiac autonomic nervous system function in type 1 diabetes mellitus: the Diabetes Control and Complications Trial/Epidemiology of Diabetes Interventions and Complications study (DCCT/EDIC). *Circulation*, 2009; Vol. 119: pp. 2886–93.
   Comments: After 13–14 years follow-up from DCCT close-out, prevalence of cardiac autonomic neuropathy significantly lower in former intensive glycemia group (28.9%) versus former conventional glycemia group (35.2%, p=0.02).

Vinik AI, Ziegler D. Diabetic cardiovascular autonomic neuropathy. *Circulation*, 2007; Vol. 115: pp. 387–97.
   Comments: An excellent recent review of the cardiac manifestations of DAN.

Boulton AJ, Vinik AI, Arezzo JC, et al. Diabetic neuropathies: a statement by the American Diabetes Association. *Diabetes Care*, 2005; Vol. 28: pp. 956–62.
   Comments: ADA position statement for DPN.

Vinik AI, Maser RE, Mitchell BD, et al. Diabetic autonomic neuropathy. *Diabetes Care*, 2003; Vol. 26: pp. 1553–79.
   Comments: An older, but still relevant general review of autonomic neuropathy in diabetes.

Valensi P, Sachs RN, Harfouche B, et al. Predictive value of cardiac autonomic neuropathy in diabetic patients with or without silent myocardial ischemia. *Diabetes Care*, 2001; Vol. 24: pp. 339–43.
   Comments: Small study that assesses the predictive value of cardiac autonomic neuropathy on major cardiac events.

Gaede P, Vedel P, Parving HH, et al. Intensified multifactorial intervention in patients with type 2 diabetes mellitus and microalbuminuria: the Steno type 2 randomised study. *Lancet*, 1999; Vol. 353: pp. 617–22.
   Comments: An important study that demonstrated that intensive multifactorial intervention reduced C-DAN by 68%.

Dyck PJ, Kratz KM, Karnes JL, et al. The prevalence by staged severity of various types of diabetic neuropathy, retinopathy, and nephropathy in a population-based cohort: the Rochester Diabetic Neuropathy Study. *Neurology*, 1993; Vol. 43: pp. 817–24.
   Comments: A widely cited natural history study of diabetic neuropathy.

Ziegler D, Gries FA, Spüler M, et al. The epidemiology of diabetic neuropathy. Diabetic Cardiovascular Autonomic Neuropathy Multicenter Study Group. *J Diabetes Complications*, 1992; Vol. 6: pp. 49–57.
   Comments: Reviews epidemiology of diabetic neuropathy.

Pfeifer MA, Weinberg CR, Cook DL, et al. Autonomic neural dysfunction in recently diagnosed diabetic subjects. *Diabetes Care*, 1984; Vol. 7: pp. 447–53.
   Comments: Reviews the evidence that subclinical autonomic neuropathy can develop early in diabetes.

COMPLICATIONS AND COMORBIDITIES

STROKE

Martinson K. Arnan, MD, and Rebecca Gottesman, MD, PhD

DEFINITION

- Results from any disruption of blood flow to the brain, prolonged enough to cause cell death and manifesting as focal neurological symptoms.
- **Hemorrhagic strokes:** caused by blood leaking from blood vessels into brain tissue.
- **Ischemic strokes:** caused by an occlusion of a blood vessel.
- Ischemic strokes further subcategorized by mechanism or etiology of the stroke. Subcategories include strokes due to large vessel atherosclerosis, cardio-embolism, and small-vessel disease.
- Other causes of strokes include hypercoagulability, dissection, sickle cell disease, as well as some undetermined causes (Adams).

EPIDEMIOLOGY

- Stroke is the third leading cause of death in the US (American Heart Association).
- Stroke is the leading cause of disability in the US.
- More than 700,000 strokes diagnosed in the US every year; more than 160,000 of these result in death (American Heart Association).
- Diabetes is a predisposing factor for large vessel atherosclerosis and small-vessel disease, both of which can cause strokes.
- Persons with diabetes may also have other cardiovascular risk factors such as hypertension, obesity, and hyperlipidemia that predispose to stroke.
- Diabetes is an independent risk factor for strokes (US Preventive Services Task Force). There is a 2- to 5-fold increased risk for stroke in patients with type 2 diabetes compared to those without diabetes (Manson; Stamler).
- About 15%–33% of patients with ischemic strokes have diabetes (Karapanayiotides; Megherbi; Woo).
- Although diabetes is often associated with small vessel, lacunar-type strokes (Karapanayiotides), the presence of diabetes is associated with increased risk of other stroke subtypes, as well as including cardioembolic and other nonlacunar types (Abbott).
- Hemorrhagic strokes are less frequent in persons with diabetes compared to those without diabetes (Jorgensen).
- Aspirin use in diabetes is not associated with an increased risk of hemorrhagic strokes, although it may be in persons without diabetes (The ETDRS Investigators).
- A history of diabetes mellitus is associated with poorer outcomes after a stroke (Lindsberg).
- On average ~1/3 of patients admitted with an acute stroke are found to be hyperglycemic (Williams; Scott).
- The presence of hyperglycemia is associated with poorer outcomes among patients with ischemic strokes (Bruno, 1999; Bruno, 2002; Alvarez-Sabin). Hyperglycemia may be a marker of the severity of a stroke (Candelise).

DIAGNOSIS

- Based on patient history, physical examination (including the NIH stroke score) and confirmatory diagnostic tests.

- **Brain imaging:** confirms location, type, size, and age of stroke. Typically, a non-contrast head CT is obtained during initial evaluation. Brain MRIs are obtained in most patients since it has a higher sensitivity/specificity for identifying strokes.
- **Vascular imaging:** done with CT angiography, MR angiography, or ultrasound to ascertain the presence of vessel occlusion.
- **Perfusion images:** also obtained with CT or MRI to acutely detect salvageable at-risk brain.
- **Echocardiogram:** obtained to rule out a cardiac source for a clot. Usually a transthoracic echocardiogram is an appropriate first test.
- **Blood tests:** performed to identify conditions that can mimic strokes, or increase risk of stroke. Routine tests include serum glucose, electrolytes, ECGs, markers of cardiac ischemia, platelet counts, and coagulation profile.
- Often an infectious workup can be completed if warranted.
- Further testing should exclude other conditions that predispose patients to having strokes (i.e., lipid profile, blood pressure measurement, continuous telemetry to rule out paroxysmal atrial fibrillation [Christensen]).

SIGNS AND SYMPTOMS

- Depend on the part of the brain that is involved.
- However, in all strokes, symptom onset is almost always sudden.
- Common symptoms include: (1) numbness and/or weakness over face, arm and/or leg; (2) trouble speaking or understanding people; (3) dizziness, gait instability or unsteadiness, and loss of coordination; (4) visual disturbance (Lloyd-Jones) including diplopia, unilateral vision loss, or a visual field cut.
- Hemorrhagic strokes more often associated with headache, nausea, and vomiting; otherwise, strokes rarely cause pain.
- Reappearance of old neurological deficits in the setting of an infection or glucose abnormalities (both hypoglycemia and hyperglycemia) can be mistaken for a stroke.
- Rarely, hypoglycemia can cause focal neurologic signs and symptoms, and can mimic stroke-like symptoms (Wallis), even in the absence of prior history of clinical stroke.

CLINICAL TREATMENT

Prevention

- **Glycemic control:** similar to other forms of macrovascular disease, long-term follow-up of the UK Prospective Diabetes Study and the Diabetes Control and Complications Trial (EDIC) suggest that glycemic control is important to reduce risk.
- **Hypertension:** high blood pressure directly related to risk of ischemic stroke (Rodgers). Risk of stroke decreases by 30%–40% with blood pressure lowering (Lawes). Among persons with diabetes, those with well-controlled blood pressure have 44% reduced risk of stroke compared to those who do not (UKPDS 38).
- **Hyperlipidemia:** goal LDL <70 mg/dl (Grundy). In the Heart Protection Study, statin use decreased risk of strokes by 28% among persons with diabetes, independent of baseline LDL, preexisting vascular disease, type or duration of diabetes, or adequacy of glycemic control (Collins).
- **Smoking cessation**
- **Lifestyle modification:** multiple large-scale prospective studies have shown that being overweight is associated with an increased risk of stroke in a dose-response fashion (Rexrode; Kurth; Song).

COMPLICATIONS AND COMORBIDITIES

- The Look AHEAD trial, a randomized trial of intensive lifestyle interventions in diabetes, will include analysis of cardiovascular outcomes such as stroke at study completion, but interim analysis has already shown significant reductions in cardiovascular risk factors (The Look AHEAD Research Group).
- Although stroke risk calculators not typically used in clinical practice, may be useful in some patients who need to fully understand their risk for stroke before implementing lifestyle changes. Available risk engines include the UKPDS 60.

Acute Stroke Management

- Decision to safely administer thrombolytics depends on duration of symptoms so knowing exact time of symptom onset is important. If a patient awakes from sleep with symptoms, the time of symptom onset is assumed to be the last time patient was seen normal.
- Administration of intravenous (IV) tissue plasminogen activator (tPA) within 4.5 hours of symptom onset significantly decreases the devastating effects of ischemic strokes (Hacke).
- Patients with an anterior circulation territory stroke who are ineligible for IV tPA but are within a 6-hour window may be candidates for intraarterial (IA) tPA (Chalela; Choi). For posterior circulation strokes, window for IA tPA may even be extended to 24 hours (Ogawa). Both treatments require coordination with interventional radiology and involvement of vascular neurologists.
- Clot retrieval devices are actively being studied as a means of reestablishing flow in an artery that is occluded by a clot (Yu, Schumacher). The MERCI device from the Mechanical Embolus Removal in Cerebral Embolism (MERCI) trial is used at some centers for clot removal, although the utility of the device in improving post-stroke outcomes remains unclear (Smith).
- Most patients with acute ischemic stroke do not require anticoagulation during hospitalization. Individuals with apical thrombus or a mechanical heart valve may require anticoagulation soon after admission.
- Initiation of aspirin 325 mg within 24–48 h of acute ischemic stroke (Coull) is recommended. Aspirin may not significantly limit the consequences of the acute stroke but can help prevent recurrent strokes.
- For acute ischemic stroke, aggressive blood pressure management is associated with poorer outcomes (Castillo). Only intervene if blood pressure is >220 mmHg systolic, or >120 mmHg diastolic. A reasonable goal is to decrease the blood pressure by 15%–25% within the first day (Grossman). However, administering tPA is contraindicated if SBP >185 mmHg or DP >110 mmHg (The National Institute of Neurological Disorders and Stroke rt-PA Stroke Study Group).
- Blood glucose should be kept in the normoglycemic range during stroke management.
- Persistent hyperglycemia in the first 24 hours of a stroke is an independent predictor of stroke volume expansion (Baird). Because hyperglycemia increases the metabolic needs of the brain and may therefore worsen any brain edema, glycemic control is particularly important in the early period after stroke.
- Because IV contrast may be needed for CT angiography or conventional angiography, metformin should be held on admission to decrease risk of lactic acidosis.

FOLLOW-UP

- Detailed interim history to exclude complications of strokes such as seizures, pain syndromes, contractures, or depression.
- Detailed physical examination can help determine the rate of recovery; most patients will regain some, if not all, function, up to 1–1.5 years after their initial event.
- Optimize glycemic control.
- Check routine labs needed for risk factor modification (i.e., lipid panel).
- Antiplatelet medication such as aspirin, unless the stroke has a cardioembolic etiology, in which case warfarin is preferred.
- Ask about ongoing behavior/lifestyle modification such as smoking cessation, physical activity, weight reduction, maintaining a low-salt diet.
- Closely follow progress in physical, occupation, and/or speech therapies.
- Stroke risk increased in individuals with history of previous stroke. Patients with prior history of stroke need education on possible stroke symptoms, and benefit of seeking immediate emergency medical treatment if they experience any symptoms.

EXPERT OPINION

- Strokes in persons with diabetes are more common than the general population and are associated with poorer outcomes.
- Ischemic strokes are more common than hemorrhagic strokes in diabetes, and may be partially related to the presence of comorbidities such as hyperlipidemia and hypertension.
- Aspirin use can be safely used in diabetes and is not associated with increased risk of hemorrhagic strokes.
- Cardiovascular risk factor modification and glycemic control can reduce the risk of stroke.
- Lifestyle interventions can also decrease the risk of stroke.
- Early recognition of stroke symptoms and presentation to the hospital determines whether a patient is a candidate for thrombolytics and can affect stroke outcomes.
- Decisions about vascular or perfusion imaging approaches may be affected by presence of coexisting renal disease in individuals with diabetes due to risk for contrast nephropathy and/or nephrogenic systemic fibrosis.
- CT angiography or CT perfusion requires IV iodinated contrast, and MR perfusion or MR angiography of the neck (but not the head) requires gadolinium.
- A multidisciplinary approach including physical therapy, occupational therapy, and speech therapy is important for successful rehabilitation following stroke.

BASIS FOR RECOMMENDATIONS

Sacco RL, Adams R, Albers G, et al. Guidelines for prevention of stroke in patients with ischemic stroke or transient ischemic attack. *Stroke*, 2006; Vol. 37: pp. 577–617.

Comments: Describes recommendations for prevention of stroke, including a section on risk factor control in persons with diabetes.

OTHER REFERENCES

Look AHEAD Research Group, Wing RR. Long-term effects of a lifestyle intervention on weight and cardiovascular risk factors in individuals with type 2 diabetes mellitus: four-year results of the Look AHEAD trial. *Arch Intern Med*, 2010; Vol. 170: pp. 1566–75.

Comments: Effect of lifestyle interventions in diabetics on cardiovascular risk factors.

COMPLICATIONS AND COMORBIDITIES

Lloyd-Jones D, Adams R, Carnethon M, et al. Heart disease and stroke statistics—2009 update: a report from the American Heart Association Statistics Committee and Stroke Statistics Subcommittee. *Circulation*, 2009; Vol. 119: pp. e21–181.
Comments: Stroke statistics and symptoms.

Hacke W, Kaste M, Bluhmki E, et al. Thrombolysis with alteplase 3 to 4.5 hours after acute ischemic stroke. *NEJM*, 2008; Vol. 359: pp. 1317–29.
Comments: Alteplase use in acute stroke is safe in the 3- to 4.5-hour window.

Ogawa A, Mori E, Minematsu K, et al. Randomized trial of intraarterial infusion of urokinase within 6 hours of middle cerebral artery stroke: the middle cerebral artery embolism local fibrinolytic intervention trial (MELT) Japan. *Stroke*, 2007; Vol. 38: pp. 2633–9.
Comments: Clot lysis interventions in the posterior circulation may be done in an extended time window.

Choi JH, Bateman BT, Mangla S, et al. Endovascular recanalization therapy in acute ischemic stroke. *Stroke*, 2006; Vol. 37: pp. 419–24.
Comments: Time window for intra-arterial tPA.

Ohira T, Shahar E, Chambless LE, et al. Risk factors for ischemic stroke subtypes: the Atherosclerosis Risk in Communities study. *Stroke*, 2006; Vol. 37: pp. 2493–8.
Comments: Stroke in diabetic patients.

Christensen H, Fogh Christensen A, Boysen G. Abnormalities on ECG and telemetry predict stroke outcome at 3 months. *J Neurol Sci*, 2005; Vol. 234: pp. 99–103.
Comments: Stroke predictors.

Smith WS, Sung G, Starkman S, et al. Safety and efficacy of mechanical embolectomy in acute ischemic stroke: results of the MERCI trial. *Stroke*, 2005; Vol, 36: pp. 1432–8.
Comments: Safety and efficacy data for MERCI clot removal.

Karapanayiotides T, Piechowski-Jozwiak B, van Melle G, et al. Stroke patterns, etiology, and prognosis in patients with diabetes mellitus. *Neurology*, 2004: Vol. 62: pp. 1558–62.
Comments: Stroke in diabetic patients.

Lindsberg PJ, Roine RO. Hyperglycemia in acute stroke. *Stroke*, 2004; Vol. 35: pp. 363–4.
Comments: Stroke prognosis in diabetic patients.

Castillo J, Leira R, García MM, et al. Blood pressure decrease during the acute phase of ischemic stroke is associated with brain injury and poor stroke outcome. *Stroke*, 2004; Vol. 35: pp. 520–6.
Comments: Blood pressure management in acute stroke management.

Alvarez-Sabín J, Molina CA, Ribó M, et al. Impact of admission hyperglycemia on stroke outcome after thrombolysis: risk stratification in relation to time to reperfusion. *Stroke*, 2004; Vol. 35: pp. 2493–8.
Comments: Post-tPA stroke prognosis in the setting of hyperglycemia on admission.

Lawes CM, Bennett DA, Feigin VL, et al. Blood pressure and stroke: an overview of published reviews. *Stroke*, 2004; Vol. 35: pp. 776–5.
Comments: Effect of reduction of blood pressure management on strokes.

Grundy SM, Cleeman JI, Merz CN, et al. Implications of recent clinical trials for the National Cholesterol Education Program Adult Treatment Panel III guidelines. *Circulation*, 2004; Vol. 110: pp. 227–39.
Comments: Management of hyperlipidemia.

Song YM, Sung J, Davey Smith G, et al. Body mass index and ischemic and hemorrhagic stroke: a prospective study in Korean men. *Stroke*, 2004; Vol. 35: pp. 831–6.
Comments: Weight as a risk factor stroke in Korean men.

American Heart Association. *Heart Disease and Stroke Statistics—2004 Update*. Dallas, TX: American Heart Association; 2003.
Comments: Stroke statistics.

Megherbi SE, Milan C, Minier D, et al. Association between diabetes and stroke subtype on survival and functional outcome 3 months after stroke: data from the European BIOMED Stroke Project. *Stroke*, 2003; Vol. 34: pp. 688–94.
Comments: Diabetes and stroke subtypes.

Yu W, Binder D, Foster-Barber A, et al. Endovascular embolectomy of acute basilar artery occlusion. *Neurology*, 2003; Vol. 61: pp. 1421–3.
Comments: Mechanical clot removal of posterior circulation strokes.

Schumacher HC, Meyers PM, Yavagal DR, et al. Endovascular mechanical thrombectomy of an occluded superior division branch of the left MCA for acute cardioembolic stroke. *Cardiovasc Intervent Radiol*, 2003; Vol. 26: pp. 305–8.
Comments: Mechanical clot removal in MCA strokes.

Baird TA, Parsons MW, Phanh T, et al. Persistent poststroke hyperglycemia is independently associated with infarct expansion and worse clinical outcome. *Stroke*, 2003; Vol. 34: pp. 2208–14.
Comments: Hyperglycemia and infarct expansion.

Collins R, Armitage J, Parish S, et al. MRC/BHF Heart Protection Study of cholesterol-lowering with simvastatin in 5963 people with diabetes: a randomised placebo-controlled trial. *Lancet*, 2003; Vol. 361: pp. 2005–16.
Comments: Benefit of statin use.

Williams LS, Rotich J, Qi R, et al. Effects of admission hyperglycemia on mortality and costs in acute ischemic stroke. *Neurology*, 2002; Vol. 59: pp. 67–71.
Comments: Hyperglycemia in acute stroke patients.

Bruno A, Levine SR, Frankel MR, et al. Admission glucose level and clinical outcomes in the NINDS rt-PA Stroke Trial. *Neurology*, 2002; Vol. 59: pp. 669–74.
Comments: Relevance of admission serum glucose levels in stroke management.

Coull BM, Williams LS, Goldstein LB, et al. Anticoagulants and antiplatelet agents in acute ischemic stroke: report of the Joint Stroke Guideline Development Committee of the American Academy of Neurology and the American Stroke Association (a division of the American Heart Association). *Stroke*, 2002; Vol. 33: pp. 1934–42.
Comments: Aspirin use in acute strokes.

Kurth T, Gaziano JM, Berger K, et al. Body mass index and the risk of stroke in men. *Arch Intern Med*, 2002; Vol. 162: pp. 2557–62.
Comments: Weight as a risk factor for stroke in men.

Chalela JA, Katzan I, Liebeskind DS, et al. Safety of intra-arterial thrombolysis in the postoperative period. *Stroke*, 2001; Vol. 32: pp. 1365–9.
Comments: Safety of IA tPA.

Woo D, Gebel J, Miller R, et al. Incidence rates of first-ever ischemic stroke subtypes among blacks: a population-based study. *Stroke*, 1999; Vol. 30: pp. 2517–22.
Comments: Strokes in black diabetic patients.

Scott JF, Robinson GM, French JM, et al. Prevalence of admission hyperglycaemia across clinical subtypes of acute stroke. *Lancet*, 1999; Vol. 353: pp. 376–7.
Comments: Hyperglycemia in different stroke subtypes.

Bruno A, Biller J, Adams HP, et al. Acute blood glucose level and outcome from ischemic stroke. Trial of ORG 10172 in Acute Stroke Treatment (TOAST) Investigators. *Neurology*, 1999; Vol. 52: pp. 280–4.
Comments: Prognosis in acute strokes in the setting of hyperglycemia.

Grossman E, Ironi AN, Messerli FH. Comparative tolerability profile of hypertensive crisis treatments. *Drug Saf*, 1998; Vol. 19: pp. 99–122.
Comments: Treatment options for blood pressure management.

COMPLICATIONS AND COMORBIDITIES

UK Prospective Diabetes Study Group. Tight blood pressure control and risk of macrovascular and microvascular complications in type 2 diabetes: UKPDS 38. *BMJ*, 1998; Vol. 317: pp. 703–13.
Comments: Blood pressure management in diabetes.

Rexrode KM, Hennekens CH, Willett WC, et al. A prospective study of body mass index, weight change, and risk of stroke in women. *JAMA*, 1997; Vol. 277: pp. 1539–45.
Comments: Weight as a risk factor for stroke in women.

US Preventive Services Task Force. *Guide to Clinical Preventive Services*. 2nd ed. Baltimore, MD: Williams & Wilkins; 1996.
Comments: Primary prevention of stroke.

Rodgers A, MacMahon S, Gamble G, et al. Blood pressure and risk of stroke in patients with cerebrovascular disease. The United Kingdom Transient Ischaemic Attack Collaborative Group. *BMJ*, 1996; Vol. 313: pp. 147.
Comments: Blood pressure as a risk factor for stroke.

The National Institute of Neurological Disorders and Stroke rt-PA Stroke Study Group. Tissue plasminogen activator for acute ischemic stroke. *NEJM*, 1995; Vol. 333: pp. 1581–7.
Comments: Checklist for administering tPA safely.

Jørgensen H, Nakayama H, Raaschou HO, et al. Stroke in patients with diabetes. The Copenhagen Stroke Study. *Stroke*, 1994; Vol. 25: pp. 1977–84.
Comments: Types of strokes in diabetic patients.

Adams HP, Bendixen BH, Kappelle LJ, et al. Classification of subtype of acute ischemic stroke. Definitions for use in a multicenter clinical trial. TOAST. Trial of Org 10172 in Acute Stroke Treatment. *Stroke*, 1993; Vol. 24: pp. 35–41.
Comments: Classifies subtypes of stroke.

Stamler J, Vaccaro O, Neaton JD, et al. Diabetes, other risk factors, and 12-yr cardiovascular mortality for men screened in the Multiple Risk Factor Intervention Trial. *Diabetes Care*, 1993; Vol. 16: pp. 434–44.
Comments: Cardiovascular risk factors in men.

ETDRS Investigators. Aspirin effects on mortality and morbidity in patients with diabetes mellitus. Early Treatment Diabetic Retinopathy Study report 14. *JAMA*, 1992; Vol. 268: pp. 1292–300.
Comments: Aspirin is safe to use in diabetes.

Manson JE, Colditz GA, Stampfer MJ, et al. A prospective study of maturity-onset diabetes mellitus and risk of coronary heart disease and stroke in women. *Arch Intern Med*, 1991; Vol. 151: pp. 1141–7.
Comments: Cardiovascular risk factors in women.

Abbott RD, Donahue RP, MacMahon SW, et al. Diabetes and the risk of stroke. The Honolulu Heart Program. *JAMA*, 1987; Vol. 257: pp. 949–52.
Comments: Stroke in diabetic patients.

Candelise L, Landi G, Orazio EN, et al. Prognostic significance of hyperglycemia in acute stroke. *Arch Neurol*, 1985; Vol. 42: pp. 661–3.
Comments: Acute stroke prognosis in the setting of hyperglycemia.

Wallis WE, Donaldson I, Scott RS, et al. Hypoglycemia masquerading as cerebrovascular disease (hypoglycemic hemiplegia). *Ann Neurol*, 1985; Vol. 18: pp. 510–2.
Comments: Focal neurological symptoms in hypoglycemia.

Ophthalmologic Diseases

RETINOPATHY

Sachin D. Kalyani, MD

DEFINITION
- Retinal vascular complications of diabetes mellitus are classified into nonproliferative and proliferative forms.
- **Nonproliferative diabetic retinopathy (NPDR):** describes the earliest retinal changes of diabetic retinopathy, resulting from damage to the small blood vessels in the retina.
- **Proliferative diabetic retinopathy (PDR):** describes a later stage of retinopathy, with new growth of abnormal blood vessels on the surface of the retina.

EPIDEMIOLOGY
- Leading cause of new cases of blindness in US population, 20–74 years of age.
- There are 5000 new cases of legal blindness each year secondary to diabetic retinopathy.
- Duration of diabetes and severity of hyperglycemia is directly associated with an increased prevalence of diabetic retinopathy in people with both type 1 and type 2 diabetes.
- In the Wisconsin Epidemiological Study of Diabetic Retinopathy, after 20 years of diabetes, nearly 99% of patients with type 1 and >60% with type 2 diabetes had some degree of diabetic retinopathy.
- Frequency of diabetic retinopathy is higher among non-Hispanic blacks (27%) and Mexican Americans (33%) than in non-Hispanic whites (18%) over 40 years of age.

DIAGNOSIS
- **Mild NPDR:** defined as microaneurysms only.
- **Moderate NPDR:** defined as more than just microaneurysms (i.e., microhemorrhages, hard exudates, or cotton wool spots), but less than the definition for severe NPDR.
- **Severe NPDR:** NPDR 4:2:1 rule defined as presence of any 1 of the following, and very severe NPDR by 2 of the following: (1) diffuse intraretinal hemorrhages and microaneurysms in 4 quadrants; (2) venous beading in 2 quadrants; or (3) intraretinal microvascular abnormalities (IRMA) in 1 quadrant.
- **PDR:** new blood vessels, which are fragile and can easily bleed, form on the retina or iris.
- Severity of NPDR is significant in that laser photocoagulation may be indicated for more severe stages.
- Some patients will never develop NPDR or PDR.
- Dilated fundoscopic examination is the best way to diagnose diabetic retinopathy.
- In areas underserved by ophthalmologists, retinal photographs can also be used to make the diagnosis.

COMPLICATIONS AND
COMORBIDITIES

SIGNS AND SYMPTOMS

- **NPDR:** microaneurysms, dot-and-blot intraretinal hemorrhages, hard exudates, retinal edema, venous beading, intraretinal microvascular abnormalities (IRMA), cotton wool spots (nerve fiber layer infarcts), areas of capillary nonperfusion.
- **PDR:** Signs of NPDR in addition to neovascularization of the disc (NVD) or elsewhere in the retina (NVE), preretinal hemorrhage, vitreous hemorrhage, fibrovascular proliferation on posterior vitreous surface, tractional retinal detachment.
- Clinically significant macular edema (p. 339) can be seen at any stage of retinopathy, although more likely to be seen as retinopathy progresses.
- Frequently asymptomatic; may cause decreased, blurry, or fluctuating vision (which may also be due to refraction errors induced by hyperglycemia or hypoglycemia), floaters, difficulty with night vision, shadows, or areas of vision missing.

CLINICAL TREATMENT

Medical Management

- Principal goal is prevention of diabetic retinopathy by good glycemic control.
- The Diabetes Control and Complications Trial (DCCT): intensive glycemic control reduced the risk of new retinopathy by 76%, and slowed progression by 54%, in type 1 diabetes.
- The United Kingdom Prospective Diabetes Study (UKPDS): intensive control of blood glucose reduced the risk of microvascular complications by 25%, mostly due to the decreased need for retinal photocoagulation, in patients with type 2 diabetes.
- Also from UKPDS: intensive blood pressure control reduced microvascular complications by 37%, reduced progression of retinopathy by 34%, and reduced moderate vision loss by 47%.
- Hypertension, carotid artery occlusive disease, advanced diabetic renal disease, and anemia may have an adverse effect on diabetic retinopathy.
- The FIELDS study: treatment with fenofibrate in type 2 diabetes reduces the need for laser treatment for DR, independent of changes in plasma lipids.
- ACCORD Eye Study Group: recently reported that among participants with type 2 diabetes at high risk for cardiovascular disease, participants receiving intensive versus standard glycemic treatment ($<$6% vs 7%–7.9%) had 33% lower rate of retinopathy progression and fenofibrate and simvastatin versus simvastatin alone had 40% lower rates of retinopathy progression. No significant effect seen with intensive blood pressure control.
- Early Treatment Diabetic Retinopathy Study (ETDRS): aspirin has neither a beneficial nor harmful effect.
- Although antivascular endothelial growth factors are used in the treatment of severe NPDR and PDR, currently evidence is insufficient to recommend its routine use.
- Intravitreal injections of steroids may be considered in eyes with persistent loss of vision when conventional treatment has failed.
- Pregnancy is associated with a transient but reversible worsening of retinopathy.

Laser Treatment

- The mainstay of treatment for severe NPDR and PDR is thermal laser photocoagulation in a panretinal pattern to induce regression.
- The Diabetic Retinopathy Study (DRS) showed a 50% or greater reduction in severe visual loss with PDR or severe NPDR treated with panretinal photocoagulation (PRP) over 5 years.

Surgical Management

- Vitreous hemorrhage and tractional retinal detachment (both complications of PDR) may be treated surgically by vitrectomy.
- The goal of vitrectomy is to relieve vitreoretinal traction and to facilitate retinal reattachment.
- Diabetic Retinopathy Vitrectomy Study (DRVS): early vitrectomy was beneficial in type 1 diabetes with severe vitreous hemorrhage; however, there was no advantage in type 2 diabetes.
- Current recommendation: if PRP has not been performed, early surgical intervention is recommended for a severe vitreous hemorrhage due to PDR.
- Vitrectomy is indicated when progression of a tractional retinal detachment threatens the macula.

Recommendations for Performing Complete Ophthalmic History and Eye Examination (Including Dilated Funduscopic Exam)

- Type 1 diabetes: examine 5 years after onset of diabetes mellitus, then annually if no retinopathy is seen.
- Type 2 diabetes: examine at diagnosis, then annually if no retinopathy is seen.
- During diabetic pregnancy: examine before pregnancy, each trimester, and 3–6 months postpartum.
- See Table 3-13 for recommended timetable of testing based on retinopathy findings.

TABLE 3-13. TIMETABLE OF TESTING BASED ON RETINOPATHY FINDINGS

Retinal Abnormality	Suggested Follow-up
Normal or rare microaneurysms	Annually
Mild NPDR	Every 9 months
Moderate NPDR	Every 6 months
Severe NPDR	Every 4 months
Clinically significant macular edema	Every 2–4 months
PDR	Every 2–3 months

Source: Regillo C. Basic and clinical science course, section 12: retina and vitreous. American Academy of Ophthalmology, 2004–2005. Reprinted with permission from the American Academy of Ophthalmology, Inc., a Minnesota nonprofit corporation.

COMPLICATIONS AND COMORBIDITIES

EXPERT OPINION

- Important: significant DR can be entirely without symptoms.
- Vision loss may or may not be seen with retinopathy.
- The key to successful management of DR is to make the diagnosis early and treat appropriately to prevent development of further ophthalmic complications.
- Cataract surgery can worsen or cause progression of diabetic retinopathy.
- Diabetic retinopathy, including macular edema, should be treated prior to performing cataract surgery (if severity of cataract does not hinder view of the retina).

BASIS FOR RECOMMENDATIONS

Fong DS, Aiello L, Gardner TW, et al. for the American Diabetes Association. Retinopathy in diabetes. *Diabetes Care*, 2004; Vol. 27: pp. s84–87.

OTHER REFERENCES

ACCORD Study Group, ACCORD Eye Study Group, Chew EY, et al. Effects of medical therapies on retinopathy progression in type 2 diabetes. *NEJM*, 2010; Vol. 363: 233–44.

  Comments: The ACCORD Eye Study Group recently reported that in 2856 participants with type 2 diabetes at high risk for cardiovascular disease, participants who had intensive versus standard glycemic treatment (<6% vs 7%–7.9%) had 33% lower rate of retinopathy progression (7.3% vs 10.4%, p = 0.003). Those who had fenofibrate and simvastatin versus simvastatin alone also had 40% lower rates of retinopathy progression (6.5% vs 10.2%, p = 0.0006). However, no significant beneficial effect was seen with intensive blood pressure control (<120 mmHg) versus standard control (<140 mmHg).

Keech AC, Mitchell P, Summanen PA, et al. Effect of fenofibrate on the need for laser treatment for diabetic retinopathy (FIELD study): a randomised controlled trial. *Lancet*, 2007; Vol. 370: pp. 1687–97.

  Comments: Study showed that treatment with fenofibrate in individuals with type 2 diabetes mellitus reduces the need for laser treatment for diabetic retinopathy.

Mohamed Q, Gillies MC, Wong TY. Management of diabetic retinopathy: a systematic review. *JAMA*, 2007; Vol. 298: pp. 902–16.

  Comments: Objective was to review the best evidence for primary and secondary intervention in the management of diabetic retinopathy, including diabetic macular edema.

American Academy of Ophthalmology. Basic and Clinical Science Course, Section 12: *Retina and Vitreous*; 2004: pp. 99–112.

  Comments: Good summary in diabetic retinopathy chapter, including epidemiology, diagnosis, and treatment of the disease.

Kaiser PK, Friedman NJ, Pineda II R. *The Massachusetts Eye and Ear Infirmary Illustrated Manual of Ophthalmology.* Philadelphia: Elsevier Science, 2004; Vol. 2: pp. 317–22.

  Comments: Good summary in diabetic retinopathy chapter, including epidemiology, diagnosis, and treatment of the disease.

Eliott D, Lee MS, Abrams GW. Proliferative diabetic retinopathy: principles and techniques of surgical treatment. In Ryan, SJ, (Ed). *Retina.* 3rd edition. St. Louis: Mosby, 2001; Vol. 3: pp. 2436–76.

  Comments: Chapter with excellent summary on diabetic retinopathy.

Harris MI, Klein R, Cowie CC, et al. Is the risk of diabetic retinopathy greater in non-Hispanic blacks and Mexican Americans than in non-Hispanic whites with type 2 diabetes? A US population study. *Diabetes Care,* 1998; Vol. 21: pp. 1230–5.

  Comments: This study compared the risk for diabetic retinopathy in non-Hispanic white, non-Hispanic black, and Mexican-American adults with type 2 diabetes in the US population.

UK Prospective Diabetes Study (UKPDS) Group. Intensive blood-glucose control with sulphonylureas or insulin compared with conventional treatment and risk of complications in patients with type 2 diabetes (UKPDS 33). *Lancet*, 1998; Vol. 352: pp. 837–53.

  Comments: Results showed that intensive blood-glucose control by either sulphonylureas or insulin substantially decreases the risk of microvascular complications, but not macrovascular disease, in patients with type 2 diabetes.

UK Prospective Diabetes Study Group. Tight blood pressure control and risk of macrovascular and microvascular complications in type 2 diabetes: UKPDS 38. *BMJ*, 1998; Vol. 317: pp. 703–13.

  Comments: Study concluded that tight blood pressure control in patients with hypertension and type 2 diabetes achieves a clinically important reduction in the risk of deaths related to diabetes, complications related to diabetes, progression of diabetic retinopathy, and deterioration in visual acuity.

American Academy of Ophthalmology, Preferred Practice Patterns Committee. Retina Panel, Diabetic Retinopathy. San Francisco; 1998.

Comments: The American Academy of Ophthalmology's recommendations for follow-up of patients with diabetes and diabetic retinopathy.

Chew EY, Mills JL, Metzger BE, et al. Metabolic control and progression of retinopathy. The Diabetes in Early Pregnancy Study. National Institute of Child Health and Human Development Diabetes in Early Pregnancy Study. *Diabetes Care,* 1995; Vol. 18: pp. 631–7.

Comments: This study evaluated the role of metabolic control in the progression of diabetic retinopathy during pregnancy.

Diabetes Control and Complications Trial Research Group. Progression of retinopathy with intensive versus conventional treatment in the Diabetes Control and Complications Trial. *Ophthalmology,* 1995; Vol. 102: pp. 647–61.

Comments: More detailed analysis regarding the effect of intensive diabetes management on retinopathy in insulin-dependent diabetes mellitus.

The Diabetes Control and Complications Trial Research Group. The effect of intensive treatment of diabetes on the development and progression of long-term complications in insulin-dependent diabetes mellitus. *NEJM,* 1993; Vol. 329: pp. 977–86.

Comments: Results showed that intensive therapy effectively delays the onset and slows the progression of diabetic retinopathy, nephropathy, and neuropathy in patients with IDDM.

Early Treatment Diabetic Retinopathy Study Research Group. Early photocoagulation for diabetic retinopathy. ETDRS report no. 9. *Ophthalmology,* 1991; Vol. 98: pp. 766–85.

Comments: This study evaluated when and with what type of laser photocoagulation should be initiated in patients with diabetic retinopathy.

The Diabetic Retinopathy Vitrectomy Study Research Group. Early vitrectomy for severe proliferative diabetic retinopathy in eyes with useful vision. Results of a randomized trial—Diabetic Retinopathy Vitrectomy Study Report 3. *Ophthalmology,* 1988; Vol. 95: pp. 1307–20.

Comments: The study showed that early vitrectomy for type 1 diabetics with advanced PDR was beneficial.

Klein R, Klein BE, Moss SE, et al. The Wisconsin epidemiologic study of diabetic retinopathy II. Prevalence and risk of diabetic retinopathy when age at diagnosis is less than 30 years. *Arch Ophthalmol,* 1984; Vol. 102: pp. 520–6.

Comments: Younger-onset persons with diabetes were examined using standard protocols to determine the prevalence and severity of diabetic retinopathy and associated risk factors.

The Diabetic Retinopathy Study Research Group. Photocoagulation treatment of proliferative diabetic retinopathy. Clinical application of Diabetic Retinopathy Study (DRS) findings, DRS Report No. 8. *Ophthalmology,* 1981; Vol. 88: pp. 583–600.

Comments: Photocoagulation reduces the risk of severe visual loss by 50% or more in eyes with severe PDR.

COMPLICATIONS AND COMORBIDITIES

MACULAR EDEMA

Sachin D. Kalyani, MD

DEFINITION

- The macula is a small and highly sensitive part of the retina, located roughly in the center of the retina and just temporal to the optic nerve.
- Macular edema occurs due to fluid and protein leaking from blood vessels within the macula causing it to swell and thicken.

- Focal macular edema is caused by foci of vascular abnormalities, primarily microaneurysms, which tend to leak fluid.
- Diffuse macular edema is caused by dilated retinal capillaries in the retina.
- Clinically significant macular edema (CSME) was defined by the Early Treatment Diabetic Retinopathy Study Group (ETDRS)—see Diagnosis section for full definition.

EPIDEMIOLOGY

- Accounts for three-quarters of visual loss associated with diabetes (Sutter).
- Prevalence of CSME reported as 5.9% and 7.5% for individuals with younger- and older-onset of diabetes ($<$30 vs $>$30 years), respectively (Hirai).
- Higher incidence of macular edema associated with male sex, severe diabetic retinopathy, higher glycosylated hemoglobin, proteinuria, higher systolic and diastolic blood pressure, and greater pack-years of smoking (Klein).
- Can occur at any stage of diabetic retinopathy, although more likely to occur as retinopathy progresses.
- CSME associated with decreased survival in persons with older-onset diabetes mellitus (Hirai).

DIAGNOSIS

- The ETDRS defined CSME as (1) retinal edema located at or within 500 μm of the center of the macula; (2) hard exudates at or within 500 μm of the center if associated with thickening of adjacent retina; or (3) a zone of thickening larger than 1 disc area if located within 1 disc diameter of the center of the macula (ETDRS).
- Diagnosis best made by ophthalmologist using slit-lamp binocular stereoscopic ophthalmoscopy of the posterior pole using a contact lens.
- Funduscopic exam with direct ophthalmoscope may reveal hard exudates and microaneurysms surrounding or within the macula; however, does not provide stereoscopic view for diagnosis.

SIGNS AND SYMPTOMS

- Blurring of vision in the middle or to the side of the central visual field.
- Visual loss can progress over a period of months.
- Visual acuity may be 20/20 in some cases of CSME.
- Patient may complain of being unable to focus clearly.
- Symptoms may be unilateral or bilateral.

CLINICAL TREATMENT

- Laser treatment considered first-line therapy: focal (for focal disease) and grid (for diffuse disease).
- ETDRS demonstrated that eyes with CSME benefited from focal argon laser photocoagulation treatment when compared to untreated eyes in controls. Treatment reduced the risk of moderate visual loss by 50%, increased the chance of visual improvement, and was associated with only minor losses of visual field (ETDRS).
- Eyes with retinal edema not meeting the criteria of CSME showed no significant difference between the treatment and control group.
- Preferable to initiate focal laser for macular edema prior to either panretinal laser treatment for high-risk proliferative diabetic retinopathy or cataract surgery because of potential risk for progression of macular edema.

- Side effects of focal laser include paracentral scotoma, transient increased edema, decreased vision, choroidal neovascularization, photocoagulation scar expansion, inadvertent foveolar burns (Kim).
- ETDRS demonstrated that subretinal fibrosis occurred less often in laser-treated eyes than in untreated control eyes.
- Intravitreal administration of corticosteroids has been shown to be useful in cases of refractory CSME; however, side effects of corticosteroid use include 2–3 times increase in cataract surgery and a 4–8 times increase in intraocular pressure (Martidis).
- Pars plana vitrectomy and detachment of the posterior hyaloid may also be useful in treating diabetic macular edema (Kaiser).
- Medical treatment including topical NSAIDs and steroid eye drops can be used, but laser treatment is preferred and more beneficial.
- Risk factor management of hypertension, hyperlipidemia, and hyperglycemia is also important to prevent macular edema progression (Ciulla).

FOLLOW-UP

- A dilated fundoscopic exam should be performed every 2–4 months until resolution of CSME.

EXPERT OPINION

- Visual acuity is not a criterion in the diagnosis and/or treatment of CSME but may be helpful in following clinical course.
- Requires stereoscopic exam by specialist for diagnosis.

REFERENCES

Klein R, Knudtson MD, Lee KE, et al. The Wisconsin Epidemiologic Study of Diabetic Retinopathy XXIII: the twenty-five-year incidence of macular edema in persons with type 1 diabetes. *Ophthalmology,* 2009; Vol. 116: pp. 497–503.

Comments: This study examined the 25-year cumulative incidence of macular edema (ME) and its relation to various risk factors.

Hirai FE, Knudtson MD, Klein BE, et al. Clinically significant macular edema and survival in type 1 and type 2 diabetes. *Am J Ophthalmol,* 2008; Vol. 145: pp. 700–6.

Comments: Investigation of the association of CSME and long-term survival in type 1 and type 2 diabetics.

Sutter FK, Gillies MC, Helbig H. In Holze FG, Spaide RF (Eds.), *Diabetic Macular Edema in Medical Retina.* Springer; 2007; pp. 131–146.

Comments: Review of current treatments for macular edema.

Ciulla TA, Amador AG, Zinman B. Diabetic retinopathy and diabetic macular edema: pathophysiology, screening, and novel therapies. *Diabetes Care,* 2003; Vol. 26: pp. 2653–64.

Comments: Review of pathophysiology and treatments for diabetic retinopathy and macular edema.

Martidis A, Duker JS, Greenberg PB, et al. Intravitreal triamcinolone for refractory diabetic macular edema. *Ophthalmology,* 2002; Vol. 109: pp. 920–7.

Comments: The purpose of this study was to determine if an intravitreal injection of triamcinolone acetonide is safe and effective in treating diabetic macular edema unresponsive to prior laser photocoagulation.

Kaiser PK, Riemann CD, Sears JE, et al. Macular traction detachment and diabetic macular edema associated with posterior hyaloidal traction. *Am J Ophthalmol,* 2001; Vol. 131: pp. 44–9.

COMPLICATIONS AND COMORBIDITIES

Comments: Reviewed the clinical, photographic, fluorescein angiographic, and optical coherence tomographic findings in patients with diabetic macular traction and edema (DMTE) associated with posterior hyaloidal traction (PHT).

Kim JW, Ai E. Diabetic retinopathy. In Regillo, CD, Brown, GC, Flynn Jr, HW, (Eds.), *Vitreoretinal Diseases: The Essentials.* New York: Georg Thieme; 1999: p. 147 (Table 3).

Comments: This table examines the side effects and complications of focal laser photocoagulation.

Early Treatment Diabetic Retinopathy Study Research Group. Focal photocoagulation treatment of diabetic macular edema. Relationship of treatment effect to fluorescein angiographic and other retinal characteristics at baseline: ETDRS Report no. 19. *Arch Ophthalmol,* 1995; Vol. 113: pp. 1144–55.

Comments: This study's objective was to determine whether the efficacy of photocoagulation treatment of diabetic macular edema may be influenced by degree of capillary closure, severity or source of fluorescein leakage, extent of retinal edema, presence of cystoid changes, or severity of hard exudates.

Early Treatment Diabetic Retinopathy Study Research Group. Photocoagulation for diabetic macular edema. ETDRS Report no. 1. *Arch Ophthalmol,* 1985; Vol. 103: pp. 1796–806.

Comments: Examined if laser photocoagulation helped reduce the risk of vision loss secondary to CSME.

CATARACTS

Sachin D. Kalyani, MD

DEFINITION

- A clouding or opacity of the natural crystalline lens of the eye.
- When glucose increases in the lens (as in hyperglycemic states), the sorbitol pathway is activated more than glycolysis; sorbitol accumulates and is retained in the lens.
- Along with sorbitol, fructose also builds up in a lens surrounded by a high glucose environment.
- These two sugars increase the osmotic pressure within the lens, drawing in water.
- The result is swelling of the lens fibers, disruption of the normal cytoskeletal architecture, and ultimately, lens opacification (Andley).

EPIDEMIOLOGY

- Persons with diabetes mellitus (DM) are at increased risk of age-related lens changes indistinguishable from nondiabetic age-related cataracts.
- The lens changes occur at a younger age than in people without DM (Flynn).
- With DM, cortical or posterior subcapsular opacities also occur earlier than in age-matched persons.
- Cataracts are present in 20% of patients with type 1 DM, associated with age, history of retina photocoagulation, higher serum creatinine values, and hypertension (Esteves).
- The number of cataract cases among adults 40 years or older with DM will likely increase 235% by 2050 (Saaddine).

DIAGNOSIS

- History to evaluate if vision is affecting patient's activities of daily living (ADLs) (e.g., driving, reading, watching TV).
- Comprehensive eye exam, including visual acuity, slit lamp examination, and a dilated funduscopic exam to evaluate the cataract.
- On examination, funduscopic exam may reveal a clouding of the lens and difficult or hazy view of the retina.

SIGNS AND SYMPTOMS

- Cloudy or blurry vision.
- Glare (headlights or sunlight may decrease vision); halos around lights.
- Poor night vision.
- Subdued colors.
- Monocular diplopia or multiple images in one eye.
- Cataracts usually present bilaterally; however, may have progressed more in one by time of presentation.

CLINICAL TREATMENT

- Symptoms of early cataract may be improved with new eyeglasses, brighter lighting, anti-glare sunglasses, or magnifying lenses.
- If these measures are not adequate, surgery is the only effective treatment, usually cataract extraction with phacoemulsification and intraocular lens implantation.
- Cataract surgery usually recommended only when vision loss interferes with ADLs.
- Other indications for cataract surgery: if the cataract prevents examination or treatment of another eye problem, such as diabetic retinopathy, or age-related macular degeneration.
- Diabetic retinopathy may progress following cataract surgery (Jaffe).
- Therefore, consider laser photocoagulation prior to cataract surgery for patients with clinically significant macular edema (CSME), severe nonproliferative diabetic retinopathy (NPDR), or proliferative diabetic retinopathy (PDR).

FOLLOW-UP

- Reevaluate all patients with preexisting diabetic retinopathy following cataract surgery.
- Patients with DM undergoing phacoemulsification cataract surgery have a doubling of diabetic retinopathy progression 12 months after surgery (Hong).
- This outcome, however, represents less progression than was previously documented with intracapsular and extracapsular cataract surgical techniques (Jaffe).

EXPERT OPINION

- Consider treatment for diabetic retinopathy prior to cataract extraction where appropriate.
- Cataracts usually present bilaterally; however, may have progressed more in one eye.
- Best corrected visual acuity after cataract extraction may be limited secondary to diabetic retinopathy.

REFERENCES

National Eye Institute: Cataracts. *http://www.nei.nih.gov/health/cataract/cataract_facts.asp*, 2009. Accessed November 1, 2009.

Comments: The National Eye Institute's website on cataracts.

Hong T, Mitchell P, de Loryn T, et al. Development and progression of diabetic retinopathy 12 months after phacoemulsification cataract surgery. *Ophthalmology,* 2009; Vol. 116: pp. 1510–4.

Comments: This study evaluated whether phacoemulsification cataract surgery exacerbates the development and progression of diabetic retinopathy.

Esteves JF, Dal Pizzol MM, Sccoco CA, et al. Cataract and type 1 diabetes mellitus. *Diabetes Res Clin Pract,* 2008; Vol. 82: pp. 324–8.

Comments: Evaluated the prevalence and possible risk factors of cataract formation in type 1 diabetics.

COMPLICATIONS AND COMORBIDITIES

Saaddine JB, Honeycutt AA, Narayan KM, et al. Projection of diabetic retinopathy and other major eye diseases among people with diabetes mellitus: United States, 2005–2050. *Arch Ophthalmol*, 2008; Vol. 126: pp. 1740–7.
Comments: Estimates the number of people with cataracts among Americans 40 years or older with diabetes for the years 2005–2050.

Flynn HW, Jr., Smiddy WE. Diabetes and ocular disease: past, present, and future therapies. *Ophthalmology Monograph 14*, American Academy of Ophthalmology: 2000; Vol. 226: pp. 49–53.
Comments: Focuses on the epidemiology of cataracts in patients with diabetes.

Andley UP, Liang JJN, Lou MF. Biochemical mechanisms of age-related cataract. Albert DM, Jakobiec FA, (Eds.), *Principles and Practice of Ophthalmology*, 2nd edition. Philadelphia: WB Saunders Publishers; 2000: pp. 1428–1449.
Comments: Describes pathophysiology of cataract formation.

Jaffe GJ, Burton TC, Kuhn E, et al. Progression of nonproliferative diabetic retinopathy and visual outcome after extracapsular cataract extraction and intraocular lens implantation. *Am J Ophthalmol*, 1992; Vol. 114: pp. 448–56.
Comments: Looked at the progression of diabetic retinopathy after cataract surgery.

Otologic Diseases

HEARING IMPAIRMENT

Nisa M. Maruthur, MD, MHS

DEFINITION

- Refers to either (1) sensorineural hearing impairment, characterized by frequency and intensity of hearing loss, or (2) conductive hearing loss.
- In diabetes, the increased prevalence of sensorineural hearing impairment is likely related to microvascular disease.

EPIDEMIOLOGY

- In those with diabetes, overall likelihood of sensorineural hearing impairment approximately 2 times that in those without diabetes (Bainbridge).
- Both low- and high-frequency hearing impairment far more common among those with diabetes.
- Age-adjusted prevalence of mild or greater high-frequency hearing impairment among those with diabetes is 54.1% (vs 32% among those without diabetes).
- Age-adjusted prevalence of mild or greater low-frequency hearing impairment among those with diabetes is 21.3%.
- Age, noise, ototoxic medications, and smoking increase risk of hearing impairment along with presence of microvascular conditions.

DIAGNOSIS

- **History:** presence or absence of subjective hearing impairment, timing, occupational history, trauma, medications, family history, and family member response.
- **Self-report:** defined by audiometry pure-tone threshold. "Yes" response has likelihood ratio (LR) positive of 2.5 (95% CI 1.7–3.6). "No" response has LR negative of 0.13 (95% CI 0.09–0.19). Family member response may have some value.
- **Whispered voice perception:** standing behind patient with untested ear occluded by examiner's finger, examiner whispers combination of 3 numbers and letters and can repeat once more. Normal if 3/6 letters or numbers repeated by patient. Inability to perceive whispered voice has LR positive of 6.1 (95% CI 4.5–8.4). Normal perception has LR negative of 0.03 (95% CI 0–0.24).
- **Weber test:** positive if tuning fork vibrating on middle of forehead perceived as louder on one side (lateralization). Suggests conductive hearing loss on loudest side or sensorineural loss on diminished side. Not useful if bilateral, symmetric hearing loss since the test depends on lateralization. Abnormal result: LR positive of 1.6 (95% CI 1.0–2.3).
- **Rinne test:** to evaluate for conductive hearing loss, place vibrating tuning fork on mastoid process (bone conduction [BC]) until sound is not heard, then move to 1 inch from external meatus (air conduction [AC]) to see if sound still heard. Normal: AC >BC. Abnormal test: LR positive 2.7–62. Normal test: LR negative 0.01–0.85.
- Evaluate for other medical causes of hearing impairment such as syphilis (i.e., fluorescent treponemal antibody absorption test).
- Otoscopy to evaluate external ear canal and tympanic membrane.

- Imaging with MRI or CT to evaluate for acoustic neuroma or other abnormality.
- Referral for audiologic examination by audiologist.

SIGNS AND SYMPTOMS

- Progressive difficulty hearing at low or high frequencies and/or different sound intensities.
- Difficulty hearing as evidenced by self-report, whispered voice perception, Weber or Rinne tests.
- May have associated vertigo or tinnitus.

CLINICAL TREATMENT

- Treatment of external and middle ear disorders (e.g., cerumen impaction and otitis media).
- Avoid/discontinue ototoxic medications (e.g., aminoglycosides, loop diuretics, salicylates, and nonsteroidal anti-inflammatories, vancomycin, and erythromycin).
- Consultation with audiologist and/or otolaryngologist for hearing aids and other hearing assistive devices.

FOLLOW-UP

- Screen by inquiring about subjective hearing impairment periodically.
- Counseling regarding hearing aids.
- Referral for formal audiologic examination if hearing impairment suspected.

EXPERT OPINION

- Inquire about subjective hearing impairment every 6 months during regular diabetes follow-up visits.
- Input from family members may be helpful in determining presence and extent of hearing impairment.
- Though there is no convincing data at this time, if diabetes-related hearing loss is indeed due to microvascular disease, blood pressure and glycemic control should play a role in prevention and treatment of this complication.
- Comparison of initial office-based tests for hearing impairment suggests that Weber and Rinne tests have limited value and that referral for audiometry should be based on patient's subjective report of hearing loss and/or abnormal whispered-voice test (Bagai).
- Severe, congenital, or maternally transmitted deafness should raise possibility of mitochondrial diabetes (see Mitochondrial Diabetes, p. 140).

REFERENCES

Arts HA. Sensorineural hearing loss: evaluation and management in adults; etiology of SNHL (pharmacologic toxicity). In Cummings CW, Haughey BH, Thomas JR, (Eds.), *Cummings Otolaryngology: Head and Neck Surgery*, 4th edition. Philadelphia: Elsevier Mosby; 2005.

> **Comments:** Preeminent reference for otolaryngology.

US Preventive Services Task Force. Screening for Hearing Impairment in Older Adults, Topic Page. US Preventive Services Task Force. Agency for Healthcare Research and Quality (AHRQ), Rockville, MD. *http://www.ahrq.gov/clinic/uspstf/uspshear.htm*, Accessed August 9, 2009.

> **Comments:** Screening guidelines for hearing impairment in the US from US Preventive Services Task Force. Update in progress.

Bainbridge KE, Hoffman HJ, Cowie CC. Diabetes and hearing impairment in the United States: audiometric evidence from the National Health and Nutrition Examination Survey, 1999 to 2004. *Ann Intern Med,* 2008; Vol. 149: pp. 1–10.

Comments: Nationally representative analysis of the relationship between diabetes and hearing impairment in the US.

Bagai A, Thavendiranathan P, Detsky AS. Does this patient have hearing impairment? *JAMA,* 2006; Vol. 295: pp. 416–28.

Comments: Systematic review of bedside clinical maneuvers to evaluate hearing impairment.

Korsch B. Commentary: screening for psychosocial problems. *Pediatrics,* 1976; Vol. 58: pp. 471–2.

Comments: Results from a cohort study of aging in Wisconsin showing a modest association between type 2 diabetes and hearing loss but no association between glycemic control and hearing loss.

COMPLICATIONS AND COMORBIDITIES

Psychiatric Diseases

DEPRESSION IN DIABETES

Sherita Hill Golden, MD, MHS

DEFINITION

- Depression is a mental disorder, diagnosed using specific criteria from the *Diagnostic and Statistical Manual of Mental Disorders* (*DSM-IV*), characterized by depressed mood and/or loss of pleasure in most activities (anhedonia), along with the signs and symptoms described in Table 3-14.
- Symptoms must be present for at least 2 weeks.

EPIDEMIOLOGY

- Depressive disorders are a significant comorbidity in diabetes; worldwide, estimated 43 million people with diabetes have symptoms of depression.
- People with diabetes are twice as likely to have depressive symptoms as those without diabetes (Anderson).
- In a meta-analysis of individuals with diabetes, the aggregate prevalence of major depressive disorder (MDD) was 11.4% while the prevalence of elevated depressive symptoms was higher, estimated at 31% (Anderson).
- Individuals with elevated depressive symptoms have an approximately 30%–60% increased risk of developing type 2 diabetes and individuals with type 2 diabetes have an approximately 12%–50% increased risk of developing elevated depressive symptoms (Mezuk; Golden).
- Depressive disorders in diabetes are associated with poor glycemic control and microvascular and macrovascular complications (Lustman; deGroot).

DIAGNOSIS

- Depressive disorders are most accurately diagnosed using a structured clinical interview based on criteria from the *DSM-IV*. Two commonly used clinical interviews are the Diagnostic Interview Scheduled (DIS) and the Structured Clinical Interview for Depression (SCID).
- Diagnostic criteria for depressive disorders based on *DSM-IV* criteria are listed in Table 3-14.
- Depressive symptoms can also be assessed by self- or interviewer-administered questionnaire. Patient Health Questionnaire-9 (PHQ-9) is most often used in primary care settings, screening for MDD, and significant depressive symptoms (Kroenke). A score of ≥10 with five symptoms (including either depressed mood or lack of pleasure in usual activities) present for more than half the days is consistent with major depression.
- Another efficient screening tool for MDD in the clinical setting is the PHQ-2, an abbreviated version of the PHQ-9 (Kroenke).

SIGNS AND SYMPTOMS

- See symptoms listed in Table 3-14.

TABLE 3-14. DIAGNOSTIC CRITERIA FOR DEPRESSIVE DISORDERS BASED ON *DSM-IV* CRITERIA

	Major Depressive Disorder	Minor Depression	Dysthymia
Requires presence of depressed mood to be one symptom			X
Requires presence of depressed mood or anhedonia to be at least one symptom	X	X	
Number of additional symptoms	At least five: Depressed mood Markedly diminished interest or pleasure in all or most activity (anhedonia) Significant weight loss or weight gain (>5% body weight within one month) or decreased or increased appetite Insomnia or hypersomnia Psychomotor agitation or retardation Fatigue or loss of energy Feelings of worthlessness or inappropriate guilt Diminished ability to think or concentrate; indecisiveness Recurrent thoughts of death or suicidal ideation	At least two but less than five symptoms of Major Depressive Disorder	Two or more: Poor appetite or overeating Insomnia or hypersomnia Low energy or fatigue Low self-esteem Poor concentration or indecisiveness Feelings of hopelessness
Symptom duration	At least 2 weeks with symptoms occurring daily	At least 2 weeks with symptoms occurring daily	At least 2 years on more days than not Never without symptoms for more than 2 months

Courtesy of Sherita Hill Golden.

COMPLICATIONS AND COMORBIDITIES

CLINICAL TREATMENT

Psychotherapies for Depression

- Psychotherapies studied to treat depressive disorders in diabetes include cognitive behavior therapy (CBT) and problem-solving therapy for depression. Both psychotherapeutic treatments improve depressive symptoms in people with diabetes (Petrak).
- In the one study of CBT, hemoglobin A1c was lower in the CBT group (9.5%) compared to the control group (10.9%) three months after discontinuation of treatment, but problem-solving therapy did not result in significant improvements in glycemic control (Petrak).

Pharmacologic Therapy for Depression

- Pharmacologic therapies that have been shown to improve depressive symptoms in people with diabetes include the selective serotonin reuptake inhibitors (SSRIs)—fluoxetine, sertraline, or paroxetine (Kroenke).
- Therapeutic effects may take 4–6 weeks, after which, if no improvement in symptoms, dose should be titrated upward until symptoms are improved. Recommended initial dosing titration and maximum dosing are included in Table 3-15.
- Common side effects of SSRIs include gastrointestinal effects (nausea, vomiting, diarrhea, xerostomia [dry mouth]), central nervous system effects (anxiety, nervousness, insomnia, drowsiness, fatigue, dizziness, tremor, headache, suicidal ideation), platelet dysfunction, and diaphoresis.
- Other effects relevant to diabetes: fluoxetine and sertraline may be associated with weight loss, improvement in hyperglycemia, and improvement in insulin sensitivity.
- Use of atypical antipsychotics in patients with bipolar disorder may be associated with weight gain and worsening of glycemic control (see Antipsychotics, p. 476).

TABLE 3-15. DOSING AND TITRATION OF SELECTIVE SEROTONIN REUPTAKE INHIBITORS FOR TREATMENT OF DEPRESSION IN DIABETES

Medicaion	Initial Dose	Titration	Maximum Dose
Fluoxetine	20 mg daily	Increase dose every month if needed by 10–20 mg.	80 mg daily (can be taken in divided doses before breakfast and lunch if total daily dose ≥80 mg daily).
Sertraline	25 mg or 50 mg daily	Titrate at intervals of at least one week.	200 mg daily.
Paroxetine	20 mg daily (10 mg daily in the elderly)	Increase dose by 10 mg weekly as needed.	50 mg daily (40 mg daily in the elderly).
Courtesy of Sherita Hill Golden.			

FOLLOW-UP

- If depressive symptoms do not improve on initial pharmacologic therapy, which can be assessed by readministering the PHQ-9, then antidepressant therapy should be titrated as outlined in Table 3-15.

EXPERT OPINION

- Clinicians should suspect a depressive disorder in patients whose glycemic control is not improving despite intensification of glucose-lowering therapy and consider screening for depression using the PHQ-2 or PHQ-9.
- Because elevated depressive symptoms are associated with poor health behaviors, such as increased caloric intake and physical inactivity, overweight and obesity can worsen and contribute to poor glycemic control.
- Behavioral treatments for depression should also address motivating patients to participate in physical activity and healthy lifestyle choices.
- Work collaboratively with a mental health provider (i.e., psychologist or psychiatrist) to treat this comorbidity of diabetes.

BASIS FOR RECOMMENDATIONS

Petrak F, Herpertz S. Treatment of depression in diabetes: an update. *Curr Opin Psychiatry,* 2009; Vol. 22: pp. 211–7.

> **Comments:** Provides an excellent overview of psychotherapies and pharmacologic treatments for depression. In summary, most depression treatments improve depressive symptoms but do not significantly improve glycemic control in diabetes.

Kroenke K, Spitzer RL, Williams JB. The Patient Health Questionnaire-2: validity of a two-item depression screener. *Med Care,* 2003; Vol. 41: pp. 1284–92.

> **Comments:** Describes the validity of using the PHQ-2 screening questionnaire to identify individuals at increased risk for having a depressive disorder.

Kroenke K, Spitzer RL, Williams JB. The PHQ-9: validity of a brief depression severity measure. *J Gen Intern Med,* 2001; Vol. 16: pp. 606–13.

> **Comments:** Describes the validity of using the PHQ-9 questionnaire to identify individuals with depressive disorders.

OTHER REFERENCES

Mezuk B, Eaton WW, Albrecht S, et al. Depression and type 2 diabetes over the lifespan: a meta-analysis. *Diabetes Care,* 2008; Vol. 31: pp. 2383–90.

> **Comments:** This is the first meta-analysis demonstrating that depression is associated with an increased risk of type 2 diabetes and that type 2 diabetes is associated with an increased risk of depression.

Golden SH, Lazo M, Carnethon M, et al. Examining a bidirectional association between depressive symptoms and diabetes. *JAMA,* 2008; Vol. 299: pp. 2751–9.

> **Comments:** Population-based study in a multiethnic cohort showing that there is a bidirectional relationship between elevated depressive symptoms and type 2 diabetes.

Anderson RJ, Freedland KE, Clouse RE, et al. The prevalence of comorbid depression in adults with diabetes: a meta-analysis. *Diabetes Care,* 2001; Vol. 24: pp. 1069–78.

> **Comments:** This is the most comprehensive study describing the prevalence of major depressive disorder and elevated depressive symptoms in diabetes.

de Groot M, Anderson R, Freedland KE, et al. Association of depression and diabetes complications: a meta-analysis. *Psychosom Med,* 2001; Vol. 63: pp. 619–30.

> **Comments:** This meta-analysis demonstrates that depression is associated with increased microvascular and macrovascular diabetes complications.

Lustman PJ, Anderson RJ, Freedland KE, et al. Depression and poor glycemic control: a meta-analytic review of the literature. *Diabetes Care,* 2000; Vol. 23: pp. 934–42.

> **Comments:** This meta-analysis demonstrates that depression is associated with poor glycemic control.

Maheux P, Ducros F, Bourque J, et al. Fluoxetine improves insulin sensitivity in obese patients with non-insulin-dependent diabetes mellitus independently of weight loss. *Int J Obes Relat Metab Disord,* 1997; Vol. 21: pp. 97–102.

COMPLICATIONS AND COMORBIDITIES

Comments: This study suggests that fluoxetine improves insulin sensitivity in diabetes patients independent of weight loss.

EATING DISORDERS IN DIABETES

Mariana Lazo, MD, ScM, PhD, and Mary Huizinga, MD, MPH

DEFINITION

- A group of psychiatric illnesses including anorexia nervosa, bulimia nervosa, and other eating disorders not otherwise specified (e.g., binge eating disorder, night eating syndrome) with potentially life-threatening health impact.
- **Anorexia nervosa** is characterized by self-starvation and excessive weight loss, and an intense fear of weight gain.
- **Bulimia nervosa** is characterized by a secretive cycle of binge eating (eating large amounts of food—more than most people would eat in one meal—in short periods of time) followed by purging (getting rid of the food and calories through vomiting, laxative abuse, or over-exercising).
- In patients with type 1 diabetes, the most common purging manifestation is deliberate insulin omission and restriction.
- Binge eating disorder (without purging) leads to excessive weight gain and may exacerbate diabetes management.

EPIDEMIOLOGY

- Eating disorders are very common among patients with type 1 diabetes. Insulin omission or restriction has been reported by ~2% among preteen girls, 11%–15% among midteen years, and 30%–39% among late teenage years and early adulthood (Nielsen; Jones; Colton).
- The prevalence of overt eating disorder syndromes in type 1 diabetes ranges from 0%–11% and the prevalence of subthreshold eating disorders ranges from 7%–35% (Colton).
- Mortality rates are much higher with combined anorexia nervosa and type 1 diabetes (10-year mortality rate = 34.6/1000 person-years) than with either condition alone (type 1 diabetes only: 10-year mortality rate = 2.2/1000 person-years; anorexia only: 10-year mortality rate = 7.3/1000 person-years) (Nielsen).
- Rates of diabetic complications (mainly retinopathy, ketoacidosis, neuropathy) are higher among people with type 1 diabetes and coexisting eating disorders (Rydall; Peveler).
- Patients with type 2 diabetes are more likely to have a binge eating disorder due to the frequent coexistence of overweight or obesity along with the need for weight control (dietary restraint) (Herpertz).
- Prevalence estimates of eating disorders in type 2 diabetes range between 6.5%–9%.
- Risk factors: female sex, family history of eating disorder, history of dieting, body dissatisfaction, higher BMI, depression and anxiety disorders, personality disorder (obsessive compulsive, perfectionist, histrionic trait, impulsive), young age (although later onset is also observed).

DIAGNOSIS

- Often patients do not present with a chief complaint of an eating disorder, and the eating disorders are well hidden.
- Deliberate insulin omission is a common behavior and patients may initially deny it.

- Refer to Table 3-16 for signs and symptoms of the most common eating disorders.
- **Anorexia:** formal diagnostic criteria based on *DSM-IV* criteria include (1) refusal to maintain body weight at or above a minimally normal weight for height, body type, age, and activity level (~less than 85% of that expected); (2) intense fear of weight gain or being "fat," or feeling "fat" or overweight despite dramatic weight loss; (3) loss of menstrual periods; (4) extreme concern with body weight and shape.
- **Bulimia nervosa:** the *DSM-IV* criteria include (1) recurrent episodes of binge eating in a discrete period of time involving more food than most people would eat, with a distinct feeling of lack of control during episode; (2) recurrent inappropriate compensatory behavior to prevent weight gain, such as self-induced vomiting, misuse of laxatives, diuretics, enemas or other medications, fasting, or excessive exercise; (3) both binge eating and inappropriate compensatory mechanisms occur on average at least twice a week for 3 months; (4) extreme concern with body weight and shape.
- Clinical warning signs: overall deterioration in psychosocial functioning, depressive symptoms, poor body image/low self-esteem, low weight, concern expressed by family member, refractory metabolic control, amenorrhea, delay in puberty, sexual maturation or growth.

TABLE 3-16. SIGNS AND SYMPTOMS FOR THE MOST COMMON EATING DISORDERS

Eating Disorder	Symptoms	Signs
Anorexia nervosa	Weakness, lassitude, fatigue, palpitations, dizziness, cold extremities and intolerance, apathy, poor concentration, abdominal bloating, constipation, hair loss, loss of libido	Low body weight, dehydration, hypothermia, cachexia, bradychardia, orthostatic hypertension, weak irregular pulse, anxious, irritable or depressed mood, hypothermia, abdominal bowel sounds, benign parotid hyperplasia, lanugo, skin abnormalities, amenorrhea, infertility, arrested sexual development
Bulimia nervosa	Weakness, palpitations, apathy, poor concentration, reflux, heartburn, abdominal discomfort and bloating, weight fluctuations, dental decay, pain in pharynx, infertility	Arrythmias, anxiousness, irritable or depressed mood, enlarged salivary glands, gastritis, blood-streaked vomitus, esophagitis, gastroesophageal reflux and erosions, pancreatitis, scarring on dorsum of hand (Russell's sign), petechia, conjunctival hemorrhages shortly after vomiting, dental caries with erosion of dental enamel (particularly the lingular surface of incisors), erythema of pharynx, palatal scratches, enlarged salivary glands, oligorrhea, or amenorrhea

Courtesy of Mariana Lazo and Mary Huizinga.

COMPLICATIONS AND COMORBIDITIES

- Specific signs relevant to diabetes: episodes of hyperglycemia and glycosuria, unexplained elevations in A1c, repeated problems with diabetic ketoacidosis (DKA).
- Other behaviors/attitudes associated with disordered eating: excessive physical activity and restrictive eating.
- Extended instruments (questionnaires) are available for the formal assessment of eating disorders. Usually performed and scored by trained interviewers and not validated in diabetes (Criego).
- Clinicians working with individuals who have diabetes should use open-ended screening questions to understand patients' current satisfaction with body weight, patterns of insulin use, and overall eating behaviours: (1) What did you eat yesterday? (2) Do you ever eat more than you want or use unprescribed laxatives, diuretics, diet pills? (3) Do you take less insulin than you should? (4) Do you think you are thin?

CLINICAL TREATMENT
General Considerations
- These diagnoses are very serious, especially with coexisting diabetes; their significance should not be ignored or minimized.
- In patients with poorly controlled diabetes, hospitalization is recommended until medically safe. In general, patients with type 1 diabetes and eating disorders may be more difficult to manage.
- An integrated inpatient team approach is the recommended model of care including the following: endocrinologist, psychologist/psychiatrist, general internist, specialized nutritionist, and diabetes educator.
- Level of care needed: consider the patient's overall physical and psychological conditions, behaviors, and social circumstances rather than simply relying on one or more physical parameters such as weight.
- Basic laboratory analyses: glucose, A1c, serum electrolytes, blood urea nitrogen, serum creatinine (interpretations must incorporate assessments of weight), thyroid-stimulating hormone test; complete blood count including differential, erythrocyte sedimentation rate, liver tests, urinalysis.
- Specialized tests: electrocardiogram, osteopenia, and osteoporosis assessments (amenorrhea for >6 months), serum estradiol in female patients, serum testosterone in male patients.
- Evidence-based treatment guidelines for the management of eating disorders exist for the general population (American Psychiatric Association). However the efficacy and effectiveness in patients with diabetes has not been clearly shown. Very few, small studies have been conducted in this population.

Diabetes Management
- Set small incremental goals for reestablishing patient on appropriate insulin dose, for improving overall blood glucose control, and for normalizing eating patterns.
- Aim for A1c levels within safe guidelines; discourage perfectionistic goals for A1c and blood glucose (pre- and postprandial) (Goebel-Fabbri, 2009).
- Anticipate insulin edema and fluid retention that may occur as blood glucose improves and could increase the risk of relapse.
- Consistent SMBG and insulin administration (type 1 diabetes). Medication adjustments and hypoglycemia prevention as weight changes.

Nutritional Rehabilitation

- Caloric intake levels should usually start at 30–40 kcal/kg per day (approximately 1000–1600 kcal/day). During the weight gain phase, intake may have to be advanced progressively to as high as 70–100 kcal/kg per day for some patients; many male patients require a very large number of calories to gain weight.
- Three meals with three snacks are usually needed to meet caloric goals.
- Regular monitoring of serum potassium levels is recommended in patients who are persistent vomiters. Hypokalemia should be treated with oral or intravenous potassium supplementation and rehydration.
- Thiamine may also be reduced in patients with vomiting.
- If severely malnourished, patients should be monitored closely for refeeding syndrome. Refeeding syndrome requires careful monitoring of electrolytes (especially for hypophosphatemia), neurologic, cardiac, and pulmonary systems.
- Supplemental calcium, vitamin D, and vitamin B12 are often recommended.
- Avoid focus on food labels, especially since this may be a trigger for food restriction.
- Long-term goal is to have an eating pattern consistent with insulin (or diabetes medication) administration.

Psychological Treatment

- Family-based interventions to promote family support in the diabetes management.
- Interventions to develop flexible approaches to food and meal planning.
- Individual or group therapies to increase self-esteem, body acceptance.
- If severe psychiatric symptoms, formal evaluation and treatments may be required.

Pharmacologic Therapy

- SSRIs are widely used in treating patients with anorexia nervosa and persistent depressive, anxiety, or obsessive compulsive symptoms and for bulimic symptoms in weight-restored patients.
- Fluoxetine is the best studied of these and is the only FDA-approved medication for bulimia (recommended dose titration to 60 mg/day with periodic reassessment of need).

Follow-up

- Monitor the patient for shifts in weight (weekly and then monthly), blood pressure, pulse, other cardiovascular parameters, glucose, and other metabolic parameters.
- Monitor patient's attitudes and behaviors to detect early signs of relapse.

Expert Opinion

- Eating disorders are more common among patients with type 1 or type 2 diabetes than among the general population, who may be concerned about weight gain associated with intensive diabetes management.
- Closer attention to food, portion control, and meal planning may influence attitude/behaviors negatively and favor the development of eating disorders.
- Be aware that people with eating disorders often go to great lengths to rationalize, deny, or hide them.
- Mortality and diabetic complications rates are higher among individuals with coexisting diabetes and eating disorders, compared to people with diabetes only, probably due to the increased risk of recurrent hypoglycemia and overall poor diabetic control.
- Early and routine screening is recommended. Eating disorders may go undetected until serious complications have developed. Physicians should be alert of clinical warning

COMPLICATIONS AND COMORBIDITIES

signs. Weight loss resulting from an eating disorder may be passed off as the result of careful diet control.

- Skipping or cutting back on insulin can mask binge eating. "Metabolic purging" refers to people failing to take insulin so that they can eat and not gain weight—a dangerous practice.
- Many patients, particularly younger patients, have combinations of eating disorder symptoms that cannot be strictly categorized as anorexia or bulimia nervosa.
- A multidisciplinary approach constitutes the model of care.

BASIS FOR RECOMMENDATIONS

American Psychiatric Association. Treatment of patients with eating disorders, Third Edition. American Psychiatric Association. *Am J Psychiatry*, 2006; Vol. 163: pp. 4–54.

Comments: This is the most recent official medical guideline by the American Psychiatric Association for the treatment of eating disorders in the general population.

OTHER REFERENCES

Colton P, Rodin G, Bergenstal R, Parkin C. Eating disorders and diabetes: introduction and overview. *Diabetes Spectrum*, 2009; Vol. 22: pp. 138–42 .

Comments: Narrative review of the topic. First invited article of a section in one of the leading journals of diabetes education.

Goebel-Fabbri AE. Disturbed eating behaviors and eating disorders in type 1 diabetes: clinical significance and treatment recommendations. *Curr Diab Rep*, 2009; Vol. 9: pp. 133–9.

Comments: Comprehensive review of the literature on type 1 diabetes and eating disorders.

Goebel-Fabbri AE, Fikkan J, Franko DL, et al. Insulin restriction and associated morbidity and mortality in women with type 1 diabetes. *Diabetes Care*, 2008; Vol. 31: pp. 415–9.

Comments: Paper that provided evidence of the role of insulin restriction as predictor of mortality.

American Psychiatric Association. Treatment of patients with eating disorders, Third Edition. American Psychiatric Association. *Am J Psychiatry,* 2006; Vol. 163: pp. 4–54.

Comments: This is the most recent official medical guideline by the American Psychiatric Association for the treatment of eating disorders in the general population.

Peveler RC, Bryden KS, Neil HA, et al. The relationship of disordered eating habits and attitudes to clinical outcomes in young adult females with type 1 diabetes. *Diabetes Care*, 2005; Vol. 28: pp. 84–8.

Comments: Provides data on complications associated with eating disorders and diabetes.

Nielsen S. Eating disorders in females with type 1 diabetes: an update of a meta-analysis. *Eur Eat Dis Rev*, 2002; Vol. 10: pp. 241–54.

Comments: Summary of the evidence of the epidemiology of eating disorders in patients with type 1 diabetes, including data on long-term mortality.

Jones JM, Lawson ML, Daneman D, et al. Eating disorders in adolescent females with and without type 1 diabetes: cross sectional study. *BMJ*, 2000; Vol. 320: pp. 1563–6.

Comments: This study provides a snapshot of the epidemiology of eating disorders in people with diabetes and nondiabetes among teenage girls.

Herpertz S, Albus C, Lichtblau K, et al. Relationship of weight and eating disorders in type 2 diabetic patients: a multicenter study. *Int J Eat Disord*, 2000; Vol. 28: pp. 68–77.

Comments: One of the few studies on the association between eating disorders and type 2 diabetes.

Rydall AC, Rodin GM, Olmsted MP, et al. Disordered eating behavior and microvascular complications in young women with insulin-dependent diabetes mellitus. *NEJM*, 1997; Vol. 336: pp. 1849–54.

Comments: This paper was one of the first to provide evidence of higher rates of microvascular complications among people with diabetes and eating disorders.

Pulmonary Diseases

CYSTIC FIBROSIS-RELATED DIABETES

Sherita Hill Golden, MD, MHS

DEFINITION
- Cystic fibrosis (CF): an autosomal recessive disease, diagnosed if (1) clinical symptoms consistent with CF in at least one organ system AND (2) evidence of CF transmembrane conductance regulator (CFTR) dysfunction, which can include elevated sweat chloride >60 mmol/L on two occasions, presence of two disease-causing mutations in the CFTR (most common mutation is delta F508), or abnormal nasal potential difference.
- Clinical manifestations: respiratory tract disease, sinus disease, exocrine pancreatic insufficiency, meconium ileus and distal ileal obstruction, biliary disease, infertility, musculoskeletal disorders (reduced bone mineral content, hypertrophic osteoarthropathy), nephrolithiasis and nephrocalcinosis, and recurrent venous thrombosis.
- Cystic fibrosis-related diabetes (CFRD): distinct from types 1 or 2 diabetes, with evidence of beta-cell dysfunction but conflicting results regarding insulin resistance. Because basal insulin secretion is retained, patients with CFRD are not ketosis prone.

EPIDEMIOLOGY
- CFRD prevalence rises steadily with age and present in 2% of children, 19% of adolescents, and 40%–50% of adults with CF (Moran).
- Incidence estimated at 2.7 cases per 100 patient-years (Moran).
- Estimated prevalence of impaired glucose tolerance (IGT) among all individuals with CF is 15%–30% (Moran).
- Risk factors for CFRD: homozygosity for the delta F508 mutation, older age, female sex, pancreatic insufficiency, more severe pulmonary disease, greater number of pulmonary exacerbations, impaired nutritional status, use of oral/implanted contraceptives, presence of *Pseudomonas aeruginosa* or *Bacteroides cepacia* complex in the sputum, liver disease, and allergic bronchopulmonary aspergillosis (ABPA) (Marshall).

DIAGNOSIS
- Diagnostic criteria for CFRD are the same as those for diabetes.
- Type 1 diabetes can occur independently of CF and should be suspected in a child who presents with ketosis prior to the age of 10 years.

SIGNS AND SYMPTOMS
- Polyuria or polydipsia in person with CF
- Failure to gain or maintain weight despite appropriate nutritional intervention
- Poor growth velocity
- Delayed progression of puberty
- Unexplained chronic decline in pulmonary function

CLINICAL TREATMENT
Pharmacologic Therapy
- Nutritional insulin initiated for postprandial hyperglycemia, which is seen most often in patients with CFRD. Dosed based on carbohydrate intake (e.g., 1 unit/10 grams

COMPLICATIONS AND COMORBIDITIES

carbohydrate). Administered as short-acting insulin (aspart or lispro). Goal is 2-hour postprandial glucose <180 mg/dl.
- If patient does not have fasting hyperglycemia, basal insulin is not necessary for initial therapy.
- Basal insulin initiated for patients with fasting hyperglycemia, providing 40%–50% of patient's total daily insulin dose. Administered as once daily basal insulin analog (glargine or detemir) or NPH in the morning and at bedtime. Goal is a fasting glucose of 80–120 mg/dl.
- Oral agents are not effective in the management of CFRD.

Medical Nutrition Therapy
- Due to increased metabolic demands of CF, total energy intake is 120%–150% of recommended daily allowance to restore growth, achieve a weight 100% of that predicted based on height, and to achieve a body mass index of at least 21 kg/m^2.
- 40% of energy intake is from fat to compensate for malabsorption.
- Intake of complex carbohydrates is promoted, and refined carbohydrates are allowed liberally (except sugary drinks between meals).
- Do not reduce protein even in setting of nephropathy.
- Fiber intake is discouraged due to malabsorption and malnutrition.
- Salt intake is increased.

FOLLOW-UP
- Hemoglobin A1c to monitor average glycemic control.
- Optimal care of CRFD requires visiting a diabetes specialist, diabetes nurse educator, and/or nutritionist every 3 months.
- CRFD without fasting hyperglycemia: start medical nutrition therapy, exercise, and screening for complications; monitor closely to detect progression to fasting hyperglycemia; and monitor glucose levels more frequently during acute illness.
- Indications for insulin therapy: weight loss, poor growth, delayed puberty, and unexplained deterioration of lung capacity.
- Nutritional insulin should be considered in patients with postprandial hyperglycemia (2-hour glucose >180 mg/dl).

EXPERT OPINION
- Unlike patients with type 1 diabetes, patients with CRFD have residual beta-cell function and often do not present with fasting hyperglycemia.
- Typically, postprandial glucoses are elevated at diagnosis so the initial insulin therapy is most often nutritional insulin, not basal.
- Nutritional requirements for CF are greatly increased, so medical nutrition therapy is different from that of most patients with diabetes.

BASIS FOR RECOMMENDATIONS

Brennan AL, Gyi KM, Wood DM, et al. Relationship between glycosylated haemoglobin and mean plasma glucose concentration in cystic fibrosis. *J Cyst Fibros*, 2006; Vol. 5: pp. 27–31.

Comments: This study determined whether hemoglobin A1c was an accurate measure of glycemic control in patients with CFRD. The study showed that hemoglobin A1c correlated with mean plasma glucose in patients with CFRD just as it does in patients with type 1 diabetes.

Moran A, Hardin D, Rodman D, et al. Diagnosis, screening and management of cystic fibrosis related diabetes mellitus: a consensus conference report. *Diabetes Res Clin Pract*, 1999; Vol. 45: pp. 61–73.

Comments: This comprehensive consensus statement provides current guidelines regarding the diagnosis, screening, and treatment of CFRD.

OTHER REFERENCES

Moran A, Dunitz J, Nathan B, et al. Cystic fibrosis-related diabetes: current trends in prevalence, incidence, and mortality. *Diabetes Care*, 2009; Vol. 32: pp. 1626–31.

Comments: This provides the most up-to-date statistics on the epidemiology (prevalence, incidence, and mortality) of CFRD.

Marshall BC, Butler SM, Stoddard M, et al. Epidemiology of cystic fibrosis-related diabetes. *J Pediatr*, 2005; Vol. 146: pp. 681–7.

Comments: This article provides an excellent summary of the epidemiology of CFRD from the Epidemiology Study of Cystic Fibrosis. This is one of the largest populations of cystic fibrosis patients and at baseline includes 8247 adolescents and adults with the disease in the United States.

Yung B, Noormohamed FH, Kemp M, et al. Cystic fibrosis-related diabetes: the role of peripheral insulin resistance and beta-cell dysfunction. *Diabet Med*, 2002; Vol. 19: pp. 221–6.

Comments: This study demonstrates beta-cell dysfunction in CFRD with similar levels of insulin resistance among CF patients with and without diabetes.

SLEEP APNEA

Naresh Punjabi, MD, PhD

DEFINITION

- Sleep apnea is a common medical comorbidity in patients with type 2 diabetes, and treatment with continuous positive airway pressure (CPAP) may improve glycemic control.

EPIDEMIOLOGY

- 25% of men and 9% of women in the general adult population have obstructive sleep apnea (OSA) (Young).
- Up to 80% of the patients with type 2 diabetes have OSA with 20% affected with severe disease (Foster).
- Patients with type 2 diabetes have increased prevalence of Cheyne-Stokes respiration (Resnick).
- Presence of autonomic neuropathy is associated with a high prevalence of sleep apnea (Bottini).
- OSA may be associated with presence of cardiovascular disease.
- Treatment of OSA with CPAP may improve glycemic control and hypertension (Babu).

DIAGNOSIS

- Overnight sleep study (polysomnography) is the gold-standard diagnostic test.
- Apnea event: complete cessation of airflow during sleep.
- Hypopnea event: decreased airflow during sleep associated with oxygen desaturation or arousal from sleep.
- Obstructive event: Diminished or no airflow with respiratory effort.
- Central event: Diminished or no airflow without respiratory effort.
- Apnea-hypopnea index (AHI): Apneas + hypopneas per hour of sleep.
- Sleep apnea: AHI >5 events/hr.
- OSA: Greater than 50% of disordered breathing events during sleep are obstructive.

COMPLICATIONS AND COMORBIDITIES

- Central sleep apnea: Greater than 50% of disordered breathing events during sleep are central.
- Techniques for monitoring sleep (e.g., oximetry, airflow) available for diagnosis in the home setting.

SIGNS AND SYMPTOMS

- Loud snoring with pauses in breathing during sleep witnessed by a bed partner or family member (Steier).
- Nocturnal episodes of choking and gasping.
- Restless sleep (tossing and turning) and awakenings for nocturia.
- Morning headache, excessive daytime sleepiness and fatigue, impotence.
- Impairments in concentration, attention, and memory.
- Personality changes (aggressiveness, irritability, anxiety, or depression).
- Neck circumference larger than 40 cm.
- Retrognathia, dental overjet (a forward extrusion of the upper incisors beyond the lower incisors).
- Small oropharynx, tonsillar enlargement, macroglossia, edema or erythema of uvula.
- Overweight or obesity (BMI >28 kg/m^2), large abdominal girth, presence of hypertension, lower extremity edema

CLINICAL TREATMENT

- CPAP first-line therapy for moderate to severe OSA.
- Weight loss essential and can be curative. Modest weight loss (10%) can relieve mild sleep-disordered breathing (Peppard).
- Oral appliances (e.g., mandibular advancement devices) for mild disease or for CPAP-intolerant patients.
- Upper airway surgery is an option for those intolerant to CPAP therapy. Lack of consensus as to the most appropriate procedures for OSA patients.
- Supplemental oxygen may be necessary with severe sleep-related hypoxemia.
- Avoidance of alcohol, sedatives, and narcotics, which can increase upper airway collapsibility during sleep.
- Optimizing habitual nighttime sleep duration to avoid sleep deprivation, which can blunt hypoxic and hypercapnic ventilatory chemoresponsiveness.
- Stimulant therapy (e.g., modafinil) approved for the treatment of residual sleepiness in OSA adequately treated with CPAP.

FOLLOW-UP

- After diagnosis, overnight CPAP titration study necessary to determine therapeutic pressure.
- Clinical improvement and compliance with CPAP assessed initially between 1–3 months.
- Yearly routine follow-up for assessing CPAP compliance.
- Repeat sleep testing indicated if sleepiness persists despite CPAP, weight increases or decreases by more than 10%–15%, and patient has upper airway surgery or fabrication of an oral appliance for treatment.

EXPERT OPINION

- Health professionals managing patients at risk for type 2 diabetes or OSA should adopt clinical practices to ensure that a patient with one condition is considered for the other.

- Patients with type 2 diabetes should be assessed for snoring, observed apneas during sleep, and daytime sleepiness.
- A low threshold for referral to diagnose OSA should be used in type 2 diabetes because of the established benefits of therapy on daytime sleepiness, quality of life, glycemic control, and hypertension.
- Management of OSA should focus initially on weight reduction.
- CPAP is the current best treatment for moderate to severe OSA.

REFERENCES

Foster GD, Sanders MH, Millman R, et al. Obstructive sleep apnea among obese patients with type 2 diabetes. *Diabetes Care*, 2009; Vol. 32: pp. 1017–9.

Comments: Demonstration of high prevalence of untreated sleep apnea in patients with type 2 diabetes.

Bazzano LA, Khan Z, Reynolds K, et al. Effect of nocturnal nasal continuous positive airway pressure in obstructive sleep apnea. *Hypertension*, 2007; Vol. 50: pp. 417–23.

Comments: This study demonstrated significant reductions in mean systolic and diastolic blood pressure of ~2 mmHg in those OSA patients treated with versus without CPAP.

Babu AR, Herdegen J, Fogelfeld L, et al. Type 2 diabetes, glycemic control, and continuous positive airway pressure in obstructive sleep apnea. *Arch Intern Med*, 2005; Vol. 165: pp. 447–52.

Comments: Treatment of obstructive sleep apnea with CPAP reduces hemoglobin A1c levels in patients with type 2 diabetes.

Stierer T, Punjabi NM. Demographics and diagnosis of obstructive sleep apnea. *Anesthesiol Clin North Am*, 2005; Vol. 23: pp. 405–20, v.

Comments: General review of the demographic factors associated with obstructive sleep apnea and the methods for diagnosis.

Resnick HE, Redline S, Shahar E, et al. Diabetes and sleep disturbances: findings from the Sleep Heart Health Study. *Diabetes Care*, 2003; Vol. 26: pp. 702–9.

Comments: Largest community-based study demonstrating the higher prevalence of periodic breathing (Cheyne-Stokes respiration) in those with type 2 diabetes.

Bottini P, Dottorini ML, Cristina Cordoni M, et al. Sleep-disordered breathing in nonobese diabetic subjects with autonomic neuropathy. *Eur Respir J*, 2003; Vol. 22: pp. 654–60.

Comments: Autonomic neuropathy in patients with type 2 diabetes associated with a higher prevalence of obstructive sleep apnea.

Shamsuzzaman AS, Gersh BJ, Somers VK. Obstructive sleep apnea: implications for cardiac and vascular disease. *JAMA*, 2003; Vol. 290: pp. 1906–14.

Comments: This systematic review describes the association of OSA with cardiovascular diseases.

Peppard PE, Young T, Palta M, et al. Prospective study of the association between sleep-disordered breathing and hypertension. *N Engl J Med*, 2000; Vol. 342: pp. 1378–4.

Comments: Describes the dose-response association of sleep-disordered breathing with presence of hypertension four years later.

Peppard PE, Young T, Palta M, et al. Longitudinal study of moderate weight change and sleep-disordered breathing. *JAMA*, 2000; Vol. 284: pp. 3015–21.

Comments: Observation longitudinal study describing the association between weight increase and decrease and the propensity for sleep apnea.

Young T, Palta M, Dempsey J, et al. The occurrence of sleep-disordered breathing among middle-aged adults. *NEJM*, 1993; Vol. 328: pp. 1230–5.

Comments: Population-based study on prevalence of obstructive sleep apnea in adult men and women. Approximately 9% of women and 25% of men have obstructive sleep apnea.

COMPLICATIONS AND COMORBIDITIES

Renal and Urinary Diseases

NEPHROPATHY

Donna I. Myers, MD

DEFINITION

- Diabetic nephropathy (DN) is one of the more common long-term, microvascular complications of diabetes.
- Characterized initially by microalbuminuria (30–300 mg albumin/gram creatinine), then macroalbuminuria ("gross" or "clinical" proteinuria) (>300 mg/gram creatinine), followed by elevated BUN and creatinine, and finally end-stage renal disease (ESRD).
- Pathologic changes in the kidney are classically nodular glomerulosclerosis, although histologic changes may include a number of other features.

EPIDEMIOLOGY

- Occurs in any type of diabetes mellitus, with a similar prevalence rate of 25%.
- The predictive value of microalbuminuria for progression is strongest in type 1 diabetes.
- Microalbuminuria within 10 years of onset of type 1 diabetes almost always progresses; after 16 years of diabetes, the onset of microalbuminuria is less predictive (30% progress).
- For type 2 diabetes the predictive value of microalbuminuria is weaker; 25% of type 2 patients have microalbuminuria at 10 years' duration, but only 20%–40% will progress to macroalbuminuria.
- Although the outcome for diabetic nephropathy has improved due to improved blood pressure (BP) management and renin angiotensin aldosterone system (RAAS) blockade, despite advances in treatment, the increased prevalence of diabetes has increased the number of patients with diabetes and ESRD.
- In type 1 diabetes, if both parents had hypertension (HTN), there is an increased risk of developing chronic kidney disease (CKD).
- The majority of type 1 diabetes patients with macroalbuminuria have some sign of diabetic retinopathy, but only ~50% of patients with type 2 diabetes and overt proteinuria have diabetic retinopathy.

DIAGNOSIS

- Chronic kidney disease (CKD) is classified by proteinuria and glomerular filtration rate (GFR) in ml/min/1.73 m^2 as follows: Stage 1 = persistent proteinuria >3 months, GFR >90; Stage 2 = GFR 60–89; Stage 3 = GFR 30–59; Stage 4 = GFR 15–29; Stage 5 = GFR <15.
- Glomerular hyperfiltration (GFR >120) occurs early in 25%–50% of patients with diabetes; this triples the risk of developing diabetic nephropathy.
- Microalbuminuria or macroalbuminuria can be diagnosed based on a random urine sample collected for both albumin and creatinine, and confirmed on a different day. Random urine samples provide relatively good approximations of daily albumin excretion; 24-hour urine collections are not routinely used for diagnosis and may be less practical (see Albuminuria, p. 597).

- Macroalbuminuria heralds a decline in glomerular filtration rate (GFR); the natural history is progression to end-stage renal disease (ESRD) within 3–5 years.
- Hypertension, or resting BP >140/90 mmHg, virtually always occurs early in the course of DN; its absence puts the diagnosis of DN in question.
- Nondiabetic renal disease should be suspected if: diabetes duration <5 years; sudden onset of macroalbuminuria; reduced GFR in the absence of proteinuria; acute renal failure; active urinary sediment; and absence of diabetic retinopathy, especially in type 1 diabetes.

SIGNS AND SYMPTOMS

- DN and stages 1–2 CKD generally have no symptoms, although HTN may be present.
- Nephrotic syndrome (>3 g albuminuria/day) causes renal sodium retention; frothy urine; weight gain with diffuse edema; progression to uncontrolled HTN and heart failure; and nocturia that may disrupt sleep.
- Imaging typically finds normal to large sized kidneys, even with advanced stages of CKD due to DN.
- Urine sediment is nephrotic (bland with lipiduria); microscopic hematuria may be present.
- Anemia, progressive metabolic acidosis, hyperphosphatemia with secondary hyperparathyroidism, and hyperkalemia may be present by stage 3 CKD.
- Late symptoms of uremia include anorexia, weight loss (often masked by fluid retention), early morning nausea, lack of energy, and hypersomnolence; a metallic taste may be noted.
- With slowly progressive CKD, symptoms are indolent and the patient may be unaware of them.
- Dialysis (see Dialysis Initiation and Management, p. 372) generally indicated earlier with DN versus other causes of ESRD (i.e., when GFR is 10–15 vs <10) because of comorbidities such as cardiovascular disease.
- Evaluate for diabetic retinopathy and other comorbidities (e.g., obesity, obstructive sleep apnea).

CLINICAL TREATMENT

Glycemic Control

- Tighter blood glucose control early in the course of diabetes reduces hyperfiltration.
- In the early stages of DN (CKD 1–3) optimizing glycemic control may stabilize or even reverse renal disease; HbA1c of 6%–7% is advised.
- Educate patients about the relationship between poor diabetic control and the potential late complications of DN.
- With CKD stages 4–5, initially there is insulin resistance and worsening glycemic control requiring higher insulin dosage; later, decreased renal degradation of insulin and hypoglycemia may ensue in ESRD requiring lower insulin dosage.
- When approaching ESRD, closely monitor for hypoglycemia and adjust; patients may come off insulin altogether.
- Metformin is contraindicated when GFR <60 and/or serum creatinine >1.5 mg/dl, because of an increased risk of lactic acidosis.

Hypertension Management

- See also Renal Diseases in Diabetes, p. 367.
- Monitor blood pressure (BP) at each clinic visit and at home.

- Target BP <130/80 mmHg.
- Restrict dietary sodium restriction to 100 mM/day (2.3 g), limit alcohol intake, promote weight loss (if needed) and exercise.
- Unilateral or bilateral renal artery stenosis (RAS) often coexists with DN; in CKD stages 1–2, RAS diagnosed with a gadolinium-enhanced magnetic resonance angiography (MRA) but in CKD stages 3–5, Doppler flow studies of the renal arteries or an unenhanced MRA is best.
- Most hypertensive diabetic patients will require multiple anti-HTN agents to achieve BP goals; thiazides or loop diuretics may be first-line therapy for many patients.
- RAAS blockade using angiotensin converting enzyme inhibitors (ACE-I) or angiotensin receptor blockers (ARBs) is useful for both blood pressure and proteinuria control and indicated for left ventricular systolic dysfunction; drug combinations of ACE-I and ARB may worsen renal outcome and, if used, require close renal monitoring. ACE-I and ARBs are contraindicated in women of child-bearing age who are trying to become pregnant, patients prone to dehydration, patients with refractory hyperkalemia, or a rise in serum creatinine >0.6 mg/dl with initiation of therapy.
- Beta-blockers are beneficial, especially in patients with a history of congestive heart failure, but should be used with caution in all patients with asthma.
- Calcium channel blockers (CCBs), both dihydropyridine (DHP) and non-DHPs, are useful; non-DHPs are more renoprotective but may depress myocardial function. CCBs may cause lower extremity edema and constipation.
- Simplify dosing schedules whenever possible to improve compliance.

Micro- and Macroalbuminuria

- A spot urine albumin to creatinine ratio is recommended to screen for microalbuminuria.
- RAAS blockade should be initiated in type 1 diabetes with microalbuminuria with or without hypertension (see previous Hypertension Management section).
- With RAAS blockade, monitor closely to avoid hypotension and dehydration. Check serum potassium and creatinine levels at baseline and 7–10 days after initiation of therapy or an increase in dosage.
- Titrate RAAS blockade if microalbuminuria progresses, as blood pressure allows.
- Macroalbuminuria management is similar to that of microalbuminuria management; however, dietary sodium restriction is usually necessary at this stage, <100 mM/day (<2.3 g).
- RAAS blockade in patients who have diabetes but no proteinuria is controversial; it may improve cardiovascular outcomes but actually worsen renal outcomes.
- Modest dietary protein reduction for CKD stages 4–5, 0.8 g/kg with protein supplements.
- At all stages of CKD, avoid weight reduction diets.
- High protein intake in CKD is associated with glomerular hyperfiltration, increased azotemia, metabolic acidosis, and fatigue.

Edema Management

- Dietary counseling with reduction of processed foods and salt.
- Fluid retention is treated initially with dietary sodium restriction to ≤2 g/day.
- Diuretics should be used only if diet fails to manage edema.
- In early CKD (stages 1–2) thiazide diuretics are used; in CKD stages 3–5, loop diuretics (furosemide) are preferred, and may require a twice-daily dosing schedule.

- For comfort, avoid diuretics in the evening.
- Patients should elevate their legs (hip height) when sitting and after taking diuretics to reduce swollen legs.
- Support stockings during day and before getting out of bed in the morning may enhance diuretics and reduce risk of skin breakdown and infection.
- Serum electrolytes, creatinine, and blood urea nitrogen should be monitored closely in all patients on diuretics.
- Mild prerenal azotemia may be tolerated, but severe prerenal failure should be avoided.
- The National Kidney Foundation website is a resource for patient education (*http://www.kidney.org*).

Nephrology Referral

- Early referral to nephrology lowers morbidity, promotes more timely placement of dialysis access, facilitates preemptive renal transplantation, lowers overall costs, and improves survival.
- Late referral means within 6 months of starting dialysis.
- See Dialysis Initiation and Management, p. 372.

FOLLOW-UP

- Check urine microalbumin annually beginning in type 1 diabetes after 5 years, and from the onset of type 2 diabetes; a positive finding requires confirmation.
- Check BP with each clinic visit; for orthostatic symptoms, check in supine, sitting, and standing positions.
- In known DN with CKD stages 1–2, monitor renal function at least every 6 months.
- In known DN with CKD stages 3–5, monitor every 3 months including serum electrolytes (sodium, potassium, chloride, CO_2), bone-mineral balance (calcium, phosphorus, intact PTH), nutrition (serum albumin, urea nitrogen), anemia (Hgb, Hct, iron studies) along with an estimate of GFR (serum creatinine) and spot urine microalbumin.
- In early DN (stages 1–2 CKD), goal is reversal of disease, achieved by tight glycemic control, BP management, and RAAS blockade, especially in type 1 diabetes.
- With intermediate diabetic nephropathy (stages 3–4 CKD) goal is slowing progression by meticulous attention to known therapeutic interventions and avoidance of nephrotoxins.
- With late diabetic nephropathy (stage 5 CKD), goal is the avoidance of acute on chronic kidney disease (e.g., by contrast studies) and smoothing the transition to maintenance dialysis or transplantation in a timely manner.

EXPERT OPINION

- Referral to nephrology should be made by stage 3 CKD to: evaluate for other causes of CKD, educate regarding management options for ESRD, arrange referral to vascular surgery for access planning, and plan for the possibility of preemptive renal transplantation.
- Potentially reversible comorbidities such as obstructive sleep apnea, cigarette smoking, morbid obesity, hyperlipidemia, RAS, bladder outlet obstruction with associated hydronephrosis and/or infection, and ongoing exposure to nephrotoxins (e.g., NSAIDs) should be addressed in all stages of DN.
- Patients considering pregnancy should be taken off RAAS blockade. Diabetic nephropathy may worsen during pregnancy, sometimes irreversibly.

COMPLICATIONS AND COMORBIDITIES

BASIS FOR RECOMMENDATIONS

KDOQI. KDOQI Clinical Practice Guidelines and Clinical Practice Recommendations for Diabetes and Chronic Kidney Disease. *Am J Kidney Dis*, 2007; Vol. 49: pp. S12–154.

Comments: The Kidney Disease Outcomes Quality Initiative (K/DOQI) has published this comprehensive reference text for the clinician involved in managing diabetic patients with chronic kidney disease. Reviews national (US) guidelines for management and the rationale for these therapies.

Chobanian AV, Bakris GL, Black HR, et al. The seventh report of the Joint National Committee on Prevention, Detection, Evaluation, and Treatment of High Blood Pressure: the JNC 7 report. *JAMA*, 2003; Vol. 289: pp. 2560–72.

Comments: A landmark report outlining stricter guidelines for blood pressure control.

OTHER REFERENCES

Magee GM, Bilous RW, Cardwell CR, et al. Is hyperfiltration associated with the future risk of developing diabetic nephropathy? A meta-analysis. *Diabetologia*, 2009; Vol. 52: pp. 691–7.

Comments: A meta-analysis of 10 cohort studies in type 1 diabetes mellitus to determine the predictive value of early glomerular hyperfiltration for future diabetic nephropathy.

Onuigbo MA. Reno-prevention vs. reno-protection: a critical re-appraisal of the evidence-base from the large RAAS blockade trials after ONTARGET—a call for more circumspection. *QJM*, 2009; Vol. 102: pp. 155–67.

Comments: An important review article outlining the need for close monitoring to avoid acute kidney injury when using RAAS blockade in advanced CKD.

Locatelli F, Del Vecchio L, Cavalli A. Inhibition of the renin-angiotensin system in chronic kidney disease: a critical look to single and dual blockade. *Nephron Clin Pract*, 2009; Vol. 113: pp. c286–c293.

Comments: A comprehensive review article of the benefits and risks of RAAS blockade in CKD patients.

Mann JF, Schmieder RE, Dyal L, et al. Effect of telmisartan on renal outcomes: a randomized trial. *Ann Intern Med*, 2009; Vol. 151: pp. 1–10, W1–2.

Comments: Summarizes the renal outcomes of the TRANSCEND trial that randomized patients with diabetes or cardiovascular disease to telmisartan versus placebo and found a positive effect of ARB therapy on cardiac outcomes but a negative impact on renal outcomes.

Parfrey PS. Angiotensin-receptor blockers in the prevention or treatment of microalbuminuria. *Ann Intern Med*, 2009; Vol. 151: pp. 63–5.

Comments: An editorial that reviews the adverse or neutral effects of ARB therapy on renal outcome in diabetic patients without baseline renal disease.

Waden J, Forsblom C, Thorn LM, et al. A1C variability predicts incident cardiovascular events, microalbuminuria, and overt diabetic nephropathy in patients with type 1 diabetes. *Diabetes*, 2009; Vol. 58: pp. 2649–55.

Comments: A Finnish study of 2107 patients with type 1 diabetes showed that increasing A1c levels were associated with microalbuminuria, progressive CKD and CVD events, confirming and expanding the original findings of the Diabetes Control and Complications Trial (DCCT).

Diabetes Control and Complications Trial/Epidemiology of Diabetes Interventions and Complications (DCCT/EDIC) Research Group, Nathan DM, Zinman B, et al. Modern-day clinical course of type 1 diabetes mellitus after 30 years' duration: the diabetes control and complications trial/epidemiology of diabetes interventions and complications and Pittsburgh epidemiology of diabetes complications experience (1983–2005). *Arch Intern Med*, 2009; Vol. 169: pp. 1307–16.

Comments: An update on the importance of the DCCT and other longitudinal trials that changed the course of type 1 diabetes over the last 25 yrs by intensive diabetic management, resulting in a 50% reduction in microvascular complications.

Kalaitzidis R, Bakris GL. Effects of angiotensin II receptor blockers on diabetic nephropathy. *J Hypertens*, 2009; Vol. 27 Suppl 5: pp. S15–21.

Comments: A comprehensive review of the importance of targeting proteinuria as a risk factor for both renal and cardiovascular disease.

Mauer M, Zinman B, Gardiner R, et al. Renal and retinal effects of enalapril and losartan in type 1 diabetes. *NEJM,* 2009; Vol. 361: pp. 40–51.

Comments: A small but meticulous study of the effects of RAAS blockade on renal and retinal outcomes in normotensive subjects with type 1 diabetes. There were no renal benefits by biopsy, but they did receive retinal benefits. Surprisingly, ARB therapy was associated with a higher incidence of developing microalbuminuria than placebo or ACE-I therapy.

Fioretto P, Caramori ML, Mauer M. The kidney in diabetes: dynamic pathways of injury and repair. The Camillo Golgi Lecture 2007. *Diabetologia,* 2008; Vol. 51: pp. 1347–55.

Comments: An elegant review of general interest regarding current and future directions for the treatment of diabetic nephropathy.

Wolf G, Müller N, Mandecka A, et al. Association of diabetic retinopathy and renal function in patients with types 1 and 2 diabetes mellitus. *Clin Nephrol,* 2007; Vol. 68: pp. 81–6.

Comments: Underscores the variability of diabetic retinopathy and renal disease in types 1 and 2 diabetes mellitus.

Atkins RC, Briganti EM, Lewis JB, et al. Proteinuria reduction and progression to renal failure in patients with type 2 diabetes mellitus and overt nephropathy. *Am J Kidney Dis,* 2005; Vol. 45: pp. 281–7.

Comments: A comparison trial (The Irbesartan Diabetic Nephropathy Trial, IDNT) of an ARB (irbesartan) and a calcium channel blocker (amlodipine) for proteinuria reduction in type 2 diabetes.

Morales E, Valero MA, Leon M, et al. Beneficial effects of weight loss in overweight patients with chronic protein-uric nephropathies. *Am J Kidney Dis,* 2003; Vol. 41: pp. 319–27.

Comments: A study that looks at the association of obesity with proteinuria, and protection by weight loss.

Adler AI, Stratton IM, Neil HA, et al. Association of systolic blood pressure with macrovascular and microvascular complications of type 2 diabetes (UKPDS 36): prospective observational study. *BMJ,* 2000; Vol. 321: pp. 412–9.

Comments: A multicentered observational study (UK Prospective Diabetes Study Group 36) of hypertension and vascular complications of type 2 diabetes.

RENAL DISEASES IN DIABETES

Donna I. Myers, MD

COMPLICATIONS AND COMORBIDITIES

DEFINITION

- Renal disease in diabetes may be caused by diabetes, or may be of other etiology, coexisting with diabetes.
- In diabetes, persistant proteinuria without other cause is the first sign of diabetic nephropathy.

EPIDEMIOLOGY

- Diabetes is the most common cause of end-stage renal disease (ESRD) in the world (Harvey).
- Only 25% of type 1 and 2 diabetes patients will develop classic diabetic nephropathy, hypertensive nephropathy; however, nephrosclerosis, atherosclerotic renal artery stenosis, nondiabetic glomerulopathies, acute and chronic pyelonephritis, papillary necrosis, and type IV renal tubular acidosis (RTA) are all more prevalent in diabetes (Mazzucco).
- The majority of proteinuric renal disease in both types 1 and 2 diabetes with a gradual onset after 10 years of diabetes is due to diabetic nephropathy (Mazzucco; Harvcy).

DIAGNOSIS

- Staging kidney disease requires only a spot urine albumin to creatinine ratio, a serum creatinine level, and a calculated GFR using the modified MDRD formula (see National Kidney Foundation GFR Calculator, *http://www.kidney.org/professionals/kdoqi/ gfr_calculator.cfm*).
- Chronic kidney disease (CKD) is classified by urinary albumin and glomerular filtration rate (GFR) in ml/min/1.73 m²: Stage 1 = proteinuria, GFR ≥90; Stage 2 = proteinuria, GFR 60–89; Stage 3 = GFR 30–59; Stage 4 = GFR 15–29; Stage 5 = GFR <15.
- Further evaluation includes a complete urinalysis, serum electrolytes, and renal ultrasound; renal biopsy may be necessary in some cases (see Renal Function, p. 593).
- Type IV RTA (hyporeninemic hypoaldosteronism) should be suspected in any patient with diabetes and hyperkalemia in the absence of advanced kidney disease, K+ supplements or K+ sparing diuretics; a mild metabolic acidosis is usually present with a normal anion gap (see Hypoaldosteronism, p. 557).
- Suspect renal artery stenosis if accelerated hypertension, severe peripheral vascular disease, abdominal and femoral bruits, asymmetric kidneys (1.5-cm discrepancy), and/or a rise in serum creatinine >0.6 mg/dl with angiotensin-converting enzyme inhibitors (ACE-I) or angiotensin receptor blockers (ARBs).

SIGNS AND SYMPTOMS

- Laboratory signs of renal disease include proteinuria, decreased glomerular filtration rate, elevated blood urea nitrogen, hyperkalemia and type 4 renal tubular acidosis.
- Physical findings of patients with early renal disease include hypertension and edema.
- Early symptoms of renal disease include anorexia, a "metal" taste in the mouth, early morning nausea, frothy urine (with >3 g proteinuria), nocturia, fatigue, and excessive sleeping.
- Intermediate symptoms include difficulty concentrating, loss of lean body mass, restless legs, and lethargy.
- Late signs include uremic fetor, asterixis, peripheral neuropathy, altered mental status, and seizures.

CLINICAL TREATMENT

Therapeutic Goals

- There are no agreed-upon guidelines for glycemic control in diabetic patients with CKD, but good control may slow progression.
- With CKD stages 1–4, follow general guidelines and maintain HbA1c between 6%–7%.
- Interference with HbA1c assay by uremia, acidosis, and shortened red blood cell survival may spuriously affect HbA1c levels in stage 5 CKD and ESRD.
- Follow blood pressure (BP) guidelines of JNC7 (<130/80 mmHg) with attention to postural changes from medications and diabetic autonomic neuropathy.
- Reduce proteinuria by renin angiotensin system (RAAS) blockade in all renal patients.
- Limit dietary sodium to 2.0 g/day (100 mM), including "hidden" dietary sodium (i.e., canned foods).
- Uncontrollable hyperkalemia and a rise in serum creatinine >0.6 mg/dl limit therapy.
- Obesity should be addressed with dieting and exercise to reduce hypertension, obstructive sleep apnea, and secondary focal and segmental glomerulosclerosis caused by hyperfiltration across glomerular capillary membranes.

- Hyperlipidemia management may reduce the burden of atherosclerotic disease, which often accompanies diabetic renal disease.
- Cigarette smoking cessation reduces proteinuria.

Pharmacology-Drug Adjustment for Declining GFR

- Patients with diabetes and progressive renal disease may develop poor glucose control due to reduced insulin sensitivity and require increasingly higher doses of insulin therapy.
- As patients approach ESRD, insulin requirements may decline due to reduced insulin clearance from the kidneys.
- Avoid metformin in stages 3, 4, and 5 CKD (increased risk of lactic acidosis). Contraindicated with creatinine >1.5 mg/dl.
- Dose-adjust all diabetes medications for reduced GFR (see Table 3-17).
- Type IV RTA should be treated with dietary K+ limitation and avoidance of K+ supplements; discontinuation of ACE-I or ARB therapy may become necessary in some patients.

TABLE 3-17. DOSING ADJUSTMENTS BY CKD STAGE FOR DRUGS USED TO TREAT HYPERGLYCEMIA*

Class	Drug	CKD Stage 3–5	Dialysis
First-generation sulfonylureas	Acetohexamide	Avoid.	Avoid.
	Chlorpropamide	Dose adjustment if GFR 50–70 ml/min; avoid with GFR <50 ml/min.	Avoid.
	Tolazamide	Avoid.	Avoid.
	Tolbutamide	Avoid.	Avoid.
Second-generation sulfonylureas	Glipizide	Oral drug of choice.	Oral drug of choice.
	Glyburide	Avoid.	Avoid.
	Glimepiride	Initiate at low dose.	Avoid.
Alpha-glucosidase inhibitors	Acarbose	Avoid if creatinine >2 mg/dl.	Avoid.
	Miglitol	Avoid if creatinine >2 mg/dl.	Avoid.

COMPLICATIONS AND COMORBIDITIES

TABLE 3-17. DOSING ADJUSTMENTS BY CKD STAGE FOR DRUGS USED TO TREAT HYPERGLYCEMIA* (CONT.)

Class	Drug	CKD Stage 3–5	Dialysis
Biguanides	Metformin	Avoid if creatinine >1.5 mg/dl (men) or >1.4 mg/dl (women).	Avoid.
Meglitinides	Repaglinide	Use with caution.	Use with caution.
	Nateglinide	Initiate at low dose.	Avoid.
Thiazolidinediones	Pioglitazone	Use with caution.	Use with caution.
	Rosiglitazone	Use with caution.	Use with caution.
Incretin mimetic	Exenatide	Avoid with GFR <30 ml/min.	Avoid.
Amylin analog	Pramlintide	Use with caution.	Not studied.
DPP-4 inhibitor	Sitagliptin	Dose adjustment required if GFR < 50 ml/min.	Dose adjustment required.

*Adapted from National Kidney Foundation. KDOQI Clinical Practice Guidelines and Clinical Practice Recommendations for Diabetes and Chronic Kidney Disease. Am J Kidney Dis, 2007; Vol. 49 Suppl 2: S1–180 (Table 22).

Hypertension Management

- Lifestyle: exercise, limited alcohol, weight loss; limit sodium to 2 g/day (100 mM).
- Check BP supine and standing.
- If diuretics needed, use thiazides diuretics in stages 1–3 CKD; loop diuretics (furosemide) in stages 4–5 CKD, may require twice-daily dosing; potassium-sparing diuretics used cautiously if at all in stages 3, 4, and 5 CKD.
- RAAS blockade with ACE-I and ARBs indicated for urinary protein reduction, reno-protection and HTN control; also improves cardiac outcome if congestive heart failure or left ventricular dysfunction.
- Combining ACE and ARB therapy may further reduce proteinuria but also worsen overall renal outcome; monitor closely.
- Initiation or increases in ACE-I or ARBs should be monitored within 7 days for hyperkalemia and acute kidney injury.
- The combination of diuretics and ACE-I or ARB therapy in a patient who becomes volume depleted may precipitate acute renal failure.
- Nonselective beta-blockers improve insulin sensitivity and reduce proteinuria in contrast to beta-1 selective blockers.
- Non-dihydropyridine agents are more effective in reducing proteinuria but may cause myocardial depression.

Avoid Nephrotoxins

- Avoid NSAIDs in all patients with CKD; with diabetes, further increases risk of papillary necrosis.
- Radiographic IV contrast is nephrotoxic in a dose-dependent manner; risk factors include diabetes, proteinuria, ineffective renal perfusion (CHF, Cirrhosis), and CKD stages 3–5.
- If contrast is essential, use low osmolar nonionic contrast and prophylactic measures one day before and the day of the dye load.
- Prophylactic measures: N-acetylcysteine 1200 mg PO twice-daily · 2 days (see Acetylcysteine, p. 531), saline hydration, and discontinuation of ACE-I/ARBs and diuretics.
- Minimizing the dye load is most important.
- Gadolinium, to enhance MRI studies, used only with caution in early CKD, and contraindicated with stages 4–5 CKD due to risk of nephrogenic systemic fibrosis.
- Bisphosphonates contraindicated in patients with a GFR <30 ml/min (stages 4–5 CKD).
- Phosphate-containing bowel preps may cause severe hyperphosphatemia and acute, irreversible kidney injury; avoid with CKD.

FOLLOW-UP

- Annual screening for CKD starting with diagnosis of T2DM and after 5 years of T1DM using spot urinary albumin:creatinine ratio, serum creatinine, estimated GFR.
- Refer patients with diabetes and stage 1–2 chronic kidney disease in whom the renal diagnosis is unclear.
- When feasible, refer to nephrology at stage 3 CKD.
- Stages 4–5 pre-ESRD patients should be followed closely by nephrology.

EXPERT OPINION

- Inform the patient of the therapeutic goals of management.
- Therapy with RAAS blockade and diuretics is a double-edged sword: risk is that these agents can cause acute kidney injury from dehydration.
- In the absence of coexisting diabetic retinopathy, diabetic nephropathy is uncommon and other etiologies for renal disease should be considered.
- Many diabetes medications including insulin and oral agents will need dose adjustment as renal disease progresses.

BASIS FOR RECOMMENDATIONS

Bakris GL, Sowers JR, American Society of Hypertension (ASH) Writing Group. ASH position paper: treatment of hypertension in patients with diabetes—an update. *J Clin Hypertens* (Greenwich), 2008; Vol. 10: pp. 707–13, discussion 714-5.

    Comments: A consensus report from the American Society of Hypertension (ASH) on managing HTN in patients with diabetes.

The Kidney Disease Outcomes Quality Initiative (K/DOQI). K/DOQI clinical practice guidelines and clinical practice recommendations for diabetes and chronic kidney disease. *Am J Kidney Dis*, 2007; Vol. 49(2 Suppl 2): S12– 154.

    Comments: The Kidney Disease Outcomes Quality Initiative (K/DOQI) has published this comprehensive reference text for the clinician involved in managing diabetic patients with chronic kidney disease; reviews national (US) guidelines for management and the rationale for these therapies.

Chobanian AV, Bakris GL, Black HR, et al. The seventh report of the Joint National Committee on Prevention, Detection, Evaluation, and Treatment of High Blood Pressure: the JNC 7 report. *JAMA*, 2003; Vol. 289: pp. 2560–72.

    Comments: A landmark report updating stricter guidelines for blood pressure control.

COMPLICATIONS AND COMORBIDITIES

Bakris GL, Williams M, Dworkin L, et al. Preserving renal function in adults with hypertension and diabetes: a consensus approach. National Kidney Foundation Hypertension and Diabetes Executive Committees Working Group. *Am J Kidney Dis,* 2000; Vol. 36: pp. 646–61.

    Comments: National guidelines on hypertension management in patients with diabetes and CKD.

OTHER REFERENCES

Appel LJ, American Society of Hypertension Writing Group, Giles TD, et al. ASH Position Paper: dietary approaches to lower blood pressure. *J Clin Hypertens (Greenwich),* 2009; Vol. 11: pp. 358–68.

    Comments: An ASH position paper on dietary management of HTN.

Wetzels JF. Renal outcomes in the ONTARGET study. *Lancet,* 2008; Vol. 372: p. 2020, author reply 2020–1.

    Comments: A trial with some evidence that the combination of ACE-I and ARB therapy may impact negatively on renal outcome in diabetes.

Bakris GL, Fonseca V, Katholi RE, et al. Differential effects of beta-blockers on albuminuria in patients with type 2 diabetes. *Hypertension,* 2005; Vol. 46: pp. 1309–15.

    Comments: A comparison of selective versus nonselective beta-blockers in diabetes.

Grossman E, Messerli FH. Are calcium antagonists beneficial in diabetic patients with hypertension? *Am J Med,* 2004; Vol. 116: pp. 44–9.

    Comments: A meta-analysis of 14 studies using calcium antagonists in hypertensive patients with diabetes and outcomes of cardiovascular protection

Harvey, John N. Trends in the prevalence of diabetic nephropathy in type 1 and type 2 diabetes. *Curr Opin Nephrol Hypertens,* 2003; Vol. 12(3): pp. 317–322.

    Comments: A concise epidemiologic review article of the increasing prevalence of diabetic nephropathy worldwide.

Ansari A, Thomas S, Goldsmith D. Assessing glycemic control in patients with diabetes and end-stage renal failure. *Am J Kidney Dis,* 2003; Vol. 41: pp. 523–31.

    Comments: A focused review of monitoring glycemic control in end-stage renal disease patients.

Mazzucco, G., Bertani T, Fortunato, M, et al. Different patterns of renal damage in type 2 diabetes mellitus: a multicentric study on 393 biopsies. *Am J Kidney Dis,* 2002; Vol. 39(4): pp. 713–720.

    Comments: An original article that underscores the prevalence of nondiabetic nephropathy in patients with diabetes.

Emslie-Smith AM, Boyle DI, Evans JM, et al. Contraindications to metformin therapy in patients with type 2 diabetes—a population-based study of adherence to prescribing guidelines. *Diabet Med,* 2001; Vol. 18: pp. 483–8.

    Comments: An article that reveals widespread prescribing of metformin against pharmaceutical precautions and yet a very low incidence of lactic acidosis.

DeFronzo RA. Pharmacologic therapy for type 2 diabetes mellitus. *Ann Intern Med,* 1999; Vol. 131: pp. 281–303.

    Comments: An article that includes precautions for using metformin in diabetic patients with CKD.

DIALYSIS INITIATION AND MANAGEMENT

Donna I. Myers, MD

DEFINITION

- Management options for all people with end-stage renal disease (ESRD) include maintenance hemodialysis (HD), peritoneal dialysis (PD), and renal transplantation (Tpl).

EPIDEMIOLOGY

- About 40%–50% of all people on dialysis have ESRD secondary to diabetic nephropathy (DN), making diabetes the most common cause of ESRD.
- Survival on dialysis is worse for patients with diabetes compared to those without diabetes.

- Survival on PD and HD are similar in most studies. Five-year survival for patients with diabetic nephropathy on PD is about 24%, on HD is about 27%, versus 33% for all patients on dialysis.
- 50% of asymptomatic patients with diabetes and advanced chronic kidney disease (CKD) have previously unsuspected coronary artery disease.
- Most deaths of patients on renal replacement therapy are from accelerated cardiovascular disease and infections.

DIAGNOSIS

- See Nephropathy (p. 362) and Renal Diseases in Diabetes (p. 367).

SIGNS AND SYMPTOMS

- Uremia refers to a constellation of multiorgan signs and symptoms due to accumulation of nitrogenous waste products.
- Signs and symptoms that constitute "hard" indications for starting dialysis include uremic or gastrointestinal bleeding, refractory fluid overload with recurrent congestive heart failure, uremic serositis (pericarditis, pleuritis, or peritonitis), uncontrollable metabolic acidosis and/or hyperkalemia, and altered mental status with no other apparent etiology.
- Less clear, "soft," indications for initiating dialysis include anorexia, nausea, metallic taste, weight loss, fluid retention, inattention, and failure to thrive in a patient with stage 5 CKD (GFR <15 ml/min/1.73 m²).

CLINICAL TREATMENT

Overall Management and Patient Preparation

- Early referral to nephrology in stages 1–3 chronic kidney disease (CKD) may allow reversal or slowing of DN progression. With continuing irreversible decline in glomular filtration rate (GFR), patient education should begin by stage 3 CKD.
- Because of comorbidities and uremic symptoms in diabetes, start dialysis with GFR <15 ml/min/1.73 m², rather than <10 ml/min/1.73 m² as in other patients.
- Selection of modality of treatment (HD, PD, Tpl) is guided by comorbidities and preferences of the patient and family.
- PD is an option in diabetes. Limiting factors: poor vision, inadequate manual dexterity in the absence of home support, uncontrolled diabetes (type 1), multiple abdominal surgeries, and morbid obesity.
- HD is also an option. Limiting factors: difficulty creating a permanent vascular access, hemodynamic instability during dialysis, and mobility problems.
- If patient is a candidate for kidney Tpl, this is preferred, particularly if there is an eligible living related or unrelated donor (see Kidney Transplantation, p. 379). Five-year all-patient survival with a kidney transplant is 69% better than for dialysis.
- Late referral to nephrology (within 6 months of starting dialysis) occurs in 25%–50% of patients and is associated with a poorer outcome.
- Patient Preparation: Pre-ESRD, inform the patient of his/her treatment options. Optimally, use a dialysis nurse, a transplant representative, renal dietician, and social worker.
- Prior to selecting HD or PD, refer to vascular surgeon, to estimate the feasibility of a native arteriovenous fistula (AVF), a fistula/graft (AVF/G), or a Tenckhoff peritoneal dialysis catheter.

COMPLICATIONS AND COMORBIDITIES

- For HD, a native fistula (using patient's own vein and artery) is far preferable to a graft, which itself is preferable to a catheter. Lead time for maturation of AVF is at least 3–6 months; for an AVF/G 4–6 weeks. A catheter may be used immediately.

General Complications

- With extensive peripheral vascular disease, increased risk for a steal syndrome (distal ischemia due to high blood flow through an AVF or AVF/G); PD may be a better option.
- Temporary or long-term tunneled HD catheters may cause central venous stenosis, thrombosis, and life-threatening infections; they should be avoided whenever possible.
- With morbid obesity or multiple abdominal procedures, abdominal PD may not be feasible but could consider pre-sternal PD. Lead time for a PD catheter is 3–4 weeks.
- Infection may complicate both HD and PD.
- Catheter-related PD complication: Bacterial peritonitis occurs about once in 30 treatment months. Signs and symptoms: abdominal pain, cloudy effluent; generally without bacteremia. Treat usually with intraperitoneal antibiotics in an outpatient setting.
- HD complication: Access-related infections may begin as undetected intermittent bacteremia, progressing to symptoms of overt sepsis (rigors, fever, nausea, and vomiting) with no other obvious source. Bacterial endocarditis (*Staphylococcal aureus*) with or without septic emboli is common. Infection rate is 10–20 times more common with a catheter versus a native AVF.
- Consider preemptive Tpl for diabetic patients with stages 4–5 CKD, if there is a suitable donor. Evaluation begins within 6 months of needing dialysis. Tpl after starting dialysis is possible if patient is a good surgical candidate.

Fluid and Electrolyte Complications in ESRD

- Hypertension in ESRD is generally volume-related. Other complications of fluid overload: CHF and hemodynamic instability during HD.
- Lower fluid gains between dialyses are achieved by dietary counseling (sodium restriction) and glycemic control to avoid excessive thirst and fluid overload.
- Intradialytic hypotension occurs in up to 30% of hemodialysis treatments. It is more common among patients who are elderly, those with autonomic dysfunction (diabetes), high fluid gains, or poor cardiac reserve.
- Therapies for recurrent intradialytic hypotension on HD include dietary counseling, cooling the dialysate, sodium modeling (varying the sodium concentration of the dialysate), and pharmacologic therapy with predialysis midodrine. Patients with this problem may benefit from a transfer to PD.
- Complications during hemodialysis include painful muscle cramps, an increased risk of stroke and myocardial ischemia; chronic fluid overload and worsening of cardiac function creates a vicious cycle.
- Many new dialysis patients are nonoliguric (urine output >500 ml/day). Preservation of residual GFR is important for survival on PD and may be beneficial in HD; thus, avoid nonemergency IV contrast and NSAIDs during PD and HD as long as the patient still makes urine.
- Ultrafiltration (UF) with conventional HD occurs 3×/week for 3–4 hrs a session. Ideal hourly fluid removal (UFR) is <500 ml to avoid hemodynamic instability. Fluid gains between dialyses often exceed this goal, requiring UFR >1L/hr. Daily home HD (not readily available) and daily PD have a lower, better-tolerated UFR.

- On PD, hyperglycemia limits the osmotic gradient to remove fluid, and fluid may actually be reabsorbed.
- Chronic hyperkalemia is a problem for oliguric HD patients; dietary potassium restriction is needed.
- Hypokalemia often occurs in PD patients; dietary potassium liberalization or supplements may be needed (confusing for previously potassium-limited patients).
- Monitor calcium, phosphate, and parathyroid hormone (PTH) in all ESRD patients. K/DOQI guidelines: serum calcium 8.4–9.5 mg/dl, phosphate 3.5–5.5 mg/dl, calcium-phosphate product <55, intact PTH 150–300 pg/ml.
- For hyperphosphatemia, nonaluminum-containing phosphate binders (calcium acetate, sevelamer, and lanthanum carbonate) are taken with meals.
- With serum phosphate <5.5 mg/dl, but iPTH still above target, vitamin D analogs are added (calcitriol, paricalcitol, and doxercalciferol). Use calcimimetics (cinacalcet) if iPTH remains >300 pg/ml and calcium is >8.4 mg/dl; these agents are very effective but not well tolerated due to gastrointestinal (GI) side effects.

Cardiovascular Disease (CVD)

- CVD accounts for 40%–50% of deaths on HD and PD.
- Coronary artery calcification is seen in even young dialysis patients. Medial calcification is seen more commonly than intimal calcifications in CKD patients.
- The cause of accelerated atherosclerosis of dialysis patients is unclear; anemia, left ventricular hypertrophy, hypertension, chronic volume overload, and mineral imbalance are all postulated.
- Predisposing to vascular calcification in ESRD is hyperphosphatemia, hyperparathyroidism, vitamin D deficiency, and chronic inflammation.
- Lower extremity peripheral vascular disease present in up to 25% of HD patients. Risk factors: cigarette smoking, diabetes, age, male gender, and hypertension.
- Some dialysis clinics schedule monthly foot checks for their diabetic patients to reduce the risk of infections and limb loss.

Nutrition and Anemia

- Unless the dialysis patient is being considered for transplantation and has a BMI >40 kg/m², weight loss is not stressed although recommended. Regular exercise is beneficial.
- Protein-calorie malnutrition correlates with mortality in ESRD. Linear relationship between serum albumin level and survival on dialysis, persisting even with normal serum albumin range. Stop the predialysis "renal diet," which limits protein, once dialysis is started.
- PD patients are prone to hypoalbuminemia due to protein wasting in dialysis effluent. Should receive 1.2 g/kg/day dietary protein. Persistent hypoalbuminemia, especially postoperatively or during chemotherapy, may require temporary or permanent transfer to HD.
- ESRD patients receive erythropoiesis stimulating agents (ESAs) with HD or PD. Poor response is seen with inflammation, chronic transplant rejection, HIV, occult infection, and severe hyperparathyroidism.
- Most dialysis patients require supplemental iron—IV iron with HD or with monthly blood draws for PD. All dialysis patients require folic acid and B and C vitamins.
- Guidelines for anemia management in CKD include target Hgb between 11–12 g/dl.

COMPLICATIONS AND COMORBIDITIES

- **Glycemic management:** Blood glucose can be checked on dialysis without finger sticks, allowing for timely insulin adjustment.
- The standard dialysis bath contains 200 mg/dl glucose.
- Large between-dialysis fluid gains requiring high hourly ultrafiltration rate (HD) or higher osmotic strengths of dialysate (PD) correlate with increased morbidity and mortality. Counsel patients to restrict dietary sodium intake and avoid uncontrolled hyperglycemia to reduce fluid gains.
- HbA1c is used to monitor long-term glucose levels even on dialysis. Falsely elevated HbA1c readings may result from nonimmunoassay methods due to elevated BUN acidosis and iron deficiency.
- Target HbA1c level 6%–7% for type 1 diabetes and 7%–8% in type 2 diabetes. If the low A1c level is not due to malnutrition, it is a good prognostic indicator.
- With ESRD, avoid metformin (risk of lactic acidosis) and rosiglitazone (cardiovascular mortality). Sulfonylureas such as glipizide may be used with caution; avoid glyburide and chlorpropamide (long-acting). Alpha-glucosidase inhibitors are not recommended in CKD (see Renal Diseases in Diabetes, p. 367).
- Although intraperitoneal insulin has been suggested for PD patients, it is difficult to dose, and adds a source of potential contamination. Consider nonglucose containing dialysate solutions (icodextrin) for PD patients with diabetes, although it is not readily available.
- PD will not properly ultrafiltrate if the blood glucose is high; in chronically poor glycemic control, HD may be a better option.
- Manage severe hyperglycemia and ketoacidosis in oliguric or anuric patients by low dose IV insulin. Fluid replacement is not warranted and potentially hazardous.
- Hyperkalemia is a potentially life-threatening complication of hyperglycemia in ESRD patients. Reverse extracellular shifts of potassium with insulin administration. Avoid routine administration of concentrated glucose to an unconscious patient without first confirming hypoglycemia. When altered consciousness is from hyperglycemia in CKD (even pre-ESRD), administering concentrated glucose solutions without insulin may worsen hyperkalemia, causing cardiac arrhythmias.

FOLLOW-UP

- Carefully define who is the primary care physician; a multidisciplinary approach in ESRD is indicated.
- Monitor the dialysis patient quarterly with HbA1c levels, reported to the patient and primary caregiver.
- Early studies suggesting more rapid progression of diabetic retinopathy on hemodialysis have not been substantiated. Routine ophthalmology visits are nevertheless imperative.
- Consider cardiology consultation given the high rate of CVD in CKD.
- Routine visits to podiatry and early referral to vascular surgery if indicated. Monthly foot checks in the dialysis unit have been shown to save limbs.

EXPERT OPINION

- Kidney Tpl yields improved survival of all patients with ESRD when compared to HD or PD, although this may in part reflect a selection bias.

- No consensus regarding the relative survival of patients with diabetes and ESRD managed on HD versus PD. Base decision on patient's personal preferences, comorbidities, availability of service, and social support network.
- Consider the malnutrition-inflammation syndrome in all dialysis patients. It is associated with poor overall prognosis.
- Survival for patients with diabetes on dialysis has improved but is still quite poor, which is a strong reason to emphasize prevention in earlier stages of diabetic nephropathy.

BASIS FOR RECOMMENDATIONS

Slinin Y, Foley RN, Collins AJ. Calcium, phosphorus, parathyroid hormone, and cardiovascular disease in hemodialysis patients: the USRDS waves 1, 3, and 4 study. *J Am Soc Nephrol*, 2005; Vol. 16: pp. 1788–93.

Comments: Using the USRDS database, this article links disorders of calcium homeostasis with cardiovascular events in HD patients.

K/DOQI Workgroup. K/DOQI clinical practice guidelines for cardiovascular disease in dialysis patients. *Am J Kidney Dis*, 2005; Vol. 45: pp. S1–153.

Comments: Practice guidelines for evaluation and management of cardiovascular disease in ESRD patients.

National Kidney Foundation. K/DOQI clinical practice guidelines for bone metabolism and disease in chronic kidney disease. *Am J Kidney Dis*, 2003; Vol. 42: pp. S1–201.

Comments: K/DOQI guidelines for mineral bone metabolism in ESRD.

OTHER REFERENCES

Kalantar-Zadeh K, Regidor DL, Kovesdy CP, et al. Fluid retention is associated with cardiovascular mortality in patients undergoing long-term hemodialysis. *Circulation*, 2009; Vol. 119: pp. 671–9.

Comments: This article stresses the importance of reducing interdialytic fluid gains in intermittent HD patients.

Kalantar-Zadeh K, Lee GH, Miller JE, et al. Predictors of hyporesponsiveness to erythropoiesis-stimulating agents in hemodialysis patients. *Am J Kidney Dis*, 2009; Vol. 53: pp. 823–34.

Comments: In maintenance HD patients, erythropoietin-stimulating agent (ESA) hyporesponsiveness was associated with high turnover bone disease, hyperparathyroidism and low iron stores.

Kovesdy CP, Kalantar-Zadeh K. Review article: biomarkers of clinical outcomes in advanced chronic kidney disease. *Nephrology* (Carlton), 2009; Vol. 14: pp. 408–15.

Comments: Markers of protein-energy wasting, especially albumin, remain the strongest predictors of survival in advanced CKD.

Kovesdy CP, Kalantar-Zadeh K. Why is protein-energy wasting associated with mortality in chronic kidney disease? *Semin Nephrol*, 2009; Vol. 29: pp. 3–14.

Comments: A discussion of the possible mechanisms why protein-energy wasting is such a strong marker for mortality on dialysis.

Ramirez SP, Albert JM, Blayney MJ, et al. Rosiglitazone is associated with mortality in chronic hemodialysis patients. *J Am Soc Nephrol*, 2009; Vol. 20: pp. 1094–101.

Comments: Association of rosiglitazone with worse outcome in 2393 HD patients.

US Renal Data System (RSRDS). Morbidity and mortality. *USRDS 2008 Annual Report*, 2008; Vol. 2, Chapter 6: pp. 269–280. Available online at *http://www.usrds.org/* (accessed 3/4/2011).

Comments: A comprehensive review of mortality trends in ESRD patients in the US from the exhaustive USRDS 2008 database.

COMPLICATIONS AND COMORBIDITIES

Cosio FG, Hickson LJ, Griffin MD, et al. Patient survival and cardiovascular risk after kidney transplantation: the challenge of diabetes. *Am J Transplant*, 2008; Vol. 8: pp. 593–9.

Comments: Compared to nondiabetic patients receiving kidney transplantation, diabetic patients had more pretransplant cardiovascular disease and worse posttransplant survival.

Ishimura E, Okuno S, Taniwaki H, et al. Different risk factors for vascular calcification in end-stage renal disease between diabetics and nondiabetics: the respective importance of glycemic and phosphate control. *Kidney Blood Press Res*, 2008; Vol. 31: pp. 10–5.

Comments: Review article of vascular calcification in pre-ESRD and ESRD diabetic patients emphasizing the role of glycemic and phosphate control.

Dinavahi R, Akalin E. Preemptive kidney transplantation in patients with diabetes mellitus. *Endocrinol Metab Clin North Am*, 2007; Vol. 36: pp. 1039–49, x.

Comments: A review article summarizing the data in favor of preemptive renal transplantation in diabetic patients with ESRD prior to starting dialysis.

Westra WM, Kopple JD, Krediet RT, et al. Dietary protein requirements and dialysate protein losses in chronic peritoneal dialysis patients. *Perit Dial Int*, 2007; Vol. 27: pp. 192–5.

Comments: PD patients using the automated cycler machine at night may have higher 24-hour protein losses than patients performing manual exchanges.

Kalantar-Zadeh K, Kopple JD, Regidor DL, et al. A1C and survival in maintenance hemodialysis patients. *Diabetes Care*, 2007; Vol. 30: pp. 1049–55.

Comments: In another large study on survival of diabetic patients on dialysis followed for 3 years, unadjusted higher A1c levels were paradoxically associated with lower death rates. However, after adjusting for anemia, malnutrition, and inflammation, glycemic control correlated with improved survival.

Berns JS, Szczech LA. What is the nephrologist's role as a primary care provider? We all have different answers. *Clin J Am Soc Nephrol*, 2007; Vol. 2: pp. 601–3.

Comments: Reviews the complex issues involved in caring for dialysis patients and coordinating care with other physicians.

Rajagopalan S, Dellegrottaglie S, Furniss AL, et al. Peripheral arterial disease in patients with end-stage renal disease: observations from the Dialysis Outcomes and Practice Patterns Study (DOPPS). *Circulation*, 2006; Vol. 114: pp. 1914–22.

Comments: Data from the Dialysis Outcomes and Practice Patterns Study (DOPPS) on >29,000 HD patients reviews associations between PVD and underlying clinical variables.

Williams ME, Lacson E, Teng M, et al. Hemodialyzed type I and type II diabetic patients in the US: characteristics, glycemic control, and survival. *Kidney Int*, 2006; Vol. 70: pp. 1503–9.

Comments: In a large population of HD patients with diabetes, survival did not vary with HbA1c at 12 months.

Vonesh EF, Snyder JJ, Foley RN, et al. The differential impact of risk factors on mortality in hemodialysis and peritoneal dialysis. *Kidney Int*, 2004; Vol. 66: pp. 2389–401.

Comments: The relative risk of hemodialysis versus peritoneal dialysis varies by time on dialysis and comorbidities.

Kalantar-Zadeh K, Rodriguez RA, Humphreys MH. Association between serum ferritin and measures of inflammation, nutrition and iron in haemodialysis patients. *Nephrol Dial Transplant*, 2004; Vol. 19: pp. 141–9.

Comments: Overview of the malnutrition-inflammation syndrome in ESRD patients.

KIDNEY TRANSPLANTATION

Bassam G. Abu Jawdeh, MD, and Nada Alachkar, MD

DEFINITION

- The surgical implantation of a kidney from one donor to a non-identical human recipient (allograft).
- Kidney transplantation that occurs between identical twins referred to as isograft.
- Simultaneous pancreas and kidney (SPK) transplantation has been a successful therapy for patients with end-stage kidney disease secondary to type 1 diabetes mellitus. Other options include pancreas or islet cell transplantation before or after kidney transplantation.
- Most patients with kidney transplantation (and all with pancreas transplantation) are allograft recipients and require lifetime immunosuppression to prevent immune-mediated graft rejection.
- Diabetes, in the context of kidney transplantation, includes both patients who have diagnosed diabetes prior to transplantation and patients who develop post-transplantation diabetes mellitus (PTDM).

EPIDEMIOLOGY

- Diabetes accounts for ~45% of new cases of chronic kidney disease diagnosed each year.
- In 2007, among newly listed adults for kidney transplantation, ~40% had diabetes.
- For most patients with history of diabetes, this is the cause of end-stage kidney disease necessitating kidney and/or pancreas transplant.
- In addition, about 5%–25% of nondiabetic kidney transplant recipients will develop post-transplant diabetes mellitus (PTDM) per year.
- Incidence of PTDM is 9%, 16%, and 24% at 3, 12, and 36 months after transplantation, respectively.
- PTDM is a strong, independent predictor of allograft failure and poor patient survival.
- Nonmodifiable risk factors for PTDM include age, family history, female gender, Hispanic ethnicity and African American race.
- Modifiable risk factors for PTDM include obesity (BMI >30 kg/m^2), hepatitis C, and tacrolimus use.

DIAGNOSIS

- Kidney transplantation remains the renal replacement therapy of choice for patients with end-stage kidney disease, particularly those who lack comorbidities that hinder surgery or complicate immunosuppression therapy.
- Patient's GFR needs to be <20 ml/min/1.73 m^2 before they can be listed in the United Network for Organ Sharing (UNOS) registry for a cadaveric renal transplant; an exception is when the combination of kidney and other organs is considered.
- Usually, patients with severe obstructive or restrictive lung disease, chronic intestinal malabsorption and diarrhea, illicit drug use, or a compromised social support system are not considered candidates for kidney transplantation.
- Obesity is a relative contraindication for kidney transplantation, associated with worse allograft outcomes and wound healing problems. Most programs exclude patients with BMI of >40 kg/m^2 from transplantation.

- Before considering a patient for kidney transplant, need to assess presence of active infections, malignancies, and cardiovascular risk.
- Transplant candidates should be screened with hepatitis B virus (HBV), hepatitis C virus (HCV), cytomegalovirus (CMV), epstein barr virus (EBV), varicella zoster virus (VZV), human immunodeficiency virus (HIV), syphilis (RPR) serologies in addition to PPD test to exclude tuberculosis.
- Potential candidates should also have annual age-appropriate cancer screening tests. This includes colonoscopy, mammography, and pap smear in females and PSA in males.
- For cardiovascular risk stratification, asymptomatic transplant candidates require a cardiac stress test. If symptomatic, often cardiac catheterization needed. In the event of unstable coronary lesions or coronary obstruction, revascularization therapy has to precede transplantation.
- This entire evaluation process is carried by transplant coordinators who are guided by transplant nephrologists.
- The final decision to approve a candidate for transplantation is achieved by a multidisciplinary committee.

SIGNS AND SYMPTOMS

- Signs and symptoms related to presence of chronic kidney disease (see Nephropathy, p. 362, and Renal Diseases in Diabetes, p. 367).

CLINICAL TREATMENT

Immunosuppression

- Transplant recipients are maintained on lifelong immunosuppression.
- Common regimens include low-dose corticosteroids; an antiproliferative agent including mycophenolate mofetil (CellCept), mycophenolic acid (Myfortic), or less commonly azathioprine (Imuran); and a calcineurin inhibitor, usually tacrolimus (Prograf) or less commonly cyclosporine (Neoral, Gengraf).
- Sirolimus (Rapamune) is an m-TOR inhibitor that is less frequently used.
- Steroid-sparing immunosuppressive regimens are associated with a higher incidence of subclinical, biopsy-proven rejection, ultimately resulting in increased fibrosis and scarring of the allograft, so these regimens are not commonly used.
- Additionally, transplant recipients receive prophylactic antibiotics with valganciclovir, trimethoprim-sulfamethoxazole and clotrimazole against CMV, *Pneumocystis carinii* pneumonia (PCP), and fungal (candidal) infections, respectively.
- Prophylaxis treatment begins one day post transplantation and continues for 3–6 months.

Post-Transplant Diabetes Mellitus (PTDM)

- Glucocorticoid use can lead to steroid-induced diabetes (see p. 149).
- Calcineurin inhibitors (commonly used for immunosuppression after transplantation), particularly tacrolimus, may be associated with beta cell injury, and can result in insulin resistance.
- Risk of PTDM is 53% greater in patients treated with tacrolimus compared to patients not treated with tacrolimus, and is dose-dependent

- Risk of PTDM also increased when sirolimus (m-TOR inhibitor) combined with a calcineurin inhibitor. Sirolimus may alter beta cell function and diminish insulin sensitivity.
- Oral hypoglycemics that are cleared by the kidney (i.e., sulfonylureas) should be avoided if possible in patients with allograft dysfunction.
- Insulin dosage may need to be lowered in patients with allograft dysfunction who have decreased insulin clearance.
- After pancreas transplantation, patients usually achieve normal fasting blood glucose and HbA1c levels. Both pancreas after kidney (PAK) and SPK transplantations halt progression of microvascular and macrovascular complications of diabetes.

Other Post-Transplant Complications

- Opportunistic infections and malignancies may occur due to immunosuppression after surgery.
- An overt infection can be primary or a reactivation of a previous infection, such as reactivation of mucosal herpes simplex virus.
- Infections are more likely to occur in the first year after transplantation. They include CMV, HSV, PCP.
- EBV infection associated with post-transplant lymphoproliferative disease.
- BK virus infection is associated with allograft nephropathy.
- Non-melanoma skin cancers most common malignancies post-transplantation and are 50-fold more common in kidney transplant recipients compared to the general population.
- Persons with diabetes have a higher risk of developing cardiovascular disease both before and after kidney transplantation compared to persons without diabetes.

FOLLOW-UP

- Transplant recipients should be followed by a transplant nephrologist or a general nephrologist with transplantation experience.
- Because of the high risk of acute rejection and opportunistic infections soon after transplantation, patients are followed closely during the first 3–6 months, after which visits become less frequent.
- Renal panel, complete blood count, urinalysis, and calcineurin inhibitor trough levels are the standard laboratory tests monitored routinely after transplantation.
- In addition, patients should have intact-PTH, 25-OH-Vitamin D (vitamin D) checked periodically. Intact-PTH usually falls to normal range shortly post-transplantation if allograft function adequate; however, can take up to 1 year in some patients.
- Serum BK virus PCR checked monthly, then quarterly and then yearly after the first year.
- Patients who report flu-like symptoms or symptoms suggestive of CMV tissue invasive disease should be tested by obtaining CMV PCR in the serum.
- Worsening allograft function may result from urinary tract obstruction and hemodynamic mediated (prerenal) azotemia.
- Biopsy of transplanted kidney may diagnose acute allograft rejection, recurrence of primary kidney disease, and other etiologies.

EXPERT OPINION

- Kidney transplantation remains the best available renal replacement modality in patients with end-stage kidney disease.
- Potential candidates for kidney transplantation should be referred to nephrology.

COMPLICATIONS AND COMORBIDITIES

- Simultaneous pancreas–kidney transplantation is a good option in patients with end-stage kidney disease from type 1 diabetes mellitus.
- Because of the relative shortage of transplantable organs in the face of a growing end-stage kidney disease population, allografts should be managed closely, emphasizing compliance with medications, laboratory testing, and clinic visits.
- Keep a very low threshold to workup signs or symptoms suspicious of infections or malignancies in transplant patients. Consider consultation with a transplant infectious disease specialist if needed.
- Caring for transplant patients is a complex lifelong process that requires a multidisciplinary team approach.

REFERENCES

Razonable RR. Strategies for managing cytomegalovirus in transplant recipients. *Expert Opin Pharmacother*, 2010; Vol. 11: pp. 1983–97.
Comments: Reviews strategies for managing cytomegalovirus in transplant recipients.

Sharif A, Baboolal K. Risk factors for new-onset diabetes after kidney transplantation. *Nat Rev Nephrol*, 2010; Vol. 6: pp. 415–23.
Comments: A recent review of risk factors associated with post-transplant diabetes mellitus.

Sis B, Mengel M, Haas M, et al. Banff '09 meeting report: antibody mediated graft deterioration and implementation of Banff working groups. *Am J Transplant*, 2010; Vol. 10: pp. 464–71.
Comments: The most recent Banff classification of renal allograft pathology.

Desai NM, Schnitzler M, Jendrisak MD, et al. Maintenance steroid therapy for kidney recipients—not ready for relegation. *Am J Transplant*, 2009; Vol. 9: pp. 1263–4.
Comments: Discusses corticosteroid withdrawal from maintenance immunosuppressive therapy; argues that it is still early to adopt this strategy.

Cimbaluk D, Pitelka L, Kluskens L, et al. Update on human polyomavirus BK nephropathy. *Diagn Cytopathol*, 2009; Vol. 37: pp. 773–9.
Comments: A comprehensive review on BK virus nephropathy.

Morath C, Schmied B, Mehrabi A, et al. Simultaneous pancreas-kidney transplantation in type 1 diabetes. *Clin Transplant*, 2009; Vol. 23 Suppl 21: pp. 115–20.
Comments: A review of simultaneous pancreas-kidney transplantation in diabetes mellitus type 1.

Evaluation of kidney transplant candidates. In: Hricik DE, ed. *Kidney Transplantation*, 2nd ed. Lincolnshire, IL: Remedica Publishing; 2007: .
Comments: Discusses the approach for evaluation of potential transplant recipients.

Ekberg H, Tedesco-Silva H, Demirbas A, et al. Reduced exposure to calcineurin inhibitors in renal transplantation. *NEJM*, 2007; Vol. 357: pp. 2562–75.
Comments: Shows that the use of a regimen that includes mycophenolate, corticosteroids, and low-dose tacrolimus is advantageous for renal function, allograft survival, and acute rejection rates.

Ciancio G, Burke GW, Gaynor JJ, et al. A randomized long-term trial of tacrolimus/sirolimus versus tacrolimus/mycophenolate versus cyclosporine/sirolimus in renal transplantation: three-year analysis. *Transplantation*, 2006; Vol. 81: pp. 845–52.
Comments: Shows better graft function and fewer endocrine side-effects in mycophenolate/tacrolimus regimen when compared to sirolimus/tacrolimus regimen.

Larsen JL, Bennett RG, Burkman T, et al. Tacrolimus and sirolimus cause insulin resistance in normal sprague dawley rats. *Transplantation*, 2006; Vol. 82: pp. 466–70.

Comments: Shows that tacrolimus and sirolimus have a synergistic effect on islet cell apoptosis in Sprague Dawley rats.

Vajdic CM, McDonald SP, McCredie MR, et al. Cancer incidence before and after kidney transplantation. *JAMA*, 2006; Vol. 296: pp. 2823–31.

Comments: Highlights the role of the interaction between the immune system and common viral infections in the etiology of cancer.

Moloney FJ, Comber H, O'Lorcain P, et al. A population-based study of skin cancer incidence and prevalence in renal transplant recipients. *Br J Dermatol*, 2006; Vol. 154: pp. 498–504.

Comments: Demonstrates a biphasic increase in skin cancer incidence following kidney transplantation; this was determined by the age at transplantation.

Ojo AO. Cardiovascular complications after renal transplantation and their prevention. *Transplantation*, 2006; Vol. 82: pp. 603–11.

Comments: Discusses risk factors that confer greater risk of CVD morbidity and mortality in the post-transplant period.

Numakura K, Satoh S, Tsuchiya N, et al. Clinical and genetic risk factors for posttransplant diabetes mellitus in adult renal transplant recipients treated with tacrolimus. *Transplantation*, 2005; Vol. 80: pp. 1419–24.

Comments: Suggests that certain genetic polymorphisms may predict patients' risk for developing post-transplant diabetes mellitus.

Webster AC, Woodroffe RC, Taylor RS, et al. Tacrolimus versus ciclosporin as primary immunosuppression for kidney transplant recipients: meta-analysis and meta-regression of randomised trial data. *BMJ*, 2005; Vol. 331: p. 810.

Comments: A meta-analysis showing a higher risk for developing post-transplant diabetes mellitus with tacrolimus compared to cyclosporine.

Teutonico A, Schena PF, Di Paolo S. Glucose metabolism in renal transplant recipients: effect of calcineurin inhibitor withdrawal and conversion to sirolimus. *J Am Soc Nephrol*, 2005; Vol. 16: pp. 3128–35.

Comments: Shows that sirolimus is associated with worsening insulin resistance.

Cosio FG, Kudva Y, van der Velde M, et al. New onset hyperglycemia and diabetes are associated with increased cardiovascular risk after kidney transplantation. *Kidney Int*, 2005; Vol. 67: pp. 2415–21.

Comments: Demonstrates a significant relationship between post-transplant hyperglycemia and cardiovascular events.

Markell M. New-onset diabetes mellitus in transplant patients: pathogenesis, complications, and management. *Am J Kidney Dis*, 2004; Vol. 43: pp. 953–65.

Comments: A review that discusses the pathogenesis, complications, and management of post-transplant diabetes mellitus.

Kasiske BL, Snyder JJ, Gilbertson DT, et al. Cancer after kidney transplantation in the United States. *Am J Transplant*, 2004; Vol. 4: pp. 905–13.

Comments: Shows that the rates for most malignancies are higher after transplantation; concludes that cancer prevention should be a main focus in kidney transplant recipients.

Kasiske BL, Snyder JJ, Gilbertson D, et al. Diabetes mellitus after kidney transplantation in the United States. *Am J Transplant*, 2003; Vol. 3: pp. 178–85.

Comments: Analyzes data from the United Renal Data System and identifies risk factors associated with post-transplant diabetes mellitus.

Montori VM, Basu A, Erwin PJ, et al. Posttransplantation diabetes: a systematic review of the literature. *Diabetes Care*, 2002; Vol. 25: pp. 583–92.

Comments: Shows that immunosuppressive regimens including high-dose calcineurin inhibitors increase risk for post-transplant diabetes mellitus.

COMPLICATIONS AND COMORBIDITIES

Harden PN, Fryer AA, Reece S, et al. Annual incidence and predicted risk of nonmelanoma skin cancer in renal transplant recipients. *Transplant Proc*, 2001; Vol. 33: pp. 1302–4.

Comments: Identifies risk factors for developing non-melanoma skin cancer post-transplantation.

Sung RS, Althoen M, Howell TA, et al. Peripheral vascular occlusive disease in renal transplant recipients: risk factors and impact on kidney allograft survival. *Transplantation*, 2000; Vol. 70: pp. 1049–54.

Comments: Shows that peripheral vascular disease after transplantation is associated with reduced survival; it appears that transplantation does not accelerate or retard its progression.

Fishman JA, Rubin RH. Infection in organ-transplant recipients. *NEJM*, 1998; Vol. 338: pp. 1741–51.

Comments: A comprehensive review on infections in organ-transplant recipients.

National Institutes of Health, National Institute of Diabetes and Digestive and Kidney Diseases. US Renal Data System. USRDS 2008 Annual Data Report: Atlas of Chronic Kidney Disease and End-Stage Renal Disease in the United States. Bethesda, MD. Available at: http://www.usrds.org/2008/view/ckd_00_intro.asp (accessed 3/4/2011).

Comments: The national data registry that collects and analyzes information on the end-stage renal disease population in the US.

U.S. Department of Health and Human Services, Health Resources and Services Administration, Healthcare Systems Bureau, Division of Transplantation, 2008 Annual Report of the U.S. Organ Procurement and Transplantation Network and the Scientific Registry of Transplant Recipients: Transplant Data 1998–2007. Rockville, MD. Available at: http://optn.transplant.hrsa.gov/ar2008/ (accessed 3/4/2011).

Comments: Organ Procurement and Transplantation Network and the Scientific Registry of Transplant Recipients.

BLADDER DISORDERS IN DIABETES

Nisa M. Maruthur, MD, MHS

DEFINITION

- Bladder dysfunction in diabetes mellitus (DM) spans a spectrum from lower urinary tract symptoms (LUTS) such as incontinence to bladder cystopathy.
- Detrusor muscle, neurologic, and urothelial dysfunction underlie bladder dysfunction in DM.
- **Urge incontinence:** involuntary loss of urine while feeling a need to urinate. Usually due to neurogenic detrusor overactivity (i.e., spastic bladder)
- **Stress incontinence:** involuntary loss of urine that occurs during physical activity, such as coughing, sneezing, laughing, or exercise. Usually due to weak pelvic floor muscles.
- **Bladder cystopathy:** decreased bladder sensation and contractility resulting in urinary retention, the most severe bladder disorder in DM. Usually due to autonomic neuropathy (also known as neurogenic bladder).

EPIDEMIOLOGY

- More than 50% of patients with DM have some bladder dysfunction (e.g., incontinence) while bladder cystopathy is rare (Brown).
- Of women with DM in the US, 35% report at least weekly incontinence, 26% at least weekly *urge* incontinence, and 30% at least weekly *stress* incontinence; corresponding prevalences in those with normal glucose (NHANES) are 17%, 8%, and 14% (Brown, Vittinghoff).

- Benign prostatic hyperplasia is a common cause of symptoms that can be indistinguishable from LUTS associated with DM bladder dysfunction in men.
- In the Diabetes Prevention Program, intensive lifestyle modification with weight loss and increased physical activity led to a decreased prevalence of weekly urinary incontinence in women at high risk for DM relative to the metformin and placebo arms (Brown, Wing, 2006).

DIAGNOSIS

- History of signs and symptoms consistent with bladder dysfunction often sufficient for diagnosis.
- Urodynamic testing can also be performed by a urologist: Cystometry, sphincter electromyography, uroflowmetry, urethral pressure.

SIGNS AND SYMPTOMS

- **LUTS:** Urinary frequency, urinary urgency, nocturia, and incontinence.
- **Diabetic cystopathy:** Decreased urge to urinate, incomplete bladder emptying, decreased frequency of urination.
- Urodynamic findings vary based on stage of bladder dysfunction but can show increased bladder capacity, decreased detrusor contractility with time, and increased post-void residual urine.
- Bladder cystopathy can lead to an atonic bladder manifested by decreased micturition reflex.
- Other signs of autonomic neuropathy (e.g., postural hypotension) may also be found.
- Bladder dysfunction may result in urinary tract infections.

CLINICAL TREATMENT

- **Stress incontinence:** bladder and pelvic muscle training in women.
- **Urge incontinence:** anti-cholinergic medications (e.g., Oxybutynin, p. 546).
- Voiding at regular, scheduled intervals.
- Glycemic control may be important since bladder dysfunction may result from neuropathy. However intensive glucose control did not decrease prevalence of LUTS in men participating in DCCT/EDIC (Van Den Eeden).
- **Diabetic cystopathy:** cholinergic receptor agonists (e.g., Bethanechol, p. 544).
- Intermittent catheterization in unusually severe cases.
- Urologic consultation.

EXPERT OPINION

- Evaluate for possible bladder dysfunction symptoms regularly.
- Patients with a sudden change in bladder symptoms should be evaluated for urinary tract infection with urinalysis and/or culture.

REFERENCES

Danforth KN, Townsend MK, Curhan GC, et al. Type 2 diabetes mellitus and risk of stress, urge and mixed urinary incontinence. *J Urol,* 2009; Vol. 181: pp. 193–7.

   Comments: Study showing that DM is associated with incident urinary incontinence (urge incontinence in particular) in the Nurses' Health Study.

Brown JS. Diabetic cystopathy—what does it mean? *J Urol,* 2009; Vol. 181: pp. 13–4.

   Comments: Editorial on meaning of diabetic cystopathy.

COMPLICATIONS AND COMORBIDITIES

Van Den Eeden SK, Sarma AV, Rutledge BN, et al. Effect of intensive glycemic control and diabetes complications on lower urinary tract symptoms in men with type 1 diabetes: Diabetes Control and Complications Trial/Epidemiology of Diabetes Interventions and Complications (DCCT/EDIC) study. *Diabetes Care,* 2009; Vol. 32: pp. 664–70.
Comments: Potentially underpowered analysis of UroEDIC cohort showing no effect of intensive glucose control on LUTS.

Brown JS, Vittinghoff E, Lin F, et al. Prevalence and risk factors for urinary incontinence in women with type 2 diabetes and impaired fasting glucose: findings from the National Health and Nutrition Examination Survey (NHANES) 2001–2002. *Diabetes Care,* 2006; Vol. 29: pp. 1307–12.
Comments: Nationally representative study (NHANES) evaluating prevalence of urinary incontinence in women with DM, impaired glucose tolerance, and normal fasting glucose.

Brown JS, Wing R, Barrett-Connor E, et al. Lifestyle intervention is associated with lower prevalence of urinary incontinence: the Diabetes Prevention Program. *Diabetes Care,* 2006; Vol. 29: pp. 385–90.
Comments: Analysis of Diabetes Prevention Program data showing decreased prevalence of weekly urinary incontinence in the lifestyle intervention relative to the metformin and placebo groups.

Brown JS, Wessells H, Chancellor MB, et al. Urologic complications of diabetes. *Diabetes Care,* 2005; Vol. 28: pp. 177–85.
Comments: Unstructured review of urologic complications of DM.

Sasaki K, Yoshimura N, Chancellor MB. Implications of diabetes mellitus in urology. *Urol Clin North Am,* 2003; Vol. 30: pp. 1–12.
Comments: Review of urologic complications in DM.

Wein, AJ. Lower urinary tract dysfunction in neurologic injury and disease. In Wein, AJ (Ed.), *Campbell-Walsh Urology,* 9th edition, Philadelphia: Saunders Elsevier; 2007: chapter 59.
Comments: Chapter from Campbell's urology reviewing bladder dysfunction in DM.

SECTION 4
MEDICATIONS

ANTICOAGULANT USE (ASPIRIN, CLOPIDOGREL, WARFARIN)

Sheldon H. Gottlieb, MD, and Paul A. Pham, PharmD

INDICATIONS

FDA

Aspirin

- **Secondary prevention:** treatment of transient transchemic attack (TIA) and ischemic stroke; prevent recurrent myocardial infarction (MI); reduce risk of MI or sudden death in unstable angina and chronic stable angina; after angioplasty, coronary artery bypass graft (CABG), and carotid endarterectomy.

Clopidogrel

- **Secondary prevention:** acute coronary syndromes (unstable angina, non-ST elevation MI), including those that are to be managed with coronary revascularization; ST elevation MI; after MI, stroke, and established peripheral vascular disease.

Warfarin

- **Secondary indication:** prophylaxis or treatment of thromboembolism in atrial fibrillation, mechanical heart valves; reduce risk of stroke or recurrent MI after MI; prophylaxis or treatment of venous thrombosis or thromboembolism in high-risk patients.

Non-FDA Approved Uses

Aspirin

- **Primary prevention** of cardiovascular events in diabetes (see Routine Preventive Care, p. 61).

Clopidogrel

- **Primary prevention:** not established.

Warfarin

- **Primary indication:** not established.

MECHANISM

- **Aspirin:** irreversibly binds to (acetylates) and inhibits cyclooxygenase, thereby preventing formation of platelet aggregating factor thromboxane A2.
- **Clopidogrel:** the active metabolite of clopidogrel irreversibly binds to the P2Y12 class of platelet ADP receptors, thereby inhibiting platelet aggregation.
- **Warfarin:** inhibits vitamin K-dependent coagulation factors, thereby inhibiting blood coagulation.

USUAL ADULT DOSING

- **Aspirin:** 75–325 mg daily.
- **Clopidogrel:** 75 mg daily. No dose adjustment in elderly.
- **Warfarin:** dose is highly individualized and depends greatly on genetic factors (CYP2C9 and VKORC1 genotypes), vitamin K intake, and coadministered drug. Usual daily dose ranges between 2–7.5 mg. Lower doses recommended in the

elderly and patients with CYP2C9 and VKORC1 genotypes. Dose adjusted to goal INR range.

FORMS

See Table 4-1.

DOSING IN SPECIAL POPULATIONS

Renal

- **Aspirin:** avoid in severe renal failure (GFR <10 ml/min).
- **Clopidogrel:** limited data, use with caution.
- **Warfarin:** lower doses in advanced renal failure. Use in dialysis patients with great caution; benefit may be low and warfarin may cause increased vascular calcifications (Bennett).

Hepatic

- **Aspirin:** avoid in severe hepatic insufficiency.
- **Clopidogrel:** no dose adjustment.
- **Warfarin:** use with caution; dosing is highly individualized; risk of bleeding complications is high in moderate to severe hepatic insufficiency.

Pregnancy

- **Aspirin:** Category C. Use only if clearly needed in the first and second trimester of pregnancy. Contraindicated after third trimester due to potential effects on fetal circulation (potential closure of ductus arteriosus) and maternal bleeding.
- **Clopidogrel:** Category B. Animal-reproduction studies have not demonstrated a fetal risk, but no human data.
- **Warfarin:** Category X. Contraindicated in woman who are or who may become pregnant. Warfarin passes placental barrier. High risk for fetal mortality and malformations.

Breastfeeding

- **Aspirin:** excreted in breast milk and should be used cautiously during breastfeeding.
- **Clopidogrel:** avoid—not known if excreted in human breast milk.
- **Warfarin:** high protein binding in maternal circulation; little excreted in milk, and considered relatively safe to use while breastfeeding.

ADVERSE DRUG REACTIONS

General

- All anticoagulants may increase risk for bleeding.

Common

- **Aspirin:** GI intolerance (dose dependent).

Occasional

- **Aspirin:** tinnitus (with high-dose and/or long-term aspirin); esophageal, gastric, peptic ulcer; nephrotoxicity (e.g., acute interstitial nephritis or prerenal acute tubular necrosis), increased uric acid (dose dependent); rebound headache (with chronic use); acid-base disturbance with overdose (e.g., metabolic acidosis or respiratory alkalosis).

Rare

- **Aspirin:** allergic reaction, rash; pancytopenia (e.g., leukopenia, thrombocytopenia, agranulocytosis, aplastic anemia); anaphylaxis reaction; Reye syndrome (following varicella infection); hepatitis.

MEDICATIONS

- **Clopidogrel:** neutropenia, TTP, allergic reactions, anaphylaxis, hepatitis.
- **Warfarin:** purple-toe syndrome secondary to cholesterol microembolization (onset between 3 and 10 weeks). Presents with purple discoloration, pain, and tenderness of the toes. If warfarin is not discontinued, may result in gangrene and tissue necrosis, rash, tracheobronchial calcification.

DRUG INTERACTIONS

- **Aspirin:** nonsteroidal anti-inflammatory drugs interfere with the platelet binding of aspirin. Most side effects are dose related.
- **Clopidogrel:** conversion to active metabolite by CYP2C19, whose inhibitors (e.g., omeprazole, esomeprazole, cimetidine, fluconazole, ketoconazole, voriconazole, etravirine, felbamate, fluoxetine, fluvoxamine) may decrease the efficacy of clopidogrel. Avoid coadministration.
- **Warfarin:** potential interactions due to impaired hemostasis or clotting factor synthesis, competitive vitamin K antagonism, pharmacokinetic interactions due to hepatic enzyme induction (e.g., rifampin) or inhibition (e.g., fluconazole), reduced plasma binding, or other comorbid medical diseases. Specific diseases include, but are not limited to, blood dyscrasias, cancer, collagen vascular diseases, heart failure, diarrhea, elevated temperature, hepatic disorders, hyperthyroidism, poor nutritional state including vitamin K deficiency, steatorrhea.
  - Warfarin's anticoagulant effect *increased* with cotrimoxazole, erythromycin, fluconazole, isoniazid, metronidazole, amiodarone, clofibrate, propafenone, propranolol, and sulfinpyrazone; phenylbutazone; piroxicam; alcohol, cimetidine, and omeprazole.
  - Warfarin anticoagulant effect *decreased* with griseofulvin, rifampin, nafcillin, barbiturates, carbamazepine, chlordiazepoxide, cholestyramine, and sucralfate.
  - Individual drug interactions with warfarin are too numerous to list. See website for additional drug interactions: http://www.drugs.com/drug-interactions/warfarin.html.
- Patients need to be educated on possible drug interactions (see Table 4-2).

PHARMACOKINETICS

TABLE 4-1. PHARMACOKINETICS AND FORMS OF ANTICOAGULANTS

Medications	Absorption	Metabolism	Excretion	Formulations†	Pricing*
Aspirin	Rapid Duration: 4–6 hours	Hydrolysis to active salicylate by esterases. Metabolism of salicylate by hepatic conjugation.	Urine t½ for parent drug: 15–20 minutes. t½ for salicylate: dose dependent. 3 hours at low (300–600 mg) doses, 5–6 hours (1 g or higher), 10 hours with higher doses. (>2–4 g)	Generic tablets available, including chewable 81 mg, regular and enteric-coated 81 mg, 325 mg, 500 mg, controlled-release 800 mg, enteric-coated 975 mg.	Many different manufacturers. Chewable 81 mg (36 tab): $11.99 325 mg (100 tab): $11.99 Controlled release 800 mg (100 tab): $125.53 Enteric-coated 975 mg (90 tab): $11.25
Clopidogrel (Plavix®)	Well absorbed	Extensively hepatic, through CYP450 mediated oxidation to active thiol metabolite.	Urine, feces. t½ = ~6 hours	Only brand available, as 75 mg and 300 mg tablets.	75 mg (30 tab): $165.99

(Continued)

TABLE 4-1. [CONT.]

Medications	Absorption	Metabolism	Excretion	Formulations†	Pricing*
Warfarin (Coumadin®)	Rapid and complete absorption. Onset of action: 24–72 hours. Full therapy effect: 5–7 days. Duration: 2–5 days.	Hepatic metabolism of S-warfarin (more potent isomer) primarily through CYP2C9. Minor metabolism through CYP2C8, 2C18, 2C19, 1A2, 3A4 (R-warfarin)	Urine t½ = 20–60 hours. Mean ~40 hours, highly variable (based on CYP2C9 and VKORC1 genetic variation).	Generic tablet form available, as 1 mg, 2 mg, 2.5 mg, 3 mg, 4 mg, 5 mg, 7.5 mg, and 10 mg.	1 mg (30 tab): $13.99 2 mg (30 tab): $14.88 2.5 mg (30 tab): $14.99 3 mg (30 tab): $15.99 4 mg (30 tab): $14.99 5 mg (30 tab): $13.99 7.5 mg (30 tab): $23.21 10 mg (30 tab): $24.24

*Prices represent cost per unit specified, are representative of "Average Wholesale Price" (AWP).

†Dosage is indicated in mg unless otherwise noted.

Courtesy of Paul Pham, PharmD, Johns Hopkins University School of Medicine.

TABLE 4-2. EXPLANATIONS TO PATIENTS TAKING COUMARINS

1. Why treatment is necessary.
2. How the drug works.
3. Why monitoring is needed.
4. Why it is important to take the drug at a fixed time daily.
5. How alcohol may affect anticoagulation and increases risk for falls.
6. How dietary changes affect therapy.
7. How drug–drug interactions might affect treatment.
8. Why clinic personnel should be notified of changes in medications.
9. What precautions should be taken to avoid bleeding.
10. How to recognize signs and symptoms of bleeding.

Source: Green D. Avoiding "sticker" shock. *Blood*, 2009; Vol. 114: pp. 930–1. Reproduced with permission of The American Society of Hematology (ASH).

EXPERT OPINION
- The evidence for benefit of aspirin in primary prevention of CVD in diabetes is inconclusive and likely greatest in persons with diabetes at high risk of future cardiovascular disease (i.e., >10%). However, aspirin remains FDA approved only for secondary (and not primary) prevention.
- Recent guidelines have recognized the potentially increased bleeding associated with aspirin therapy and narrowed the criteria for persons who may benefit from primary prevention of CVD with aspirin therapy.
- The use of aspirin therapy needs to be individualized for each patient.
- Clopidogrel and warfarin may be preferred for thromboembolic disease, or if aspirin is not considered appropriate.

REFERENCES

Würtz M, Grove EL, Kristensen SD, et al. The antiplatelet effect of aspirin is reduced by proton pump inhibitors in patients with coronary artery disease. *Heart*, 2010; Vol. 96: pp. 368–71.
  Comments: Proton pump inhibitors (PPI) may reduce aspirin effect on platelet aggregation. This topic remains controversial; PPI use should be monitored and dose adjusted to effect.

Pignone M, Alberts MJ, Colwell JA, et al. Aspirin for primary prevention of cardiovascular events in people with diabetes: a position statement of the American Diabetes Association, a scientific statement of the American Heart Association, and an expert consensus document of the American College of Cardiology Foundation. *Diabetes Care*, 2010; Vol. 33: pp. 1395–402.
  Comments: This position statement by the ADA, AHA, and ACC outlines recommendations for use of low dose ASA (75–162 mg/day) in the primary prevention of cardiovascular disease in diabetes.

De Berardis G, Sacco M, Strippoli GF, et al. Aspirin for primary prevention of cardiovascular events in people with diabetes: meta-analysis of randomised controlled trials. *BMJ*, 2009; Vol. 339: p. b4531.

MEDICATIONS

Comments: This meta-analysis of 6 trials found that though ASA reduced risk of cardiovascular outcomes by 6–17%, no significant difference was found compared to placebo. Increased risk of bleeding and GI symptoms was noted in a few studies but not significant. ASA significantly reduced MI risk in men but not women.

Antithrombotic Trialists' (ATT) Collaboration, Baigent C, Blackwell L, et al. Aspirin in the primary and secondary prevention of vascular disease: collaborative meta-analysis of individual participant data from randomised trials. *Lancet*, 2009; Vol. 373: pp. 1849–60.

Comments: The use of aspirin in primary prevention remains controversial; the authors recommend that guidelines be "relaxed" until more information is available. See Expert Opinion section.

Haynes R, Bowman L, Armitage J. Aspirin for primary prevention of vascular disease in people with diabetes. *BMJ*, 2009; Vol. 339: p. b4596.

Comments: A review of the uncertainty surrounding the use of aspirin for prevention of CV events, and a call to encourage patients to enroll in clinical trials to help determine who should receive aspirin.

Price HC, Holman RR. Primary prevention of cardiovascular events in diabetes: is there a role for aspirin? *Nat Clin Pract Cardiovasc Med*, 2009; Vol. 6: pp. 168–9.

Comments: This article summarizes the evidence for use of aspirin in primary prevention of CVD.

Connolly SJ, Ezekowitz MD, Yusuf S, et al. Dabigatran versus warfarin in patients with atrial fibrillation. *NEJM*, 2009; Vol. 361: pp. 1139–51.

Comments: This was a non-inferiority trial of dabigatran, an oral direct thrombin inhibitor, versus warfarin, in patients with atrial fibrillation. Outcomes were similar. Dabigatran scheduled to be reviewed by the FDA in the summer of 2010.

Singer DE, Chang Y, Fang MC, et al. The net clinical benefit of warfarin anticoagulation in atrial fibrillation. *Ann Intern Med*, 2009; Vol. 151: pp. 297–305.

Comments: Study documents risks and benefits of warfarin use in patients with atrial fibrillation, based on CHADS(2) score. Older high-risk patients benefit the most, despite risk of hemorrhage.

Green D. Avoiding "sticker" shock. *Blood*, 2009; Vol. 114: pp. 930–1.

Comments: Practical review of laboratory monitoring of anticoagulation with useful patient information.

Singla A, Antonino MJ, Bliden KP, et al. The relation between platelet reactivity and glycemic control in diabetic patients with cardiovascular disease on maintenance aspirin and clopidogrel therapy. *Am Heart J*, 2009; Vol. 158: pp. 784.e1–6.

Comments: In patients with type 2 diabetes treated with dual antiplatelet agents, poor glycemic control is associated with greater platelet reactivity; these patients may require adjustment of antiplatelet regimen.

Bennett WM. Should dialysis patients ever receive warfarin and for what reasons? *Clin J Am Soc Nephrol*, 2006; Vol. 1: pp. 1357–1359.

Comments: This article reviews the use of warfarin in dialysis patients.

Vane JR, Botting RM. The mechanism of action of aspirin. *Thromb Res*, 2003; Vol. 110: pp. 255–8.

Comments: Vane won the Nobel Prize for his studies of aspirin effects.

Savi P, Nurden P, Nurden AT, et al. Clopidogrel: a review of its mechanism of action. *Platelets*, 1998; Vol. 9: pp. 251–5.

Comments: In-depth review of important drug.

US Food and Drug Administration (FDA). Aspirin: Questions and Answers. Available online at *http://www.fda.gov/Drugs/ResourcesForYou/Consumers/QuestionsAnswers/ucm071879.htm* (accessed 7/15/2010).

Complementary and Alternative Medicines

COMPLEMENTARY AND ALTERNATIVE MEDICINE: HERBALS

Todd T. Brown, MD, PhD, and Paul A. Pham, PharmD

DEFINITION
- Herbals refers to use of a plant or part of a plant for medicinal purposes.
- Also called botanical medicine or phytomedicine.
- Many different herbal preparations used for treatment of diabetes mellitus (DM) in different cultures.
- Few have been systematically evaluated for efficacy and safety.
- Compounds that have had some scientific evaluation are discussed in this section.

EPIDEMIOLOGY
- In the US, over a third of diabetes patients use herbal or traditional therapies (Egede).

CLINICAL TREATMENT

Ginseng
- One of the most widely used medicinal herbs.
- Two major types: Asian Ginseng (*Panax ginseng*) and American Ginseng (*Panax quinquefolius*).
- Active compounds thought to be ginsenosides (20–30 different types present in a single plant, depending on species); non-ginsenoside components may also have physiologic properties (Attele, 1999).
- **Mechanisms:** preclinical data suggest ginsenosides improve insulin resistance (Attele, 2002).
- **Efficacy:** clinical data limited. Use of ground root most common (Vuksan), in doses of 1–3 g/day. Other parts of ginseng plants have also been tested (berries, leaves, etc.).
- **Adverse effects:** hypertension, nausea, headache, insomnia, nervousness.
- **Herb–drug interactions:** concomitant administration with warfarin reduces warfarin's therapeutic effect (Yuan).

Cinnamon (*Cinnamon cassia*)
- **Mechanism:** may enhance insulin signaling, increase glycogen synthase activity (Qin).
- **Efficacy:** human trials have investigated 1–6 g per day. Modest effect on reducing fasting blood glucose (5%–24%) with short-term administration, but results are mixed (Kirkham).
- **Safety:** no reported adverse effects.
- **Herb–drug interactions:** none known.

Bitter melon (*Momordica charantia*)
- Traditional diabetes remedy in many cultures, including Ayurvedic medicine.
- **Mechanism:** may improve insulin resistance through activation of AMP kinase (Miura; Cheng).
- **Clinical efficacy:** some benefit in large case series, but two randomized controlled trials showed no effect (Leung). Positive studies reported using juice or fresh, rather than dried, fruit. Recent review found insufficient evidence to recommend for treatment of type 2 diabetes (Ooi).

MEDICATIONS

- **Adverse effects:** some gastrointestinal distress reported; ingestion of seeds can cause favism in G6PD deficiency.
- **Herb–drug interactions:** none known.

Fenugreek (*Trigonella foenum-graecum*)

- Traditional plant used in Asian and Mediterranean cultures. Leaves and seeds used in Ayurvedic medicine.
- **Mechanism:** contains 4-hydroxyisoleucine, which may enhance insulin secretion (Sauvarie). Also, rich in fiber.
- **Efficacy:** limited, short-term data, mixed results. Doses of powdered seed 10–100 g with meals (Basch).
- **Adverse effects:** transient diarrhea, flatulence, dizziness (Basch).
- **Herb–drug interactions:** none known.

Gymnema (*Gymnema sylvestre*)

- Leaves used in Ayurvedic medicine to treat diabetes, cholesterol, and obesity. Also known as gurmar (sugar destroyer) in Hindi.
- **Mechanism:** unclear. Some evidence suggests effect on insulin secretion (Liu).
- **Efficacy:** some benefit noted in small trials of limited quality (decrease of ~0.6% HbA1c). Doses used: 200–400 mg twice daily of leaf extract (Leach).
- **Adverse effects:** none reported.
- **Herb–drug interactions:** none known.

EXPERT OPINION

- Herbal-derived compounds are used in many cultures for the treatment of diabetes.
- Although benefits of some of these compounds have been described, currently there are insufficient data to recommend any herbal remedies in the treatment of diabetes.
- Although generally well-tolerated at the doses used, some compounds have significant herb–drug interactions (e.g., ginseng-warfarin), which require further investigation.

REFERENCES

Ooi CP, Yassin Z, Hamid TA. *Momordica charantia* for type 2 diabetes mellitus. *Cochrane Database Syst Rev,* 2010; Vol. 2: CD007845.
  Comments: Cochrane review of 3 randomized trials found insufficient evidence to recommend *Momordica charantia* for treatment of type 2 diabetes.

Kirkham S, Akilen R, Sharma S, et al. The potential of cinnamon to reduce blood glucose levels in patients with type 2 diabetes and insulin resistance. *Diabetes Obes Metab,* 2009; Vol. 11: pp. 1100–13.
  Comments: Good review of human cinnamon/diabetes studies.

Leung L, Birtwhistle R, Kotecha J, et al. Anti-diabetic and hypoglycaemic effects of *Momordica charantia* (bitter melon): a mini review. *Br J Nutr,* 2009; Vol. 102: pp. 1703–8.
  Comments: Good review of human bitter melon/diabetes studies.

Liu B, Asare-Anane H, Al-Romaiyan A, et al. Characterisation of the insulinotropic activity of an aqueous extract of *Gymnema sylvestre* in mouse beta-cells and human islets of Langerhans. *Cell Physiol Biochem,* 2009; Vol. 23: pp. 125–32.
  Comments: New study investigating the mechanisms underlying fenugreek.

Cheng HL, Huang HK, Chang CI, et al. A cell-based screening identifies compounds from the stem of *Momordica charantia* that overcome insulin resistance and activate AMP-activated protein kinase. *J Agric Food Chem,* 2008; Vol. 56: pp. 6835–43.
  Comments: This paper provides some evidence that *Momoridica charantia* may improve insulin resistance.

Vuksan V, Sievenpiper JL. Herbal remedies in the management of diabetes: lessons learned from the study of ginseng. *Nutr Metab Cardiovasc Dis*, 2005; Vol. 15: pp. 149–60.

Comments: Good review of clinical effect by research team who have completed many of the human studies.

Yuan CS, Wei G, Dey L, et al. Brief communication: American ginseng reduces warfarin's effect in healthy patients: a randomized, controlled trial. *Ann Intern Med*, 2004; Vol. 141: pp. 23–7.

Comments: Identifies important interaction between ginseng and warfarin.

Qin B, Nagasaki M, Ren M, et al. Cinnamon extract (traditional herb) potentiates in vivo insulin-regulated glucose utilization via enhancing insulin signaling in rats. *Diabetes Res Clin Pract*, 2003; Vol. 62: pp. 139–48.

Comments: Shows potential mechanism of cinnamon.

Basch E, Ulbricht C, Kuo G, et al. Therapeutic applications of fenugreek. *Altern Med Rev*, 2003; Vol. 8: pp. 20–7.

Comments: Good review of clinical studies on fenugreek.

Egede LE, Ye X, Zheng D, et al. The prevalence and pattern of complementary and alternative medicine use in individuals with diabetes. *Diabetes Care*, 2002; Vol. 25: pp. 324–9.

Comments: Survey of CAM usage among patients with diabetes.

Attele AS, Zhou YP, Xie JT, et al. Antidiabetic effects of Panax ginseng berry extract and the identification of an effective component. *Diabetes*, 2002; Vol. 51: pp. 1851–8.

Comments: Shows effect of ginseng on insulin resistance.

Miura T, Itoh C, Iwamoto N, et al. Hypoglycemic activity of the fruit of the *Momordica charantia* in type 2 diabetic mice. *J Nutr Sci Vitaminol (Tokyo)*, 2001; Vol. 47: pp. 340–4.

Comments: Further evidence that *Momoridica charantia* may improve insulin resistance.

Attele AS, Wu JA, Yuan CS. Ginseng pharmacology: multiple constituents and multiple actions. *Biochem Pharmacol*, 1999; Vol. 58: pp. 1685–93.

Comments: Good review of ginseng pharmacology.

Sauvaire Y, Petit P, Broca C, et al. 4-Hydroxyisoleucine: a novel amino acid potentiator of insulin secretion. *Diabetes*, 1998; Vol. 47: pp. 206–10.

Comments: Identifies a potential active compound and mechanism for fenugreek.

COMPLEMENTARY AND ALTERNATIVE MEDICINE: NONHERBAL SUPPLEMENTS

Todd T. Brown, MD, PhD, and Paul A. Pham, PharmD

DEFINITION

- Nonherbal supplements are non-plant based complementary and/or alternative medicines used for treatment of diabetes mellitus (DM).
- Few have been systematically evaluated for efficacy and safety.
- Nonherbal compounds that have had controlled evaluation are discussed in this section.

CLINICAL TREATMENT

Chromium

- Essential trace element with an important role in carbohydrate and lipid metabolism. Chromium deficiency leads to reversible insulin resistance and diabetes.
- Most common forms are chromium picolinate and Brewer's yeast.
- Doses of 200–1000 g for 6–26 weeks reduced HbA1c levels by an average of 0.6% (95% CI –0.9 to 0.2) and FBG levels by an average of 1 mmol/L (95% CI –1.4 to 0.5) in a

MEDICATIONS

recent meta-analysis. More than half of the studies examined were deemed poor quality (Pittler).
- May have modest effect on weight in randomized trials (1.1 kg reduction over 6–14 weeks) (Pittler) and may attenuate sulfonylurea-related weight gain (Martin).
- No significant adverse effects were reported in any of the reviewed trials.
- There are no known interactions with other medications.
- Although initial clinical trials appear promising, larger, well-designed clinical studies are needed before chromium can be recommended.

Vanadium

- Trace element that may inhibit phosphotyrosine phosphatase enzymes that affect the insulin receptor (Verma).
- Vanadyl sulfate or sodium metavanadate 50–300 mg/d given over 3–6 weeks have shown reductions in fasting blood glucose of 13–40 mg/dl and HgbA1c of 0.4%–0.8% in small, uncontrolled trials (Smith). One recent study (Jacques-Camerena), showed no benefit on insulin sensitivity, but increases in triglycerides.
- Side effects were common including gastrointestinal upset, bloating, and nausea.
- Vanadium cannot be recommended for the treatment of diabetes.

Calcium/Vitamin D

- Observational studies demonstrate an association between type 2 diabetes and vitamin D deficiency.
- Possible mechanisms supporting causal association include a role of vitamin D in beta-cell function, insulin action, and reduction of systemic inflammation. Calcium may also affect insulin action and secretion.
- Clinical trials have no demonstrated clear benefit of either calcium or vitamin D supplementation for the treatment of hyperglycemia. One post hoc analysis of a randomized clinical trial showed that daily doses of vitamin D3 700 IU and calcium 500 mg attenuated the rise in glycemia and insulin resistance over 3 years in patients with baseline impaired glucose tolerance (Pittas).
- Further studies are needed to confirm a benefit of vitamin D and calcium in the management of diabetes and determine the optimal dosing. Because osteoporosis and fractures are common in patients with diabetes, daily doses of 1000–1200 mg of calcium and 800–1000 IU of vitamin D should be recommended for bone health.
- See Vitamin D (p. 553).

EXPERT OPINION

- Chromium may show some benefit for improving glucose metabolism in patients with diabetes. Larger studies of longer duration are needed before chromium can be recommended for routine use.

REFERENCES

Jacques-Camerena O, González-Ortiz M, Martz-Abundis E, et al. Effect of vanadium on insulin sensitivity in patients with impaired glucose tolerance. *Ann Nutr Metab*, 2008; Vol. 53: pp. 195–8.
  Comments: Well-designed negative study on effect of vanadium on insulin sensitivity.

Smith DM, Pickering RM, Lewith GT. A systematic review of vanadium oral supplements for glycaemic control in type 2 diabetes mellitus. *QJM*, 2008; Vol. 101: pp. 351–8.
  Comments: Good review of existing evidence of safety and efficacy of vanadium on diabetes and insulin resistance.

Smith DM, Pickering RM, Lewith GT. A systematic review of vanadium oral supplements for glycaemic control in type 2 diabetes mellitus. *QJM*, 2008; Vol. 101: pp. 351–8.

Comments: Review of vanadium effect on glycemia.

Pittas AG, Lau J, Hu FB, et al. The role of vitamin D and calcium in type 2 diabetes. A systematic review and meta-analysis. *J Clin Endocrinol Metab*, 2007; Vol. 92: pp. 2017–29.

Comments: Well-designed meta-analysis summarizing the data on the effect of calcium and vitamin D on glucose outcomes.

Martin J, Wang ZQ, Zhang XH, et al. Chromium picolinate supplementation attenuates body weight gain and increases insulin sensitivity in subjects with type 2 diabetes. *Diabetes Care*, 2006; Vol. 29: pp. 1826–32.

Comments: Well-designed randomized trial of chromium's effect on insulin sensitivity.

Pittler MH, Stevinson C, Ernst E. Chromium picolinate for reducing body weight: meta-analysis of randomized trials. *Int J Obes Relat Metab Disord*, 2003; Vol. 27: pp. 522–9.

Comments: Good meta-analysis of chromium's effect on glucose and weight.

Verma S, Cam MC, McNeill JH. Nutritional factors that can favorably influence the glucose/insulin system: vanadium. *J Am Coll Nutr*, 1998; Vol. 17: pp. 11–8.

Comments: Review about potential mechanisms of vanadium on glucose metabolism.

MEDICATIONS

Dyslipidemia

BILE ACID SEQUESTRANTS

Simeon Margolis, MD, PhD, and Paul A. Pham, PharmD

INDICATIONS

FDA

- **Hypercholesterolemia:** to prevent cardiovascular disease or its complications.
- **Poorly controlled type 2 diabetes:** to lower HbA1c (colesevelam).
- Relief of pruritus associated with partial biliary obstruction (cholestyramine).

MECHANISM

- Binds bile acids in the intestine and removes them in the stools. In compensation, the liver converts more cholesterol to bile acids.
- The fall in liver-free cholesterol leads to synthesis of the hepatic LDL receptor, increases the removal of LDL from the blood, and lowers serum levels of total and LDL cholesterol.

USUAL ADULT DOSING

- **Cholestyramine powder:** administer 1 or 2 packets or 1 or 2 level scoopfuls once or twice a day. Maintenance dose: 2 to 4 packets or scoopfuls daily (8–16 grams anhydrous cholestyramine resin), divided into two doses; take with meals.
- **Colestid tablets:** 2 to 16 g (2 to 16 tabs) daily given once or in divided doses. Starting dose: 2 grams once or twice daily. Titrate by 2 grams over a 1- or 2-month intervals to maintenance dose, OR Colestid granules: 5 to 30 g (one to six packets or level scoopfuls given once or in divided doses). Treatment should be started with one dose once or twice daily.
- **Colesevelam hydrochloride:** 6 tablets (3.75 g) once daily or 3 tablets (1.875 g) twice daily with a meal or liquid.
- Thoroughly stir or use Waring blender to mix powder before ingestion.

FORMS

Brand Name (mfr)	Preparations	Forms†	Cost*
Questran (multiple generic manufacturers)	cholestyramine	oral powder 4 g	$2.12
Colestid (Pfizer and generic manufacturers)	colestipol	oral granules 5 g oral granules (flavored) 7.5 g oral tablet 1 g	$2.70 $3.17 $0.84
WelChol (SANKYO PHARMA INC)	colesevelam hydrochloride	oral tablet 625 mg	$1.36

*Prices represent cost per unit specified, are representative of "Average Wholesale Price" (AWP).
†Dosage is indicated in mg unless otherwise noted.

DOSING IN SPECIAL POPULATIONS

Renal
- No data. Likely usual dose.

Hepatic
- No data. Likely usual dose.

Pregnancy
- Category B

Breastfeeding
- Not found in breast milk; however, bile acid sequestrants interfere with absorption of fat-soluble vitamins and should be used with caution in nursing women.

ADVERSE DRUG REACTIONS

General
- Except for causing constipation, bile acid sequestrants are well tolerated.

Common
- Constipation

Occasional
- Belching, bloating

Rare
- Stomach pain
- Nausea and vomiting

DRUG INTERACTIONS
- Can interfere with the absorption of many orally administered medications.
- To minimize drug interactions, administer all drugs at least 1 hour before or at least 4–6 hours after the administration of cholestyramine. Medications should be taken 4 hours before a dose of colesevelam.
- Drug–drug interactions with the following medications, causing potential lost of therapeutic efficacy: thiazide diuretic, furosemide, glipizide, propranolol, oral penicillin, oral vancomycin, tetracyclines, fat-soluble vitamins (e.g., ADEK), iron supplement, levothyroxine, raloxifene, digoxin, methotrexate, ursodiol, imipramine, valproic acid, certain NSAIDs, gemfibrozil, and fenofibrate.
- **Warfarin:** may increase or decrease INR with coadministration.
- **Ezetimibe:** efficacy may be decreased. Ezetimibe should be administered at least 2 hours before or 4 hours after administration of a bile acid sequestrant.

PHARMACOKINETICS
- **Absorption:** Bile acid sequestrants are not absorbed. All of their actions take place within the intestine.
- **Metabolism:** Not hydrolyzed by digestive enzymes.
- **Excretion:** Primarily fecal, as a complex bound to bile acids; renal <1%.

EXPERT OPINION
- Bile acid sequestrants can lower LDL cholesterol by 15% to 25% depending on the amount taken, and may raise HDL cholesterol by about 2%.
- Can raise triglyceride levels (Crouse), and should not be taken by people with hypertriglyceridemia.
- The powders and granules are inconvenient because they must be thoroughly mixed with a liquid. Colestid pills are large and may be difficult to swallow.

MEDICATIONS

- Colesevelam is the form most commonly used, is more convenient to take, and is associated with fewer side effects (Davidson).
- To avoid interference with absorption of other medications by cholestyramine or Colestid, take them one hour before or 4 to 6 hours after taking the sequestrant. Or take medications 4 hours before colesevelam.
- Sequestrants may particularly interfere with the absorption of fat-soluble vitamins.
- Colesevelam can lower HbA1c slightly in patients with type 2 diabetes (Fonseca; Bays).
- Do not use bile acid sequestrants with biliary or intestinal obstruction, gastroparesis, or other problems with gastrointestinal motility.
- Colesevelam and colestid tablets should be used with caution in people with dysphagia or swallowing disorders.
- Colesevelam can lower HbA1c slightly in patients with type 2 diabetes (Fonseca; Bays).

REFERENCES

Fonseca VA, Rosenstock J, Wang AC, et al. Colesevelam HCl improves glycemic control and reduces LDL cholesterol in patients with inadequately controlled type 2 diabetes on sulfonylurea-based therapy. *Diabetes Care,* 2008; 31: 1479–84.

   Comments: Colesevelam improved glycemic control and reduced LDL cholesterol levels in patients with type 2 diabetes receiving sulfonylurea-based therapy.

Bays HE, Goldberg RB. The "forgotten" bile acid sequestrants: is now a good time to remember? *Am J Ther,* 2007; 14: 567–80.

   Comments: Bile acid sequestrants should be considered for the treatment of patients with type 2 diabetes to lower LDL cholesterol and improve diabetic control.

Davidson MH, Dillon MA, Gordon B, et al. Colesevelam hydrochloride (cholestagel): a new, potent bile acid sequestrant associated with a low incidence of gastrointestinal side effects. *Arch Intern Med,* 1999; 159: 1893–900.

   Comments: Colesevelam has fewer gastrointestinal side effects than the other bile acid sequestrants.

Crouse JR. Hypertriglyceridemia: a contraindication to the use of bile acid binding resins. *Am J Med,* 1987; 83: 243–8.

   Comments: Bile acid sequestrants can raise triglyceride levels and should not be used in patients with elevated triglycerides.

[No authors listed]. The Lipid Research Clinics Coronary Primary Prevention Trial results. II. The relationship of reduction in incidence of coronary heart disease to cholesterol lowering. *JAMA,* 1984; 251: 365–74.

   Comments: The Lipid Research Clinics clearly demonstrated for the first time that lowering cholesterol levels significantly reduced the number of coronary events in men with elevated cholesterol levels.

EZETIMIBE

Simeon Margolis, MD, PhD, and Paul A. Pham, PharmD

INDICATIONS

FDA

- Reduce total and LDL cholesterol to prevent cardiovascular disease or events.

MECHANISM

- Ezetimibe selectively inhibits absorption of cholesterol and related phytosterols in the small intestine.

USUAL ADULT DOSING

- 10 mg daily with or without food.
- Can be used as monotherapy, but is usually added to a statin.

FORMS

Brand Name (mfr)	Preparations	Forms†	Cost*
Zetia (Merck & Co., Inc.)	ezetamibe	oral tab 10 mg	$4.03

*Prices represent cost per unit specified, are representative of "Average Wholesale Price" (AWP).
†Dosage is indicated in mg unless otherwise noted.

DOSING IN SPECIAL POPULATIONS

Hepatic
• Not recommended in patients with moderate to severe hepatic impairment.

Pregnancy
• Category C

Breastfeeding
• Not recommended unless the potential benefit justifies the possible risk to the fetus.

ADVERSE DRUG REACTIONS

General
• No significant adverse drug reactions (ADR) unless ezetimibe is taken with a statin.
• Generally well tolerated with ADR comparable to placebo.

Rare
• Arthalgias
• Dizziness

DRUG INTERACTIONS
• **Cyclosporine:** cyclosporine and ezetimibe concentration may be increased. Cyclosporine AUC was increased by 15%. Monitor cyclosporine concentrations closely with coadministration.
• **Fibrates:** fenofibrate and gemfibrozil increased total ezetimibe concentrations by approximately 50% or 70%, respectively. Limited data on the coadministration; use with close monitoring for potential increased risk of cholelithiasis.
• **Cholestyramine and other bile acid sequestrants:** ezetimibe serum concentrations (AUC) decreased by 55%. Administered ezetimibe at least 2 hours before or 4 hours after bile acid sequestrant.
• **Coumarin anticoagulants:** case report of increased international normalized ratio (INR). Monitor INR closely with ezetimibe coadministration.
• When combined with a statin, adverse effects and contraindications are the same as for the statin.

PHARMACOKINETICS
• **Absorption:** Although large amounts of ezetimibe are rapidly absorbed and glucuronidated, the known action of the drug takes place only in the intestine.
• **Metabolism and excretion:** Metabolized via glucuronidation in small intestine and liver. About 80% found in the feces, 10% of administered dose in the urine as glucuronide.
• **Cmax, Cmin, and AUC:** Cmax for unmodified ezetimibe is 3.4–5.5 ng/ml at 4–12 hours after dose. Cmax for glucuronide 45–71 ng/ml between 1 and 2 hours.
• $T\frac{1}{2}$: 20–30 hrs.

MEDICATIONS

EXPERT OPINION

- The addition of ezetimibe to a statin can decrease LDL cholesterol by an additional ~15%; however, regression of carotid artery intima/media thickness in patients with type 2 diabetes is not affected (Fleg).
- Since ezetimibe is very well tolerated, it is reasonable to add ezetimibe in patients who fail to meet their LDL cholesterol targets despite maximal use of statins (Brown).
- Ezetimibe does not inhibit absorption of triglycerides, fat soluble vitamins, ethinyestradiol or progesterone (van Heek).
- Ezetimibe inhibits the absorption of plant sterols like sitosterol and campesterol and is useful in treatment of sitosterolemia.

REFERENCES

Fleg JL, Mete M, Howard BV, et al. Effect of statins alone versus statins plus ezetimibe on carotid atherosclerosis in type 2 diabetes: the SANDS (Stop Atherosclerosis in Native Diabetics Study) trial. *J Am Coll Cardiol*, 2008; Vol. 52: pp. 2198–205.

Comments: Reducing LDL-C to aggressive targets resulted in similar regression of carotid artery intima-media thickness in patients with type 2 diabetes who attained equivalent LDL-C reductions from a statin alone or statin plus ezetimibe.

Kastelein JJ, Akdim F, Stroes ES, et al. ENHANCE Investigators. Simvastatin with or without ezetimibe in familial hypercholesterolemia. *NEJM*, 2008; Vol. 358: pp. 1431–43.

Comments: In patients with familial hypercholesterolemia, combined therapy with Vytorin (ezetimibe and simvastatin) did not result in a significant difference in changes in carotid intima-media thickness, as compared with simvastatin alone, despite greater decreases in levels of LDL cholesterol and C-reactive protein in those treated with Vytorin.

Brown BG, Taylor AJ. Does ENHANCE diminish confidence in lowering LDL or in ezetimibe? *NEJM*, 2008; Vol. 358: pp. 1504–7.

Comments: In response to the disappointing findings of ENHANCE: continue to use ezetimibe in patients who fail to meet their LDL cholesterol targets despite maximal use of other cholesterol-lowering drugs, and await the outcomes of further studies.

Pearson T, Ballantyne C, Sisk C, et al. Comparison of effects of ezetimibe/simvastatin versus simvastatin versus atorvastatin in reducing C-reactive protein and low-density lipoprotein cholesterol levels. *Am J Cardiol*, 2007; Vol. 99: pp. 1706–1713.

Comments: Ezetimibe plus simvastatin (Vytorin) was significantly more effective than simvastatin alone in lowering LDL cholesterol, 53% versus 38%, and in lowering C-reactive protein levels.

Clarenbach JJ, Reber M, Lütjohann D, et al. The lipid-lowering effect of ezetimibe in pure vegetarians. *J Lipid Res*, 2006; Vol. 47: pp. 2820–4.

Comments: Ezetimibe 10 mg lowered LDL cholesterol by 17% in vegetarians who had a very low cholesterol intake.

Patrick JE, Kosoglou T, Stauber KL, et al. Disposition of the selective cholesterol absorption inhibitor ezetimibe in healthy male subjects. *Drug Metab Dispos*, 2002; Vol. 30: pp. 430–7.

Comments: Although known actions of ezetimibe are limited to the intestine, most of the administered drug is rapidly absorbed. It is possible that absorbed ezetimibe may exert additional benefits.

van Heek M, Farley C, Compton DS, et al. Ezetimibe selectively inhibits intestinal cholesterol absorption in rodents in the presence and absence of exocrine pancreatic function. *Br J Pharmacol*, 2001; Vol. 134: pp. 409–17.

Comments: Ezetimibe selectively inhibited the absorption of cholesterol, with no effect on the absorption of triglycerides, fat-soluble vitamins, ethinylestradiol, or progesteron.

Bays HE, Moore PB, Drehobl MA, et al. Effectiveness and tolerability of ezetimibe in patients with primary hyper-cholesterolemia: pooled analysis of two phase II studies. *Clin Ther,* 2001; Vol. 23: pp. 1209–30.
Comments: Ezetimibe 10 mg lowered LDL cholesterol by 15% or more and raised HDL cholesterol slightly.

FIBRIC ACID DERIVATIVES

Simeon Margolis, MD, PhD, and Paul A. Pham, PharmD

INDICATIONS

FDA

- **Hypertriglyceridemia:** to prevent cardiovascular disease and events (Buse).
- **Mixed dyslipidemia:** to prevent cardiovascular disease and events (Buse).

Non-FDA Approved Uses

- Prevention of acute pancreatitis secondary to severe hypertriglyceridemia.

MECHANISM

- Activation of PPAR alpha reduces the synthesis of apo AIII, an inhibitor of the action of lipoprotein lipase (van Dijk), the enzyme that breaks down circulating triglycerides (Hertz).
- Activation of PPAR alpha also stimulates the formation of apoAV, which lowers blood levels of triglycerides (Prieur).

USUAL ADULT DOSING

- **Fenofibrate (Tricor):** 48–145 mg daily.
- **Fenofibrate (Fenoglide):** 20–120 mg daily.
- **Fenofibrate, micronized (Antara, Lofibra):** Antara 43–130 mg daily; Lofibra 67–200 mg daily; Trilipix 45–135 mg daily. Administer with food.
- **Gemfibrozil (Lopid):** 120 mg twice daily.
- Start with maximal dose in patients with triglycerides >500 mg/dl
- In others, dose titrations are based on patient responses when assessed at the end of 4–6 weeks.

FORMS

Brand Name (mfr)	Preparations	Forms[†]	Cost*
Tricor (Fournier Pharmaceuticals [fenofibrate is available as generic])	fenofibrate	oral nanocrystallized tab 145 mg	$4.51
		oral nanocrystallized tab 48 mg	$1.50
Lofibra (Gate Pharmaceuticals)	fenofibrate micronized	oral micronized cap 67 mg	$1.04
		oral micronized cap 134 mg	$2.00
		oral micronized cap 200 mg	$3.12
Fenoglide (Sciele Pharmaceuticals, Inc.)	fenofibrate	oral tab 40 mg	$1.60
		oral tab 120 mg	$4.80
Antara (Oscient Pharmaceuticals)	fenofibrate micronized	oral micronized tab 43 mg	$1.57
		oral micronized tab 130 mg	$4.70

(Continued)

MEDICATIONS

FORMS *(CONT.)*

Brand Name (mfr)	Preparations	Forms†	Cost*
Lopid (Pfizer and generic manufacturers)	gemfibrozil	oral tab 600 mg	$1.25
Trilipix (Abbott Laboratories)	fenofibrate delayed release	oral delayed release capsule 45 mg	$1.62
		oral delayed release capsule 135 mg	$4.92

*Prices represent cost per unit specified, are representative of "Average Wholesale Price" (AWP).
†Dosage is indicated in mg unless otherwise noted.

DOSING IN SPECIAL POPULATIONS
Renal
- Contraindicated with severe renal disease (GFR <30 ml/min) or on dialysis
- Reduced dose with moderate renal disease, GFR between 30 and 60 ml/min

Hepatic
- Contraindicated for active liver disease or primary biliary cirrhosis

Pregnancy
- Category C

Breastfeeding
- Contraindicated

ADVERSE DRUG REACTIONS
General
- Major concern is development of severe myositis and rhabdomyolysis when used in combination with a statin.

Common
- There are no common side effects.

Occasional
- Abnormal liver function tests
- Abdominal pain
- Upset stomach
- Myositis
- Headache, dizziness

Rare
- Severe myositis, rabdomyolysis, and renal failure when used in combination with a statin
- Gallstones
- Bone marrow suppression

DRUG INTERACTIONS
- **Statins:** may increase risk of rhabdomyolysis. Monitor for sign and symptoms of rhabdomyolysis. Gemfibrozil increases rosuvastatin AUC by 90% (use fenofibrate with rosuvastatin).

- **Warfarin:** may increase INR. Monitor closely with coadministration.
- **Bile acid sequestrants** can reduce fibrate absorption. Fibrates should be taken 1 hour before or 4–6 hours after a sequestrant.
- **Glyburide:** case report of increased hypoglycemic effect with glyburide and gemfibrozil coadministration. Use with close monitoring.
- **Repaglinide:** gemfibrozil increased repaglinide serum concentrations 8.1-fold increase; therefore, coadministration is contraindicated. No significant interaction between fenofibrate and repaglinide.
- **Pioglitazone and rosiglitazone :** coadministration with fibric acid derivatives may increase hypoglycemic effect. Gemfibrozil increases pioglitazone and rosiglitazone AUC by 226% and 130%, respectively.
- **Ursodiol:** efficacy may be decreased.

PHARMACOKINETICS

- **Absorption:** Gemfibrozil: 97% absorbed; fenofibrate: 60%–90% absorbed.
- **Metabolism and excretion:** Gemfibrozil: hepatic metabolism and excreted unchanged both renally (70%) and by the fecal route (6%). Fenofibrate: extensive glucuronidation, also renal conversion to fenofibric acid before excretion (60%–90%) with fecal excretion (10%–25%).
- **T$\frac{1}{2}$:** Gemfibrozil 1.3 hours; fenofibrate 20 hours.

EXPERT OPINION

- Fibrates lower triglycerides by 25%–50% and raise HDL cholesterol by about 8%, but may raise LDL cholesterol in patients with triglycerides >500 mg/dl.
- Severe myositis occurs most commonly when a fibrate is taken in combination with a statin.
- The risk of myositis is greater with gemfibrozil than with fenofibrate.
- When triglyceride levels are between 200 and 500 mg/dl and LDL is elevated, begin treatment with a statin. If triglycerides are still >200 mg/dl, consider adding fenofibrate. The target is a non-HDL cholesterol <100 mg/dl (non-HDL cholesterol = total cholesterol –HDL cholesterol (NCEP Expert panel).
- Fibrates can be used as monotherapy in patients with normal LDL cholesterol and triglycerides between 200 and 500 mg/dl and in patients with triglycerides >500 mg/dl (NCEP Expert panel).
- Fenofibrate has not been shown to reduce coronary heart disease mortality or morbidity in a large trial of patients with type 2 diabetes (Keech).
- Fenofibrate lowers the incidence of laser treatment for diabetic retinopathy (Keech).
- Weight loss and improved glycemic control lower triglyceride levels and should always be attempted before and during treatment with a fibrate.
- Recent trial (ACCORD) tested effect of fenofibrate added to simvastatin in 5518 people with diabetes at high risk for cardiovascular events. LDL-cholesterol was low (about 80 mg/dl) in both fenofibrate and placebo treated groups, and fenofibrate had no additional benefit to simvastatin alone (Ginsberg).

REFERENCES

ACCORD Study Group, Ginsberg HN, Elam MB, et al. Effects of combination lipid therapy in type 2 diabetes mellitus. *NEJM*, 2010; Vol. 362: pp. 1563–74.
Comments: The ACCORD Study tested the effect of intensive glucose control, intensive blood pressure control, and addition of fenofibrate. In this report, patients starting with triglyceride >200 mg/dl and low HDL had

MEDICATIONS

benefit from fenofibrate—not surprising, since the fibrates are generally used to tread hypertriglyceridemia. However, no overall benefit observed with addition of fenofibrate to statin therapy on the risk of cardiovascular outcomes.

Buse JB, Ginsberg HN, Bakris GL, et al. Primary prevention of cardiovascular diseases in people with diabetes mellitus: a scientific statement from the American Heart Association and the American Diabetes Association. *Circulation,* 2007; Vol. 115: pp. 114–26.

Comments: Recommendations from AHA and ADA for the primary prevention of cardiovascular heart disease in patients with diabetes.

Keech AC, Mitchell P, Summanen PA, et al. Effect of fenofibrate on the need for laser treatment for diabetic retinopathy (FIELD study): a randomised controlled trial. *Lancet,* 2007; Vol. 370: pp. 1687–97.

Comments: Treatment with fenofibrate in individuals with type 2 diabetes mellitus reduced the need for laser treatment for diabetic retinopathy.

Sarwar N, Danesh J, Eiriksdottir G, et al. Triglycerides and the risk of coronary heart disease: 10,158 incident cases among 262,525 participants in 29 Western prospective studies. *Circulation,* 2007; Vol. 115: pp. 450–8.

Comments: Prospective studies in Western populations consistently indicate moderate and highly significant associations between triglyceride values and coronary heart disease risk.

Keech A, Simes RJ, Barter P, et al. Effects of long-term fenofibrate therapy on cardiovascular events in 9795 people with type 2 diabetes mellitus (the FIELD study): randomised controlled trial. *Lancet,* 2005; Vol. 366: pp. 1849–61.

Comments: Fenofibrate did not significantly reduce the risk of the primary outcome of coronary events. It did reduce total cardiovascular events.

Grundy SM, Vega GL, Yuan Z, et al. Effectiveness and tolerability of simvastatin plus fenofibrate for combined hyperlipidemia (the SAFARI trial). *Am J Cardiol,* 2005; Vol. 95: pp. 462–8.

Comments: The combination of a statin and fenofibrate is beneficial in the treatment of combined hyperlipidemia.

van Dijk KW, Rensen PC, Voshol PJ, et al. The role and mode of action of apolipoproteins CIII and AV: synergistic actors in triglyceride metabolism? *Curr Opin Lipidol,* 2004; Vol. 15: pp. 239–46.

Comments: Apo CIII raises triglyceride levels by inhibiting lipoprotein lipase activity. Apo AV lowers plasma triglyceride levels.

Prieur X, Coste H, Rodriguez JC. The human apolipoprotein AV gene is regulated by peroxisome proliferator-activated receptor-alpha and contains a novel farnesoid X-activated receptor response element. *J Biol Chem,* 2003; Vol. 278: pp. 25468–80.

Comments: Apo AV formation is stimulated by activation of PPAR alpha.

Expert Panel on Detection, Evaluation, and Treatment of High Blood Cholesterol in Adults Executive Summary of The Third Report of The National Cholesterol Education Program (NCEP) Expert Panel on Detection, Evaluation, And Treatment of High Blood Cholesterol In Adults (Adult Treatment Panel III). *JAMA,* 2001; Vol. 285: pp. 2486–97.

Comments: General guidelines for management of blood lipid abnormalities—risk factors, normal and abnormal cholesterol levels, when to initiate treatments, targets for treatment.

Hertz R, Bishara-Shieban J, Bar-Tana J. Mode of action of peroxisome proliferators as hypolipidemic drugs. Suppression of apolipoprotein C-III. *J Biol Chem,* 1995; Vol. 270: p. 134705.

Comments: Fibrates exert their effects by activating PPAR alpha, which inhibits the formation of apo CIII.

NIACIN

Simeon Margolis, MD, PhD, and Paul A. Pham, PharmD

INDICATIONS

FDA

- Hyperlipidemia (especially in patients with low HDL cholesterol)
- Atherosclerosis prevention and myocardial infarction prophylaxis
- Niacin deficiency and pellagra

MECHANISM

- Niacin binds to a specific G-protein-coupled receptor in adipocytes and immune cells (Tunaru).
- When receptor is activated, it lowers cAMP levels, reducing the activity of hormone-sensitive lipase that releases fatty acids from triglycerides in adipose tissue (Tunaru).
- Niacin decreases production of plasma free fatty acids (FFA) used by the liver to form the triglycerides (Tunaru) carried on very low-density lipoproteins (VLDL), which is converted in the circulation to LDL.
- Binding of niacin to the receptor on immune cells also causes the flushing and itching side effects of the drug.

USUAL ADULT DOSING

- **Niaspan ER (extended-release niacin) or Slo-Niacin (controlled release):** 500–2000 mg at bedtime. Titration schedule: 500 mg at bedtime (wks 1–4); increase to 1 g at bedtime (wks 5–8). May increase by 500 mg/4-wk (max: 2 g/d).
- **Niacor (immediate-release niacin):** 500–1000 mg 2–3 times a day. Titration schedule: initiate with 100 mg 3 times a day with gradual increase over 5–8 wks to average dose of 1 g 3 times a day (max: 6 g/d).
- **Niacin SR:** 500 mg at bedtime titrate to maintenance of 1–2 g 3 times a day.
- Take with food to reduce GI distress and consider aspirin (ASA) for flushing (Guyton).

FORMS

Brand Name (mfr)	Preparation	Forms†	Cost*
Niaspan ER (Abbott Laboratories)	Extended release niacin	ER tablet 500 mg ER tablet 750 mg ER tablet 1000 mg	$2.49 $3.55 $4.40
Slo-niacin (available over-the-counter) (Upsher-Smith)	Controlled release niacin	oral CR tablet 250 mg oral CR tablet 500 mg oral CR tablet 750 mg	$0.09 $0.13 $0.18
Niacor (Upsher-Smith)	Crystalline or immediate acting niacin	oral tablet 500 mg	$0.28

(Continued)

MEDICATIONS

FORMS *(CONT.)*

Brand Name (mfr)	Preparation	Forms†	Cost*
Niacin (available over-the-counter) (Generic manufacturers)	Crystalline or immediate acting niacin	oral tablet 50 mg 100 mg; 125 mg 250 mg; 500 mg 1000 mg	$0.01–0.06
Niacin SR (Generic manufacturers)	Sustained release niacin	oral SR tablet 250 mg oral SR tablet 500 mg	$0.04 $0.05

*Prices represent cost per unit specified, are representative of "Average Wholesale Price" (AWP).
†Dosage is indicated in mg unless otherwise noted.

DOSING IN SPECIAL POPULATIONS

Renal
- Use with caution in patients with significant renal disease, GFR <50.

Hepatic
- Active liver disease or unexplained elevations in liver transaminases are contraindications to niacin use.
- Use with caution in people with past history of liver disease or who drink alcohol to excess.

Pregnancy
- Category C

Breastfeeding
- Contraindicated. Either stop breastfeeding or discontinue the niacin.

ADVERSE DRUG REACTIONS

Common
- Flushing (occurs in the early course of therapy but generally improves with continued use). Pretreatment 30 min before niacin with aspirin may help with flushing (Guyton).
- Abnormal liver enzymes.
- Increased uric acid levels.
- Itching (consider using antihistamine).

Occasional
- Exacerbate peptic ulcer disease
- Nausea, vomiting; abdominal pain
- Gout
- Elevation of alkaline phosphatase; decreased phosphorous (mean 13% decrease)
- Raise blood glucose levels (Elam)

Rare
- Hepatotoxicity (incidence may be higher with sustained-release niacin)
- Acanthosis nigricans
- Rhabomyolysis when taken with a statin
- Thrombocytopenia
- Rash

DRUG INTERACTIONS

- **Statins:** simvastatin and lovastatin may increase risk of myopathy with coadministration, although a prospective trial did not find a higher incidence of myopathy when niacin 1 g was coadministered with lovastatin 40 mg/d (Bays). Consider holding dose at simvastatin 10 mg or lovastatin 20 mg/d with coadministration.
- **Oral hypoglycemics:** effect may be decreased by niacin. Monitor for therapeutic efficacy.
- **Cholestyramine:** may decrease niacin absorption. Separate administration time by 4–6 hrs.
- **Alcohol and hot drinks:** may increase flushing and pruritus. If so, avoid with niacin (Guyton).

PHARMACOKINETICS

- **Absorption:** 60%–76% absorbed.
- **Metabolism and excretion:** Metabolized extensively in liver and 90% excreted in urine as metabolites
- **T$\frac{1}{2}$:** 20–45 minutes.

EXPERT OPINION

- Niacin is the most effective drug for raising HDL cholesterol.
- It can raise HDL by 20%–35%, lower total and LDL cholesterol by 15%–25%, and decrease triglycerides by 30%–50% (Pan). Some reports indicate that niacin also lowers lipoprotein(a).
- Preparations are available over-the-counter, but should only be taken under the supervision of a physician due to risk of major adverse effects.
- Slo-Niacin has been associated with greater liver toxicity than other niacin preparations (Myers).
- Niacin can be beneficial in patients with type 2 diabetes by reducing LDL cholesterol and triglycerides, and increasing HDL cholesterol, but may worsen glycemic control in few patients (Elam).
- Flushing often minimized by taking an aspirin or other NSAID 30 minutes before niacin dose (Guyton).
- Flushing may be more severe if niacin dose is accompanied by hot drinks or food. Tends to wane with long-term use of niacin (Guyton).
- While many experts have recommended raising HDL cholesterol levels, there is no clear evidence of cardiovascular benefit from raising HDL cholesterol levels with niacin (Briel).

REFERENCES

Briel M, Ferreira-Gonzalez I, You JJ, et al. Association between change in high density lipoprotein cholesterol and cardiovascular disease morbidity and mortality: systematic review and meta-regression analysis. *BMJ*, 2009; Vol. 338: p. b92.

    Comments: Conclusions of the authors: "Available data suggest that simply increasing the amount of circulating HDL cholesterol does not reduce the risk of coronary heart disease events, coronary heart disease deaths, or total deaths. The results support reduction in LDL cholesterol as the primary goal for lipid modifying interventions."

Guyton JR, Bays HE. Safety considerations with niacin therapy. *Am J Cardiol*, 2007; Vol. 99: pp. 22C–31C.

    Comments: This article describes ways to overcome the side effects of niacin, including the use of aspirin to prevent or reduce flushing. The authors argue that niacin is underused because of excessive concern about side effects. No-flush niacin does not cause flushing, but it has no effects on blood lipids or lipoproteins.

Tunaru S, Kero J, Schaub A, et al. PUMA-G and HM74 are receptors for nicotinic acid and mediate its anti-lipolytic effect. *Nat Med*, 2003; Vol. 9: pp. 352–5.

MEDICATIONS

Comments: Activation of a niacin receptor in adipose tissue is responsible for the lipid-lowering effect of the drug.

Meyers CD, Carr MC, Park S, et al. Varying cost and free nicotinic acid content in over-the-counter niacin preparations for dyslipidemia. *Ann Intern Med*, 2003; Vol. 139: pp. 996–1002.
Comments: This review identified the following formulations of over-the-counter niacins: 10 immediate-release, 9 slow (sustained)-release, and 10 "no-flush" formulations.

Bays HE, Dujovne CA, McGovern ME, et al. Comparison of once-daily, niacin extended-release/lovastatin with standard doses of atorvastatin and simvastatin (the ADvicor Versus Other Cholesterol-Modulating Agents Trial Evaluation [ADVOCATE]). *Am J Cardiol*, 2003; Vol. 91: pp. 667–72.
Comments: No drug-induced myopathy was seen in a trial using Niaspan and lovastatin.

Pan J, Lin M, Kesala RL, et al. Niacin treatment of the atherogenic lipid profile and Lp(a) in diabetes. *Diabetes Obes Metab*, 2002; Vol. 4: pp. 255–61.
Comments: In this small study of patients with type 2 diabetes, HDL cholesterol rose by 31% while the following decreased: LDL cholesterol (20%), triglycerides (52%), and lipoprotein a (40%). The percentage of small dense LDL also fell.

Elam MB, Hunninghake DB, Davis KB, et al. Effect of niacin on lipid and lipoprotein levels and glycemic control in patients with diabetes and peripheral arterial disease: the ADMIT study: A randomized trial. Arterial Disease Multiple Intervention Trial. *JAMA*, 2000; Vol. 284: pp. 1263–70.
Comments: Niacin can be safely used in people with diabetes, but the drug may result in worsening of glycemic control in some patients.

Capuzzi DM, Guyton JR, Morgan JM, et al. Efficacy and safety of an extended-release niacin (Niaspan): a long-term study. *Am J Cardiol*, 1998; Vol. 82: pp. 74U–81U; discussion 85U–86U.
Comments: Niaspan is equally effective and associated with fewer side effects than other forms of niacin.

McKenney JM, Proctor JD, Harris S, et al. A comparison of the efficacy and toxic effects of sustained vs immediate-release niacin in hypercholesterolemic patients. *JAMA*, 1994; Vol. 271: pp. 672–7.
Comments: Slow-release niacin is associated with an increased risk of severe hepatotoxicity compared with other forms of niacin.

Brown G, Albers JJ, Fisher LD, et al. Regression of coronary artery disease as a result of intensive lipid-lowering therapy in men with high levels of apolipoprotein B. *NEJM*, 1990; Vol. 323: pp. 1289–98.
Comments: Treatment with colestipol plus large doses of niacin was associated with reduced frequency of coronary artery disease progression and increased frequency of regression compared with conventional treatment.

OMEGA-3 FATTY ACIDS (FISH OILS)

Simeon Margolis, MD, PhD, and Paul A. Pham, PharmD

INDICATIONS

FDA

- To reduce very high (>500 mg/dl) triglyceride (TG) levels in adults (as an adjunct to diet).

Non-FDA Approved Uses

- Prevention of cardiovascular events and sudden death in patients with known cardiovascular disease (secondary prevention) (GISSI; Rupp; Oikawa).
- Prevention of arrhythmias (Rupp).

MECHANISM

- Unknown mechanism, but omega-3 fatty acids appear to lower blood triglyceride levels by inhibiting triglyceride formation in the liver and reducing the release of very low-density lipoproteins (VLDL) (Chan; Harris).

FORMS

Brand Name (mfr)	Preparation	Forms†	Cost*
Lovaza (Glaxo SmithKline)	Omega-3 fatty acids	oral soft gel capsule 1 g	$1.52 per capsule
Fish oil (Several major pharmaceutical and other supplement manufacturers)	Omega-3 fatty acids	oral capsules 1 g	$0.10 per capsule

*Prices represent cost per unit specified, are representative of "Average Wholesale Price" (AWP).
†Dosage is indicated in mg unless otherwise noted.

USUAL ADULT DOSING
- Lovaza: 4 g (4 capsules) once daily or 2 g (2 capsules) twice daily
- Fish oil capsules 4–12 capsules per day

DOSING IN SPECIAL POPULATIONS
Renal
- No special dosing needed
Hepatic
- No data
Pregnancy
- Category C: not teratogenic in animal studies
Breastfeeding
- No data

ADVERSE DRUG REACTIONS
General
- Generally well tolerated
- Weight gain
Common
- Increase LDL cholesterol (Balk)
Occasional
- GI: nausea, abdominal pain, and eructation (belching)
- Taste perversion
- Rash
- Increased ALT levels

DRUG INTERACTIONS
- Limited data and no human studies.
- **Aspirin:** may increase bleeding time.
- **Warfarin:** may increase bleeding time. Although in clinical studies omega-3 fatty acid did not produce clinically significant bleeding episodes, patients should be closely monitored.
- **Clopidogrel:** may increase bleeding time.
- **Propranolol:** may enhance antihypertensive effect.
- **Lopinavir:** did not affect lopinavir plasma concentrations.

MEDICATIONS

PHARMACOKINETICS

- **Absorption:** eicosapentaenoic acid (EPA) and docosahexaenoic acid (DHA) are absorbed after oral administration.

EXPERT OPINION

- Fish oils are a safe and effective way to lower triglyceride levels in patients with diabetes, although no Phase I studies have been performed using fish oils.
- They can lower triglycerides by about 30%–50% in patients with severe hypertriglyceridemia (>500 mg/dl) compared to placebo (Balk; Harris).
- Lovaza: nearly 90% long-chain omega-3 fatty acids. More expensive, but taking smaller amounts of fatty acids in Lovaza than in standard fish oil capsules reduces potential weight gain and the likelihood of unpleasant upper GI symptoms.
- Convincing evidence that fish oil is effective in preventing cardiovascular events in secondary prevention (GISSI; Oikawa).
- In combination with fibrate and/or statins, Lovaza can further decrease serum TG levels, but may increase LDL by 6 mg/dl (Balk; Davidson).
- The major coronary heart disease benefit: prevention of sudden death, probably by stabilizing or preventing dangerous arrhythmias (GISSI; Rupp; Oikawa).

REFERENCES

Rupp H. Omacor(R) (prescription omega-3-acid ethyl esters 90): from severe rhythm disorders to hypertriglyceridemia. *Adv Ther,* 2009; Vol. 26: pp. 675–90.
  Comments: In addition to lowering triglycerides, Omacor can improve rhythm disorders and reduce cardiovascular events in secondary prevention.

Oikawa S, Yokoyama M, Origasa H, et al. Suppressive effect of EPA on the incidence of coronary events in hypercholesterolemia with impaired glucose metabolism: sub-analysis of the Japan EPA Lipid Intervention Study (JELIS). *Atherosclerosis,* 2009; Vol. 206: pp. 535–9.
  Comments: A randomized study involving over 18,000 patients found that treatment with the fish oil eicosapentaenoic acid (EPA) plus statin over a 4.5-year period reduced the incidence of coronary artery disease by 22% in hypercholesterolemic individuals with impaired fasting glucose or diabetes.

Davidson MH, Stein EA, Bays HE, et al. Efficacy and tolerability of adding prescription omega-3 fatty acids 4 g/d to simvastatin 40 mg/d in hypertriglyceridemic patients: an 8-week, randomized, double-blind, placebo-controlled study. *Clin Ther,* 2007; Vol. 29: pp. 1354–67.
  Comments: Compared with those taking statin plus placebo, the group taking omega-3 plus statin had significantly lower non-HDL cholesterol and triglyceride levels along with higher HDL cholesterol.

Balk EM, Lichtenstein AH, Chung M, et al. Effects of omega-3 fatty acids on serum markers of cardiovascular disease risk: a systematic review. *Atherosclerosis,* 2006; Vol. 189: pp. 19–30.
  Comments: In this review of 21 trials fish oil lowered triglycerides by 27 mg/dl and increased HDL cholesterol by 1.6 mg/dl, but increased LDL cholesterol by 6 mg/dl.

Harris WS, Bulchandani D. Why do omega-3 fatty acids lower serum triglycerides? *Curr Opin Lipidol,* 2006; Vol. 17: pp. 387–93.
  Comments: Fish oils reduce triglyceride synthesis in the liver.

Chan DC, Watts GF, Barrett PH, et al. Regulatory effects of HMG CoA reductase inhibitor and fish oils on apolipoprotein B-100 kinetics in insulin-resistant obese male subjects with dyslipidemia. *Diabetes,* 2002; Vol. 51: pp. 2377–86.
  Comments: Fish oils reduce secretion of VLDL in obese men with insulin resistance.

Gruppo Italiano per lo Studio della Sopravvivenza nell'Infarto miocardico (GISSI). Dietary supplementation with n-3 polyunsaturated fatty acids and vitamin E after myocardial infarction: results of the GISSI-Prevenzione trial. *Lancet,* 1999; Vol. 354: pp. 447–55.

Comments: During a 3.5-year follow-up, fish oil supplementation, started in patients after an acute myocardial infarction, significantly decreased the risk for overall and cardiovascular disease death, particularly for sudden death.

Harris WS. n-3 fatty acids and serum lipoproteins: human studies. *Am J Clin Nutr,* 1997; Vol. 65: pp. 1645S–1654S.
Comments: This review found that fish oils lowered triglycerides by 25%–30% while increasing both HDL and LDL cholesterol levels by small amounts.

STATINS AND COMBINATION PILLS

Simeon Margolis, MD, PhD, and Paul A. Pham, PharmD

INDICATIONS

FDA

- Hypercholesterolemia
- Atherosclerosis (primary and secondary prevention)
- Cardiovascular events (primary and secondary prevention)

MECHANISM

- By inhibiting the enzyme HMG CoA reductase, which controls the route of cholesterol synthesis, the statins reduce the amount of free cholesterol in the liver.
- The result is activation of the gene that forms the LDL receptor, especially in the liver.
- Increased membrane levels of the LDL receptor leads to removal of more LDL from the blood, which lowers blood levels of total and LDL cholesterol.

USUAL ADULT DOSING

- **Atorvastatin:** 10–80 mg once daily at any time
- **Fluvastatin:** 20–80 mg without regard to meals OR fluvastatin (Lescol) XL 80 mg daily
- **Lovastatin:** 20–80 mg once daily at bedtime
- **Pitavastatin:** 1–4 mg once daily
- **Pravastatin:** 10–80 mg once daily at any time, with or without food
- **Rosuvastatin:** 5–40 mg once daily at any time
- **Simvastatin:** 10–40 mg once daily at bedtime
- **Ezetimibe + simvastatin** are coformulated as Vytorin 10/10 mg, 10/20 mg, 10/40 mg, and 10/80 mg. Vytorin dose: 1 tablet once daily at bedtime
- **Niacin + lovastatin** are coformulated as Advicor 500/20 mg, 750/20 mg, 1000/20 mg, and 1000/40 mg. Advicor dose: 500/20 mg–2000/40 mg once daily
- **Niacin + simvastatin** are coformulated as Simcor 500/20 mg, 750/20 mg, and 500/20 mg. Simcor dose 500/20 mg–2000/40 mg once daily
- **Amlodopine + atorvastatin** are coformulated as Caduet 2.5/10 mg, 5/10 mg, 10/10 mg, 2.5/20 mg, 5/20 mg, 10/20 mg, 2.5/40 mg, 5/40 mg, 10/40 mg, 5/80 mg, 10/80 mg. Caduet dose: 1 tablet daily.

FORMS

Brand Name (mfr)	Preparation	Forms†	Cost*
Lipitor (Pfizer)	atorvastatin	oral tablet 10 mg	$3.19
		oral tablet 20 mg, 40 mg, 80 mg	$4.54

(Continued)

MEDICATIONS

Brand Name (mfr)	Preparation	Forms†	Cost*
Lescol, Lescol XL (Novartis)	fluvastatin	oral ER tablet 80 mg oral capsule 20 mg, 40 mg	$3.66 $2.86
Mevacor; Altocor (Merck and generic manufacturers)	lovastatin	oral Altoprev (time release tablet) 20 mg, 40 mg, 60 mg oral tablet 10 mg oral tablet 20 mg oral tablet 40 mg	$5.00 $0.71 $1.26 $2.21
Livalo (Kowa Pharmaceuticals America)	pitavastatin	oral tablet 1 mg, 2 mg, 4 mg	$3.62
Pravachol (Bristol-Myers and generic manufacturers)	pravastatin	oral tablet 5 mg oral tablet 10 mg oral tablet 20 mg oral tablet 40 mg, 80 mg	$2.00 $2.79 $4.73 $4.92
Crestor (AstraZenica)	rosuvastatin	oral tablet 5 mg, 10 mg, 20 mg, 40 mg	$3.97
Zocor (Merck and generic manufactures)	simvastatin	oral tablet 5 mg oral tablet 10 mg oral tablet 20 mg, 40 mg, 80 mg	$2.00 $2.79 $4.92
Vytorin (Schering Corporation and Merck/Schering-Plough)	simvastatin plus ezetimibe	oral tab 10/10 mg, 10/20 mg, 10/40 mg, 10/80 mg	$4.08
Simcor (Abbott Laboratories)	simvastatin and extended-release niacin	oral tab 500/20 mg oral tab 750/20 mg oral tab 1000/20 mg	$2.49 $3.56 $4.41
Caduet (Pfizer)	amlodipine + atorvastatin	oral tab 10/10 mg, 2.5/10 mg oral tab 5/20 mg, 5/40 mg, 5/80 mg, 2.5/20 mg, 2.5/40 mg, 10/20 mg, 10/40 mg, 10/80 mg oral tab 5/10 mg	$4.37 $5.98 $3.21

Brand Name (mfr)	Preparation	Forms†	Cost*
Advicor ER (Kos Pharmacueticals)	lovastatins and extended-release niacin	oral tab 500/20 mg	$2.74
		oral tab 750/20 mg	$2.94
		oral tab 1000/20 mg	$3.16
		oral tab 1000/40 mg	$3.67

*Prices represent cost per unit specified, are representative of "Average Wholesale Price" (AWP).
†Dosage is indicated in mg unless otherwise noted.

DOSING IN SPECIAL POPULATIONS

Renal
- No special dosing needed.

Hepatic
- Active liver disease or unexplained persistent elevations of serum transaminases are contraindications for statin use.

Pregnancy
- Statins are contraindicated in pregnant women: Category X.
- Statins should be administered to women of childbearing age only with adequate birth control methods and after being informed of the potential hazards.

Breastfeeding
- Women should not breastfeed if they are taking a statin.

ADVERSE DRUG REACTIONS

General
- Muscle pain and/or weakness are the most common symptoms.
- Severe myositis is uncommon but dangerous.

Common
- Myalgia

Occasional
- Abdominal pain
- Nausea
- Insomnia
- Dizziness
- Abnormal liver transaminases

Rare
- Severe myositis, rhabdomyolysis, and renal failure (Joy).

DRUG INTERACTIONS

- Simvastatin, lovastatin, and atorvastatin are CYP3A4 substrates. Atorvastatin also undergoes glucuronidation. CYP3A4 inhibitors (e.g., macrolides antibiotics, amiodarone, azole antifungals, HIV-protease inhibitors) can significantly increase serum levels of these statins.
- Pravastatin undergoes extensive first-pass metabolism via multiple metabolic pathways, particularly glucuronidation (independent of CYP3A4); fluvastatin metabolized primarily by CYP2C9; and rosuvastatin minimally metabolized by the liver;

MEDICATIONS

therefore, pravastatin, rosuvastatin, and fluvastatin are less likely to interact with CYP3A4 inhibitors.

- **Fibrates, especially gemfibrozil, and niacin:** may increase risk of myopathy. Coadminister with close monitoring for myopathy (Joy).
- **Antibiotics:** erythromycin and clarithromycin may significantly increase simvastatin and lovastatin serum concentrations. Consider alternative statins such as pravastatin and rosuvastatin.
- **HIV-protease inhibitors:** contraindicated with simvastatin and lovastatin. Consider low-dose atorvastatin (10 mg), rosuvastatin (5 mg), or pravastatin.
- **Itraconazole, ketoconazole, voriconazole, and posaconazole:** may significantly increase simvastatin and lovastatin serum concentrations. Consider alternative statins such as pravastatin and rosuvastatin.
- **Coumarin anticoagulants:** INR may be increased. Monitor INR closely with coadministration.
- **Diltiazem:** may significantly increase simvastatin and lovastatin serum concentrations. Consider alternative statins such as pravastatin and rosuvastatin.
- **Oral contraceptives:** rosuvastatin increases ethinyl estradiol and norgestrel by 26% and 34%, respectively. Monitor for potential ADR.

PHARMACOKINETICS

- **Absorption:** Pravastatin: 34% absorption with 17% bioavailability. Lovastatin: 30% absorption with 5% bioavailability (take with food). Simvastatin: 5% bioavailability. Fluvasatin: 95% absorption with 20%–30% bioavailability. Atorvastatin: rapidly absorbed with 14% bioavailability. Rosuvastatin: 50% absorption with 20% bioavailability.
- **Metabolism and excretion:** Pravastatin: extensive first-pass metabolism in liver with 20% renal and 71% in biliary excretion. Lovastatin: extensive liver hydrolysis to an active metabolite with 10% renal and 83% biliary excretion. Simvastatin: is a prodrug that undergoes extensive liver metabolism via CYP3A4 with 13% renal and 60% biliary excretion. Fluvastatin: metabolized by CYP2C9 (75%), 3A4(20%), and 2D6 with 5% renal and 95% biliary excretion. Atorvastatin: metabolized by CYP3A4, and excreted in bile. Rosuvastatin: minimally metabolized by liver with 10% renal and 90% biliary excretion.
- **Protein binding:** Pravastatin: 43%–55%. Lovastatin: >95%. Simvastatin: 95%. Fluvastatin: 98%. Atorvastatin: 98%. Rosuvastatin: 88%.
- **Cmax, Cmin, and AUC:** Cmax for pravastatin: 15 ng/ml; lovastatin: 5.8 ng/ml; fluvastatin: 287 ng/ml; atorvastatin: 25 ng/ml; rosuvastatin: 37 ng/ml.
- **$T_{\frac{1}{2}}$:** Pravastatin, Simvastatin: ~3 hrs. Fluvastatin: <3 hrs. Atorvastatin: 7–14 hrs. Lovastatin: 4.5 hrs. Rosuvastatin: 13–20 hrs.

EXPERT OPINION

- The statins are by far the most effective and best-tolerated class of drugs for lowering total and LDL cholesterol levels and also decrease triglycerides by 10%–25% and raise HDL-C by about 5%–10%.
- At recommended dose range, the potency of statins is as follows: pitavastatin > rosuvastatin > atorvastatin > lovastatin > simvastatin > pravastatin > fluvastatin, with mean LDL reduction of 55%–60%, 48%–52%, 48%, 39%–41%, 32%, and 23%, respectively (Jones, 1998; Jones, 2003).

- Due to lack of drug–drug interaction, pravastatin is often recommended in patients on drugs that are potent inhibitors of CYP3A4 (e.g., macrolides, HIV-protease inhibitors, azole antifungals), but more potent agents including atorvastatin (use with caution at lowest dose of 10 mg with slow titration up to maximum of 40 mg/d) or rosuvastatin (start with 5 mg/d) may be considered; lovastatin and simvastatin contraindicated in patients taking CYP3A4 inhibitors.
- Patients should be counseled about symptoms of rhabdomyolysis (e.g., muscle ache, weakness) especially with concurrent fibrate therapy (Joy).
- Statins have beneficial effects other than lowering LDL cholesterol; these pleiotropic effects include lowering blood levels of inflammatory markers such as C-reactive protein and improved function of endothelial cells, which likely contribute to its role in cardiovascular disease prevention.
- Ingestion of a statin and grapefruit juice (>1 quart/day) can increase blood concentrations of the statins (Li).
- Statins lower the incidence of cardiovascular events in individuals who do or do not have diabetes (Pedersen; Heart Protection Study Collaborative Group).
- Statin therapy is associated with a 9% increased risk of development of diabetes, but the risk is low when compared with the reduction in cardiovascular events (Sattar).

REFERENCES

Sattar N, Preiss D, Murray HM, et al. Statins and risk of incident diabetes: a collaborative meta-analysis of randomised statin trials. *Lancet*, 2010; Vol. 375 Suppl 9716: pp. 735–42.

   Comments: The increased risk of developing diabetes is very small compared with the reduction in cardiovascular events achieved with statins.

Shaw SM, Fildes JE, Yonan N, et al. Pleiotropic effects and cholesterol-lowering therapy. *Cardiology*, 2009; Vol. 112: pp. 4–12.

   Comments: This review provides a critical evaluation of the proposed pleiotropic effects of the statins.

Joy TR, Hegele RA. Narrative review: statin-related myopathy. *Ann Intern Med*, 2009; Vol. 150: pp. 858–68.

   Comments: Myalgia is common; rhabdomyolysis is rare. This review discusses the management of myalgia and the prevention of rhabdomyolysis.

Golomb BA, Evans MA Statin adverse effects: a review of the literature and evidence for a mitochondrial mechanism. *Am J Cardiovasc Drugs*, 2008; Vol. 8: pp. 373–418.

   Comments: This review considers some of the less common adverse effects of statins and the relationship of these effects to statin interactions with mitochondrial mechanisms.

Li P, Callery PS, Gan LS, et al. Esterase inhibition by grapefruit juice flavonoids leading to a new drug interaction. *Drug Metab Dispos*, 2007; Vol. 35: pp. 1203–8.

   Comments: Flavenoids in grapefruit juice interfere with the breakdown of statins in the intestine and can raise blood levels of ingested statin.

Pedersen TR, Kjekshus J, Berg K, et al. Randomised trial of cholesterol lowering in 4444 patients with coronary heart disease: the Scandinavian Simvastatin Survival Study (4S). 1994. *Atheroscler Suppl*, 2004; Vol. 5: pp. 81–7.

   Comments: This study (4S) enrolled nearly 4500 subjects with known coronary heart disease. Simvastatin reduced the number of major coronary events and the need for angioplasty or bypass surgery by more than 35% in both men and women.

Jones PH, Davidson MH, Stein EA, et al. Comparison of the efficacy and safety of rosuvastatin versus atorvastatin, simvastatin, and pravastatin across doses (STELLAR* Trial). *Am J Cardiol*, 2003; Vol. 92: pp. 152–60.

   Comments: The STELLAR trial showed that rosuvastatin was more potent than the other available statins.

MEDICATIONS

Heart Protection Study Collaborative Group. MRC/BHF Heart Protection Study of cholesterol lowering with simvastatin in 20,536 high-risk individuals: a randomised placebo-controlled trial. *Lancet*, 2002; Vol. 360: pp. 7–22.
  Comments: This, the largest randomized, controlled trial of statin therapy, enrolled subjects with known cardiovascular disease, diabetes, or hypertension. The simvastatin group exhibited a 38% fall in nonfatal heart attacks, about a 25% reduction in the rates of stroke and revascularization procedures, and a 13% lower incidence of all cause mortality. The benefits extended to women, subjects over the age of 70, and those with a baseline LDL cholesterol less than 100 mg/dl.

Jones P, Kafonek S, Laurora I, et al. Comparative dose efficacy study of atorvastatin versus simvastatin, pravastatin, lovastatin, and fluvastatin in patients with hypercholesterolemia (the CURVES study). *Am J Cardiol*, 1998; Vol. 81: pp. 582–7.
  Comments: The CURVES trial determined the relative potencies of five statins.

Erectile Dysfunction

SILDENAFIL

Ari Eckman, MD, and Paul A. Pham, PharmD

INDICATIONS

FDA

- Treatment of erectile dysfunction (ED).
- Treatment of pulmonary arterial hypertension (WHO Group I) to improve exercise ability and delay clinical worsening.

MECHANISM

- Phosphodiesterase (PDE) type 5 inhibitor is an enzyme found in trabecular smooth muscle, that promotes erection through smooth muscle relaxation.
- PDE-5 catalyzes the degradation of cGMP, resulting in an elevated cytosolic calcium concentration and smooth-muscle contraction.

USUAL ADULT DOSING

- 50 mg once daily 1 hour (range: 30 minutes to 4 hours) before sexual activity; dosing range: 25–100 mg once daily. Maximum dose 100 mg/dose, 1 dose/day.
- Start 25 mg once if >65 years old, with renal or hepatic impairment, or with the coadministration of CYP3A4 inhibitors (see drug interaction section).
- May be administered without regard to meals but may take longer to be effective after a high-fat meal.

FORMS

Brand Name (mfr)	Preparation	Forms†	Cost*
Viagra (Pfizer)	sildenafil	oral tablet 25 mg; 50 mg; 100 mg	$18.22
Revatio (Pfizer)	sildenafil	oral tablet 20 mg	$17.35

*Prices represent cost per unit specified, are representative of "Average Wholesale Price" (AWP).
†Dosage is indicated in mg unless otherwise noted.

DOSING IN SPECIAL POPULATIONS

Renal

- CrCl ≥30 ml/min: no dosage adjustment needed.
- CrCl <30 ml/min: reduce starting dose to 25 mg.

Hepatic

- Cirrhosis (Child-Pugh Class A and B): reduce starting dose to 25 mg. Do not exceed a maximum single dose of 25 mg sildenafil in a 48-hour period.

MEDICATIONS

Pregnancy

- Classified as FDA pregnancy risk Category B. Animal studies have shown no evidence of teratogenicity of sildenafil during organogenesis, but no information on the use of sildenafil in humans during pregnancy. Not indicated for use in pregnant women.

Breastfeeding

- No information on the use of sildenafil in humans during breastfeeding. Not indicated for use in lactating women.

ADVERSE DRUG REACTIONS

General

- Headache, flushing, dyspepsia, and visual disturbances (including sudden decrease in vision, photosensitivity, or seeing a "bluish tinge").
- Caution should be used with cardiac disease.
- CONTRAINDICATED IN PATIENTS TAKING NITRATES.

Occasional

- Nasal congestion, urinary tract infection, diarrhea, dizziness and rash.
- Rare
- Priapism, palpitations, hypotension, serious cardiovascular events (myocardial infarction, cardiac arrest, angina pectoris), allergic reaction.
- Unclear association: respiratory tract infection, back pain, flu syndrome, arthralgia, asthenia, chills, angioedema, pain, and shock.
- Sudden hearing loss.

DRUG INTERACTIONS

- Potent inhibitors of hepatic CYP3A4 or 2C9 isoenzymes decrease sildenafil clearance and metabolism, increasing sildenafil concentration. Use with caution or dose reduction if sildenafil required (maximum dose 25 mg q48h) with the coadministration of the following drugs: conivaptan, erythromycin, fluconazole, imatinib, itraconazole, ketoconazole, posaconazole, mibefradil, nefazodone, other macrolide antibiotics (clarithromycin, troleandomycin), quinidine, ranolazine, sparfloxacin (withdrawn from the US market), voriconazole, zafirlukast, zileuton, delavirdine, HIV protease inhibitors (ritonavir, saquinavir, indinavir, darunavir, fosamprenavir, atazanavir, nelfinavir, lopinavir, tipranavir).
- Moderate inhibitors of hepatic CYP3A4 or 2C9 isoenzymes, decrease sildenafil clearance and metabolism, increasing sildenafil concentration. Use with caution or decrease dose to 25 mg q48 hrs with increased monitoring for adverse reactions with coadministration of the following: cimetidine, diltiazem, grapefruit juice, mifepristone, tacrilomus, monoamine oxidase inhibitors (MAOIs), nilotinib, ciprofloxacin, aprepitant, fosaprepitant, fluoxetine, fluvoxamine, verapamil.
- Inducers of hepatic CYP3A4 or 2C9 isoenzymes, increase sildenafil clearance and metabolism, decreasing sildenafil concentration: etravirine, efavirenz, bosentan, barbiturates, carbamazepine, dexamethasone, phenytoin, phosphenytoin, nevirapine, rifabutin, rifampin, troglitazone (withdrawn from the US market), nebivolol.
- **Alpha-blockers:** may increase risk of hypotension. Use with close blood pressure monitoring. Patients should be stable on their alpha-blocker prior to initiating low-dose sildenafil.
- **Nitrates:** CONTRAINDICATED. Coadministration with sildenafil is contraindicated due to significant hypotension.

- **Amlodipine:** additional blood pressure reduction of 8 mmHg systolic and 7 mmHg diastolic were noted with sildenafil coadministration.
- **Cisapride** (no longer on the US market) is substrate for CYP3A4; avoid concurrent sildenafil and cisapride use as sildenafil (weak inhibitor of CYP3A4) could increase concentration of cispride, leading to cardiac arrhythmias.
- Prolonged erections may be seen with sildenafil and dihydrocodeine; use caution.
- No significant interactions noted with aspirin, ethanol, thiazide diuretics, ACE inhibitors, warfarin, antacids, or tolbutamide.
- **Sapropterin** acts as cofactor in synthesis of nitric oxide, may cause vasorelaxation; use with caution as may decrease blood pressure.

PHARMACOKINETICS

- **Absorption:** Rapidly absorbed after oral administration, with a mean absolute bioavailability of about 41% (25%–63%).
- **Metabolism and excretion:** Metabolized by hepatic cytochrome CYP3A4 (major) and CYP2C9 (minor). One active metabolite with properties similar to parent drug has been identified, accounting for about 20% of the pharmacologic effects of sildenafil. The metabolite is further metabolized to inactive compounds. 80% excreted as metabolites in feces and in about 13% in urine.
- **Protein binding:** 96% bound to plasma proteins. Independent of total drug concentrations.
- **Cmax, Cmin, and AUC:** Cmax reached within 30–120 minutes (median 60 minutes) of oral dosing in the fasted state. Taken with a high-fat meal, absorption is reduced, with median Tmax of 120 minutes and a mean reduction in Cmax of 29%.
- **T$\frac{1}{2}$:** Both sildenafil and its active metabolite have half-life of about 4 hours.
- **Distribution:** Mean steady state volume of distribution for sildenafil is 105 L, indicating widespread tissue distribution.

EXPERT OPINION

- Sildenafil potentiates hypotensive effects of nitrates; concurrent use contraindicated.
- Use with caution in patients with left ventricular outflow obstruction (e.g., aortic stenosis, idiopathic hypertrophic subaortic stenosis) and those with severely impaired autonomic control of blood pressure.
- Expected response to sildenfil is less compared to patients without diabetes, but 50%–80% of patients with diabetes still report benefit (Ng; Price; Blonde; Stuckey).
- Newer PDE-5 inhibitors such as vardenafil (Levitra) (Ishii; Goldstein) and tadalafil (Cialis) (Sáenz de Tejada) are also effective in the treatment of ED for patients with diabetes but have not been studied as extensively.
- Vardenafil has a peak effect at 1 hour and may last up to 4–6 hours.
- Tadalafil has a peak effect at 2 hours and may last up to 36–48 hours.

REFERENCES

Blonde L. Sildenafil citrate for erectile dysfunction in men with diabetes and cardiovascular risk factors: a retrospective analysis of pooled data from placebo-controlled trials. *Curr Med Res Opin*, 2006; Vol. 22: pp. 2111–20. **Comments:** Retrospective analysis showing 62% of patients with DM had improvement in erections with sildenafil, compared to 18% with placebo.

Ishii N, Nagao K, Fujikawa K, et al. Vardenafil 20-mg demonstrated superior efficacy to 10-mg in Japanese men with diabetes mellitus suffering from erectile dysfunction. *Int J Urol*, 2006; Vol. 13: pp. 1066–72.

MEDICATIONS

Comments: Randomized, controlled, 12-week study demonstrating that in Japanese men with DM and ED, vardenafil 10 mg and 20 mg were effective in improving erectile function with comparable safety profiles. Vardenafil 20 mg demonstrated superior efficacy compared with 10 mg, suggesting incremental clinical benefit in using the higher dose in this difficult-to-treat population.

Jackson G. Sexual dysfunction and diabetes. *Int J Clin Pract,* 2004; Vol. 58: pp. 358–62.

Comments: Reviews common agents used for ED in patients with DM.

Stuckey BG, Jadzinsky MN, Murphy LJ, et al. Sildenafil citrate for treatment of erectile dysfunction in men with type 1 diabetes: results of a randomized controlled trial. *Diabetes Care,* 2003; Vol. 26: pp. 279–84.

Comments: Randomized, double-blinded clinical study focusing on sildenafil use for ED in patients with T1DM, showing 66% of patients had improvement in erections with sildenafil, compared to 29% in placebo group.

Goldstein I, Young JM, Fischer J, et al. Vardenafil, a new phosphodiesterase type 5 inhibitor, in the treatment of erectile dysfunction in men with diabetes: a multicenter double-blind placebo-controlled fixed-dose study. *Diabetes Care,* 2003; Vol. 26: pp. 777–83.

Comments: Prospective, randomized, multicenter double-blind placebo-controlled fixed-dose parallel-group phase III trial, 452 patients with type 1 or type 2 DM and ED taking 10 or 20 mg vardenafil or placebo as needed for 12 weeks. Vardenafil statistically improved erectile function and was generally well tolerated in these diabetic patients with ED.

Eardley I, Ellis P, Boolell M, et al. Onset and duration of action of sildenafil for the treatment of erectile dysfunction. *Br J Clin Pharmacol,* 2002; Vol. 53 Suppl 1: pp. 61S–65S.

Comments: Sildenafil is an effective oral treatment for ED that acts relatively quickly and has a duration of action lasting at least 4 h.

Ng KK, Lim HC, Ng FC, et al. The use of sildenafil in patients with erectile dysfunction in relation to diabetes mellitus—a study of 1,511 patients. *Singapore Med J,* 2002; Vol. 43: pp. 387–90.

Comments: 78% of patients with DM reported success with sildenafil, compared to 86.5% of patients without DM.

Sáenz de Tejada I, Anglin G, Knight JR, et al. Effects of tadalafil on erectile dysfunction in men with diabetes. *Diabetes Care,* 2002; Vol. 25: pp. 2159–64.

Comments: Randomized study suggesting that tadalafil therapy significantly enhanced erectile function and was well tolerated by men with diabetes and ED.

Price DE, Gingell JC, Gepi-Attee S, et al. Sildenafil: study of a novel oral treatment for erectile dysfunction in diabetic men. *Diabet Med,* 1998; Vol. 15: pp. 821–5.

Comments: Improved erections reported by 50% and 52% of patients with DM treated with sildenafil 25 mg and 50 mg, respectively, compared with 10% of those receiving placebo.

Gastroparesis

DOMPERIDONE

Lipika Samal, MD, MPH, and Paul A. Pham, PharmD

INDICATIONS

FDA
- Not FDA approved.
- FDA encourages physicians who would like to prescribe domperidone for their patients with severe gastrointestinal disorders that are refractory to standard therapy to open an Investigational New Drug (IND) application.

Non-FDA Approved Uses
- Diabetic gastroparesis
- Gastroesophageal reflux disease (GERD)
- Antiemetic

MECHANISM
- Domperidone is a dopamine antagonist (blocking both D1 and D2 receptors).
- Domperidone facilitates gastrointestinal smooth muscle activity by inhibiting dopamine at the D1 receptors and inhibiting neuronal release of acetylcholine by blocking D2 receptors.

USUAL ADULT DOSING
- Treatment of gastric hypomotility: 10–20 milligrams up to 3 times daily, before meals and at night.

FORMS

Brand Name (mfr)	Preparation	Form†	Cost*
Domperidone maleate (available under a treatment IND. Call the FDA [301] 796-3400)	domperidone	oral tablet 10 mg	n/a

*Prices represent cost per unit specified, are representative of "Average Wholesale Price" (AWP).
†Dosage is indicated in mg unless otherwise noted.

DOSING IN SPECIAL POPULATIONS

Renal
- Renal excretion is low so dose adjustment may not be necessary.

Hepatic
- Extensive liver metabolism. Avoid or use with caution in severe liver disease.

Pregnancy
- Contraindicated

Breastfeeding
- Excreted in breast milk; the FDA advises against use in breastfeeding women.

MEDICATIONS

ADVERSE DRUG REACTIONS

General

- Most studies have reported minimal side effects with repeated doses of domperidone, usually between 30 and 60 mg daily, for several weeks.
- Occasional reported side effects include dry mouth, transient skin rash or itching, headache, thirst, abdominal cramps, diarrhea, drowsiness, and nervousness.

Common

- **CNS:** somnolence, akathisia, asthenia, anxiety, depression, and reduced mental acuity
- **Endocrine:** hyperprolactinemia, gynecomastia, mastalgia, menstrual disturbances, galactorrhea

Occasional

- **Cardiac:** ventricular fibrillation (reported with high-dose IV administration), prolonged QT interval

Rare

- **CNS:** extrapyramidal symptoms (EPS), neuroleptic malignant syndrome (NMS), seizures are rare since domperidone has low CNS penetration.
- **Cardiac:** Torsades de pointes.

DRUG INTERACTIONS

- Lithium may interact with dopamine antagonists, particularly haldol, and may also interact with domperidone. Weakness, dyskinesias, increased extrapyramidal symptoms, and encephalopathy may occur with coadministration and should be avoided. Lithium levels should be monitored and titrated to the low therapeutic range.

PHARMACOKINETICS

- **Absorption:** (13%–17%); bioavailability is increased by preadministration of cimetidine or NaHCO3 solution. Does not readily pass the blood–brain barrier.
- **Metabolism and excretion:** Extensive first-pass hepatic and gut wall metabolism.
- **Protein binding:** 91%–93%.
- **T$\frac{1}{2}$:** 7–9 hours.

EXPERT OPINION

- Not currently FDA approved for treatment of diabetic gastroparesis but often used off-label for this indication.
- For the management of diabetic gastroparesis, domperidone can be considered in cases unresponsive to metoclopramide or low-dose erythromycin.
- Domperidone and metoclopramide likely have similar effects in alleviating symptoms of diabetic gastroparesis, but domperidone results in less CNS side effects (Patterson).
- Potentially serious side effects include cardiac arrest and arrhythmias.
- The FDA does not recommend the use of domperidone to stimulate lactation.

REFERENCES

Sugumar A, Singh A, Pasricha PJ. A systematic review of the efficacy of domperidone for the treatment of diabetic gastroparesis. *Clin Gastroenterol Hepatol,* 2008; Vol. 6: pp. 726–33.

    Comments: A good review on the safety and efficacy of domperidone.

Patterson D, Abell T, Rothstein R, et al. A double-blind multicenter comparison of domperidone and metoclopramide in the treatment of diabetic patients with symptoms of gastroparesis. *Am J Gastroenterol,* 1999; Vol. 94: pp. 1230–4.

    Comments: Domperidone and metoclopramide were equally effective in alleviating symptoms of diabetic gastroparesis, but domperidone resulted in less CNS side effects.

Heykants J, Knaeps A, Meuldermans W, et al. On the pharmacokinetics of domperidone in animals and man. I. Plasma levels of domperidone in rats and dogs. Age related absorption and passage through the blood brain barrier in rats. *Eur J Drug Metab Pharmacokinet*, 1981a; Vol. 6: pp. 27–36.

Comments: Pharmacokinetics were described in the 1980s.

ERYTHROMYCIN

Lipika Samal, MD, MPH, and Paul A. Pham, PharmD

INDICATIONS

FDA

- Multiple antiinfective indications

NON-FDA APPROVED USES

- Diabetic gastroparesis (low-dose erythromycin)

MECHANISM

- Enhances gastrointestinal motility especially during the between-meal period, probably due to agonism at the motilin receptors, which are found mainly in the gastric antrum and proximal duodenum.
- Increases gastric emptying.

USUAL ADULT DOSING

- Diabetic gastroparesis: 150–250 mg PO 3–4 times per day, 30 minutes before meals

FORMS

Brand Name (mfr)	Preparation	Forms†	Cost*
Erythromycin base (Abbott Pharmaceuticals and other generic manufacturers)	erythromycin	oral tablet 250 mg; 500 mg oral suspension 200 mg/5 ml; 400 mg/5 ml	$0.27 $0.41–$0.65

*Prices represent cost per unit specified, are representative of "Average Wholesale Price" (AWP).
†Dosage is indicated in mg unless otherwise noted.

DOSING IN SPECIAL POPULATIONS

Renal

- Usual dose

Pregnancy

- Category B

Breastfeeding

- Excreted in breast milk. American Academy of Pediatrics considers erythromycin to be compatible with breastfeeding.

ADVERSE DRUG REACTIONS

General

- GI: side effects are dose related; therefore, erythromycin dose should be titrated based on clinical response and side effects.

Common

- GI: abdominal pain, diarrhea, loss of appetite, nausea, vomiting

Occasional

- GI: liver function test (LFT) elevation, acquired hypertrophic pyloric stenosis, pseudomembranous enterocolitis secondary to *Clostridium difficile*
- Rash (reversible)
- Cardiac: prolonged QTc (generally observed with high-dose IV or coadministration of erythromycin with potent CYP3A4 inhibitor)
- Ototoxicity (generally observed with high-dose IV)

Rare

- *Pancreatitis*
- Dermatologic: erythema multiforme, Stevens-Johnson syndrome, toxic epidermal necrolysis
- Exacerbation of symptoms of myasthenia gravis and new onset of symptoms of myasthenic syndrome have been reported.
- Cholestatic hepatitis (1:1000 especially with estolate salt formulation, reversible)
- Torsades de pointes (especially in women)

DRUG INTERACTIONS

- Erythromycin is a substrate and known inhibitor of cytochrome P450-3A4 and 1A2; there are multiple drug–drug interactions and ANY CYP3A4 substrate will be significantly increased with erythromycin coadministration. Potent inhibitors of CYP3A4 (e.g., HIV protease inhibitors, azole antifungal) will significantly increase erythromycin concentrations and should be avoided.
- Cisapride, terfenadine, astemizole, pimozide, ergot alkaloids, and ziprasidone coadministration with erythromycin is contraindicated.
- **Some statins** (simvastatin, lovastatin) should be avoided due to increased risk of myopathy and rhabdomyolysis; atorvastatin, pravastatin, and rosuvastatin can be considered with close monitoring.
- Colchicine, digoxin, diltiazem, verapamil, amiodarone, cyclosporine, tacrolimus, sirolimus, corticosteroid, buprenorphine, buspirone, and theophylline serum concentrations may be increased with erythromycin coadministration; use with close monitoring.
- Carbamazepine, clozapine, diazepam, sertraline, ranolazine, and tramadol serum concentrations may be increased; avoid coadministration or use with caution.
- **Midazolam and fentanyl:** avoid coadministration; severe sedation and respiratory depression have been reported with coadministration.
- **Calcium channel blockers** (e.g., diltiazem, amlodipine, nifedipine): serum concentration may be increased; lower calcium channel blocker dose may be needed.

PHARMACOKINETICS

- **Absorption:** 20%–50%
- **Metabolism and excretion:** Partially metabolized to N-demethylation metabolite. Excreted primarily in feces as unchanged drug and metabolite via biliary excretion. Only small amount excreted in urine.
- **Protein binding:** 75%–90%
- $T\frac{1}{2}$: 1–1.5 hours

EXPERT OPINION

- Commonly used as a chronic treatment for gastroparesis, but should be used with caution in the elderly and those with comorbid conditions.
- Checking for drug–drug interaction is critical before using erythromycin.

- May reduce fasting glucose levels in patients with type 2 diabetes, but the mechanism is unclear (Ueno).

REFERENCES

Arts J, Caenepeel P, Verbeke K, et al. Influence of erythromycin on gastric emptying and meal related symptoms in functional dyspepsia with delayed gastric emptying. *Gut*, 2005; Vol. 54: pp. 455–60.

    Comments: Describes the effect of erythromycin on gastric emptying.

Maganti K, Onyemere K, Jones MP. Oral erythromycin and symptomatic relief of gastroparesis: a systematic review. *Am J Gastroenterol*, 2003; Vol. 98: pp. 259–63.

    Comments: A good review of low-dose erythromycin for the symptomatic relief of gastroparesis.

Boivin MA, Carey MC, Levy H. Erythromycin accelerates gastric emptying in a dose-response manner in healthy subjects. *Pharmacotherapy*, 2003; Vol. 23: pp. 5–8.

    Comments: Mechanism of action of low-dose erythromycin.

Ueno N, Inui A, Asakawa A, et al. Erythromycin administration before sleep is effective in decreasing fasting hyperglycemia in type 2 diabetic patients. *Diabetes Care*, 2001; Vol. 24: p. 607.

    Comments: Erythromycin may reduce fasting glucose levels in patients with type 2 diabetes.

Ueno N, Inui A, Asakawa A, et al. Erythromycin improves glycaemic control in patients with Type II diabetes mellitus. *Diabetologia*, 2000; Vol. 43: pp. 411–15.

    Comments: Low doses of erythromycin significantly improved glycemic control over 4 weeks and lowered fasting blood glucose and fructosamine concentrations.

METOCLOPRAMIDE

Lipika Samal, MD, MPH, and Paul A. Pham, PharmD

INDICATIONS

FDA

- Diabetic gastroparesis (PO and IV).
- Stimulation of gastric emptying and intestinal transit of barium in cases where delayed emptying interferes with radiological examination (IV).
- Gastroesophageal reflux disease (GERD) (PO).
- Nausea/vomiting (postop and chemotherapy induced) (IV).
- Small bowel intubation if tube does not pass the pylorus with conventional maneuvers (IV).

NON-FDA APPROVED USES

- Lactation induction.
- Singultus (hiccups).
- Migraine.
- Radiation sensitizer in combination with radiation therapy in the treatment of patients with non-small cell lung cancer (NSCLC).

MECHANISM

- Metoclopramide augments cholinergic activity either by causing release of acetylcholine from postganglionic nerve endings or by sensitizing muscarinic receptors on smooth muscle.
- It increases the tone and amplitude of gastric contractions, relaxes the pyloric sphincter and duodenal bulb, and enhances peristalsis of the duodenum and jejunum.
- It also inhibits central and peripheral dopamine reception.

MEDICATIONS

USUAL ADULT DOSING

- 10 mg per orally (PO), intravenously (IV), or intramuscularly (IM) 4 times per day, 30 minutes before meals and at bedtime for 2–8 weeks. Up to 10 days may be required before symptoms subside.

FORMS

Brand Name (mfr)	Preparation	Forms†	Cost*
Reglan (Invamed Inc. and other generic manufacturers)	metoclopramide hydrochloride	oral tablet 5 mg; 10 mg oral solution 5 mg/ml IM/IV vial 5 mg/ml	$0.27–$0.32 $19.27 per 16 oz $5.58

*Prices represent cost per unit specified, are representative of "Average Wholesale Price" (AWP).
†Dosage is indicated in mg unless otherwise noted.

DOSING IN SPECIAL POPULATIONS

Renal

- CrCl <40 ml/min: initiate with 50% of normal dose, then titrate to effect.

Hepatic

- No dosage adjustments are needed.

Pregnancy

- Pregnancy Category B. No impairment of fertility or significant harm to the fetus in animal studies. Limited clinical data on the safe use of metoclopramide for the treatment of hyperemesis gravidarum.

Breastfeeding

- Metoclopramide is distributed into breast milk. The American Academy of Pediatrics continues to recommend caution during the use of metoclopramide in breastfeeding secondary to the potential for CNS effects from the use of the drug.

ADVERSE DRUG REACTIONS

General

- Adverse CNS effects: black box warning regarding the risk of tardive dyskinesia.

Common

- Neurologic: somnolence (oral: 2.1%–10%; IV: up to 70% with high dose 1–2 mg/kg/dose)
- Fatigue

Occasional

- Reversible extrapyramidal effects, pseudoparkinsonism (dose-related occurs more commonly with doses >40 mg/d)
- Hyperprolactinemia, erectile dysfunction, menstrual irregularity
- Headache (4.2%–5.2%)
- Gastrointestinal: nausea and vomiting (association unclear)

Rare

- Neuroleptic malignant syndrome
- Insomnia, restlessness, and depression

- Hypotension, hypertension, AV block, sinus bradycardia, and supraventricular tachycardia (SVT)
- Hypersensitivity reaction

DRUG INTERACTIONS

- **Posaconazole:** may decrease posaconazole serum concentrations. Take posaconazole with a high-fat meal and monitor for therapeutic efficacy.
- **Venlafazine:** may increase risk of serotonin syndrome, but this is rare. Monitor with coadministration.
- **Sedatives, benzodiazepines, opiates:** somnolence may be increased with metoclopramide coadministration.
- **MAOI:** use with close monitoring.
- **Digoxin:** digoxin serum concentration may be decreased. Monitor digoxin serum concentrations with metoclopramide coadministration.
- **Dopamine agonist** (e.g., ropinirole, amantadine, bromocriptine, levodopa, pergolide, and pramipexole): metoclopramide may antagonize dopamine agonist activities. Use with close monitoring.
- **Cyclosporine and tacrolimus:** serum concentrations of cyclosporine and tacrolimus may be increased. Use with close therapeutic drug monitoring.

PHARMACOKINETICS

- **Absorption:** Tmax for oral: 1–2 hr; IV: 15 minutes.
- **Metabolism and excretion:** Minimal hepatic metabolism, 85% renal clearance.
- **Protein binding:** alpha-1-acid glycoprotein: approximately 30%.
- **T$\frac{1}{2}$:** 5–6 hr, approximately.
- **Distribution:** 3.5 L/kg.

EXPERT OPINION

- Metoclopramide is the only FDA approved medication for gastroparesis.
- Short-term (2–8 weeks) use of metoclopramide can be beneficial for diabetic gastroparesis; however, somnolence can be problematic for some patients.
- Small prospective randomized studies in diabetic patients found improved gastric emptying time with the use of metoclopramide.

REFERENCES

Lata PF, Pigarelli DL. Chronic metoclopramide therapy for diabetic gastroparesis. *Ann Pharmacother*, 2003; Vol. 37: pp. 122–6.

    Comments: Literature review through 2002 concluding that there is limited evidence of long-term efficacy of metoclopramide for diabetic gastroparesis.

Patterson D, Abell T, Rothstein R, et al. A double-blind multicenter comparison of domperidone and metoclopramide in the treatment of diabetic patients with symptoms of gastroparesis. *Am J Gastroenterol*, 1999; Vol. 94: pp. 1230–4.

    Comments: Prospective randomized trial found metoclopramide to be as effective as domperidone for the treatment diabetic gastroparesis; however, CNS side effects were more severe and more common with metoclopramide (49% vs 29% after 4 weeks of metoclopramide 40 mg/d).

Ricci DA, Saltzman MB, Meyer C, et al. Effect of metoclopramide in diabetic gastroparesis. *J Clin Gastroenterol*, 1985; Vol. 7: pp. 25–32.

    Comments: Randomized double-blind crossover design—13 patients received 10 mg metoclopramide 4 times a day. Overall mean symptom reduction of 52.6% for nausea, vomiting, anorexia, fullness, and bloating. 7 patients had improved gastric retention on gastric emptying studies, though these results did not correlate with symptom relief.

McCallum TW, Ricci DA, Rakatansky H, et al. A multicenter placebo-controlled clinical trial of oral metoclopramide in diabetic gastroparesis. *Diabetes Care,* 1983; Vol. 6: p. 463.

Comments: 40 patients with diabetic gastroparesis were randomized in a double-blind study to metoclopramide 10 mg tablet 4 times daily or placebo. Treatment significantly reduced postprandial fullness. Mean gastric emptying assessed by radionuclide scintigraphy was significantly improved in the metoclopramide-treated group when compared with their baseline.

Snape WJ, Battle WM, Schwartz SS, et al. Metoclopramide to treat gastroparesis due to diabetes mellitus: a double-blind, controlled trial. *Ann Intern Med,* 1982; Vol. 96: pp. 444–6.

Comments: Randomized, double-blind, controlled trial—10 patients received 10 mg metoclopramide 4 times a day for 3 weeks. Treatment resulted in an increase in the rate of gastric emptying ($56.8\% \pm 7.4\%$) in contrast to the response to placebo ($37.6\% \pm 7.7\%$) ($p < 0.01$).

Glucose-Lowering

ALPHA GLUCOSIDASE INHIBITORS

Nadeen Hosein, MD, MS, and Brian Pinto, PharmD, MBA

INDICATIONS

FDA

- Type 2 diabetes mellitus

Mechanism

- Competitively and reversibly inhibit the enzymes (alpha glucoside hydrolases), which break down complex sugars in the small intestinal brush border.
- Cause delayed absorption of simple sugars from the gut, thus reducing postprandial hyperglycemia.
- Inhibit lactase only minimally and therefore do not cause lactose intolerance.

USUAL ADULT DOSING

- Before alpha glucosidase inhibitor (AGI) initiation, check baseline liver enzymes, then every 3 months for the first year of use, and periodically thereafter.
- AGIs must be always be taken with the first bite of a meal. This applies to the dosing information listed below.
- **Acarbose initiation:** 25 mg orally once daily; titrate up to 25 mg 3 times per day.
- **Acarbose maintenance:** 50–100 mg 3 times per day; maximum dose 50 mg 3 times per day (if body weight <60 kg) or 100 mg 3 times per day (if body weight >60 kg).
- **Miglitol initiation:** 25 mg orally 3 times per day.
- **Miglitol maintenance:** 50 mg 3 times per day (maximum dose 100 mg 3 times per day).

FORMS

Brand Name (mfr)	Preparation	Forms†	Cost*
Precose (Cobalt, Roxane, Bayer, and others)	acarbose	oral tablet 25 mg	$82 for 100 generic tabs
		oral tablet 50 mg	$88 for 100 generic tabs
		oral tablet 100 mg	$90 for 100 generic tabs
Glyset (Pfizer)	miglitol	oral tablet 25 mg;	$88 for 90 brand name tabs
		oral tablet 50 mg;	$97 for 90 brand name tabs
		oral tablet 100 mg	$110 for 90 brand name tabs
*Prices represent cost per unit specified, are representative of "Average Wholesale Price" (AWP).			
†Dosage is indicated in mg unless otherwise noted.			

MEDICATIONS

DOSING IN SPECIAL POPULATIONS

Renal
- Do not use if GFR <25 ml/min or if serum creatinine >2 mg/dl.

Hepatic
- Acarbose is absolutely contraindicated in cirrhosis of the liver.

Pregnancy
- FDA Category B.

Breastfeeding
- Thomson Lactation Ratings: infant risk cannot be ruled out.

ADVERSE DRUG REACTIONS

General
- Not for use in renal failure (GFR <25 ml/min or serum creatinine >2 mg/dl).
- Contraindicated in GI conditions such as inflammatory bowel disease, intestinal obstruction/ileus, conditions potentially exacerbated by increased intestinal gas, conditions associated with decreased digestion or absorption, or colonic ulcerations.
- If used with an insulin secretagogue (sulfonylureas or meglitinides), can result in hypoglycemia. This hypoglycemia must be corrected with oral glucose (monosaccharide), not with sucrose (table sugar; a disaccharide whose breakdown will be inhibited).
- Acarbose is absolutely contraindicated in cirrhosis of the liver.
- Not for use in diabetic ketoacidosis.

Common
- Many patients (up to 74%) will experience GI disturbances (flatulence, diarrhea, bloating, abdominal pain).

Occasional
- Miglitol can cause a transient skin rash.
- Miglitol can decrease serum iron levels.

Rare
- Dose-dependent hepatotoxicity. Therefore, check liver enzymes every 3 months for the first year of use, then periodically thereafter.

DRUG INTERACTIONS
- Somatropin may decrease the efficacy of oral antidiabetic agents such as acarbose and miglitol (see Table 4-3).

PHARMACOKINETICS

TABLE 4-3. PHARMACOKINETICS OF ALPHA GLUCOSIDASE INHIBITORS

	Acarbose	Miglitol
Absorption	<2% absorbed	25-mg dose is 100% absorbed; 100-mg dose is 50%–70% absorbed
Metabolism	Gastrointestinal	Not metabolized; excreted unchanged
Excretion	51% fecal, 34% renal	Renal
Protein Binding	Negligible	Minimal

	Acarbose	**Miglitol**
$T\frac{1}{2}$	2 hrs	2 hrs
Volume of Distribution	0.32 L/kg	0.18 L/kg

Courtesy of Paul Pham, PharmD, Johns Hopkins University School of Medicine.

Expert Opinion

- Expected HbA1c reduction is 0.5% to 0.7%.
- Weight neutral.
- No hypoglycemia when used as monotherapy.
- If hypoglycemia occurs with concomitant sulfonylurea use, must be corrected with oral glucose, not sucrose.
- Multiple daily dosing regimen can create compliance issues.
- GI disturbances (flatulence, diarrhea, bloating, abdominal pain) are the main reason why these medications have never become popular in the US.
- Acarbose may be useful in the prevention of diabetes and cardiovascular complications among individuals with impaired glucose tolerance.

References

Chiasson JL, Josse RG, Gomis R, et al. Acarbose treatment and the risk of cardiovascular disease and hypertension in patients with impaired glucose tolerance: the STOP-NIDDM trial. *JAMA*, 2003; Vol. 290: pp. 486–94.
  Comments: Patients with impaired glucose tolerance who were treated with acarbose had significant reductions in risk for experiencing future myocardial infarctions and for developing hypertension.

Chiasson JL, Josse RG, Gomis R, et al. Acarbose for prevention of type 2 diabetes mellitus: the STOP-NIDDM randomised trial. *Lancet*, 2002; Vol. 359: pp. 2072–7.
  Comments: In this prospective study, 1429 patients with impaired glucose tolerance were randomized to either acarbose or placebo therapy. After 3.3 years, the acarbose group had a statistically significant 25% reduction in risk for developing type 2 diabetes mellitus.

Campbell LK, Baker DE, Campbell RK. Miglitol: assessment of its role in the treatment of patients with diabetes mellitus. *Ann Pharmacother*, 2000; Vol. 34: pp. 1291–301.
  Comments: Overview of the pharmacology of miglitol and its use in treating patients with type 2 diabetes mellitus.

DPP-IV INHIBITORS

Nadeen Hosein, MD, MS, and Brian Pinto, PharmD, MBA

Indications

FDA

- Type 2 diabetes mellitus

Mechanism

- Inhibits the degradation of incretins such as GLP-1 by inhibiting the enzyme dipeptidyl peptidase IV (DPP-IV). The incretin effect is prolonged, enhancing glycemic control through various mechanisms.

Usual Adult Dosing

- **Sitagliptin:** recommended dose is 50–100 mg once a day. Can be taken with or without food.
- **Saxagliptin:** recommended dose is 2.5 or 5 mg once a day. Can be taken with or without food.

MEDICATIONS

- **Sitagliptin + metformin:** Coformulated as Janumet 50/500 mg twice a day, with meals. Can increase to 50/1000 mg twice a day, with meals (maximum dose).
- **Saxagliptin + metformin XR:** coformulated as Kombiglyze. 2.5/1000 mg, 5/1000 mg, or 5/2000 mg once daily with evening meal.
- If adding sitagliptin or saxagliptin to sulfonylurea therapy, consider decreasing the sulfonylurea dose to reduce hypoglycemia risk.
- Both are FDA approved for use as monotherapy in type 2 diabetes (T2DM).
- Sitagliptin or saxagliptin can be added to patients already on metformin or thiazolidinediones.
- In the United States, DPP-IV inhibitors have not been studied for use in combination with insulin.

Forms

Brand Name (mfr)	Preparation	Forms†	Cost*
Januvia (Merck)	sitagliptin phosphate	oral tablet 25 mg oral tablet 50 mg oral tablet 100 mg	$214 for 30 tabs $214 for 30 tabs $214 for 30 tabs
Onglyza (Bristol-Myers Squibb)	saxagliptin	oral tablet 2.5 mg oral tablet 5 mg	$190 for 30 tabs $190 for 30 tabs
Janumet (Merck Sharp & Dohme Corporation)	sitagliptin phosphate + metformin hydrochloride	oral tablet 50/500 mg oral tablet 50/1000 mg	$197 for 60 tabs $196 for 60 tabs

*Prices represent cost per unit specified, are representative of "Average Wholesale Price" (AWP).
†Dosage is indicated in mg unless otherwise noted.

Dosing in Special Populations
Renal
Sitagliptin
- GFR ≥50 ml/min, no dosage adjustment needed.
- GFR 30–50 ml/min, do not exceed 50 mg daily.
- GFR <30 ml/min, do not exceed 25 mg daily.
- For patients on hemodialysis or peritoneal dialysis, do not exceed 25 mg daily.

Saxagliptin
- GFR >50 ml/min, no dosage adjustment needed.
- GFR ≤50 ml/min, do not exceed 2.5 mg once daily.
- For patients on hemodialysis, administer 2.5 mg once daily, following hemodialysis.

Janumet
- CONTRAINDICATED if GFR ≤60 ml/min, or if serum creatinine ≥1.4 mg/dl (women) or ≥1.5 mg/dl (men).

Hepatic
- No dose adjustments needed, except for Janumet: avoid use if liver disease is present, due to increased risk of lactic acidosis.

Pregnancy
- FDA Category B

Breastfeeding
- Thomson Lactation Ratings: infant risk cannot be ruled out.

Adverse Drug Reactions

General
- Contraindicated in patients with hypersensitivity reaction to sitagliptin or saxagliptin.
- Do not use in diabetic ketoacidosis.
- Do not use as therapy for type 1 diabetes mellitus.
- Cases of acute pancreatitis have been reported with sitagliptin—physician should monitor patients closely for signs and symptoms of pancreatitis when starting sitagliptin, or increasing dose.
- Due to metformin component in Janumet, it is contraindicated in renal disease (see previous).

Occasional
- Hypoglycemia, more common when used in conjunction with a sulfonylurea
- Nasopharyngitis or upper respiratory tract infections
- Headache
- Nausea, diarrhea, abdominal pain
- Urinary tract infections
- Peripheral edema
- **Janumet:** GI disturbance initially (nausea, vomiting, diarrhea) due to metformin; lessened if taken with meals

Rare
- Acute pancreatitis with sitagliptin
- Stevens-Johnson syndrome, urticaria, exfoliative dermatitis, and other hypersensitivity skin reactions
- Anaphylaxis
- Angioedema
- Rhabdomyolysis
- Acute renal failure
- Bone fractures with saxagliptin
- Lactic acidosis with Janumet, due to metformin component

Drug Interactions
- Digoxin: oral sitagliption caused small (11%) increase in AUC and plasma Cmax (18%) of digoxin at 0.25 mg/day. Dose adjustment of digoxin not recommended, but monitor closely.

Pharmacokinetics
- **Absorption:** Sitagliptin: 87% bioavailability; time to peak concentration 1–4 hours. Saxagliptin: time to peak concentration 2 hours.
- **Metabolism and excretion:** Sitagliptin: hepatic metabolism; 87% renal and 13% fecal excretion; dialyzable, with 13.5% removed. Saxagliptin: hepatic metabolism; 60% renal and 22% fecal excretion; dialyzable, with 23% removed.
- **Protein binding:** Sitagliptin: 38%. Saxagliptin: negligible.
- **Cmax, Cmin, and AUC:** Sitagliptin: following a single oral 100-mg dose to healthy volunteers, mean plasma AUC of sitagliptin was 8.52 µM*hr; Cmax was 950 nM.
- **T$\frac{1}{2}$:** Sitagliptin: 12.4 hours. Saxagliptin: 2.5 hours.
- **Distribution:** Sitagliptin: Vd 2.8 L/kg

MEDICATIONS

EXPERT OPINION

- Overall HbA1c reduction for maximum dose sitagliptin (100 mg daily) as monotherapy is only about 0.6% after 18 weeks (range 0.5%–0.8%) (Raz). This and the high cost have led many endocrinologists to use DPP-IV inhibitors as second- or third-line drugs when baseline HbA1c is <8%.
- Sitagliptin is weight-neutral.
- Long-term safety data are not known for sitagliptin, as it was only released in October 2006.
- In July 2009, FDA approved a new DPP-IV inhibitor, saxagliptin (Onglyza), for T2DM.
- Other DPP-IV inhibitors (such as vildagliptin and alogliptin), are not yet FDA approved.
- In Europe, vildagliptin is widely approved, and sitagliptin was recently approved as add-on therapy to insulin.

REFERENCES

Rosenstock J, Aguilar-Salinas C, Klein E, et al. Effect of saxagliptin monotherapy in treatment-naïve patients with type 2 diabetes. *Curr Med Res Opin*, 2009; Vol. 25: pp. 2401–11.

Comments: In this double-blind trial, 401 patients were randomized to 2.5 mg, 5 mg, 10 mg of saxagliptin or placebo for 24 weeks. Patients in the saxagliptin groups taking 2.5 mg, 5 mg and 10 mg achieved hemoglobin A1C reductions of 0.43%, 0.46% and 0.54%, respectively, compared to a 0.19% reduction in the placebo group.

Chia CW, Egan JM. Incretin-based therapies in type 2 diabetes mellitus. *J Clin Endocrinol Metab*, 2008; Vol. 93: pp. 3703–16.

Comments: Overview of the role of DPP-IV inhibitors and GLP-1 agonists in treating type 2 diabetes mellitus.

Nauck MA, Meininger G, Sheng D, et al. Efficacy and safety of the dipeptidyl peptidase-4 inhibitor, sitagliptin, compared with the sulfonylurea, glipizide, in patients with type 2 diabetes inadequately controlled on metformin alone: a randomized, double-blind, non-inferiority trial. *Diabetes Obes Metab*, 2007; Vol. 9: pp. 194–205.

Comments: In this noninferiority study, 1172 patients on metformin monotherapy and baseline HbA1c of 7.5% were randomly assigned to receive either sitagliptin 100 mg/day or glipizide 5–20 mg/day. After 1 year, both groups showed a 0.67% HbA1c reduction, demonstrating noninferiority.

Raz I, Hanefeld M, Xu L, et al. Efficacy and safety of the dipeptidyl peptidase-4 inhibitor sitagliptin as monotherapy in patients with type 2 diabetes mellitus. *Diabetologia*, 2006; Vol. 49: pp. 2564–71.

Comments: Sitagliptin monotherapy reduced HbA1c by 0.6% after 18 weeks at its maximum daily dose of 100 mg.

INCRETIN MIMETICS AND AMYLIN ANALOGUES

Ana Emiliano, MD, and Brian Pinto, PharmD, MBA

INDICATIONS

FDA

- **Incretin mimetics (exenatide and liraglutide):** type 2 diabetes (T2DM), although not approved for use with insulin therapy.
- **Amylin analogues (pramlintide):** type 1 diabetes (T1DM) or T2DM on insulin therapy.

Mechanism

- **Incretin mimetics (exenatide, liraglutide):** stimulate glucose-dependent insulin secretion, slow gastric emptying; inhibit glucagon secretion; and suppress appetite.
  - These agents (exenatide, liraglutide) are glucagon-like peptide agonists, binding to the GLP-1 receptor, as the mechanism for stimulating glucose-dependent insulin release.
- **Amylin analogue (pramlintide):** slows gastric emptying; suppresses an exaggerated postprandial rise of glucagon (as seen in T2DM); induces satiety.

  – This agent (pramlintide): acts as the naturally occurring gastric protein amylin, which is cosecreted with insulin by pancreatic beta cells.

USUAL ADULT DOSING

- Evaluate renal function prior to starting an incretin mimetic.
- **Exenatide:** start at 5 mcg subcutaneously twice daily (within 60 minutes prior to a meal) and, after one month, increase to 10 mcg twice daily if tolerated (maximum daily dose).
- **Liraglutide:** start at 0.6 mg subcutaneously once daily for one week and then increase to 1.2 mg once daily (maximum dose 1.8 mg once daily).
- **Pramlintide:** in T1DM, start at 15 mcg subcutaneously immediately before each meal and reduce insulin dose by 50% to avoid hypoglycemia. If no significant nausea, titrate at 15-mcg increments as tolerated every 3–7 days, recommended dose 60 mcg immediately before meals. In T2DM, start at 60 mcg subcutaneously immediately before each meal; titrate to recommended dose of 120 mcg twice daily with each meal.
- Can be administered subcutaneously using a pen-injector or vials: to convert mcg (pen-injector) to units (vials), divided dose in mcg by 6 (i.e., 120 mcg = 20 units).

FORMS

Brand Name (mfr)	Preparation	Forms†	Cost*
Byetta (Amylin Pharmaceuticals, Inc.)	exenatide	subcutaneous injection solution 10 mcg/0.04 ml; 5 mcg/0.02 ml	$271 for 30 days $265 for 30 days
Victoza (Novo Nordisk, Inc.)	liraglutide	subcutaneous injection solution 18 mg/3 ml	$280 for two 3 ml pens; $400 for three 3 ml pens
Symlin (Amylin Pharmaceuticals, Inc.)	pramlintide	subcutaneous injection solution 600 mcg/ml; 1000 mcg/ml	$228 for 5 ml vial $312 for a box with two 2.7 ml pens

*Prices represent cost per unit specified, are representative of "Average Wholesale Price" (AWP).
†Dosage is indicated in mg unless otherwise noted.

DOSING IN SPECIAL POPULATIONS

Renal

- **Exenatide:** do not use in patients with GFR <30 ml/min. Monitor serum creatinine in patients with GFR between 30–50 ml/min after medication initiation or dose titration.
- **Liraglutide:** use with caution in patients with renal impairment.
- **Pramlintide:** no dose adjustment for moderate to severe kidney disease (GFR 20–50 ml/min). Unknown if pramlintide is safe in dialysis patients.

Hepatic

- **Exenatide and liraglutide:** no need for adjustment but caution recommended.
- **Pramlintide:** no studies assessing safety of use in liver disease.

Pregnancy
- Exenatide, liraglutide, and pramlintide are Category C.

Breastfeeding
- **Incretin mimetics and pramlintide:** excretion in human breast milk unknown. Caution when contemplating use in nursing mothers as infant risk cannot be ruled out.

ADVERSE DRUG REACTIONS

General
- **Incretin mimetics:** pancreatitis uncommon. If severe abdominal pain develops, discontinue medication and exclude pancreatitis. Severe, necrotizing, and hemorrhagic pancreatitis have been rarely reported per FDA reports.
- **Liraglutide:** increases risk of medullary thyroid cancer in rodents. Unclear if liraglutide poses same risk to humans, but should not be used in patients with a personal or family history of medullary thyroid cancer or patients with multiple endocrine neoplasia type 2 (MEN-2) (*http://dailymed.nlm.nih.gov/dailymed/about*).
- **Pramlintide, exenatide and liraglutide:** avoid in patients with gastroparesis, due to the drugs' effect in slowing gastric emptying.
- **Pramlintide:** black box warning regarding the need to reduce the insulin dosage with drug initiation to avoid severe hypoglycemia. Avoid use in patients with hypoglycemia unawareness.

Common
- **Incretin mimetics and pramlintide:** nausea, which usually improves over time
- **Pramlintide:** hypoglycemia

Occasional
- **Exenatide, liraglutide:** diarrhea, headache
- **Pramlintide:** abdominal pain, arthralgia

Rare
- **Exenatide:** angioedema, rash
- **Liraglutide:** angioedema

DRUG INTERACTIONS
- Hypoglycemia when combined with hypoglycemic agents.
- **Exenatide and liraglutide:** slow gastric emptying and may impact absorption of oral medications.
- **Pramlintide:** may enhance the anticholinergic effects of anticholinergic drugs.

PHARMACOKINETICS

TABLE 4-4. PHARMACOKINETICS OF INCRETIN MIMETICS AND AMYLIN ANALOGUES

Drug	Absorption	Metabolism	Elimination	Half-life
Exenatide	Peak plasma ~2 hours	Minimal systemic	Urine	2.4 hours
Liraglutide	Peak plasma 8–12 hours	Endogenously by DPP-IV	Urine, feces	~13 hours
Pramlintide	Peak plasma 20 minutes	Renal to active metabolite	Urine	~48 minutes

Courtesy of Paul Pham, PharmD, Johns Hopkins University School of Medicine.

EXPERT OPINION

- Exenatide causes a dose-dependent weight loss averaging ~1.4 kg; may be preferred for patients with comorbid obesity (DeFronzo; Kendall).
- Average weight loss with pramlintide is 0.5–1.4 kg (Ratner; Hollander).
- Liraglutide reported to cause weight reduction of 2–2.5 kg (Nauck).
- Thus, the weight loss effect of these agents is a major aspect of their attractiveness.
- HbA1c reduction with exenatide and liraglutide ~1% (Nauck), proportional to starting HbA1c.
- In individual studies, HbA1c reduction with pramlintide use in T2DM was 0.62% (Hollander) and in T1DM was 0.3% (Ratner).
- Incretin mimetics and amylin analogues not generally used as monotherapy.
- Both incretin mimetics and amylin analogues are administered through subcutaneous injection only; may not be preferred in patients who are fearful of injections.
- Recent study found that combination of exenatide and insulin glargine effective in achieving normal blood glucose without significant hypoglycemia (Buse).

BASIS FOR RECOMMENDATIONS

Nauck M, Frid A, Hermansen K, et al. Efficacy and safety comparison of liraglutide, glimepiride, and placebo, all in combination with metformin, in type 2 diabetes: the LEAD (liraglutide effect and action in diabetes)-2 study. *Diabetes Care*, 2009; Vol. 32: pp. 84–90.

Comments: A double-blind, double-dummy, placebo and active-controlled trial for 26 weeks, including 1091 type 2 diabetes patients randomly assigned to 0.6 mg, 1.2 mg, and 1.8 mg daily of liraglutide added to metformin, or placebo added to metformin, or glimepiride added to metformin. While patients in the 1.8-mg and 1.2-mg liraglutide and in the glimepiride groups achieved a hemoglobin A1c reduction of 1%, only patients taking liraglutide achieved a significant weight loss (1.8–2.8 kg), whereas patients in the glimepiride group gained on average 1.0 kg.

DeFronzo RA, Ratner RE, Han J, et al. Effects of exenatide (exendin-4) on glycemic control and weight over 30 weeks in metformin-treated patients with type 2 diabetes. *Diabetes Care*, 2005; Vol. 28: pp. 1092–100.

Comments: Double-blind, randomized, placebo-controlled trial involving 336 subjects with type 2 diabetes, who were given 0 mcg, 5 mcg, or 10 mcg of exenatide for 30 weeks. There was a mean hemoglobin A1c reduction of 0.78 (0.1%) and an average weight loss of 2.8 (0.5 kg) in the group receiving exenatide 10 mcg twice daily.

Kendall DM, Riddle MC, Rosenstock J, et al. Effects of exenatide (exendin-4) on glycemic control over 30 weeks in patients with type 2 diabetes treated with metformin and a sulfonylurea. *Diabetes Care*, 2005; Vol. 28: pp. 1083–91.

Comments: This 30-week double-blind, randomized, placebo-controlled trial including 733 subjects showed that patients on 10 mcg of exenatide twice daily achieved better glycemic control (mean hemoglobin A1c reduction of 0.8 [0.1%]) than patients taking 5 mcg or taking placebo. The weight loss was significant in both 5- and 10-mcg arms of exenatide therapy, averaging 1.6 kg (0.2%).

Ratner RE, Dickey R, Fineman M, et al. Amylin replacement with pramlintide as an adjunct to insulin therapy improves long-term glycaemic and weight control in type 1 diabetes mellitus: a 1-year, randomized controlled trial. *Diabet Med*, 2004; Vol. 21: pp. 1204–12.

Comments: Double-blind, placebo-controlled, randomized, multicenter, 52-week trial of 651 patients with type 1 diabetes, to which placebo injections 3–4 times a day or various doses of pramlintide 3–4 times daily were added to their baseline insulin regimen. Patients taking pramlintide 60 mcg 3–4 times a day achieved a hemoglobin A1c reduction of 0.29% and 0.34%, respectively, compared to the placebo group. The pramlintide group as a whole lost an average of 0.4 kg versus a gain of 0.8 kg in the placebo group.

OTHER REFERENCES

Buse JB, Bergenstal RM, Glass LC, et al. Use of twice-daily exenatide in basal insulin-treated patients with type 2 diabetes: a randomized, controlled trial. *Ann Intern Med*, 2010; Vol. 154: pp. 103–12.

    Comments: In a multicenter trial of 261 patients with uncontrolled type 2 diabetes receiving insulin glargine, adding twice-daily exenatide injections significantly improves glycemic control without increased hypoglycemia or weight gain compared to placebo (−0.69%).

Joy SV, Rodgers PT, Scates AC. Incretin mimetics as emerging treatments for type 2 diabetes. *Ann Pharmacother*, 2005; Vol. 39: pp. 110–8.

    Comments: Review of the physiology, mechanism of action, pharmacology, efficacy, and side effect profile of exenatide and liraglutide.

Hollander PA, Levy P, Fineman MS, et al. Pramlintide as an adjunct to insulin therapy improves long-term glycemic and weight control in patients with type 2 diabetes: a 1-year randomized controlled trial. *Diabetes Care*, 2003; Vol. 26: pp. 784–90.

    Comments: In this double-blind, placebo-controlled, 52-week trial, 656 patients with type 2 diabetes on insulin (some patients were also on a sulfonylurea or metformin), were randomized to receive pramlintide 60 mcg, 90 mcg, or 120 mcg twice daily versus placebo. The patients taking 120 mcg of pramlintide had a significant hemoglobin A1c reduction of 0.62% over the placebo group and lost on average 1.4 kg, while patients in the placebo group gained 0.7 kg.

US Food and Drug Administration (FDA). Information for Healthcare Professionals: Exenatide (marketed as Byetta). *www.fda.gov/Drugs/DrugSafety/PostmarketDrugSafetyInformationforPatientsandProviders/ucm124713.htm*, 8/2008 Update. Accessed June 16, 2010.

    Comments: Exenatide prescribing information for patients with pancreatitis; recommends that exenatide be discontinued if pancreatitis is suspected.

METFORMIN

Nadeen Hosein, MD, MS, and Brian Pinto, PharmD, MBA

INDICATIONS

FDA

- Type 2 diabetes mellitus

Non-FDA Approved Uses

- Polycystic ovarian syndrome (PCOS)
- Prevention of type 2 diabetes mellitus in selected patients with impaired fasting glucose (IFG) and/or impaired glucose tolerance (IGT) (prediabetes)
- Prevention against gestational diabetes mellitus

MECHANISM

- Decreases hepatic glucose production.
- Decreases intestinal absorption of glucose.
- Increases peripheral glucose uptake and utilization.

USUAL ADULT DOSING

- **Immediate-release tablet:** "start low, go slow" and take with or after meals to reduce risk of GI upset.
- Up to 20% of patients will experience GI upset if metformin is not initiated at a low dose, not titrated upwards slowly, or given on an empty stomach.

- Recommend initiation with 500 mg with dinner × 2 weeks, then 500 mg with breakfast and 500 mg with dinner × 2 weeks, then 500 mg with breakfast and 1 g with dinner × 2 weeks, then 1 g twice a day with breakfast and dinner if no side effects.
- Usual maintenance dose for immediate release: 1000 mg–2550 mg daily, split among 2 to 3 divided doses. Maximum total daily dose 2550 mg.
- **Extended-release tablet:** 500 mg XR once daily, then increase dosage by 500 mg weekly. Maximum total daily dose 2500 mg (Fortamet), or 2000 mg (Glucophage XR and Glumetza).

FORMS

Brand Name (mfr)	Preparation	Forms†	Cost*
Metformin (generic) (Sandoz, Ivax, Mylan, and others)	metformin hydrochloride	oral tablet 500 mg oral tablet 850 mg oral tablet 1000 mg	$13 for 60 tabs $52 for 60 tabs $36 for 60 tabs
Glucophage (Bristol-Myers Squibb)	metformin hydrochloride	oral tablet 500 mg oral tablet 850 mg oral tablet 1000 mg	$70 for 60 tabs $113 for 60 tabs $141 for 60 tabs
Riomet (Ranbaxy Laboratories)	metformin hydrochloride	oral solution 500 mg per 5 ml (118 ml, 473 ml)	$100 for 473 ml
Metformin extended release (generic) (Amneal, Ranbaxy, Watson, and others)	metformin hydrochloride extended release	oral tablet 500 mg oral tablet 750 mg	$19 for 90 tabs $99 for 90 tabs
Glucophage XR (Bristol-Myers Squibb)	metformin hydrochloride extended release	oral tablet 500 mg oral tablet 750 mg	$70 for 60 tabs $108 for 60 tabs
Fortamet (Sciele Pharmaceutical)	metformin hydrochloride extended release	oral tablet 500 mg oral tablet 1000 mg	$134 for 60 tabs $302 for 60 tabs
Glumetza (Depomed)	metformin hydrochloride extended release	oral tablet 500 mg oral tablet 1000 mg	$175 for 100 tabs $382 for 90 tabs

*Prices represent cost per unit specified, are representative of "Average Wholesale Price" (AWP).
†Dosage is indicated in mg unless otherwise noted.

MEDICATIONS

DOSING IN SPECIAL POPULATIONS

Renal

- Contraindicated if creatinine >1.4 mg/dl in women, or >1.5 mg/dl in men, due to increased risk of lactic acidosis.

Hepatic

- Avoid due to increased risk of lactic acidosis.

Pregnancy

- FDA Category B.

Breastfeeding

- Thomson Lactation Ratings: infant risk is minimal.
- In a study by Glueck et al. (2006), the use of metformin (2550 mg total daily dose) by mothers breastfeeding their infants for 6 months did not affect growth, motor, or social development; the effects beyond 6 months were not studied.

ADVERSE DRUG REACTIONS

General

- Generally well tolerated if taken with or after meals (reduces GI upset).
- Contraindicated in renal impairment (creatinine ≥1.4 mg/dl for women, and creatinine ≥1.5 mg/dl for men) due to increased risk of lactic acidosis.
- If patients are having radiologic studies requiring intravenous iodinated contrast dye, stop metformin prior to or at the time of the procedure and resume it 48 hours after dye administration only if renal function is normal.
- Avoid excessive alcohol use (increases risk of lactic acidosis).
- Do not use in diabetic ketoacidosis or as antihyperglycemic therapy for type 1 diabetes mellitus.

Common

- Nausea, vomiting, diarrhea, flatulence, indigestion; incidence can be decreased by drug initiation at a low dose, with slow upwards titration of dose, as described previously.
- Cobalamin (vitamin B12) deficiency.
- Asthenia (physical weakness or loss of strength).

Rare

- Megaloblastic anemia due to vitamin B12 deficiency. Metformin appears to decrease the absorption of vitamin B12 from the gut.
- Lactic acidosis—rare, but fatal in about 50% of cases. More common in patients with predisposing conditions including renal insufficiency, dehydration, excessive alcohol intake, liver disease, sepsis, congestive heart failure, cardiovascular collapse, acute myocardial infarction, the elderly (especially >80 years old), and any other condition causing tissue hypoxemia and hypoperfusion (excess lactate production or decreased lactate clearance). Metformin increases blood lactate levels as a result of enhanced lactate production.

DRUG INTERACTIONS

- **Iodinated contrast agents** may enhance the adverse/toxic effect of metformin-associated lactic acidosis. Metformin should be temporarily stopped in patients receiving iodinated contrast agents prior to or at the time of the procedure and for at least 48 hours after administration of any iodinated contrast agent. Adequate renal function should be documented prior to restarting metformin.

- **Dofetilide** (an antiarrhythmic drug) is eliminated by both glomerular filtration and active tubular secretion via the cation transport system. Because metformin may compete with dofetilide for this pathway, the elimination of dofetilide may be decreased, resulting in increased dofetilide plasma concentrations, which increases risk of cardiac toxicity. Metformin and dofetilide should be used in combination with caution.
- Caution when using metformin with other drugs that may increase serum creatinine; discontinue metformin if serum creatinine exceeds above recommendations.

PHARMACOKINETICS

- **Absorption:** 50%–60% bioavailability if fasting. Food increases AUC for extended release tablets by 38%–73%.
- **Metabolism and excretion:** Not metabolized. 90% renal excretion. Dialyzable.
- **Protein binding:** Negligible.
- **Cmax, Cmin, and AUC:**
  - **Glucophage XR:** food increases the extent of absorption for extended-release tablets (as per AUC) by approximately 50%, although Cmax and Tmax are unaltered.
  - **Fortamet:** When administered with food, the extent of absorption is increased by approximately 60%; Cmax is increased by 30% and Tmax is prolonged (6.1 hours vs 4 hours).
  - **Glumetza:** Low-fat and high-fat meals increase systemic exposure (as per AUC) by 38% and 73%, respectively, relative to fasting. Both meal types prolong Tmax by approximately 3 hours, but Cmax is not affected. Time to peak concentration 7 hours for extended-release tablet.
- **T$\frac{1}{2}$:** 6.2 hours for immediate-release tablets
- **Distribution:** Vd 654L ± 358L.

EXPERT OPINION

- After at least 3 months on maximal dose metformin monotherapy, overall HbA1c reduction is about 1%–2%.
- Metformin is effective, has a long track record, has a desirable weight loss effect in most patients, does not cause hypoglycemia when used as monotherapy, and is cheap. Thus, it remains a drug of first choice for most newly diagnosed overweight type 2 diabetic patients if no contraindications exist.
- Overweight patients with type 2 diabetes mellitus on insulin therapy often require lower doses of insulin if metformin is also on board, due to metformin's insulin-sensitizing effects. If discontinuing metformin, expect to increase insulin dose.
- If patients are having radiologic studies requiring intravenous iodinated contrast dye, stop metformin prior to or at the time of the procedure and resume it 48 hours after dye administration only if renal function is normal.
- In hospitalized patients, consider holding metformin and temporarily substituting insulin therapy; resume metformin upon hospital discharge only if creatinine meets criteria listed previously.

MEDICATIONS

- Caution in using metformin in the elderly, who may have normal serum creatinine levels despite impaired renal function, and who may also be subject to polypharmacy which might contribute to renal dysfunction and increased risk of lactic acidosis.
- Check hematologic indices and vitamin B12 levels in patients on chronic metformin therapy, especially those receiving higher doses for longer durations. Replace vitamin B12 if necessary.

REFERENCES

Mathur R, Alexander CJ, Yano J, et al. Use of metformin in polycystic ovary syndrome. *Am J Obstet Gynecol*, 2008; Vol. 199: pp. 596–609.

    Comments: Metformin has a defined role in treating some women with PCOS.

Nathan DM, Davidson MB, DeFronzo RA, et al. Impaired fasting glucose and impaired glucose tolerance: implications for care. *Diabetes Care*, 2007; Vol. 30: pp. 753–9.

    Comments: This consensus statement from the ADA (American Diabetes Association) defines and describes IFG and IGT, and gives specific recommendations on which patients with both IFG and IGT should be selected to receive metformin therapy.

Ting RZ, Szeto CC, Chan MH, et al. Risk factors of vitamin B(12) deficiency in patients receiving metformin. *Arch Intern Med*, 2006; Vol. 166: pp. 1975–9.

    Comments: Patients on chronic metformin therapy are at increased risk of developing vitamin B12 deficiency.

Glueck CJ, Salehi M, Sieve L, et al. Growth, motor, and social development in breast- and formula-fed infants of metformin-treated women with polycystic ovary syndrome. *J Pediatr*, 2006; Vol. 148: pp. 628–632.

    Comments: In nursing infants of mothers who were taking metformin (mean 2550 mg/day) for PCOS, there was no growth retardation or delayed motor/social development, and there was also no difference in intercurrent illnesses, when compared to formula-fed babies. This study only followed the babies up to 6 months of age, however. Thus, metformin during lactation appears to be safe at least up to 6 months of infancy.

UK Prospective Diabetes Study (UKPDS) Group 34. Effect of intensive blood-glucose control with metformin on complications in overweight patients with type 2 diabetes (UKPDS 34). *Lancet*, 1998; Vol. 352: pp. 854–65.

    Comments: Landmark study: metformin is an excellent first-line drug for treating patients with type 2 diabetes mellitus due to its favorable effects on glycemic control and diabetic complications, and decreased incidence of weight gain and hypoglycemia when compared to sulfonylureas or insulin.

Bailey CJ, Turner RC. Metformin. *NEJM*, 1996; Vol. 334: pp. 574–9.

    Comments: Overview of the use of metformin in treating type 2 diabetes mellitus.

Gan SC, Barr J, Arieff AI, et al. Biguanide-associated lactic acidosis. Case report and review of the literature. *Arch Intern Med*, 1992; Vol. 152: pp. 2333–6.

    Comments: Lactic acidosis occurs very rarely if metformin is used according to its prescribing guidelines.

SULFONYLUREAS AND OTHER SECRETAGOGUES

Nadeen Hosein, MD, MS, and Brian Pinto, PharmD, MBA

INDICATIONS

FDA

- Type 2 diabetes mellitus

Non-FDA Approved Uses

- Chlorpropamide: central diabetes insipidus

MECHANISM
- Sulfonylureas and meglitinides (repaglinide and nateglinide) stimulate first-phase insulin secretion from functioning beta cells in the pancreas.
- Both classes of drugs bind to and cause closure of potassium-ATP channels on pancreatic beta-cell membranes. This results in membrane depolarization, calcium influx, and insulin exocytosis.
- Sulfonylureas bind to a different membrane site than meglitinides, but the intracellular effects are the same.

USUAL ADULT DOSING
- **Chlorpropamide:** 100 mg–500 mg once daily. Maximum total daily dose (TDD) 750 mg.
- **Tolbutamide:** 250 mg–3 g daily, once or in divided doses. Maximum TDD 3 g.
- **Glipizide:** 5 mg–40 mg daily. If TDD >15 mg, divide into at least 2 doses. Maximum TDD 40 mg.
- **Glipizide XL:** 5 mg–10 mg once daily. Maximum 20 mg daily.
- **Glyburide:** 1.25 mg–20 mg once daily or in 2 divided doses. Maximum TDD 20 mg.
- **Glyburide micronized:** 0.75 mg–12 mg once daily or in 2 divided doses. Maximum TDD 12 mg.
- **Glimepiride:** 1 mg–4 mg once daily. Maximum TDD 8 mg daily.
- **Repaglinide:** 0.5 mg–4 mg with each meal. Maximum TDD 16 mg.
- **Nateglinide:** 60 mg–120 mg to be given 1–30 minutes before meals. Maximum 180 mg 3 times per day.
- **Combination pills:** coformulated with metformin as glyburide + metformin (Glucovance), glipizide + metformin (Metaglip) and repaglinide + metformin (PrandiMet). Generic combination pills also available.
- Reduce dose or entirely eliminate sulfonylurea once insulin therapy is started.

FORMS

Brand Name (mfr)	Preparation	Forms†	Cost*
Diabinese (Mylan, Pliva, UDL Laboratories)	chlorpropamide	oral tablet 100 mg oral tablet 250 mg	$17 for 60 generic tabs $21 for 60 generic tabs
Orinase, Tol-Tab (Mylan, UDL Laboratories)	tolbutamide	oral tablet 500 mg	$26 for 60 generic tabs
Glucotrol (Apotex, Ivax, Sandoz, and others)	glipizide	oral tablet 5 mg oral tablet 10 mg	$20 for 100 generic tabs $19 for 90 generic tabs

(Continued)

FORMS *(CONT.)*

Brand Name (mfr)	Preparation	Forms†	Cost*
Glucotrol XL (Watson, Greenstone, Pfizer, and others)	glipizide extended release	oral tablet 2.5 mg	$19 for 30 generic tabs
		oral tablet 5 mg	$15 for 30 generic tabs
		oral tablet 10 mg	$20 for 30 generic tabs
DiaBeta (Sanofi-Aventis, Sandoz, Teva, and others)	glyburide	oral tablet 1.25 mg	$13 for 30 generic tabs
		oral tablet 2.5 mg	$13 for 30 generic tabs
		oral tablet 5 mg	$12 for 30 generic tabs
Glynase PresTabs (Pfizer, Teva, Mylan, and others)	glyburide micronized	oral tablet 1.5 mg	$26 for 90 generic tabs
		oral tablet 3 mg	$15 for 90 generic tabs
		oral tablet 6 mg	$17 for 90 generic tabs
Amaryl (Sanofi-Aventis, Mylan, Ranbaxy, and others)	glimepiride	oral tablet 1 mg	$13 for 30 generic tabs
		oral tablet 2 mg	$19 for 90 generic tabs
		oral tablet 4 mg	$15 for 30 generic tabs
Prandin (Novo Nordisk)	repaglinide	oral tablet 0.5 mg	$72 for 30 brand name tabs
		oral tablet 1 mg	$73 for 30 brand name tabs
		oral tablet 2 mg	$193 for 90 brand name tabs
Starlix (Novartis)	nateglinide	oral tablet 60 mg	$56 for 30 brand name tabs
		oral tablet 120 mg	$60 for 30 brand name tabs

*Prices represent cost per unit specified, are representative of "Average Wholesale Price" (AWP).
† Dosage is indicated in mg unless otherwise noted.

DOSING IN SPECIAL POPULATIONS

Renal

- Patients with renal insufficiency are at increased risk for hypoglycemia due to the predominant renal excretion of the sulfonylureas, and prolongation of drug effects in this setting.
- It is recommended to avoid these drugs entirely or to use very conservative dosing due to increased risk for hypoglycemia with renal disease.
- If a sulfonylurea must be used in renal insufficiency, glipizide (inactive metabolites) or glimepiride (substantial fecal excretion) are preferred. Avoid glyburide due to accumulation of partially active metabolites, which may lead to profound hypoglycemia.
- The meglitinides are generally well tolerated in all stages of renal insufficiency.

Hepatic

- Conservative dosing is recommended (i.e., start at 50% of the usual starting dose). This is due to the increased risk for hypoglycemia, as most of these drugs are metabolized by the liver.

Pregnancy

- Glyburide is the only sulfonylurea to be rated as FDA Category B.
- All of the other sulfonylureas are rated as FDA Category C.
- Both meglitinides are rated as FDA Category C.

Breastfeeding

- Thomson Lactation Ratings: infant risk cannot be ruled out.

ADVERSE DRUG REACTIONS

General

- Contraindicated in diabetic ketoacidosis or known hypersensitivity to the drug.
- Not to be used for therapy in type 1 diabetes mellitus.
- BLACKBOX WARNING of increased risk of cardiovascular mortality based on results of the University Group Diabetes Program (UGDP) (see Key Studies in Diabetes Care: Efficacies of Therapies, p. 29).
- Patients should avoid excessive alcohol use (increased risk for hypoglycemia).

Common

- Hypoglycemia, more common in those with renal insufficiency, hepatic impairment, and in the elderly.
- Exercising without prior caloric intake also increases risk for hypoglycemia.
- Weight gain.
- Chlorpropamide-alcohol flushing: Up to 15% of people taking chlorpropamide note a distinct facial flush upon alcohol ingestion.

Occasional

- Nausea, vomiting, diarrhea, flatulence, abdominal pain
- Hyponatremia with chlorpropamide
- Elevated liver transaminases

Rare

- Hypersensitivity skin reactions

DRUG INTERACTIONS

- Agents that enhance sulfonylurea action: NSAIDs, warfarin, salicylates, sulfonamides, allopurinol, probenecid, guanethidine, MAOIs, chloramphenicol, alcohol, beta-blockers.

MEDICATIONS

PHARMACOKINETICS

TABLE 4-5. PHARMACOKINETICS OF SULFONYLUREAS AND OTHER SECRETAGOGUES

	Chlorprop-amide	Tolbuta-mide	Glipizide	Glyburide	Glime-piride	Repa-glinide	Nateg-linide
Absorption	TTPC 2–4 hrs	TTPC 3–4 hrs	100% BA 90% for XL	TTPC 4 hrs	100% BA	TTPC 1 hr 56% BA	73% BA
Metabolism	Hydroxylation	Oxidation	Hepatic	Hepatic	Hepatic	Hepatic	Hepatic
Excretion	80%–90% renal	75% renal	80% renal	50% renal, 50% fecal	60% renal, 40% fecal	90% fecal, 8% renal	83% renal, 10% fecal
Protein Binding	60%–90%	95%	98%–99%	99%	99.5%	98%	98%
T$\frac{1}{2}$	36 hrs	4.5–6.5 hrs	2–4 hrs 2–5 hrs for XL	10 hrs	5–9.2 hrs	1 hr	1.5 hrs
Distribution (Vd)	Not fully characterized	Not fully characterized	10–11 L	Not fully characterized	8.8 L	31 L	10 L

TTPC = time to peak concentration; BA = bioavailability; M = metabolism; E = excretion; Vd = volume of distribution, expressed in liters (L).

Courtesy of Paul Pham, PharmD, Johns Hopkins University School of Medicine.

- Agents that decrease sulfonylurea action: glucocorticoids, diuretics, niacin, levothyroxine, estrogens, progestins, phenytoin, diazoxide, isoniazid, rifampin, phenothiazines, sympathomimetics.

Pharmacokinetics
- See Table 4-5.

EXPERT OPINION
- Overall HbA1c reduction with the sulfonylureas is about 1%–2% after at least 3 months.
- Overall HbA1c reduction with the meglitinides is about 1%–1.5%; repaglinide (Prandin) is more potent that nateglinide (Starlix). These agents are quite effective in patients who have isolated postprandial hyperglycemia but not necessarily impaired fasting glucose.
- Side effects include weight gain and hypoglycemia due to increased insulin secretion.
- Second-generation sulfonylureas are preferred over first-generation sulfonylureas (chlorpropamide and tolbutamide), as the latter tend to have more drug interactions and adverse effects.
- Though a blackbox warning of increased cardiovascular risk with sulfonylurea treatment is based on results of the UGDP study, these drugs have been used safely in many studies since and continue to be widely used in clinical practice.
- Each year, about 5%–10% of diabetic patients on sulfonylureas need to be switched over to insulin due to secondary failure of sulfonylurea therapy.

REFERENCES

Black C, Donnelly P, McIntyre L, et al. Meglitinide analogues for type 2 diabetes mellitus. *Cochrane Database Syst Rev,* 2007; CD004654.
    Comments: Overview of the role of meglitinides in treating type 2 diabetes mellitus.

Inzucchi SE. Oral antihyperglycemic therapy for type 2 diabetes: scientific review. *JAMA,* 2002; Vol. 287: pp. 360–72.
    Comments: Review of different types of oral antidiabetic agents, including sulfonylureas and other secretagogues.

Matthews DR, Cull CA, Stratton IM, et al. UKPDS 26: Sulphonylurea failure in non-insulin-dependent diabetic patients over six years. UK Prospective Diabetes Study (UKPDS) Group. *Diabet Med,* 1998; Vol. 15: pp. 297–303.
    Comments: In this UKPDS analysis of 1305 newly diagnosed diabetics placed on sulfonylurea monotherapy, 44% experienced sulfonylurea failure by 6 years and had to be switched over to other therapy. Risk factors for secondary sulfonylurea failure included lower pancreatic beta cell reserve to begin with, more hyperglycemia, and younger age.

Skillman TG, Feldman JM. The pharmacology of sulfonylureas. *Am J Med,* 1981; Vol. 70: pp. 361–72.
    Comments: Overview of the pharmacology of first- and second-generation sulfonylureas.

THIAZOLIDINEDIONES

Nadeen Hosein, MD, MS, and Brian Pinto, PharmD, MBA

INDICATIONS
FDA
- Type 2 diabetes mellitus

Non-FDA Approved Uses
- Polycystic ovarian syndrome (PCOS)
- NASH (Non-alcoholic steatohepatitis/fatty liver)

MEDICATIONS

MECHANISM

- The thiazolidinediones (TZDs) are PPAR (peroxisome proliferator activated receptor) gamma agonists.
- They increase insulin-dependent glucose disposal and decrease hepatic glucose output by decreasing insulin resistance in the liver and in the periphery.
- They also affect fatty acid metabolism.

USUAL ADULT DOSING

- Prior to starting a TZD, check liver enzyme levels. Do not use if active liver disease is present, or if ALT (a.k.a. SGPT) is elevated by more than 2.5 times the upper limit of normal.
- **Pioglitazone:** 15–30 mg by mouth once a day. Maximum dose is 45 mg once daily.
- **Rosiglitazone:** 2–4 mg by mouth once or twice per day. Maximum total daily dose is 8 mg daily.
- **Combination pills:** coformulated as pioglitazone + metformin (Actoplus Met or Actoplus Met XR), pioglitazone + glimepiride (Duetact), rosiglitazone + metformin (Avandamet), and rosiglitazone + glimepiride (Avandaryl).

FORMS

Brand Name (mfr)	Preparation	Forms†	Cost*
Actos (Takeda, PD-Rx Pharmaceuticals)	pioglitazone hydrochloride	oral tablet 15 mg	$149 for 30 brand name tabs
		oral tablet 30 mg	$213 for 30 brand name tabs
		oral tablet 45 mg	$233 for 30 brand name tabs
Avandia (GlaxoSmithKline)	rosiglitazone maleate	oral tablet 2 mg	$82 for 30 brand name tabs
		oral tablet 4 mg	$129 for 30 brand name tabs
		oral tablet 8 mg	$239 for 30 brand name tabs

*Prices represent cost per unit specified, are representative of "Average Wholesale Price" (AWP).
†Dosage is indicated in mg unless otherwise noted.

DOSING IN SPECIAL POPULATIONS

Renal

- No dosage adjustment necessary

Hepatic

- Not recommended in patients with active liver disease or with ALT (a.k.a. SGPT) elevation more than 2.5 times the upper limit of normal

Pregnancy

- FDA Category C

Breastfeeding
- Thomson Lactation Ratings: infant risk cannot be ruled out.

ADVERSE DRUG REACTIONS

General
- **Pioglitazone:** BLACK BOX WARNING for CONGESTIVE HEART FAILURE: may cause or worsen congestive heart failure. Monitor patients for signs and symptoms of heart failure; if they develop, consider discontinuing drug. Contraindicated in NYHA Class III or IV heart failure.
- **Rosiglitazone:** BLACK BOX WARNING for CONGESTIVE HEART FAILURE: may cause or worsen congestive heart failure. Monitor patients for signs and symptoms of heart failure; if they develop, consider discontinuing drug. Contraindicated in NYHA Class III or IV heart failure.
- **Rosiglitazone:** BLACKBOX WARNING for MYOCARDIAL ISCHEMIA. From the package insert: "A meta-analysis of 42 clinical studies ... showed [rosiglitazone] to be associated with an increased risk of myocardial ischemic events such as angina or myocardial infarction. Three other studies ... have not confirmed or excluded this risk. In their entirety, the available data on the risk of myocardial ischemia are inconclusive."
- Not to be used as antihyperglycemic therapy for type 1 diabetes mellitus or in patients with diabetic ketoacidosis.
- Monitor liver enzymes in all patients, as hepatitis and liver failure have been reported (though rare).
- Dose-related anemia may also occur.

Common
- Weight gain due both to fluid retention and to increased adipose tissue, with evidence that the increased fat is peripheral (i.e., subcutaneous), not central (i.e., visceral).
- Edema due to fluid retention

Occasional
- Ovulation in previously anovulatory women with PCOS
- Increased risk of fracture, especially in women

Rare
- Fulminant hepatitis leading to liver failure
- Macular edema
- Pulmonary edema or pleural effusions

DRUG INTERACTIONS
- **Bile acid sequestrants** may decrease the absorption of TZDs. Separate the dosing of these agents by at least 2 hours.
- **Nitrates** may enhance the adverse/toxic effect of rosiglitazone. Specifically, a greater risk of myocardial ischemia was reported for users of this combination in a meta-analysis of 42 rosiglitazone clinical trials. Though not contraindicated in the rosiglitazone prescribing information, the combination of rosiglitazone and a nitrate is not recommended.
- **CYP2C8 inhibitors** (i.e., gemfibrozil) and inducers (i.e., rifampin) may increase or decrease levels of thiazolidinediones.

MEDICATIONS

PHARMACOKINETICS

TABLE 4-6. PHARMACOKINETICS OF THIAZOLIDINEDIONES

	Pioglitazone	Rosiglitazone
Absorption	Time to peak concentration within 2 hrs	Time to peak concentration 1 hr. Bioavailability 99%
Metabolism	Extensive hepatic; some nonhepatic	Extensive hepatic
Excretion	Renal and fecal	64% renal, 23% fecal
Protein Binding	>99%	>99%
$T\frac{1}{2}$	16–24 hrs (longer in the elderly)	3–4 hrs (+2 hrs in hepatic impairment)
Volume of Distribution	0.63 L/kg ± 0.41 L/kg	17.6 L

Courtesy of Paul Pham, PharmD, Johns Hopkins University School of Medicine.

EXPERT OPINION
- Overall HbA1c reduction with the TZDs is about 1%–1.5%.
- Weight gain is common and often disturbing to patients.
- Fluid retention also common. Risk for heart failure increased by approximately two-fold.
- Pioglitazone has a beneficial effect on lipids (decreased TG and increased HDL) compared to rosiglitazone.
- Controversy exists about increased risk for myocardial ischemia with rosiglitazone, but not pioglitazone.
- In September 2010, the FDA announced a decision to severely reduce access to rosiglitazone after an updated meta-analysis of 52 studies demonstrated ~28% increased risk of myocardial ischemia with rosiglitazone (Nissen). Patients will be required to document that they understand risks of continuing on this medication once the legislation is implemented and/or that no other medications for diabetes are effective for them.
- In women, can lead to increased risk of bone fractures, especially in the distal upper limb and distal lower limb (forearm, hand, wrist, foot, ankle, tibia, fibula). Early evidence of decreased bone formation activity (Home; Dormuth).
- Reports of increased risk of bladder cancer in preclinical studies with pioglitazone therapy, but clinical studies have not provided definitive evidence and are ongoing (Lewis).
- No hypoglycemia unless used in conjunction with insulin or insulin secretagogues.
- Generic tablets are not available in US, so cost may be an issue.
- TZDs may offer particular benefits in patients with HIV-associated dyslipidemia/lipodystrophy and diabetes.

BASIS FOR RECOMMENDATIONS

Nissen SE, Wolski K. Rosiglitazone revisited: an updated meta-analysis of risk for myocardial infarction and cardiovascular mortality. *Arch Intern Med*, 2010; Jun 28 [Epub ahead of print].

Comments: This updated meta-anaylsis of 52 trials found that rosiglatizone was associated with significant 28% increased risk of myocardial infarction but not cardiovascular mortality. This article was the basis of the recent FDA decision to severely restrict access to rosiglitazone in September 2010.

OTHER REFERENCES

Lewis JD, Ferrara A, Peng T, et al. Risk of bladder cancer among diabetic patients treated with pioglitazone: interim report of a longitudinal cohort study. *Diabetes Care*, 2011; Vol. 34: pp. 916–22.

Comments: A preliminary report describing no association of pioglitazone therapy with increased incidence of bladder cancer, although a slightly increased risk with pioglitazone use for more than 2 years was found.

Home PD, Pocock SJ, Beck-Nielsen H, et al. Rosiglitazone evaluated for cardiovascular outcomes in oral agent combination therapy for type 2 diabetes (RECORD): a multicentre, randomised, open-label trial. *Lancet*, 2009; Vol. 373: pp. 2125–35.

Comments: In this prospective, randomized, open-blind trial which enrolled 4447 patients, after a mean of 5.5 years, those randomly assigned to rosiglitazone had a statistically significant increased risk for developing heart failure, with a hazard ratio of 2.1. Women in the rosiglitazone group also had more distal upper and lower limb bone fractures. This study was not able to demonstrate a statistically significant increase in myocardial infarctions in those using rosiglitazone. Since the publication of this study, re-adjudication of case records by the FDA suggest that the initially reported results of this trial may have been biased in favor of rosiglitazone.

Dormuth CR, Carney G, Carleton B, et al. Thiazolidinediones and fractures in men and women. *Arch Intern Med*, 2009; Vol. 169: pp. 1395–402.

Comments: This prospective cohort study compared peripheral fractures in 10,476 patients exposed to TZDs versus 73,863 patients exposed to sulfonylureas over a period of 1998–2007. The mean age of patients was 59, and 43% were women. There was a statistically significant 28% higher incidence of peripheral fractures in men and women exposed to TZDs compared with sulfonylureas (95% CI, 1.10–1.48). When exposure to each TZD was estimated separately, pioglitazone was associated with a significant increase in peripheral fractures in women compared with sulfonylureas (adjusted HR, 1.77; 95% CI, 1.32–2.38), but rosiglitazone was not (adjusted HR, 1.17; 95% CI, 0.91–1.50).

Selvin E, Bolen S, Yeh HC, et al. Cardiovascular outcomes in trials of oral diabetes medications: a systematic review. *Arch Intern Med*, 2008; Vol. 168: pp. 2070–80.

Comments: In this meta-analysis of 40 articles, rosiglitazone was associated with an increased risk of cardiovascular morbidity and mortality, but it was a statistically nonsignificant finding (OR 1.68, 95% CI, 0.92–3.06).

Grey A, Bolland M, Gamble G, et al. The peroxisome proliferator-activated receptor-gamma agonist rosiglitazone decreases bone formation and bone mineral density in healthy postmenopausal women: a randomized, controlled trial. *J Clin Endocrinol Metab*, 2007; Vol. 92: pp. 1305–10.

Comments: In this randomized, double-blind placebo controlled trial of 50 postmenopausal women initiated on rosiglitazone 8 mg/day, there was a significant decrease in bone formation, as evidenced by a reduction in osteoblast markers: procollagen type 1 N-terminal propeptide by 13% (p <0.005), and osteocalcin by 10% (p = 0.04), when compared to placebo. Changes were seen as early as 4 weeks into rosiglitazone treatment, and persisted for the entire 14-week duration of the study.

Nissen SE, Wolski K. Effect of rosiglitazone on the risk of myocardial infarction and death from cardiovascular causes. *NEJM*, 2007; Vol. 356: pp. 2457–71.

Comments: This meta-analysis using pooled data from 42 trials (15,565 patients randomly assigned to receive rosiglitazone versus 12,282 patients randomly assigned to receive comparator drugs), included studies with a duration of at least 24 weeks. The mean age of subjects was 56 years, with a baseline HbA1c of approximately 8.2%. This meta-analysis found an increased risk for myocardial infarction with rosiglitazone, with a statistically significant odds ratio of 1.43 (95% CI, 1.03–1.98, p = 0.03). This article was the basis for the revised FDA black box warning for rosiglitazone, which now includes myocardial ischemia.

Yki-Järvinen H. Thiazolidinediones. *NEJM*, 2004; Vol. 351: pp. 1106–18.

Comments: Overview of the mechanism of action and use of TZDs in patients with type 2 diabetes mellitus.

Fonseca V. Effect of thiazolidinediones on body weight in patients with diabetes mellitus. *Am J Med*, 2003; Vol. 115 Suppl 8A: pp. 42S–48S.

MEDICATIONS

Comments: Mechanism of weight gain in patients with diabetes using TZDs, and strategies to manage/minimize the weight gain.

INSULINS (BASAL): INTERMEDIATE- AND LONG-ACTING

Nadeen Hosein, MD, MS, and Brian Pinto, PharmD, MBA

INDICATIONS

FDA

- Type 1 diabetes mellitus (DM1)
- Type 2 diabetes mellitus (DM2)
- NPH insulin: gestational diabetes mellitus (GDM)

Mechanism

- Basal insulins are long acting due to prolonged absorption following subcutaneous injection.
- Facilitates glucose uptake into muscle and fat.
- Reduces hepatic glucose output.
- Inhibits lipolysis.
- Inhibits protein breakdown and promote protein synthesis.

USUAL ADULT DOSING

- TDD = total daily dose; U = units of insulin; SQ = subcutaneously.
- **Long-acting basal insulins (glargine, detemir):** given SQ once or twice a day.
- **Intermediate-acting basal insulin (Neutral Protamine Hagadorn [NPH] insulin):** given SQ twice a day.
- In general, for basal-bolus insulin regimens, 50% of the TDD is given as basal insulin, and 50% of the TDD is given as bolus insulin (divided among the three meals).
- **Type 1 diabetes:** typical TDD for initiation is 0.2–0.5 U/kg/day and ranges from 0.4–1 U/kg/day, or more, for maintenance (see Type 1 Diabetes: Insulin Treatment, p. 155).
- **Type 2 diabetes:** typical TDD for initiation is 0.1–0.2 U/kg/day, usually given all as basal insulin for the first few weeks/months before introducing bolus insulin. For maintenance, the TDD typically ranges from 0.2–1.5 U/kg/day or more, depending on the degree of insulin resistance (see Type 2 Diabetes: Insulin Treatment, p. 173).
- If initiating insulin using weight-based formulas, adjust doses further based on the patient's glycemic response.
- An alternative method for starting insulin in an insulin naive patient is to start with 10 units basal insulin SQ every 24 hrs and titrate up by 2 units every 2–3 days until fasting blood sugar is at goal.
- If switching from twice daily NPH to once-daily glargine or detemir insulin, calculate total daily NPH dose and reduce by 20% to arrive at a glargine or detemir insulin dose to be given SQ every 24 hrs.
- Some patients using glargine or detemir achieve better glycemic control with a twice-daily regimen, especially at higher doses of basal insulin (i.e., more than 50 units daily).
- For use in treating GDM, refer to Gestational Diabetes Mellitus, p. 121.

FORMS

Brand Name (mfr)	Preparation	Forms†	Cost*
Lantus (Sanofi-Aventis US)	glargine insulin (recombinant analog)	SQ solution, 100 U/ml, vial 10 ml vial (1000 U)	$104
		SQ solution, 100 U/ml, Lantus SoloStar disposable prefilled pens box of five 3-ml pens (15 ml, 1500 U)	$188
		SQ solution, 100 U/ml, Lantus cartridges, for use in the OptiClik reusable pen, which must be obtained separately box of five 3-ml cartridges (15 ml, 1500 U)	$191
Levemir (Novo Nordisk)	detemir insulin (recombinant analog)	SQ solution, 100 U/ml, vial 10 ml vial (1000 U)	$103
		SQ solution, 100 U/ml, Levemir FlexPen disposable prefilled pens box of five 3-ml pens (15 ml, 1500 U)	$191
Humulin N (Eli Lilly)	NPH insulin (recombinant human insulin, isophane suspension)	SQ suspension, 100 U/ml, vial 10-ml vial (1000 U)	$57
		SQ suspension, 100 U/ml, Humulin N disposable prefilled pens box of five 3-ml pens (15 ml, 1500 U)	$154
Novolin N (Novo Nordisk)	NPH insulin (recombinant human insulin, isophane suspension)	SQ suspension, 100 U/ml, vial 10 ml vial (1000 U)	$58

*Prices represent cost per unit specified, are representative of "Average Wholesale Price" (AWP).
†Dosage is indicated in mg unless otherwise noted.

DOSING IN SPECIAL POPULATIONS
Renal
- Dose reductions may be needed since insulin is metabolized by the kidneys, and may have a longer half life in patients with renal impairment.
- Glargine insulin has active metabolites which may result in enhanced hypoglycemia for patients with renal impairment.

MEDICATIONS

Hepatic
- Dose reductions may be needed, since insulin is metabolized by the liver and also because most gluconeogenesis occurs in the liver.

Pregnancy
- Glargine and detemir insulins: FDA Category C
- NPH insulin: FDA Category B. This is the only basal insulin that has received FDA approval for use in treating GDM

Breastfeeding
- Glargine and detemir insulins: Thomson Lactation Ratings: infant risk cannot be ruled out
- NPH insulin: unknown risk

ADVERSE DRUG REACTIONS

General
- Contraindicated for intravenous administration
- Not for use in insulin pumps

Common
- Hypoglycemia
- Injection site pain, noted particularly with glargine insulin since it is an acidic solution
- Weight gain

Occasional
- Local injection site reactions (redness, itching, swelling).
- Lipoatrophy (loss of subcutaneous adipose tissue) at injection site; to avoid, rotate injection sites frequently.
- Lipohypertrophy (accumulation of subcutaneous adipose tissue) at injection site; to avoid, rotate injection sites frequently.

Rare
- Immune hypersensitivity reactions
- Hypokalemia

DRUG INTERACTIONS
- Any drug that also lowers blood glucose (e.g., sulfonylureas) when used in a patient on insulin may result in additive hypoglycemia.

PHARMACOKINETICS
- **Absorption:** Affected by many factors (dose, recent exercise, temperature, massage at injection area, lipodystrophy, etc.).
- **Metabolism and excretion:** Metabolism and excretion occurs via both hepatic and renal routes.
- **Protein binding:** Clinically insignificant.

TABLE 4-7. PHARMACOKINETICS OF BASAL INSULINS

	Glargine	Detemir	NPH
Onset	2–3 hrs	1–3 hrs	1–3 hrs
Peak	Theoretically peakless	6–8 hrs	4–10 hrs
Effective Duration	Usually 20–24 hrs	6–24 hrs	10–16 hrs
Courtesy of Paul Pham, PharmD, Johns Hopkins University School of Medicine.			

EXPERT OPINION

- NPH (the "cloudy" insulin) can be safely mixed with rapid-acting insulins. To do so, advise patient to (1) draw up the clear rapid acting insulin into the syringe, then (2) draw up the cloudy NPH insulin. Tell patients to draw up "clear first, then cloudy second," in that order.
- Glargine and detemir must never be mixed with other insulins, as the change in pH will affect their potency.
- The choice of basal insulin may be influenced by cost, frequency of administration, or patient preference.
- NPH insulin is an older and cheaper basal insulin that may be preferred when finances are a consideration.
- While NPH insulin used to be animal (porcine) based, all the currently available basal insulins are synthetic insulins that are either structurally identical (NPH) or analogues (glargine, detemir) of human insulin.
- Most patients prefer using insulin pens (disposable ones, or reusable ones with replaceable insulin cartridges) to drawing up insulin from traditional vials using syringes. Insulin pen needles must be prescribed and purchased separately, as they do not come packaged with the insulin pens. Refer to the preceding Forms table to see which basal insulin preparations are available in pen form.
- Alcohol may have a hypoglycemic effect in people taking insulin, and should be used (if at all) in moderation and with caution.
- The "peakless" character of long-acting insulins such as glargine is, in clinical practice, not always the case. There may be a distinct maximum time of action, potentially at higher doses, and insulin may not last 24 hours.
- Detemir insulin has on average a duration of action <20 hours, so is generally used twice daily.
- Older basal insulins include lente and ultralente and have been discontinued in the US but may still be available in other countries.

REFERENCES

Holman RR, Farmer AJ, Davies MJ, et al. Three-year efficacy of complex insulin regimens in type 2 diabetes. *NEJM*, 2009; Vol. 361: pp. 1736–47.

    Comments: In this 3-year open-label multicenter trial, 708 patients with suboptimal HbA1c while taking metformin and sulfonylurea therapy were randomly assigned to receive biphasic insulin aspart insulin twice daily, prandial insulin aspart 3 times daily, or basal insulin detemir once (or twice, if needed) daily. After 3 years, median HbA1c levels were similar for all three groups, but fewer patients had a HbA1c of <6.5% in the biphasic group than in the prandial or basal groups. There were also fewer hypoglycemic episodes and less weight gain in patients adding basal insulin.

Mooradian AD, Bernbaum M, Albert SG. Narrative review: a rational approach to starting insulin therapy. *Ann Intern Med*, 2006; Vol. 145: pp. 125–34.

    Comments: Suggestions for how to start insulin in patients with diabetes, depending on their individual blood glucose profiles.

Riddle MC. Timely initiation of basal insulin. *Am J Med*, 2004; Vol. 116 Suppl 3A: pp. 3S–9S.

    Comments: This article makes a good case for why basal insulin should be started early in patients with type 2 diabetes mellitus.

DeWitt DE, Hirsch IB. Outpatient insulin therapy in type 1 and type 2 diabetes mellitus: scientific review. *JAMA*, 2003; Vol. 289: pp. 2254–64.

MEDICATIONS

Comments: Overview of the different types of insulins available, their pharmacokinetics, and different types of insulin regimens.

Riddle MC, Rosenstock J, Gerich J, et al. The treat-to-target trial: randomized addition of glargine or human NPH insulin to oral therapy of type 2 diabetic patients. *Diabetes Care*, 2003; Vol. 26: pp. 3080–6.

Comments: In this open-label, parallel, multicenter trial, 756 overweight patients with HbA1c >7.5% on one or two oral agents were randomized to have either bedtime glargine insulin or once-daily NPH insulin added to their oral therapy. After 24 weeks, mean fasting plasma glucose and HbA1c were similar in both groups. However, patients on NPH experienced more episodes of symptomatic hypoglycemia than did those receiving glargine.

INSULINS (BOLUS): RAPID- AND SHORT-ACTING

Nadeen Hosein, MD, MS, and Brian Pinto, PharmD, MBA

INDICATIONS

FDA

- Type 1 diabetes mellitus (T1DM).
- Type 2 diabetes mellitus (T2DM).
- Gestational diabetes mellitus (GDM).
- Diabetic ketoacidosis (DKA).
- Use in insulin pumps.
- Use subcutaneously or intravenously.

Non-FDA Approved Uses

- Diabetes mellitus with hyperosmolar hyperglycemic coma
- Hyperkalemia

MECHANISM

- Facilitates glucose uptake into muscle and fat
- Reduces hepatic glucose output
- Inhibits lipolysis
- Inhibits protein breakdown and promotes protein synthesis

USUAL ADULT DOSING

- TDD = total daily dose; U = units of insulin; SQ = subcutaneously.
- **Rapid-acting insulins (aspart, lispro, and glulisine):** administer SQ 0–15 mins before meals (preferred), or within 20 minutes after starting meal (for patients with unpredictable food intake).
- **Short-acting insulin (regular):** recommend using SQ 30 mins before meals.
- Refer to Type 2 Diabetes: Insulin Initiation, p. 177, and Type 1 Diabetes: Insulin Treatment, p. 159, for specific insulin dosing information.
- In general, for basal-bolus regimens, 50% of the TDD is given as basal insulin, and 50% of the TDD is given as bolus insulin (divided among the three meals).
- May be used for patients with diabetes who are NPO and receiving total parenteral nutrition; refer to Hospital Management of Diabetes, p. 73, for specific insulin dosing information.
- Refer to GDM (p. 122), DKA (p. 40), or Hyperosmolar Hyperglycemic Coma (p. 45) for further insulin dosing information in these conditions.

- If using U-500 insulin instead of U-100 insulin, be sure to divide the normal dose by 5, as the U-500 insulin is 5 times more concentrated than the U-100 insulin.

FORMS

Brand Name (mfr)	Preparation	Forms†	Cost*
NovoLog (Novo Nordisk)	aspart insulin (recombinant analog)	SQ solution, 100 U/ml, vial 10-ml vial (1000 U)	$112
		SQ solution, 100 U/ml, NovoLog FlexPen disposable prefilled pens box of five 3-ml pens (15 ml, 1500 U)	$219
		SQ solution, 100 U/ml, NovoLog cartridges, for use in any reusable Novo-Pen, which must be obtained separately in box of five 3-ml cartridges (15 ml, 1500 U)	$201
Humalog (Eli Lilly)	lispro insulin (recombinant analog)	SQ solution, 100 U/ml, vial 10-ml vial (1000 U)	$104
		SQ solution, 100 U/ml, Humalog KwikPen disposable prefilled pens box of five 3-ml pens (15 ml, 1500 U)	$198
		SQ solution, 100 U/ml, Humalog original Pen disposable prefilled pens box of five 3-ml pens (15 ml, 1500 U)	$208
		SQ solution, 100 U/ml, Humalog cartridges, for use in the HumaPen Memoir reusable pen or the HumaPen Luxura HD reusable pen, which must be obtained separately in box of five 3-ml cartridges (15 ml, 1500 U)	$199

(Continued)

MEDICATIONS

FORMS *(CONT.)*

Brand Name (mfr)	Preparation	Forms†	Cost*
Apidra (Sanofi-Aventis US)	glulisine insulin (recombinant analog)	SQ solution, 100 U/ml, vial 10-ml vial (1000 U)	$102
		SQ solution, 100 U/ml, Apidra SoloStar disposable prefilled pens box of five 3-ml pens (15 ml, 1500 U)	$207
		SQ solution, 100 U/ml, Apidra cartridges, for use in the OptiClik reusable pen, which must be obtained separately in box of five 3-ml cartridges (15 ml, 1500 U)	$196
Novolin R (Novo Nordisk)	regular insulin (recombinant human insulin)	SQ solution, 100 U/ml, vial 10-ml vial (1000 U)	$58
Humulin R (Eli Lilly)	regular insulin (recombinant human insulin)	SQ solution, 100 U/ml, vial 10-ml vial (1000 U)	$57
Humulin R Concentrated U-500 (Eli Lilly)	concentrated regular insulin (recombinant human insulin)	SQ solution, 500 U/ml, vial 20-ml vial (10,000 U)	$261

*Prices represent cost per unit specified, are representative of "Average Wholesale Price" (AWP).
†Dosage is indicated in mg unless otherwise noted.

DOSING IN SPECIAL POPULATIONS

Renal

- Dose reductions may be needed since insulin is metabolized by the kidneys, and may have a longer half-life in patients with renal impairment.

Hepatic

- Dose reductions may be needed, since insulin is metabolized by the liver and also because most gluconeogenesis occurs in the liver.

Pregnancy

- **Aspart insulin:** FDA Category B
- **Lispro insulin:** FDA Category B
- **Glulisine insulin:** FDA Category C
- **Regular insulin:** FDA Category B

Breastfeeding
- **Aspart, lispro, and glulisine insulins:** infant risk cannot be ruled out (Thomson Lactation Ratings).
- **Regular insulin:** unknown.

ADVERSE DRUG REACTIONS

Common
- Hypoglycemia
- Weight gain
- Injection site pain, minimized by thin needle and/or use of pens

Occasional
- Local injection site reactions (redness, itching, swelling).
- Lipoatrophy (loss of adipose tissue) at injection site; to avoid, rotate sites frequently.
- Lipohypertrophy (area of fat hypertrophy) at injection site; to avoid, rotate sites frequently.

Rare
- Immune hypersensitivity reactions.
- Hypokalemia.
- Increased risk for overdose and irreversible "insulin shock" with regular insulin U-500 concentration (500 U/ml); use carefully.

DRUG INTERACTIONS
- Any drug that also lowers blood glucose (e.g., sulfonylureas), when used in a patient on insulin, could result in additive hypoglycemia.

PHARMACOKINETICS
- **Absorption:** Affected by many factors (dose, recent exercise, temperature, massage at injection area, lipodystrophy, etc.).
- **Metabolism and excretion:** Metabolism and excretion occurs via both hepatic and renal routes.

TABLE 4-8. PHARMACOKINETICS OF BOLUS INSULINS

	Aspart	Lispro	Glulisine	Regular
Onset	5–15 mins	5–15 mins	5–15 mins	30 mins–1 hr
Peak	1–2 hrs	1–2 hrs	1–2 hrs	2–4 hrs
Effective Duration	3–5 hrs	3–5 hrs	3–5 hrs	5–8 hrs

Courtesy of Paul Pham, PharmD, Johns Hopkins University School of Medicine.

EXPERT OPINION
- Bolus insulins may be used to correct for hyperglycemia and/or cover carbohydrate content of a meal.
- Due to their relatively faster onset, rapid-acting subcutaneous insulins are often preferred but regular subcutaneous insulin may be preferred if cost is a consideration.
- Avoid giving bolus insulin injections too close together (i.e., within 3–4 hours of a preceding dose) to prevent overlapping durations of action or "insulin stacking," which may predispose patients to hypoglycemia.

MEDICATIONS

- At higher doses, regular insulin may have a duration of action lasting up to 8 hours, which may also predispose to insulin stacking.
- Aspart, lispro, glulisine insulins are commonly used in insulin pumps.
- Most patients prefer using insulin pens (disposable or reusable ones with replaceable insulin cartridges) to drawing up insulin from traditional vials using syringes. Insulin pen needles must be prescribed and purchased separately, as they do not come packaged with the insulin pens. Refer to the preceding Forms table to see which bolus insulin preparations are available in pen form.
- Alcohol can have a hypoglycemic effect in people taking insulin and should be used, if at all, in moderation and with caution.
- All of the currently available bolus insulins are synthetic insulins that are either structurally identical (regular) or analogues (aspart, lispro, glulisine) of human insulin.

REFERENCES

Horton ES. Defining the role of basal and prandial insulin for optimal glycemic control. *J Am Coll Cardiol,* 2009; Vol. 53: pp. S21–7.
   Comments: Review of the available preparations of bolus and basal insulins, and recommendations for glycemic goals in patients at risk for cardiovascular disease.

DeWitt DE, Hirsch IB. Outpatient insulin therapy in type 1 and type 2 diabetes mellitus: scientific review. *JAMA,* 2003; Vol. 289: pp. 2254–64.
   Comments: Overview of the different types of insulins available, their pharmacokinetics, and different types of insulin regimens.

Gerich JE. Novel insulins: expanding options in diabetes management. *Am J Med,* 2002; Vol. 113: pp. 308–16.
   Comments: Discussion of the use of recombinant insulins as bolus and basal therapy for patients with diabetes mellitus.

PREMIXED INSULIN PREPARATIONS

Nadeen Hosein, MD, MS, and Brian Pinto, PharmD, MBA

INDICATIONS

FDA

- Type 1 diabetes mellitus (T1DM)
- Type 2 diabetes mellitus (T2DM)
- NPH/regular premixed insulin: gestational diabetes mellitus (GDM)

Mechanism

- Premixed insulins combine, in the vial, a short-acting insulin (regular) or fast-acting insulin analog, with an intermediate-acting insulin (NPH) or long-acting insulin analog.
- Insulin promotes glucose uptake into muscle and fat, and protein synthesis; reduces hepatic glucose output; and inhibits lipolysis and protein breakdown.
- Premixed insulin covers the increasing glucose after a meal as well as providing a longer between-meal insulin coverage.
- NPH and regular insulin mixed physically combines NPH with regular insulin; the analog mixes (i.e., lispro, aspart) combine the fast-acting insulin preparation with a protomine-modified longer acting preparation of the same insulin.

USUAL ADULT DOSING

- TDD = total daily dose; U = units of insulin; SQ = subcutaneously.
- **For NovoLog Mix 70/30, Humalog Mix 75/25, and Humalog Mix 50/50:** initiate treatment with one injection SQ every 24 hrs, given 0–15 minutes before the biggest meal of the day. Then increase to 2 injections per day, the first one 0–15 minutes before breakfast, and the second 0–15 minutes before dinner.
- **For NPH/regular premixed insulin:** administer 30 minutes before breakfast and 30 minutes before dinner.
- **T1DM:** typical initial TDD is 0.2 U/kg/day. Maintenance TDD typically ranges from 0.2–0.5 U/kg/day, or more. Most patients are maintained on at least 2 injections per day.
- **T2DM:** typical initial TDD is either 10 U or 0.2 U/kg/day. Maintenance TDD typically exceeds 1 U/kg/day or more, depending on the degree of insulin resistance. Most patients on insulin are maintained on at least 2 injections per day.
- Weight-based dosing will require further adjustment based on the patient's glycemic response.
- If 2 daily injections do not provide adequate glycemic control, consider adding a rapid acting insulin analog (e.g., aspart, lispro, or glulisine) 0–15 mins before lunch.

FORMS

Brand Name (mfr)	Preparation	Forms†	Cost*
Novolin 70/30 (Novo Nordisk)	NPH insulin 70% with Regular insulin 30% (recombinant human insulin)	SQ suspension, 100 U/ml, vial 10-ml vial	$58
Humulin 70/30 (Eli Lilly)	NPH insulin 70% with Regular insulin 30% (recombinant human insulin)	SQ suspension, 100 U/ml, vial 10-ml vial	$56
		SQ suspension, 100 U/ml, Humulin 70/30 disposable prefilled pens box of ten 3-ml pens (30 ml, 3000 U)	$291
NovoLog Mix 70/30 (Novo Nordisk)	Aspart protamine insulin 70% with Aspart insulin 30% (recombinant analog)	SQ suspension, 100 U/ml vial, 10-ml vial	$110
		SQ suspension, 100 U/ml NovoLog mix 70/30 FlexPen disposable prefilled pens box of five 3-ml pens (15 ml, 1500 U)	$206

(Continued)

MEDICATIONS

FORMS *(CONT.)*

Brand Name (mfr)	Preparation	Forms†	Cost*
Humalog Mix 75/25 (Eli Lilly)	Lispro protamine insulin 75% with Lispro insulin 25% (recombinant analog)	SQ suspension, 100 U/ml, vial 10-ml vial	$111
		SQ suspension, 100 U/ml, Humalog Mix 75/25 Kwikpen disposable prefilled pens box of five 3-ml pens (15-ml, 1500 U)	$200
		SQ suspension, 100 U/ml, Humalog Mix 75/25 original Pen disposable prefilled pens box of five 3-ml pens (15 ml, 1500 U)	$188
Humalog Mix 50/50 (Eli Lilly)	Lispro protamine insulin 50% with Lispro insulin 50% (recombinant analog)	SQ suspension, 100 U/ml, vial 10-ml vial;	$107
		SQ suspension, 100 U/ml, Humalog Mix 50/50 KwikPen disposable prefilled pens box of five 3-ml pens (15 ml, 1500 U)	$200
		SQ suspension, 100 U/ml, Humalog Mix 50/50 original Pen disposable prefilled pens box of five 3-ml pens (15 ml, 1500 U)	$209

*Prices represent cost per unit specified, are representative of "Average Wholesale Price" (AWP).
†Dosage is indicated in mg unless otherwise noted.

DOSING IN SPECIAL POPULATIONS

Renal
- Dose reductions may be needed since insulin is excreted by the kidneys, and may have a longer half-life in patients with renal impairment.

Hepatic
- Dose reductions may be needed since insulin is metabolized by the liver and patients with liver disease may have impaired gluconeogenesis.

Pregnancy

- **NPH/regular (Novolin 70/30 and Humulin 70/30):** FDA Category B. This is the only premixed insulin preparation that has received FDA approval for use in treating GDM.
- **NovoLog Mix 70/30:** FDA Category C.
- **Humalog Mix 75/25 and Humalog Mix 50/50:** FDA Category B.

Breastfeeding

- Maternal insulin requirements may decrease during breastfeeding due to effective increased caloric expenditure.
- **NPH/regular (Novolin 70/30 and Humulin 70/30):** unknown.
- **NovoLog Mix 70/30:** infant risk cannot be ruled out (Thomson Lactation Ratings).
- **Humalog Mix 75/25 and Humalog Mix 50/50:** infant risk cannot be ruled out (Thomson Lactation Ratings).

ADVERSE DRUG REACTIONS

Common

- Hypoglycemia, especially if meals are skipped or activity is increased
- Weight gain

Occasional

- Local injection site reactions (redness, itching, swelling).
- Lipodystrophy at injection site; to avoid, rotate sites frequently.

Rare

- Immune hypersensitivity reactions
- Hypokalemia

DRUG INTERACTIONS

- Any drug that also lowers blood glucose (e.g., sulfonylureas), when used in a patient on insulin, could result in additive hypoglycemia.

PHARMACOKINETICS

- **Absorption:** Highly variable; affected by many factors (dose, recent exercise, temperature, massage at injection area, lipodystrophy, etc.).
- **Metabolism and excretion:** Metabolism and excretion occurs via both hepatic and renal routes.
- See Table 4-9.

TABLE 4-9. PHARMACOKINETICS OF PREMIXED INSULINS

	Novolin 70/30	Humulin 70/30	Novo-log Mix 70/30	Huma-log Mix 75/25	Huma-log Mix 50/50
Onset	30–60 mins	30–60 mins	5–15 mins	5–15 mins	5–15 mins
Peak	Biphasic	Biphasic	Biphasic	Biphasic	Biphasic
Effective Duration	10–16 hrs	10–16 hrs	10–16 hrs	10–16 hrs	10–16 hrs
Courtesy of Paul Pham, PharmD, Johns Hopkins University School of Medicine.					

MEDICATIONS

EXPERT OPINION

- The premixed insulin analogs (NovoLog Mix and Humalog Mix) have a similar action profile to NPH/regular premixed insulin except with a more rapid onset of action and higher peak insulin levels. Thus, the premixed insulin analogs are more effective at controlling postprandial blood glucose spikes than premixed NPH/regular insulin.
- Adding protamine to the rapid-acting insulin analogs (aspart and lispro) prolongs their action, and the resulting protaminated insulins (aspart protamine insulin and lispro protamine insulin) take on a pharmacokinetic insulin profile similar to NPH insulin.
- Given the rapid onset of the analog premixed insulin, it should be given shortly before a meal is ingested, and not at bedtime.
- Given the longer action of the protaminated component, the presupper insulin may cause overnight lows, in which case fast-acting insulin only at suppertime and longer-acting insulin at bedtime is necessary.
- Premixed insulin regimens (which typically require 2 injections per day) are best suited for patients who decline to use the more physiologic basal-bolus insulin regimens (which require up to 4 injections per day) due to patient preference and/or cost.
- Patients who choose to use the premixed insulin preparations should have fairly routine lifestyles (eat regular meals and exercise consistently around the same times each day, and do not skip meals).
- An additional dose of rapid-acting insulin at lunchtime may be beneficial for patients on premixed insulin regimens with elevated blood glucoses in midday.
- Patients with highly variable or unpredictable lifestyles (skipping meals, exercising at different times, large variations in meal types and quantities) may be better treated using basal-bolus insulin regimens.
- Patients may prefer using insulin pens (disposable, reusable, and with replaceable insulin cartridges) but insulin pen needles must be prescribed and purchased separately, as they do not come packaged with the insulin pens. Refer to the preceding Forms table to see which premixed insulin preparations are available in pen form.
- Evidence is inconsistent in randomized trials as to whether basal alone, prandial alone, or premixed insulins are more effective (Holman; Lasserson).

REFERENCES

Holman RR, Farmer AJ, Davies MJ, et al. Three-year efficacy of complex insulin regimens in type 2 diabetes. *NEJM*, 2009; Vol. 361: pp. 1736–47.

    Comments: In this open-label, multicenter trial, 708 patients who had suboptimal HbA1c levels while taking metformin and sulfonylurea therapy were randomly assigned to receive biphasic insulin aspart twice daily, prandial insulin aspart 3 times daily, or basal insulin detemir once daily (twice if required). After 3 years, the median HbA1c level was 6.9% (no statistical difference between the groups). However, fewer patients had an HbA1c <6.5% in the biphasic group (31.9%) than in the prandial group (44.7%, p = 0.006) or in the basal group (43.2%, p = 0.03). Thus, more patients who added a basal or prandial insulin-based regimen to oral therapy were able to achieve HbA1c <6.5% than those who added a biphasic insulin-based regimen.

Lasserson DS, Glasziou P, Perera R, et al. Optimal insulin regimens in type 2 diabetes mellitus: systematic review and meta-analyses. *Diabetologia*, 2009; Vol. 52: pp. 1990–2000.

    Comments: Found significantly greater reduction in HbA1c in patients with type 2 diabetes when insulin treatment was initiated using a biphasic or prandial insulin rather than basal insulin alone.

Garber AJ. Premixed insulin analogues for the treatment of diabetes mellitus. *Drugs*, 2006; Vol. 66: pp. 31–49.

    Comments: Thorough review of the premixed insulin analogs, including their development, pharmacokinetics, efficacy, dosing regimen considerations, and comparison to more traditional insulins.

Rolla AR, Rakel RE Practical approaches to insulin therapy for type 2 diabetes mellitus with premixed insulin analogues. *Clin Ther*, 2005; Vol. 27: pp. 1113–25.

Comments: Suggestions for initial dosing regimens and subsequent dosage titrations, including titration parameters, when using premixed insulin analogs.

Rubin RR, Peyrot M. Quality of life, treatment satisfaction, and treatment preference associated with use of a pen device delivering a premixed 70/30 insulin aspart suspension (aspart protamine suspension/soluble aspart) versus alternative treatment strategies. *Diabetes Care*, 2004; Vol. 27: pp. 2495–7.

Comments: In this study of the delivery device used with a premixed insulin analog (NovoLog 70/30), insulin pens were overwhelmingly preferred over conventional insulin syringes with vials; patients reported significant improvements in their quality of life with the pens, citing convenience and flexibility.

INSULINS: OTHER FORMS AND IMPLANTABLE INSULIN INFUSION PUMPS

Christopher D. Saudek, MD, and Brian Pinto, PharmD, MBA

INDICATIONS

FDA

- There are no insulin preparations currently approved other than subcutaneous or intravenous insulin administration.

Non-FDA Approved Uses

- Only in research studies.

MECHANISM

- **Inhaled insulin** is absorbed across the alveolar membrane.
- Microsphere encapsulation has been developed to enhance absorption (Technosphere).
- **Implanted insulin pumps** have been extensively studied in human trials.
- **Oral, nasal, and rectal** absorption of insulin has been demonstrated in animal and limited human studies when bound to certain carriers such as bile acids or when encapsulated.

PHARMACOKINETICS

- **Absorption:** Varies by preparation, but in general, pulmonary absorption is far less efficient than with subcutaneously administered insulin. Absorption of inhaled insulin is 8%–16%. Insulin delivered intraperitoneally by implanted pump is rapidly absorbed.
- **Metabolism and excretion:** Once absorbed, insulin delivered by alternative routes appears to be metabolized similar to insulin delivered subcutaneously. Insulin delivered intraperitoneally by an implanted pump is preferentially absorbed to the hepatic portal system, similar to the route of normal pancreatic insulin delivery.
- **Protein binding:** Probably not different from subcutaneously delivered insulin.

EXPERT OPINION

- The FDA approval and commercial launching of inhaled insulin, Exubera, in September 2006 followed extensive preclinical trials demonstrating efficacy.
- The main side effect of inhaled insulin was a small decrease in pulmonary function, specifically FEV1.
- The delivery device was cumbersome, insulin was delivered in mg rather than unit doses, and regular pulmonary function tests were required.
- For these and other reasons, the company, Pfizer, decided in October 2007, to stop production, and it is no longer available.

MEDICATIONS

- Subsequently, in April 2008, the FDA issued a letter noting a possible association of Exubera with lung cancer; of 4740 patients on Exubera, 6 developed lung cancer versus 1 of 4292 on placebo.
- MannKind, Inc., developed a microencapsulation technique (Technoshpere), and submitted a new drug application to the FDA in March 2009.
- Implanted insulin infusion pumps have been used for up to 20 years, in over 400 humans, the majority in France.
- Manufacturer is not currently proceeding with FDA application for market approval in the US, although approval has been granted in France.
- Other insulin delivery routes (particularly oral and encapsulated preparations for GI absorption) are in earlier stages of development.

REFERENCES

Hollander PA, Cefalu WT, Mitnick M, et al. Titration of inhaled human insulin (Exubera) in a treat-to-target regimen for patients with type 2 diabetes. *Diabetes Technol Ther,* 2010; Vol. 12: pp. 185–91.

Comments: 24-week treat-to-target comparison of 2-dose escalation schemes. Either lowered A1c from mean 8.6% to 6.8%, with Exubera.

Skyler JS, Hollander PA, Jovanovic L, et al. Safety and efficacy of inhaled human insulin (Exubera) during discontinuation and readministration of therapy in adults with type 1 diabetes: a 3-year randomized controlled trial. *Diabetes Res Clin Pract,* 2008; Vol. 82: pp. 238–46.

Comments: A safety study of pulmonary function changes from Exubera treating type 1 diabetes. Found decreased FEV(1) on the inhaled insulin to be reversible when stopping it.

Rosenstock J, Bergenstal R, Defronzo RA, et al. Efficacy and safety of Technosphere inhaled insulin compared with Technosphere powder placebo in insulin-naive type 2 diabetes suboptimally controlled with oral agents. *Diabetes Care,* 2008; Vol. 31: pp. 2177–82.

Comments: 12-week demonstration that the Technosphere delivery of inhaled insulin does lower glucose, A1c dropping by 0.72%.

Rosenstock J, Cefalu WT, Hollander PA, et al. Two-year pulmonary safety and efficacy of inhaled human insulin (Exubera) in adult patients with type 2 diabetes. *Diabetes Care,* 2008; Vol. 31: pp. 1723–8.

Comments: 2-year study of 635 patients with type 2 diabetes treated with Exubera versus subcutaneous insulin. FEV1 decreased in nonprogressive manner on Exubera. A1c decrease was maintained on Exubera.

McMahon GT, Arky RA. Inhaled insulin for diabetes mellitus. *NEJM,* 2007; Vol. 356: pp. 497–502.

Comments: An unbiased clinical review of Exubera, describing the pros and cons of using inhaled insulin.

Rave K, Heise T, Pfützner A, et al. Coverage of postprandial blood glucose excursions with inhaled technosphere insulin in comparison to subcutaneously injected regular human insulin in subjects with type 2 diabetes. *Diabetes Care,* 2007; Vol. 30: pp. 2307–8.

Comments: Pharmacokinetic evaluation of Technosphere, demonstrating a far quicker peak insulin concentration (15 minutes) than for regular human insulin (120 minutes). Did not compare to fast-acting insulin analogs, and 19% of patients reported a cough.

Saudek CD, Duckworth WC, Giobbie-Hurder A, et al. Implantable insulin pump vs multiple-dose insulin for non-insulin-dependent diabetes mellitus: a randomized clinical trial. Department of Veterans Affairs Implantable Insulin Pump Study Group. *JAMA,* 1996; Vol. 276: pp. 1322–7.

Comments: The only industry-independent randomized clinical trial of implanted insulin pump (IIP) versus subcutaneously (SC) delivered insulin, in the VA system. Designed to lower A1c to equal levels, IIP had less glycemic variability, less hypoglycemia, and less weight gain than SC insulin.

Duckworth WC, Saudek CD, Henry RR. Why intraperitoneal delivery of insulin with implantable pumps in NIDDM? *Diabetes,* 1992; Vol. 41: pp. 657–61.

Comments: A description of the rationale for intraperitoneally delivered insulin.

Glucose-Raising

ANTIMICROBIALS WITH SPECIAL PRECAUTIONS IN DIABETES

Paul Auwaerter, MD, and Paul A. Pham, PharmD

DEFINITION
- Certain antibiotics (ABX) may produce undesired changes in glycemic control when used in persons with diabetes (Table 4-10).
- No apparent interactions are described between antibiotics and insulins.
- Serum concentrations of hypoglycemic agents may change due to inhibition or induction of oxidative metabolism (i.e., cytochrome P450 system) including meglitinides (repaglinide, nateglinide), sulfonylureas (glyburide, glipizide), and glitizones (pioglitazone, rosiglitazone).
- Specific cytochrome P450 substrates: repaglinide (2C8, 3A4); nateglinide (2C9 > 3A4); glyburide and glipizide (2C9); pioglitazone (3A4 > 2C8); rosiglitazone (2C8 > 2C9).
- Limited number of potential drug–drug interactions observed with metformin.

EPIDEMIOLOGY
- Both outpatients and inpatients are at risk. Elderly and more severely ill may be at higher risk of dysglycemic reactions.
- Patients with diabetes under treatment for tuberculosis may be at higher risk for treatment failure due to lowered serum concentrations of rifampin, especially if high BMI.
- Obese people with diabetes may be at higher risk for treatment failure if weight-based dosing is not followed for certain antimicrobials (e.g., vancomycin, daptomycin, fluconazole, caspofungin, penicillins, trimethoprim/sulfamethoxazole, cephalosporins, aminoglycosides, and rifamycins).

DIAGNOSIS
- Hypo- or hyperglycemia in severely ill patients may be a consequence of systemic complications (e.g., from sepsis, liver disorders) and therefore be difficult to separate from a potential drug interaction.

CLINICAL TREATMENT
All Antimicrobials
- Exenatide may slow movement of antibiotics through digestive tract.
- Recommended to take antibiotics at least 1 hour prior to exenatide injection.

Fluoroquinolones (Gatifloxacin, Levofloxacin, Moxifloxacin, Ciprofloxacin)
- Both hypo- and hyperglycemia reported, but effect may be variable within the class and appears dose dependent. Often difficult to sort out between drug effect or underlying systemic disorder.
- Gatifloxacin was withdrawn from US market (2006) due to occurrence of hypo- and hyperglycemia, especially in elderly diabetic patients on oral hypoglycemics. Seen with other fluoroquinolones, some have argued that it is a class effect.

MEDICATIONS

- Hypo- and hyperglycemia effects: gatifloxacin > levofloxacin >> ciprofloxacin and azithromycin (as a comparator)(Aspinall). Although moxifloxacin reported less dysglycemia than gatifloxacin or levofloxacin, this may be due to usage issues.
- Mechanism may be due to fluoroquinolone effect in enhancing release of insulin by interference with ATP-sensitive K+ channels of pancreatic ß cells (Saraya).
- Consider using alternative to levofloxacin in unstable people with diabetes or severely ill. Ciprofloxacin appears to have usually minimal effects and can be safely used. Moxifloxacin likely also with less dysglycemic effect, but less well studied.

Macrolides (Erythromycin, Clarithromycin, Azithromycin) and Ketolide (Telithromycin)
- Clarithromycin increased repaglinide area under the inhibitory curve (AUC) by 40%. Consider decreasing repaglinide dose to avoid hypoglycemia.
- Class may increase concentrations of pioglitazone, effect unclear.
- Class may increase sulfonylureas serum concentration. Consider decreasing sulfonylurea dose with coadministration to avoid hypoglycemia.
- Azithromycin, specifically, can be considered without regard to use of repaglinide and sulfonylureas coadministration.

Azoles (Ketoconazole, Itraconazole, Fluconazole)
- Repaglinide AUC increased 15% with ketoconazole coadministration. Nateglinide AUC increased 48% with fluconazole coadministration. Consider decreasing meglitinides dose with azole coadministration to avoid causing hypoglycemia.
- May increase level of sulfonylureas. Fluconazole increased glyburide AUC 44%. Consider dose adjustment with azoles coadministration.
- Rosiglitazone AUC increased 47% with ketoconazole coadministration. Consider decreasing rosiglitazone with azole coadministration.
- May increase levels of pioglitazone.

Rifamycins (Rifampin, Rifapentine, Rifabutin)
- Rifamycin class significantly induces cytochrome P450. Always review drug interactions when prescribing this class of drugs.
- May significantly decrease drug concentrations of nateglinide, pioglitazone, rosiglitazone, repaglinide, and sulfonylureas.
- Rifampin decreased repaglinide and nateglinide AUC by 31% and 24%, respectively. Rifampin also decreased rosiglitazone and pioglitazone AUC by 66% and 54%, respectively.
- If used for tuberculosis, consider higher dose for continuation phase of treatment especially in patients with high BMI due to increased treatment failure risk ascribed to lower rifampin levels in this population (Nijland; Ruslami). No recommendations for dose, but consider adding 300–600 mg to usual amount given.

Other Antimicrobials
- **Cephalexin:** increased metformin AUC 24%. Clinical significance unknown.
- **Isoniazid:** reports in both experimental animal studies and humans for altered insulin secretion and hypoglycemia; this remains controversial, especially given the infrequency of the observation.
- **Pentamidine:** systemic administration may cause hyper- or hypoglycemia due to toxic effect on beta-cell function and inappropriate insulin secretion. This is seen more in patients with prolonged and high doses of the drug or in patients with reduced renal function leading to drug accumulation (Assan). Aerosolized drug not likely to cause this degree effect.

TABLE 4-10. INTERACTIONS OF ANTIMICROBIALS AND DIABETES MEDICATIONS

Antimicrobial	Interacting Diabetes Medication	Effect on Blood Glucose	Recommendations
All antimicrobials	Exenatide	No effect on glucose, but may delay abx absorption	Take abx one hour prior to exenatide.
Azoles (ketoconazole, itraconazole, fluconazole),	Repaglinide, nateglinide, pioglitazone rosiglitazone, sulfonylureas	Hypoglycemia	Consider lower anti-diabetic drug dose with coadministration.
Cephalexin	Metformin	Potential hypoglycemia	Clinical significance unclear. Monitor blood glucose closely with coadministration.
Clarithromycin	Repaglinide, pioglitazone, sulfonylureas	Hypoglycemia	Consider lower anti-diabetic drug dose or use azithromycin as an alternative antibiotic.
Gatifloxacin	—	Hypo- and hyperglycemia	Avoid (pulled from US market).
Lefloxacin > ciprofloxacin	—	Hypo- and hyperglycemia	If indicated ciprofloxacin may be preferred in brittle diabetics.
Isoniazid	—	Hypoglycemia	Rare observation.
Pentamidine	—	Hypo- and hyperglycemia	Hypoglycemia more common after initiation of therapy followed by hyperglycemia.
Rifampin	Repaglinide, nateglinide, pioglitazone, rosiglitazone, sulfonylureas	Hyperglycemia	Higher antidiabetic drug dose may be needed.
Trimethoprim	Metformin	Potential hypoglycemia	Clinical significance unclear. Monitor blood glucose closely with coadministration.

Courtesy of Paul Pham, PharmD, Johns Hopkins University School of Medicine.

MEDICATIONS

- **Trimethoprim:** may increase metformin serum concentrations by inhibition of tubular secretion; increased repaglinide AUC 61%; increased rosiglitazone AUC 31%. Consider dose adjustment.
- **Vancomycin:** tissue penetration of antibiotic decreased in diabetic patients (Skhirtladze). Important to use actual body weight (ABW) when dosing vancomycin. Recommended vancomycin dose, for normal renal function: 15 mg/kg IV of ABW q12h.

EXPERT OPINION

- People with diabetes and high BMI may need adjusted doses of antibiotics when treating serious infections. Consult references, pharmacists, or infectious disease specialists for assistance when dosing drugs such as vancomycin, daptomycin, fluconazole, caspofungin, penicillins, cephalosporins, trimethoprim/sulfamethoxazole, aminoglycosides, and rifamycins.
- Fluoroquinolones are frequently employed in the treatment of infections in diabetes, including UTIs and diabetic foot infections. Ciprofloxacin likely has minimal chances of significant alteration in glucose homeostasis; however, levofloxacin may and should be used with some caution. Uncertain whether moxifloxacin has significant dysglycemic effects, but no good data have yet been suggested.
- Worse outcomes in the treatment of tuberculosis have been seen in diabetic populations. Some good evidence suggests that this may be due to altered drug concentrations, especially rifampin. No formal recommendations yet exist for different dosing in diabetes; however, some argue that rifampin doses should be increased when switched from daily therapy.

REFERENCES

Ruslami R, Nijland HM, Adhiarta IG, et al. Pharmacokinetics of antituberculosis drugs in pulmonary tuberculosis patients with type 2 diabetes. *Antimicrob Agents Chemother,* 2010; Vol. 54: pp. 1068–74.

    Comments: Authors in follow-up to their 2006 paper (Nijland et al, CID) suggest that treatment failures in diabetic patients may be due to lower rifampin concentrations in continuation rather than acute/daily dosing. Why this occurs is unclear, but may be due to increased body mass or differences in hepatic induction of enzymes in these patients.

Aspinall SL, Good CB, Jiang R, et al. Severe dysglycemia with the fluoroquinolones: a class effect? *Clin Infect Dis,* 2009; Vol. 49: pp. 402–8.

    Comments: Large cohort study of outpatients within the VA system regarding >1.2 million patients receiving a FQ between 2001–2005. For patients with diabetes, the odds ratio for azithromycin were 4.3 (95% CI, 2.7–6.6) for gatifloxacin, 2.1 (95% CI, 1.4–3.3) for levofloxacin, and 1.1 (95% CI, 0.6–2.0) for ciprofloxacin. The odds ratios for hyperglycemia were 4.5 (95% CI, 3.0–6.9) for gatifloxacin, 1.8 (95% CI, 1.2–2.7) for levofloxacin, and 1.0 (95% CI, 0.6–1.8) for ciprofloxacin. The authors conclude that the odds of either hypo- and hyperglycemia were significantly greater with gatifloxacin and levofloxacin, but not ciprofloxacin or azithromycin. It is important to note that this is an outpatient study, and that more severely ill patients may respond differently.

Hall RG, Leff RD, Gumbo T. Treatment of active pulmonary tuberculosis in adults: current standards and recent advances. Insights from the Society of Infectious Diseases Pharmacists. *Pharmacotherapy,* 2009; Vol. 29: pp. 1468–81.

    Comments: TB in diabetes often has worse outcomes. Accumulating data suggest that pharmacokinetic/pharmacodynamic factors should be considered when treating these patients. As of yet, there are no formal recommendations in this regard from the American Thoracic Society.

Lewis RJ, Mohr JF. Dysglycaemias and fluoroquinolones. *Drug Saf,* 2008; Vol. 31: pp. 283–92.

    Comments: Review of available data suggests that likelihood of glycemic dysregulation is dose dependent.

Khamaisi M, Leitersdorf E. Severe hypoglycemia from clarithromycin-repaglinide drug interaction. *Pharmacotherapy*, 2008; Vol. 28: pp. 682–4.

Comments: Case described with severe hypoglycemia occuring within 2 days of instituting the macrolide clarithromycin for *H. pylori* treatment.

Scheen AJ. Drug-drug and food-drug pharmacokinetic interactions with new insulinotropic agents repaglinide and nateglinide. *Clin Pharmacokinet*, 2007; Vol. 46: pp. 93–108.

Comments: Review article highlights that rifampin reduced the repaglinide area under the plasma concentration-time curve (AUC) by 32%–85% and reduced nateglinide AUC by almost 25%. It should be expected that use of rifampin with these agents will moderate their antihypoglycemic effects. In contrast, azoles, macrolides, and trimethoprim increased the AUC of drugs by 15%–77%. It appears that CYP3A4 impact of the glinides is modest, but that CYP2C8 is most for repaglinide and CYP2C9 is important for nateglinide.

Skhirtladze K, Hutschala D, Fleck T, et al. Impaired target site penetration of vancomycin in diabetic patients following cardiac surgery. *AAC*, 2006; Vol. 50: p. 1372.

Comments: This observational study compared vancomycin tissue penetration in 6 diabetics and 6 nondiabetics. Vancomycin tissue concentrations in diabetic patients were significantly lower compared to nondiabetics (3.7 mg/L vs 11.9 mg/L; p = 0.002). The authors hypothesize that the decreased vancomycin tissue concentrations may be due to impaired microcirculation associated with diabetes.

Nijland HM, Ruslami R, Stalenhoef JE, et al. Exposure to rifampicin is strongly reduced in patients with tuberculosis and type 2 diabetes. *Clin Infect Dis*, 2006; Vol. 43: pp. 848–54.

Comments: Initial report from Indonesia, suggesting a decreased rifampin plasma concentration in diabetics. Authors suggest that diabetics with increased BMI may need higher doses than the standard 600 mg of rifampin.

Saraya A, Yokokura M, Gonoi T, et al. Effects of fluoroquinolones on insulin secretion and beta-cell ATP-sensitive K+ channels. *Eur J Pharmacol*, 2004; Vol. 497: pp. 111–7.

Comments: Study found that gatifloxacin and temafloxacin had greater effect on stimulating insulin secretion than levofloxacin in this murine model.

Gavin JR, Kubin R, Choudhri S, et al. Moxifloxacin and glucose homeostasis: a pooled-analysis of the evidence from clinical and postmarketing studies. *Drug Saf*, 2004; Vol. 27: pp. 671–86.

Comments: Analysis of 32 studies using moxifloxacin with over 14,731 patients, found 7 pts (<0.1%) receiving moxifloxacin with a hyperglycemic adverse reaction. There were no moxifloxacin hypoglycemic-related events noted.

Kilby JM, Tabereaux PB Severe hyperglycemia in an HIV clinic: preexisting versus drug-associated diabetes mellitus. *J Acquir Immune Defic Syndr Hum Retrovirol*, 1998; Vol. 17: pp. 46–50.

Comments: Study performed in a Birmingham, AL, HIV clinic found that 2% of their HIV patients suffered from severe hyperglycemia, although this was evenly split between those who had preexisting diabetes and those who had drug-induced explanations. Not surprisingly, corticosteroids and megestrol acetate (with weight-related changes) were among the most common medication-related causes. One patient developed hyperglycemia while receiving pentamidine (plus prednisone) for PCP pneumonia, a not unusual combination and complication of therapy in this era. Pentamidine is now rarely used for treatment, but has been effective for visceral leishmania, although toxicity of the drug now has diminished use, including reports of provoking permanent diabetes in patients receiving the compound (*Rev Soc Bras Med Trop*, 1995; Vol. 28[4]: pp. 405–7 and *J Infect Chemother*, 2004; Vol. 10[6]: pp. 307–15).

Assan R, Perronne C, Assan D, et al. Pentamidine-induced derangements of glucose homeostasis. Determinant roles of renal failure and drug accumulation. A study of 128 patients. *Diabetes Care*, 1995; Vol. 18: pp. 47–55.

Comments: Although not a commonly used drug, pentamidine can cause dysglycemia especially due to drug-accumulation (either inordinately high or prolonged dosing) or secondary to renal insufficiency. The drug has toxicity to islet beta-cells and may cause dysfunctional insulin release.

MEDICATIONS

Uzzan B, Bentata M, Campos J, et al. Effects of aerosolized pentamidine on glucose homeostasis and insulin secretion in HIV-positive patients: a controlled study. *AIDS*, 1995; Vol. 9: pp. 901–7.

Comments: No longer a popular approach to PCP prophylaxis, aerosolized pentamidine in this study was not found to significantly affect glucose homeostasis, compared to receiving the drug systemically.

Villaume C, Dollet JM, Beck B, et al. Hyperinsulinemia associated with normal C-peptide levels in a woman treated with isoniazide. *Biomed Pharmacother,* 1982; Vol. 36: pp. 32–5.

Comments: Among several reports attributing INH to altered insulin secretion and hypoglycemia that bolster prior observations including animal studies (*BMJ*, 1953; Vol. 1: pp. 296–9 and *Ind J Physiol Pharmac*, 1989; Vol. 33: pp. 277–8). It is not clear from any of these reports that diabetics are more prone to this problem.

Cameron SJ, Crompton GK. Severe hypoglycaemia in the course of treatment with streptomycin, isoniazid and ethionamide. *Tubercle,* 1967; Vol. 48: pp. 307–10.

Comments: Antitubercular agents have been implicated in causing hypoglycemia, mostly in nondiabetic patients. In this report, ethionamide is argued as the cause. Others include less commonly used drugs such as PAS (para-aminosalicylic acid) (*Postgrad Med J*, 1980; Vol. 56(652): p. 135 and *J Pharm Sci*, 1968; Vol. 57: pp. 2111–6) and INH (see Villaume ref). One should keep in mind that adrenal insufficiency due to TB would be another explanation (*Korean J Intern Med,* 2004; Vol. 19[1]: pp. 70–3).

ANTIPSYCHOTICS

Paul A. Pham, PharmD

Indications
FDA
- Schizophrenia
- Bipolar disorder
- Psychotic depression
- Agitation
- Anxiety
- See Table 4-11 for specific FDA indications for each antipsychotic.

Non-FDA Approved Uses
- Hiccups
- ICU delirium

Mechanism
- Both typical (i.e., phenothiazines) and atypical antipsychotics block postsynaptic dopamine receptors in the mesolimbic system resulting in depolarization blockade of dopamine tracts, which has been correlated with antipsychotic effect.
- Atypical antipsychotics (aripiprazole, clozapine, olanzapine, risperidone, quetiapine, ziprasidone) also block serotonin receptors.

Forms
- See Table 4-11.

Usual Adult Dosing
- Elderly patients and patients with renal or hepatic disease should initiate antipsychotics at the lowest dose with slow titration.
- See Table 4-12.

TABLE 4-11. SPECIFIC FDA INDICATIONS, FORMS, AND PHARMACOKINETICS OF ANTIPSYCHOTICS

Typical Antipsychotics	FDA Indications	Metabolism/ Excretion/$T_{\frac{1}{2}}$	Pregnancy/ Breastfeeding	Brands/ Generics/ Dosage Forms
Chlorpromazine	Acute intermittent porphyria Acute psychosis Nausea/vomiting Psychotic depression Schizophrenia Singultus (hiccups) Tetanus	Metabolism: Hepatic P450 enzyme CYP2D6, >100 metabolites have been identified predominantly via enterohepatic-recirculation. Excretion: Urine, partially via the biliary tract and feces. $T_{\frac{1}{2}}$: 23–37 hours	Pregnancy Category C Not recommended for use in lactating women due to excretion into breast milk.	Generic chlorpromazine • Injection Solution: 25 mg/ml • Oral Solution: 100 mg/ml • Oral Tablet: 10 mg, 25 mg, 50 mg, 100 mg, 200 mg 60 × 10 mg tabs = $22 60 × 25 mg tabs = $26 60 × 50 mg tabs = $18 60 × 100 mg tabs = $16 60 × 200 mg tabs = $27 Thorazine • Oral Tablet: 200 mg
Fluphenazine	Acute psychosis Psychotic depression Schizophrenia	Metabolism: Hepatic, 50% of metabolites contribute to antipsychotic activity predominantly via enterohepatic-recirculation.	Pregnancy Category C Not recommended for use in lactating women due to excretion into breast milk.	Generic Fluphenazine Decanoate • Injection Solution: 25 mg/ml 5 ml = $65.99 10 ml = $125.98 Fluphenazine HCl • Intramuscular Solution: 2.5 mg/ml

(Continued)

TABLE 4-11. SPECIFIC FDA INDICATIONS, FORMS, AND PHARMACOKINETICS OF ANTIPSYCHOTICS (CONT.)

Typical Antipsychotics	FDA Indications	Metabolism/ Excretion/$T\frac{1}{2}$	Pregnancy/ Breastfeeding	Brands/ Generics/ Dosage Forms
		Excretion: Urine, partially via bile and feces. $T\frac{1}{2}$: 16 hours; 7–10 days (decanoate)		• Oral Elixir: 2.5 mg/5 ml • Oral Solution: 5 mg/ml • Oral Tablet: 1 mg, 2.5 mg, 5 mg, 10 mg 90 × 1 mg tabs = $18 60 × 2.5 mg tabs = $16 60 × 5 mg tabs = $19 60 × 10 mg tabs = $25
Perphenazine	Acute psychosis Nausea/vomiting Psychotic depression Schizophrenia Singultus (hiccups)	Metabolism: Gastric mucosa and first-pass metabolism through the liver Excretion: Biliary tract and feces. $T\frac{1}{2}$: 9 hours	Pregnancy Category C Not recommended for use in lactating women due to excretion into breast milk.	Generic perphenazine • Oral Tablet: 2 mg, 4 mg, 8 mg, 16 mg 60 × 2 mg tabs = $42 60 × 4 mg tabs = $56 60 × 8 mg tabs = $60 60 × 16 mg tabs = $83
Thioridazine	Agitation	Metabolism: Gastric mucosa and first-pass metabolism through the liver	Pregnancy Category C	Generic thioridazine • Oral Tablet: 10 mg, 15 mg, 25 mg, 50 mg, 100 mg, 150 mg, 200 mg

	Anxiety	Excretion: Urine, partially via bile and feces.	Not recommended for use in lactating women due to excretion into breast milk.
	Depression		
	Psychotic depression	$T\frac{1}{2}$: 24 hours	
	Schizophrenia		
Trifluoperazine	Anxiety	Metabolism: Hepatic through oxidation, which results in various active metabolites.	Pregnancy Category C
	Schizophrenia		Not recommended for use in lactating women due to excretion into breast milk.
		Excretion: Urine	
		$T\frac{1}{2}$: 24 hours	
Haloperidol	Schizophrenia	Metabolism: Hepatic with evidence of partial extrahepatic metabolism.	Pregnancy Category C
		Excretion: Urine, partially via feces.	Not recommended for use in lactating women due to excretion into breast milk.
		$T\frac{1}{2}$: 21 hours	

	90 × 10 mg tabs = $22
	90 × 15 mg tabs = $12
	90 × 25 mg tabs = $26
	90 × 50 mg tabs = $30
	90 × 100 mg tabs = $35
	90 × 150 mg tabs = $56
	90 × 200 mg tabs = $82
Generic trifluoperazine	
• Oral Tablet: 1 mg, 2 mg, 5 mg, 10 mg	
	60 × 1 mg tabs = $26
	60 × 2 mg tabs = $30
	60 × 5 mg tabs = $35
	60 × 10 mg tabs = $47
Generic	
• Oral Tablet: 0.5 mg, 1 mg, 2 mg, 5 mg, 10 mg, 20 mg	
	90 × 0.5 mg tabs = $26
	90 × 1 mg tabs = $20
	90 × 2 mg tabs = $19
	90 × 5 mg tabs = $26
	60 × 10 mg tabs = $72
	60 × 20 mg tabs = $125

(Continued)

MEDICATIONS

TABLE 4-11. SPECIFIC FDA INDICATIONS, FORMS, AND PHARMACOKINETICS OF ANTIPSYCHOTICS *(CONT.)*

Typical Antipsychotics	FDA Indications	Metabolism/ Excretion/$T_{\frac{1}{2}}$	Pregnancy/ Breastfeeding	Brands/ Generics/ Dosage Forms
Loxapine	Schizophrenia	Metabolism: Hepatic Excretion: Urine, partially via feces. $T_{\frac{1}{2}}$: 4–12 hours	Pregnancy Category C Not recommended for use in lactating women due to excretion into breast milk.	Generic loxapine • Oral Capsule: 5 mg 90 × 5 mg caps = $56
Molindone	Schizophrenia	Metabolism: Hepatic Excretion: Urine, partially via feces. $T_{\frac{1}{2}}$: <24 hours	Pregnancy Category C Not recommended for use in lactating women due to excretion into breast milk.	Moban tablet: 5 mg, 10 mg, 25 mg, 50 mg
Thiothixene	Psychotic disorder Schizophrenia	Metabolism: Hepatic Excretion: Urine, partially via feces. $T_{\frac{1}{2}}$: 34 hours	Pregnancy Category C Not recommended for use in lactating women due to excretion into breast milk.	Generic thiothixene • Oral Capsule: 1 mg, 2 mg, 5 mg, 10 mg 90 × 1 mg tabs = $23 90 × 2 mg tabs = $27 90 × 5 mg tabs = $26 60 × 10 mg tabs = $50 Navane • Oral Capsule: 2 mg, 5 mg, 10 mg, 20 mg

Atypical Antipsychotics	FDA Indications	Metabolism/ Excretion/$T\frac{1}{2}$	Pregnancy/ Breastfeeding	Brands/ Generics/ Dosage Forms
Aripiprazole	Autistic disorder Bipolar disorder Major depressive disorder Psychomotor agitation Schizophrenia	Metabolism: Hepatic CYP2D6, CYP3A4 Excretion: Urine (25%) and feces (55%). $T\frac{1}{2}$: 75 hours (parent drug); 94 hours (metabolite)	Pregnancy Category C Not recommended for use in lactating women due to excretion into breast milk.	Abilify Discmelt • Oral Tablet, Disintegrating: 10 mg, 15 mg 30 × 10 mg tabs = $570 90 × 10 mg tabs = $1676 Abilify • Oral Solution: 1 mg/ml • Oral Tablet: 2 mg, 5 mg, 10 mg, 15 mg, 20 mg, 30 mg
Clozapine	Schizoaffective disorder—Suicidal behavior, Recurrent Schizophrenia	Metabolism: Hepatic CYP1A2, N-demethyl-ation, and N-oxidation Excretion: Urine (50%), partially via feces (30%). $T\frac{1}{2}$: 12 hours	Pregnancy Category B Not recommended for use in lactating women due to excretion into breast milk.	Generic clozapine • Oral Tablet: 25 mg, 50 mg, 100 mg, 200 mg Clozaril • Oral Tablet: 25 mg, 100 mg FazaClo • Oral Tablet, Disintegrating: 12.5 mg, 25 mg, 100 mg
Olanzapine	Agitation—Bipolar I disorder	Metabolism: Hepatic CYP450 oxidation and glucuronidation	Pregnancy Category C	Generic olanzapine • Oral Tablet: 10 mg

(Continued)

TABLE 4-11. SPECIFIC FDA INDICATIONS, FORMS, AND PHARMACOKINETICS OF ANTIPSYCHOTICS (CONT.)

Atypical Antipsychotics	FDA Indications	Metabolism/ Excretion/$T_{\frac{1}{2}}$	Pregnancy/ Breastfeeding	Brands/ Generics/ Dosage Forms
	Agitation— Schizophrenia	Excretion: Urine (57%), partially via feces (30%). $T_{\frac{1}{2}}$: 30 hours	Not recommended for use in lactating women due to excretion into breast milk.	Zyprexa IntraMuscular • Intramuscular Powder for Solution: 10 mg Zyprexa • Oral Tablet: 2.5 mg, 5 mg, 7.5 mg, 10 mg, 15 mg, 20 mg 30 × 2.5 mg tabs = $245 30 × 5 mg tabs = $296 30 × 7.5 mg tabs = $358 30 × 10 mg tabs = $440 30 × 15 mg tabs = $639 30 × 20 mg tabs = $856 Zyprexa Zydis • Oral Tablet, Disintegrating: 5 mg, 10 mg, 15 mg, 20 mg
	Bipolar I disorder, Acute mixed or manic episodes			
	Bipolar I disorder, Maintenance therapy			
	Schizophrenia			
Quetiapine	Bipolar disorder, depressed phase Bipolar disorder, maintenance	Metabolism: Hepatic CYP3A4 Excretion: Urine (73%), partially via feces (20%).	Pregnancy Category C Not recommended for use in lactating women due to excretion into breast milk.	Generic quetiapine • Oral Tablet: 25 mg, 100 mg, 200 mg Seroquel • Oral Tablet: 25 mg, 50 mg, 100 mg, 200 mg, 300 mg, 400 mg

Major depressive disorder, Adjunct Manic bipolar I disorder Schizophrenia	$T\frac{1}{2}$: 6 hours	60 × 25 mg tabs = $182 100 × 50 mg tabs = $501 60 × 100 mg tabs = $325 60 × 200 mg tabs = $560 60 × 300 mg tabs = $788 30 × 400 mg tabs = $482 Seroquel XR • Oral Tablet, Extended Release: 50 mg, 150 mg, 200 mg, 300 mg, 400 mg 60 × 50 mg tabs = $291 60 × 150 mg tabs = $500 30 × 200 mg tabs = $560
Risperidone	Schizophrenia	Metabolism: Hepatic Excretion: Urine, partially via feces. $T\frac{1}{2}$: 34 hours	Pregnancy Category C Not recommended for use in lactating women due to excretion into breast milk.	Generic risperidon • Oral Solution: 1 mg/ml 1 mg/ml, 30 ml = $126 Oral Tablet: 0.25 mg, 0.5 mg, 1 mg, 2 mg, 3 mg, 4 mg 60 × 0.25 mg tabs = $145 60 × 0.5 mg tabs = $180 60 × 1 mg tabs = $196 60 × 2 mg tabs = $300 60 × 3 mg tabs = $300 60 × 4 mg tabs = $400

(Continued)

TABLE 4-11. SPECIFIC FDA INDICATIONS, FORMS, AND PHARMACOKINETICS OF ANTIPSYCHOTICS (CONT.)

Atypical Antipsychotics	FDA Indications	Metabolism/ Excretion/$T_{\frac{1}{2}}$	Pregnancy/ Breastfeeding	Brands/ Generics/ Dosage Forms
Risperidone (CONT.)				• Oral Tablet, Disintegrating: 0.25 mg, 0.5 mg, 1 mg, 2 mg, 3 mg, 4 mg Risperdal Consta • Intramuscular Powder for Suspension, Extended Release: 12.5 mg, 25 mg, 37.5 mg, 50 mg Risperdal M-Tab • Oral Tablet, Disintegrating: 0.5 mg, 1 mg, 2 mg Risperdal M-TAB • Oral Tablet, Disintegrating: 3 mg, 4 mg Risperdal • Oral Solution: 1 mg/ml 1 mg/ml, 60 ml = $375 • Oral Tablet: 0.25 mg, 0.5 mg, 1 mg, 2 mg, 3 mg, 4 mg 30 × 0.25 mg tabs = $137 30 × 0.5 mg tabs = $165 30 × 1 mg tabs = $175 30 × 2 mg tabs = $271 30 × 3 mg tabs = $350 30 × 4 mg tabs = $435

				Risperidone M-Tab • Oral Tablet, Disintegrating: 0.5 mg, 1 mg, 2 mg, 3 mg, 4 mg
Ziprasidone	Bipolar I disorder, Acute manic or mixed episodes, monotherapy Bipolar I disorder, to lithium or valpro- ate, Adjunct Schizophrenia	Metabolism: Hepatic Excretion: Urine (20%), mainly via feces (66%). $T\frac{1}{2}$: 7 hours PO; 2–5 hours (IM)	Pregnancy Category C Not recommended for use in lactating women due to excretion into breast milk.	Geodon • Oral Capsule: 20 mg, 40 mg, 60 mg, 80 mg 60 × 1 mg caps = \$458 60 × 2 mg caps = \$463 60 × 3 mg caps = \$550 60 × 4 mg caps = \$550

Courtesy of Paul Pham, PharmD, Johns Hopkins University School of Medicine.

TABLE 4-12. DOSING FOR ANTIPSYCHOTICS

Agent	Starting Dose	Maintenance Dose	Maximum Dose
Typical Antipsychotics			
Fluphenazine	2.5–10 mg/day; 12.5–25 mg/dose IM or SC	20 mg/day; 50 mg/dose IM or SC	40 mg/day PO; 100 mg/dose IM or SC of decanoate or enanthate depot injections
Perphenazine	20–100 mg/day PO	200–400 mg/day PO	24 mg/day PO
Thioridazine	30–150 mg/day	300 mg/day PO	300 mg/day
Trifluoperazine	4–10 mg/day PO	15–20 mg/day PO	40 mg/day PO
Haloperidol	1–6 mg/day PO	6–15 mg/day	30 mg/day PO
Loxapine	10–25 mg/day PO	60–100 mg/day PO	250 mg/day PO
Molindone	50–75 mg/day PO	15–100 mg/day PO	225 mg/day PO
Thiothixene	15 mg/day PO	20–30 mg/day PO	60 mg/day PO
Atypical Antipsychotics			
Aripiprazole	10–15 mg/day PO	30 mg/day PO (greater efficacy has not been established for doses exceeding 15 mg/day)	30 mg/day PO
Clozapine	25–50 mg/day PO	300–450 mg/day PO	600–900 mg/day PO
Olanzapine	5–10 mg/day PO; 210–300 mg IM q2wk, or 405 mg q4wk IM	10–20 mg/day PO; 150–300 mg IM q2wk, or 300–405 mg IM q4wk	20 mg/day PO
Quetiapine	50 mg/day PO	300–400 mg/day PO	800 mg/day PO
Risperidone	1–3 mg/day PO	1–6 mg/day PO; 6 mg/day IM	16 mg/day PO
Ziprasidone	40 mg/day PO	20–80 mg/day PO	200 mg/day PO

Courtesy of Paul Pham, PharmD, Johns Hopkins University School of Medicine.

DOSING IN SPECIAL POPULATIONS

Renal

- With severe renal impairment, initiate risperidone 0.5 mg twice daily with slower titration.
- No dose adjustment needed for other antipsychotics, but should be initiated at the lowest dose (especially in patients with concurrent hepatic impairment).

Hepatic

- Initiate with the lowest dose and slow dose titration.

Pregnancy

- Antipsychotics are FDA Category C (except clozapine, which is FDA Category B). Limited human clinical data; use only if benefit outweighs risk.

Breastfeeding

- Not recommended for use in lactating women due to excretion into breast milk.

ADVERSE DRUG REACTIONS

General

- Newer atypical antipsychotics are generally better tolerated compared to phenothiazines, but have been associated with weight gain and development of diabetes.
- All antipsychotics should be avoided or used with caution in patients with acute altered mental status.

Common

- Weight gain: at 10 weeks of therapy, estimated average weight gain with drug treatment compared with placebo varies from 0.5–5.0 kg.
- Olanzapine and clozapine are associated with greater weight gain and lipid elevation.
- Anticholinergic side effects (e.g., dry mouth, constipation, urinary retention). More frequently observed with thioridazine > chlorpromazine > loxapine compared to other agents. Risperidone associated with the lowest rate of anticholinergic side effects.
- Dose-related sedation with initial treatment, but improves over time.
- Dose-related extrapyramidal syndrome (e.g., dystonia and akathisia, tardive dyskinesia). More common with high-potency (e.g., phenothiazines, haloperidol, and thiothixene) compared to low-potency phenothiazines (e.g., chlorpromazine and thioridazine) and the atypical "second-generation" antipsychotics (e.g., aripiprazole, quetiapine, olanzapine, risperidone, ziprasidone).

Occasional

- New onset diabetes: associated more commonly with olanzapine compared to quetiapine, risperidone, and haloperidol.
- Increased prolactin levels.
- Orthostatic hypotension (secondary to alpha-1 blockade) ± reflex tachycardia. More common with chlorpromazine and thioridazine compared to haloperidol.
- Sexual dysfunction including loss of libido and anorgasmia.
- Impaired cognition.
- LFT elevations and hepatitis.

Rare

- Neuroleptic malignant syndrome (NMS) presenting as confusion, fever, tachycardia, muscle rigidity, and labile blood pressure.

- QTc and PR interval prolongation. Associated more frequently with ziprasidone, thioridazine, and clozapine.
- Benign pigmentary deposits on the retina associated with thioridazine and chlorpromazine.
- Agranulocytosis reported in 0.8% (1-year risk) of patients treated with clozapine during the first 4–6 month of therapy. Monitor weekly CBC for the first 6 months in clozapine treated patients. Transient leukopenia also reported with phenothiazines.
- Hyperpyrexia (more commonly reported in hot weather or during exercise).
- Seizure: use with caution in patients with a seizure history.

DRUG INTERACTIONS

- Phenothiazines and haloperidol are primarily metabolized via CYP2D6. Atypical antipsychotics are metabolized primarily via CYP2D6, CYP3A4, and CYP1A2. Potent inducers and inhibitors of these isoenzymes may decrease and increase atypical antipsychotic serum concentrations, respectively. Dose may need to be adjusted based on toxicity and therapeutic response.
- **CYP450 inducers** (e.g., carbamazepine, phenobarbital, primidone, and rifampin): may decrease serum concentrations of atypical antipsychotics, phenothiazines, and haloperidol.
- **Cimetidine:** may increase serum concentrations of clozapine, risperidal, olanzapine, quetiapine, and ziprasidone.
- **CYP1A2 inhibitors** (e.g., ciprofloxacin, cimetidine, fluvoxamine, fluoxetine): may increase serum concentration of clozapine and olanzapine. May increase risk of seizure with clozapine coadministration. Use with caution.
- **CYP3A4 inhibitors** (e.g., erythromycin, clarithromycin, azole antifungal [ketoconazole, itraconazole, voriconazole, posaconazole], HIV-protease inhibitors): may increase serum concentrations of clozapine, quetiapine, and ziprasidone.
- **CYP2D6 inhibitors** (e.g., bupropion, fluoxetine, paroxetine, duloxetine, quinidine, ritonavir): may increase thioridazine, risperidone, and haloperidol.
- **Antihypertensive agents:** may increase risk of orthostatic hypotension with antipsychotics coadministration. Coadminister with close monitoring.
- **Benzodiazepines:** may increase risk of oversedation (especially clozapine). Coadminister with close monitoring.
- **Agents with anticholinergic side effects** (e.g., tricyclic antidepressants, antihistamines): may increase risk of anticholinergic side effects and impair cognition with antipsychotic coadministration.
- **Agents known to increase QTc** (e.g., high-dose methadone, clarithromycin, erythromycin, tricyclic antidepressants): may increase risk of QTc prolongation (especially ziprasidone). Avoid coadministration with baseline QTc prolongation.
- **Metoclopramide:** may increase risk of akathisia and other extrapyramidal side effects with antipsychotic coadministration.
- Antipsychotics have not been found to significantly interact with oral hypoglycemic agents.

PHARMACOKINETICS

- **Absorption:** Well absorbed.
- **Metabolism and Excretion:** Metabolized primarily via CYP2D6, CYP3A4, and CYP1A2. Chlorpromazine, haloperidol, olanzapine, quetiapine, and risperidone have active metabolites.

- **Protein Binding:** Moderate to high protein binding.
- **Cmax, Cmin, and AUC:** Plasma concentrations not routinely performed in clinical practice. Limited data suggest some association between clozapine concentrations >350 mcg/ml and treatment response.
- **T$\frac{1}{2}$:** Long half-life range of 10–40 hours. Except quetiapine (6 hrs), ziprasidone (7 hrs), and perphenazine (9 hrs).
- **Distribution:** Wide volume of distribution with tissue accumulation.
- See Table 4-11 for pharmacokinetics of each antipsychotic.

EXPERT OPINION

- Atypical antipsychotics are now considered first line due to lower rates of extrapyramidal symptoms and tardive dyskinesia but are associated with weight gain, lipid abnormalities, and incident diabetes.
- Olanzapine and clozapine are associated with greater weight gain and increased risk of type 2 diabetes (Lambert).
- Weight gain, diabetes, and lipid abnormalities: clozapine, olanzapine > risperidone, quetiapine > ziprasidone, and aripiprazole (Lieberman).
- In obese patients with diabetes, ziprasidone may be considered since it is associated with less weight gain compared to the other atypical antipsychotics (Komossa).
- Baseline diabetes screening should be obtained before, or as soon as clinically feasible after, the initiation of any antipsychotic medication. Reassessment at 4, 8, and 12 weeks after initiating or changing atypical antipsychotic therapy and quarterly thereafter at the time of routine visits is recommended (Consensus Statement).
- Typical antipsychotics (e.g., haloperidal) are less likely to cause weight gain and diabetes compared to atypical antipsychotics (e.g., olanzapine).
- Although patients who gain weight during antipsychotic therapy are at higher risk of developing diabetes, hyperglycemia has also been reported in patients without significant weight gain (Lindenmayer).
- Evidence is lacking as to whether these drugs worsen diabetic control in people with preexisting diabetes, but diabetic patients newly started on atypical antipsychotics (e.g., olanzapine) should have their blood sugar monitored closely.

BASIS FOR RECOMMENDATIONS

American Diabetes Association. American Psychiatric Association, American Association of Clinical Endocrinologists, and North American Association for the Study of Obesity Consensus Development Conference on Antipsychotic Drugs and Obesity and Diabetes. *Diabetes Care,* 2004; Vol. 27: pp. 596–601.

Comments: Consensus recommendation on monitoring of blood glucose for patients on antipsychotics.

OTHER REFERENCES

Komossa K, Rummel-Kluge C, Hunger H, et al. Ziprasidone versus other atypical antipsychotics for schizophrenia. *Cochrane Database Syst Rev,* 2009; CD006627.

Comments: In a review of nine randomized controlled trials involving 3361 patients ziprasidone produced less weight gain and cholesterol increase than olanzapine, quetiapine, and risperidone. However, ziprasidone may be less effective with more patients leaving studies early due to low efficacy compared to olanzapine and risperidone.

Citrome LL, Holt RI, Zachry WM, et al. Risk of treatment-emergent diabetes mellitus in patients receiving antipsychotics. *Ann Pharmacother,* 2007; Vol. 41: pp. 1593–603.

Comments: Attributable risk for atypical antipsychotics relative to first-generation antipsychotics (e.g., phenothiazines, haloperidol) ranged from 40–50 new cases of diabetes per 1000 patients. However, few studies controlled for body weight, race, or ethnicity, or the presence of other diabetogenic medications.

MEDICATIONS

Lambert MT, Copeland LA, Sampson N, et al. New-onset type 2 diabetes associated with atypical antipsychotic medications. *Prog Neuropsychopharmacol Biol Psychiatry*, 2006; Vol. 30: pp. 919–23.

Comments: This retrospective analysis evaluated the one-year risk of developing type-2 diabetes between olanzapine, quetiapine, and risperidone when compared to haloperidol. Patients treated with olanzapine, but not quetiapine and risperidone, were significantly at higher risk of developing type-2 diabetes compared to haloperidol (odds ratio 8.4, 95% CI 1.8–38.7).

Lieberman JA, Stroup TS, McEvoy JP, et al. Effectiveness of antipsychotic drugs in patients with chronic schizophrenia. *NEJM*, 2005; Vol. 353: pp. 1209–23.

Comments: 1493 patients with schizophrenia were randomized to receive olanzapine, quetiapine, ziprasidone, and perphenazine. Compared to the other antipsychotics, olanzapine was the most effective, but was associated with the highest rates of discontinuation due to greater weight gain and increases in measures of glucose and lipid.

Lindenmayer JP, Czobor P, Volavka J, et al. Changes in glucose and cholesterol levels in patients with schizophrenia treated with typical or atypical antipsychotics. *Am J Psychiatry*, 2003; Vol. 160: pp. 290–6.

Comments: In this prospective randomized trial involving 157 hospitalized patients, clozapine, olanzapine, and haloperidol were all associated with an increase of plasma glucose level (>125 mg/dl) over 14 weeks.

BETA-BLOCKERS

See Beta Blockers, p. 509.

CALCIUM CHANNEL BLOCKERS

See Calcium Channel Blockers, p. 521.

DIURETICS

See Diuretics, p. 525.

NIACIN

See Niacin, p. 409.

STATINS AND COMBINATION PILLS

See Statins and Combination Pills, p. 415.

STEROID-INDUCED DIABETES

See Steroid-Induced Diabetes, p. 149.

Hypertension

ANGIOTENSIN CONVERTING ENZYME (ACE) INHIBITORS

Lipika Samal, MD, MPH, and Paul A. Pham, PharmD

INDICATIONS

FDA

- Diabetic nephropathy (captopril).
- Hypertension (HTN).
- Congestive heart failure (CHF).
- See Table 4-13 for ACE inhibitor-specific FDA indications.

Mechanism

- High affinity for angiotensin converting enzyme competing with angiotensin I, the natural substrate, to block its conversion to angiotensin II. Angiotensin II is a potent vasoconstrictor and a negative feedback mediator for renin activity. Thus, as a result of lower angiotensin II plasma levels, blood pressure decreases and plasma renin activity increases.

FORMS

- See Table 4-13.

USUAL ADULT DOSING

- **Benazepril:** 10 mg once daily in patients initial dose (not on a diuretic). Usual dose: 20–40 mg in a single or 2 divided doses.
- **Captopril:** CHF/HTN: 6.25–12.5 mg 3 times a day (with diuretic) with goal of 50 mg 3 times a day. Diabetic nephropathy: 25 mg 3 times a day.
- **Enalapril:** CHF/HTN: 2.5–5 mg daily increased up to 40 mg/day every 1–2 weeks in 2.5-mg intervals. IV: 1.25 mg/dose every 6 hours for up to 36 hours.
- **Fosinopril:** CHF/HTN: 10 mg daily initially, then titrate to effect (max dose 40 mg daily). Usual dose: 20–40 mg daily.
- **Lisinopril:** HTN: 10 mg daily (no diuretic) or 5 mg daily (if on diuretic) initially. Dose range: 10–40 mg daily. CHF: Initial: 2.5–5 mg once daily; titrate by 10-mg increments every 2 weeks to target of 20–40 mg/day.
- **Moexipril:** HTN: 7.5 mg once daily (not on a diuretic) or 3.75 mg once daily (when combined with a diuretic). Administer 1 hr prior to meal. Maintenance: 7.5–30 mg daily in 1–2 divided doses
- **Perindopril erbumine:** HTN: Initial: 4 mg daily; titrate to desired effect every 1–2 weeks to a max dose of 16 mg/day. Usual dose 4–8 mg/day in 2 divided doses. Stable coronary artery disease (CAD): Initial: 4 mg once daily for 2 weeks then increase to 8 mg once daily as tolerated.
- **Quinapril:** HTN: 10–20 mg daily initially. Initial dose may be reduced to 5 mg daily (if patient on a diuretic). Range: 10–40 mg once daily. CHF: 5 mg once or twice daily; titrate to desired effect every week to a dose of 20–40 mg daily in 2 divided doses.
- **Ramipril:** HTN: 2.5–5 mg once daily (max dose of 20 mg/day). Left ventricular dysfunction (LVD) post-MI: 2.5 mg twice daily; titrate to 5 mg twice daily as tolerated. Reduced risk of stoke, MI and death: initial: 2.5 mg once daily for 1st week, then 5 mg once daily for weeks 2–4, then titrate to 10 mg once daily as tolerated.

MEDICATIONS

- **Trandolapril:** CHF/LVD Initial: 1 mg/day, titrate to 4 mg/day as tolerated. HTN: 1 mg/day initially (may use 2 mg/day in black patients); titrate to desired effect in 1-week intervals.

DOSING IN SPECIAL POPULATIONS

Renal

- CrCl 10–50 ml/min: reduce initial recommended dose by 25%, then titrate to effect.
- CrCl <10 ml/min: reduce initial recommended dose by 50%, then titrate to effect.

Hepatic

- No dosage adjustment needed.

Pregnancy

- FDA Category D. Avoid in pregnancy.
- ACE inhibitors are teratogenic and have resulted in neonatal morbidity (cardiovascular and CNS) and mortality.

Breastfeeding

- Concentration in milk is about 1% of serum concentration. Avoid ACE inhibitors during breastfeeding.

ADVERSE DRUG REACTIONS

Common

- Cardiovascular: edema, hypotension (use low dose and titrate slowly in volume contracted patients).

Occasional

- Drug-related cough (0.5%–2%)
- Endocrine/metabolic: gynecomastia, hyperkalemia
- Rash
- Renal failure
- Dermatologic: angioedema of face, lips, and throat (0.1%)
- Metallic taste (captopril)

Rare

- Hematologic: agranulocytosis, neutropenia
- Gastrointestinal: intestinal angioedema
- Eosinophilic pneumonitis
- Photosensitivity

DRUG INTERACTIONS

- ACE inhibitors may increase the hypoglycemic effects of insulin or other antidiabetic agents.
- **Potassium-sparing diuretics** (e.g., spironolactone) **and trimethoprim:** may increase risk of hyperkalemia.
- **Potassium salt:** monitor for hyperkalemia with ACE-inhibitor coadministration.
- **ARBs** (e.g., losartan, telmisartan): may increase risk of renal failure, diarrhea, hypotension, syncope, and hyperkalemia. Monitor renal function closely with ACE inhibitor and ARBs coadministration.
- **Lithium:** lithium concentration may be increased. Monitor concentrations with ACE inhibitor coadministration.
- **Pregabalin:** may increase risk of angioedema associated with ACE inhibitors. Use with close monitoring.
- **Antacid:** may decrease ACE inhibitor absorption. Separate administration time.
- **Nephrotic agents** (e.g., contrast, NSAIDs, aminoglycosides, amphoB): may increase risk of nephrotoxicity. Monitor renal function closely with coadministration.

PHARMACOKINETICS
TABLE 4-13. SPECIFIC FDA INDICATIONS, FORMS, AND PHARMACOKINETICS OF ACE INHIBITORS

Generic Name	Brand Name	FDA Indications	Formulation (tab, caps, IV)	Cost per Dose	Half-Life	Onset/ Time to Peak	Metabolism/Excretion	Protein Binding
Benazepril	Lotensin	Hypertension alone or in combination with other medications	Benazepril/ Losentin 5 mg tab, 10 mg tab, 20 mg tab, 40 mg tab	Benazepril 5 mg tab $1.05 10 mg tab $0.95 20 mg tab $0.95 40 mg tab $1.05 Lotensin 5 mg tab $1.73 10 mg tab $1.73 20 mg tab $1.73 40 mg tab $1.73	10–11 hrs	Onset/time to peak: 1–2 hrs	**Metabolism:** Pro-drug (benazepril): hepatic cleavage Active metabolite (benazeprilat): hepatic glucuronide conjugates **Excretion:** Pro-drug (benazepril): 4% renal as glucurondine conjugates. Active metabolite (benazeprilat): 11%–12% biliary & 8% renal	Benazepril: ~97%; Benazeprilat: ~95%

(Continued)

TABLE 4-13. SPECIFIC FDA INDICATIONS, FORMS, AND PHARMACOKINETICS OF ACE INHIBITORS (CONT.)

Generic Name	Brand Name	FDA Indications	Formulation (tab, caps, IV)	Cost per Dose	Half-Life	Onset/Time to Peak	Metabolism/Excretion	Protein Binding
Captopril	Capoten	Congestive heart failure, diabetic nephropathy, hypertension, and left ventricular dysfunction with myocardial dysfunction	Captopril 12.5 mg tab, 25 mg tab, 50 mg tab, 100 mg tab	Captopril 12.5 mg tab $0.69 25 mg tab $0.79 50 mg tab $1.56 100 mg tab $1.50	1.9 hrs in healthy patients; 2.06 hrs in heart failure; 20–40 hrs in anuria	Onset/time to peak: 1 hr	**Excretion:** >95% in urine with 40–50% unchanged	25%–30%
Enalapril	Vasotec	Treatment of hypertension, asymptomatic left ventricular dysfunction, and symptomatic heart failure	Enalaprilat IV 1.25 mg/ml Enalapril/Vasotec 2.5 mg tab, 5 mg tab, 10 mg tab, 20 mg tab	Enalaprilat IV 1.25 mg/ml (2 ml vial) $3.50 Enalapril 2.5 mg tab $0.89 5 mg tab $1.02 10 mg tab $1.19 20 mg tab $1.69	Pro-drug (Enalapril) healthy adults: 2 hrs; Congestive heart failure: 3.4–5.8 hrs; Active metabolite (enalaprilat): 35–38 hrs	Onset: 1 hr Time to peak: Oral: 0.5–1.5 hr; IV: 3–4.5 hr	**Metabolism:** Pro-drug hepatically metabolized to enalaprilat **Excretion:** 60%–80% urine and some in feces	50%–60%

			Vasotec 2.5 mg tab $2.17 5 mg tab $2.51 10 mg tab $2.77 20 mg tab $2.51			
Fosinopril	Monopril	Treatment of heart failure and hypertension either alone or in combination with other medications	Fosinopril 10 mg tab, 20 mg tab, 40 mg tab Monopril 10 mg tab, 20 mg, 40 mg tab	Fosinopril 10 mg tab $1.19 20 mg tab $1.19 40 mg tab $1.19 Monopril 10 mg tab $1.53 20 mg tab $1.53 40 mg tab $1.70	Active metabolite (fosinoprilat): 12 hrs	Onset: 1 hr Time to peak: 3 hrs	**Metabolism:** 95% Pro-drug (fosinopril) hydrolyzed in intestinal wall to active metabolite fosinoprilat; also undergoes hepatic metabolism **Excretion:** Urine 45% & feces 50%

(Continued)

TABLE 4-13. **SPECIFIC FDA INDICATIONS, FORMS, AND PHARMACOKINETICS OF ACE INHIBITORS** *(CONT.)*

Generic Name	Brand Name	FDA Indications	Formulation (tab, caps, IV)	Cost per Dose	Half-Life	Onset/ Time to Peak	Metabolism/Excretion	Protein Binding
Lisinopril	Zestril	Treatment of hypertension either alone or in combination with other medications, left ventricular dysfunction after MI, acute MI within 24 hrs in stable patients and adjunctive treatment with heart failure	Lisinopril/ Zestril 2.5 mg tab, 5 mg tab, 10 mg tab, 30 mg tab, 40 mg tab	Lisinopril 2.5 mg tab $0.65 5 mg tab $0.97 10 mg tab $1.00 20 mg tab $1.07 30 mg tab $1.51 40 mg tab $1.56 Zestril 2.5 mg tab $1.02 5 mg tab $1.53 10 mg tab $1.58 20 mg tab $1.69 30 mg tab $2.40 40 mg tab $2.48	11–12 hrs	Onset: 1 hr Time to peak: ~7 hrs	**Metabolism:** Not metabolized **Excretion:** Unchanged in urine	95%

Perindopril erbumine	Aceon	Perindopril erbumine/Aceon: Aceon 2 mg tab, 4 mg tab, 8 mg tab	Perindopril erbumine 2 mg tab $1.90, 4 mg tab $2.21, 8 mg tab $2.69; Aceon 2 mg tab $2.11, 4 mg tab $2.45, 8 mg tab $2.98	Treatment of hypertension and reduce mortality/nonfatal MI in patients with stable CAD	Pro-drug: 1.5–3 hrs; Metabolite: 3–10 hrs; Terminal: 30–120 hrs	Onset/time to peak: 1–2 hrs	**Metabolism:** Hepatically hydrolyzed to active metabolite perindoprilate and other active metabolites **Excretion:** 75% Urine (4%–12% unchanged)	Perindopril: 60%; Perindoprilat: 10%–20%
Quinapril	Accupril	Quinapril/Accupril 5 mg tab, 10 mg tab, 20 mg tab, 40 mg tab	Quinapril 5 mg tab $1.22, 10 mg tab $1.22, 20 mg tab $1.22, 40 mg tab $1.22	Treatment of hypertension and heart failure	Pro drug (Quinopril): 0.8 hrs; Quinaprilat: 3 hrs; however half-life may be increased with increased CrCl	Onset/time to peak: 1–2 hrs	**Metabolism:** Hydrolyzed to quinaprilat **Excretion:** 50%–60% in urine	Quinapril: 97%; Quinaprilat: 97%

(Continued)

MEDICATIONS

TABLE 4-13. SPECIFIC FDA INDICATIONS, FORMS, AND PHARMACOKINETICS OF ACE INHIBITORS *(CONT.)*

Generic Name	Brand Name	FDA Indications	Formulation (tab, caps, IV)	Cost per Dose	Half-Life	Onset/Time to Peak	Metabolism/Excretion	Protein Binding
				Accupril 5 mg tab $2.05 10 mg tab $2.05 20 mg tab $2.05 40 mg tab $2.05				
Ramipril	Altace	Treatment of hypertension alone or in combination with another medication, left ventricular dysfunction after MI, and reduce risk of stroke, MI, and death	Ramipril/Altace 1.25 mg cap, 2.5 mg cap, 5 mg cap,10 mg cap	Ramipril 1.25 mg cap $1.53 2.5 mg cap $1.71 5 mg cap $2.04 10 mg cap $2.10 Altace 1.25 mg cap $1.99 2.5 mg cap $2.35 5 mg cap $2.47 10 mg cap $2.88	Ramiprilat: 13–17 hrs Terminal: >50 hrs	Onset: 1–2 hrs Time to peak: ramipril ~ 1 hr Ramiprilat 44%	**Metabolism:** Hepatic metabolism of parent drug to active metabolite ramiprilat **Excretion:** Parent and active metabolite: 60% urine and 40% feces	Ramipril: 73%; Ramiprilat: 56%

| Trandol-april | Mavik | Treatment of hypertension alone or in combination with another medication and left ventricular dysfunction after MI | Trandolapril/ Mavik 1 mg tab, 2 mg tab, 4 mg tab | Trandolapril 1 mg tab $1.20 2 mg tab $1.20 4 mg tab $1.20 Mavik 1 mg tab $1.40 2 mg tab $1.40; 4 mg tab $1.40 | Parent drug (trandolapril): 6 hrs Active metabolite (trandolaprilat): 10 hrs Terminal: 24 hrs | Onset: 1–2 hrs Time to peak: Parent: 1hr; Active metabolite: 4–10 hrs | **Metabolism:** Hepatic metabolism of parent drug to active metabolite trandolaprilat **Excretion:** 33% urine & 66% feces | 80% |

Courtesy of Paul Pham, PharmD, Johns Hopkins University School of Medicine.

EXPERT OPINION

- Good blood pressure control is advantageous regardless of agent used.
- Our usual practice is to begin an ACE inhibitor or ARB in people with diabetes found to be hypertensive, proteinuric, or both.
- We do not use ACE inhibitors to "protect the kidneys" in all people with diabetes.
- Frequently, other antihypertensives must be added to control blood pressure.
- Numerous trials have shown that ACE inhibitors decrease microalbuminuria and slow progression of diabetic nephropathy in patients with both type 1 and type 2 diabetes (Viberti; Microalbuminaria Captopril Study group; Ravid).
- Captopril is the only FDA-approved ACE inhibitor for diabetic nephropathy although other ACE inhibitors are likely also effective.
- Several studies demonstrated that lisinopril is effective in the reducing urinary albumin excretion in diabetes (Schjoedt). Lisinopril is superior to hydrochlorothiazide in lowering blood pressure, approximately equal to atenolol and metoprolol in lowering systolic blood pressure, and equivalent to atenolol and metoprolol in lowering diastolic blood pressure.
- In a well-controlled trial of normotensive patients with type 1 diabetes and normoalbuminuria, enalapril 20 mg did not slow progression of nephropathy when compared to placebo, but progression of retinopathy was slowed (Mauer). However, other trials have shown benefit of enalapril in reducing progression of diabetic nephropathy (Ravid).
- Patients with diabetic nephropathy randomized to fosinopril achieved reduced 24-hour urine protein excretion, serum creatinine and BUN (Huang).
- Trandalopril alone and in combination with verapamil decreased the incidence of microalbuminuria over verapamil alone and placebo in type 2 diabetes with hypertension (Ruggenenti).

REFERENCES

Mauer M, Zinman B, Gardiner R, et al. Renal and retinal effects of enalapril and losartan in type 1 diabetes. *NEJM*, 2009; Vol. 361: pp. 40–51.

  Comments: Multicenter, controlled trial of 285 normotensive patients with type 1 diabetes and normoalbuminuria randomly assigned to receive losartan (100 mg daily), enalapril (20 mg daily), or placebo for 5 years. Authors found that enalapril did not slow nephropathy progression but slowed the progression of retinopathy.

Schjoedt KJ, Astrup AS, Persson F, et al. Optimal dose of lisinopril for renoprotection in type 1 diabetic patients with diabetic nephropathy: a randomised crossover trial. *Diabetologia*, 2009; Vol. 52: pp. 46–9.

  Comments: At the Steno Diabetes Center, 49 type 1 diabetic patients with diabetic nephropathy participated in double-masked randomised crossover trial with initial washout period followed by three treatment periods of 2 months each, receiving lisinopril 20, 40, and 60 mg once daily in randomised order in addition to slow-release furosemide. Compared with lisinopril 20 mg there was a further reduction in urinary albumin excretion rate of 23% with lisinopril 40 mg and 19% with 60 mg, $p < 0.05$.

Ruggenenti P, Fassi A, Ilieva AP, et al. Preventing microalbuminuria in type 2 diabetes. *NEJM*, 2004; Vol. 351: pp. 1941–51.

  Comments: Multicenter double-blind, randomized Bergamo Nephrologic Diabetes Complications Trial (BENEDICT) in subjects with hypertension, type 2 diabetes mellitus, and normal urinary albumin excretion. 1204 subjects randomly assigned to 3 years of trandalapril plus verapamil, trandalapril alone, verapamil alone or placebo. Trandolapril plus verapamil and trandolapril alone decreased the incidence of microalbuminuria to a similar extent.

Arauz-Pacheco C, Parrott MA, Raskin P, et al. Hypertension management in adults with diabetes. *Diabetes Care,* 2004; Vol. 27 Suppl 1: pp. S65–7.

Comments: American Diabetes Association recommendations for management of hypertension in diabetes.

Huang YH, Wang HT, Zhu QZ, et al. Combination therapy with losartan and fosinopril for early diabetic nephropathy. *Di Yi Jun Yi Da Xue Xue Bao,* 2003; Vol. 23: pp. 963–5.

Comments: Fifty-seven patients with diabetic nephropathy were divided equally into group A with treatment with losartan (50 mg) and fosinopril (10 mg) daily, group B with daily losartan treatment (50–100 mg), and group C with fosinopril treatment at the daily dose of 10–20 mg for 6 months. Combined use of losartan and fosinopril decreased blood pressure, 24-h urine protein excretion, serum creatinine, and BUN to a greater extent than the use of either alone.

ACE Inhibitors in Diabetic Nephropathy Trialist Group. Should all patients with type 1 diabetes mellitus and microalbuminuria receive angiotensin-converting enzyme inhibitors? A meta-analysis of individual patient data. *Ann Intern Med,* 2001; Vol. 134: pp. 370–9.

Comments: Meta-analysis concluding that ACE inhibitors improve microalbuminuria in normotensive patients with type 1 diabetes mellitus.

UK Prospective Diabetes Study Group (UKPDS). Tight blood pressure control and risk of macrovascular and microvascular complications in type 2 diabetes: UKPDS 38. *BMJ,* 1998; Vol. 317: pp. 703–13.

Comments: Captopril was administered to one of the "tight control" arms of UKPDS and this group had significantly reduced progression of diabetic retinopathy, deterioration in visual acuity, and mortality.

The Microalbuminuria Captopril Study Group. Captopril reduces the risk of nephropathy in IDDM patients with microalbuminuria. *Diabetologia,* 1996; Vol. 39: pp. 587–93.

Comments: 235 normotensive IDDM patients with microalbuminuria participated in double-blind, randomised, placebo-controlled trials to assess the effects of captopril 50 mg twice daily on the progression to overt clinical albuminuria. The risk of progression over 24 months was significantly reduced by captopril (p = 0.004) with a risk reduction of 69.2% (31.7%–86.1%).

Viberti G, Mogensen CE, Groop LC, et al. Effect of captopril on progression to clinical proteinuria in patients with insulin-dependent diabetes mellitus and microalbuminuria. European Microalbuminuria Captopril Study Group. *JAMA,* 1994; Vol. 271: pp. 275–9.

Comments: Randomized, double-blind, placebo-controlled clinical trial of 2 years' duration including 92 patients with insulin-dependent diabetes mellitus and persistent microalbuminuria but no hypertension. Patients randomly allocated to receive either captopril, 50 mg, or placebo twice per day. Progression to clinical proteinuria was significantly reduced by captopril therapy (p = .03 by log-rank test).

Lewis EJ, Hunsicker LG, Bain RP, et al. The effect of angiotensin-converting-enzyme inhibition on diabetic nephropathy. The Collaborative Study Group. *NEJM,* 1993; Vol. 329: pp. 1456–62.

Comments: Captopril protects against deterioration in renal function in insulin-dependent diabetic nephropathy as compared to other similarly effective treatments.

Ravid M, Savin H, Jutrin I, et al. Long-term stabilizing effect of angiotensin-converting enzyme inhibition on plasma creatinine and on proteinuria in normotensive type II diabetic patients. *Ann Intern Med,* 1993; Vol. 118: pp. 577–81.

Comments: 94 normotensive, type 2 diabetic patients with microalbuminuria and normal renal function randomly assigned to receive enalapril, 10 mg per day, or placebo. Difference in rate of change in proteinuria between two groups favored enalapril (p $<$0.05).

MEDICATIONS

ANGIOTENSIN RECEPTOR BLOCKERS (ARBs)

Lipika Samal, MD, MPH, and Paul A. Pham, PharmD

INDICATIONS

FDA

- Diabetic nephropathy (Irbesartan, Losartan).
- Hypertension.
- Stroke and cardiovascular risk reduction.
- Congestive heart failure.
- See Table 4-14 for ARB-specific FDA indications.

Mechanism

- Angiotensin receptor blockers (ARBs) are selective blockers of AT1 angiotensin receptors and work by blocking the binding of angiotensin II causing a decrease in systemic vascular resistance.

USUAL ADULT DOSING

- **Candesartan:** hypertension: 4–32 mg once daily initially and titrate to effect. Heart failure: Initial: 4 mg once daily. Titrate to effect by doubling dose every 3 weeks. Max dose 32 mg.
- **Eprosartan:** 600 mg once daily initially (dose should individualized). Limited data on doses greater than 800 mg.
- **Irbesartan:** hypertension: 150 mg once daily initially. Titrate to 300 mg once daily. Nephropathy: Target dose 300 mg once daily.
- **Losartan:** hypertension: 50 mg once or twice daily, dose range 25–100 mg. Diabetic nephropathy: Initial: 50 mg once daily. Dose can be increased to 100 mg once daily based on blood pressure response. Stroke reduction: Initial: 50 mg once daily. Max dose 100 mg.
- **Olmesartan:** 20 mg once daily initially. Titrate to effect after 2 weeks, the dose may be increased to 40 mg once daily.
- **Telmisartan:** hypertension: 40 mg once daily initially. Usual dose 20–80 mg daily. Cardiovascular risk reduction: Initial: 80 mg daily
- **Valsartan:** hypertension: 80–160 mg once daily initially. Max dose 320 mg daily. Cardiovascular risk reduction: 20 mg twice daily. Target dose 160 mg twice daily. Heart failure: Initial: 40 mg twice daily. Typical doses between 80–160 mg twice daily. Max dose 320 mg daily.

FORMS

- See Table 4-14 for further information.

DOSING IN SPECIAL POPULATIONS

Renal

- CrCl ≥30 ml/min: no dosage adjustment is needed.
- For adults, no dosage adjustment needed, unless the patient is also volume-depleted.

Hepatic

- Initiate therapy with 25 mg PO once daily.

Pregnancy

- FDA Category D. Avoid in pregnancy.

- Black box warning: can cause injury or death to a developing fetus when used during the second and third trimesters.

Breastfeeding

- It is not known if losartan or its metabolite are excreted into breast milk; however, significant levels are present in rat milk. Breastfeeding is not recommended during losartan therapy because of the potential for adverse effects in the infant.

ADVERSE DRUG REACTIONS

General

- Generally well tolerated.

Occasional

- Hypotension
- Dyspepsia and diarrhea
- Dizziness
- Myalgia and muscle cramps
- Renal failure (CHF and volume depletion are risk factors)
- Malaise

Rare

- Rhabdomyolysis
- Cough (less likely compared to ACE inhibitors)
- Anaphylaxis and angioedema (less likely compared to ACE inhibitors)
- Impotence
- Allergic reactions

DRUG INTERACTIONS

- Losartan and irbesartan are CYP1A2, CYP2C9, and CYP3A4 substrates. Valsartan and candesartan are only CYP2C9 substrates. Inhibitors and inducers of these CYP isoenzymes may increase and decrease the serum concentrations of these ARBs.
- **ACE inhibitors** combination therapy has been associated with an increased risk of diarrhea, hypotension, syncope, hyperkalemia, and renal dysfunction resulting in dialysis, and doubling of serum creatinine.
- **Eplerenone, potassium-sparing diuretics, and potassium** supplements coadministration may result in hyperkalemia.
- **Rifampin and phenobarbital** may decrease all ARBs serum concentrations. Monitor for therapeutic efficacy and titrate to effect.
- **CYP2C9 inhibitors** (e.g., azole antifungals, fluoxetine, sertraline, amiodarone, cimetidine) may increase serum concentrations of valsartan and candesartan. Use lowest dose and monitor closely with coadministration.
- **CYP1A2 inhibitors** (e.g., ciprofloxacin and fluvoxamine) may increase serum concentrations of losartan and irbesartan. Use lowest dose and monitor closely with coadministration.
- **CYP3A4 inhibitors** (e.g., HIV protease inhibitors, azole antifungals, macrolide antibiotics) may increase serum concentrations of losartan and irbesartan. Use lowest dose and monitor closely with coadministration.

MEDICATIONS

PHARMACOKINETICS

TABLE 4-14. SPECIFIC FDA INDICATIONS, FORMS, AND PHARMACOKINETICS OF ARBs

Generic Name	Brand Name	FDA Indications	Formulation & U.S. Cost per Unit Dose	Half-Life	Onset/Time to Peak	Metabolism/Excretion	Protein-Binding
Candesartan	Atacand	Treatment of hypertension either alone or in combination with other medications, treatment of NYHA class II–IV heart failure	Atacand 4-mg tabs ($2.32), 8-mg tabs ($2.32), 16-mg tab ($2.32), 32-mg tab ($3.13)	5–9 hrs	Onset: 2–3 Peak: 6–8	Metabolized to candesartan by intestinal wall cells Excretion: urine	99%
Eprosartan	Teveten	Treatment of hypertension either alone or in combination with other medications	Teveten 400-mg tab ($2.82), 600-mg tab ($3.30)	5–9 hrs	Peak: 1–2 hrs	Metabolized: minimal hepatic Excretion: Feces (90%), urine (7%)	98%

					Onset/		

| Irbesartan | Avapro | Treatment of hypertension either alone or in combination with other medications, treatment of Type 2 diabetic nephropathy | Avapro 75-mg tab ($3.08), 150-mg tab ($2.50), 300-mg tab ($3.00) | 11–15 hrs | Onset/Peak: 1–2 hrs | Metabolism: hepatic CYP2C9 Excretion: feces (80%) and urine (20%) | 90% |
| Losartan | Cozaar | Treatment of hypertension either alone or in combination with other medications. Treatment of Type 2 diabetic nephropathy, stroke risk reduction in hypertension and left ventricular hypertension | Cozaar 25-mg tab ($1.86), 50-mg tab ($2.39), 100-mg tab ($3.26) | Losartan 1.5–2 hrs and E 3174 (active metabolite) 6–9 hrs | Onset: 6 hrs Peak: Losartan 1 hr E 3174 (active metabolite) 6–9 hrs | Metabolism: hepatic (14%) via CYP2C9 and 3A4 to active metabolite E 3174 Excretion: Urine | Highly protein bound to albumin |

(Continued)

TABLE 4-14. SPECIFIC FDA INDICATIONS, FORMS, AND PHARMACOKINETICS OF ARBs (CONT.)

Generic Name	Brand Name	FDA Indications	Formulation & U.S. Cost per Unit Dose	Half-Life	Onset/ Time to Peak	Metabolism/ Excretion	Protein-Binding
Olmesartan	Benicar	Treatment of hypertension either alone or in combination with other medications	Benicar 5-mg tab ($2.11), 20-mg tab ($2.29), 40-mg tab ($2.89)	13 hrs	Peak: 1–2 hrs	Metabolism: hydrolysis in the GI tract to active olmesartan Excretion: Feces (50–65%) and urine (35–50%)	99%
Telmisartan	Micardis	Treatment of hypertension either alone or in combination with other medications, cardiovascular risk reduction in pts > 55 years old at risk for a major cardiovascular event	Micardis 20-mg tab ($3.00), 40-mg tab ($3.00), 80-mg tab ($3.00)	24 hrs	Onset: 1–2 hrs Peak: 0.5–1 hrs	Metabolism: Hepatic via conjugation to inactive metabolites Excretion: 97% feces	99.5%

| Valsartan | Diovan | Treatment of hypertension either alone or in combination with other medication, cardiovascular risk reduction in patients with left ventricular dysfunction post-MI and treatment of heart failure NYHA class II–IV | Diovan 40-mg tab ($2.12), 80-mg tab ($2.54), 160-mg tab ($2.73) | 6 hrs | Onset: 2 hrs Peak: 2–4 hrs | Metabolism: To inactive metabolites Excretion: 83% feces and 13% urine | 95% |

Courtesy of Paul Pham, PharmD, Johns Hopkins University School of Medicine.

EXPERT OPINION

- Only irbesartan and losartan are FDA approved for use in diabetic nephropathy, however, most ARBs are effective in the treatment of diabetic nephropathy (Lewis; Parving; Viberti; Brenner) and offer good alternatives for patients intolerant to ACE inhibitor (i.e., cough).
- Although more renal protection data are available with ACE inhibitors, a meta-analysis found that ARBs and ACE inhibitors have comparable efficacy (Sarafidis).
- Compared with ACE inhibitors, ARBs have less common occurrence of cough as a side effect, so are a reasonable alternative either as first choice or, if patients develop cough after using ACE inhibitors.

REFERENCES

Bilous R, Chaturvedi N, Sjølie AK, et al. Effect of candesartan on microalbuminuria and albumin excretion rate in diabetes: three randomized trials. *Ann Intern Med,* 2009; Vol. 151: pp. 11–20, W3–4.

Comments: In a placebo controlled study for the treatment of diabetic nephropathy in normotensive type 1 and type 2 diabetics, 32 mg/day of candesartan did not prevent microalbuminuria after 4.7 years of follow-up, but may be due to recruitment of mainly patients with well-controlled hypertension who were at low overall vascular risk, which resulted in a low rate of microalbuminuria.

Tomino Y, Kawamura T, Kimura K, et al. Antiproteinuric effect of olmesartan in patients with IgA nephropathy. *J Nephrol,* 2009; Vol. 22: pp. 224–31.

Comments: In an observational study, patients were found to have a reduction in urinary protein after a 16-week trial of olmesartan. The reduction in urinary protein was independent of BP-lowering properties.

Sarafidis PA, Stafylas PC, Kanaki AI, et al. Effects of renin-angiotensin system blockers on renal outcomes and all-cause mortality in patients with diabetic nephropathy: an updated meta-analysis. *Am J Hypertens,* 2008; Vol. 21: pp. 922–929.

Comments: A meta-analysis of 24 studies (20 using ACE inhibitors and 4 using ARBs) found that the use ACE inhibitors was associated with a trend toward reduction of ESRD incidence (RR 0.70; 0.46–1.05) and use of ARBs with significant reduction of ESRD risk (RR 0.78; 0.67–0.91). Both drug classes were associated with reduction in the risk of doubling serum creatinine.

Kaliuzhina EV, Zibnitskaia LI, Surkova LG, et al. The effectiveness of eprosartan in patients with chronic glomerulonephritis. *Klin Med* (Mosk), 2007; Vol. 85: pp. 58–61.

Comments: Limited data of eprosartan in diabetic nephropathy. A small open label study of 15 patients over 12 weeks showed a potential renal protective (defined as an antiproteinuric and antihematuric) effect at a dose of 600 mg daily.

Arauz-Pacheco C, Parrott MA, Raskin P. The treatment of hypertension in adult patients with diabetes. *Diabetes Care,* 2002; Vol. 25: pp. 134–47.

Comments: ARBs can be considered in the management of HTN in adult patients with diabetes.

Viberti G, Wheeldon NM, MicroAlbuminuria Reduction With VALsartan (MARVAL) Study Investigators. Microalbuminuria reduction with valsartan in patients with type 2 diabetes mellitus: a blood pressure-independent effect. *Circulation,* 2002; Vol. 106: pp. 672–8.

Comments: 332 patients with type 2 diabetes and microalbuminuria were randomized to receive valsartan or amlodipine, and the valsartan group reverted to normoalbuminuria at a higher rate (29.9% vs 14.5%; <0.001).

Lewis EJ, Hunsicker LG, Clarke WR, et al. Renoprotective effect of the angiotensin-receptor antagonist irbesartan in patients with nephropathy due to type 2 diabetes. *NEJM,* 2001; Vol. 345: pp. 851–60.

Comments: Irbesartan is effective in protecting against the progression of nephropathy in patients with type 2 diabetes.

Parving HH, Lehnert H, Bröchner-Mortensen J, et al. The effect of irbesartan on the development of diabetic nephropathy in patients with type 2 diabetes. *NEJM,* 2001; Vol. 345: pp. 870–8.

Comments: Irbesartan is renoprotective in patients with type 2 diabetes and microalbuminuria.

Bakris G, Gradman A, Reif M, et al. Antihypertensive efficacy of candesartan in comparison to losartan: the CLAIM study. *J Clin Hypertens* (Greenwich), 2001; Vol. 3: pp. 16–21.

> **Comments:** When given at the maximum dose, there were statistically significantly (p <0.05) higher proportions of responders in the candesartan treated patients (62.4% and 56.0%, respectively) than in the losartan group.

Brenner BM, Cooper ME, de Zeeuw D, et al. Effects of losartan on renal and cardiovascular outcomes in patients with type 2 diabetes and nephropathy. *NEJM,* 2001; Vol. 345: pp. 861–9.

> **Comments:** Reduction of Endpoints in NIDDM with the Angiotensin II Antagonist Losartan (RENAAL) study randomized 1513 patients to losartan or placebo, and the losartan group had lower primary endpoint of combined doubling of the creatinine concentration, end-stage renal disease, or death.

BETA-BLOCKERS

Paul A. Pham, PharmD

INDICATIONS

FDA

- With or without diabetes, treatment of hypertension (HTN) alone or in conjunction with other antihypertensive agents.
- Management of angina pectoris.
- Secondary prevention of post-myocardial infarction (MI).
- Supraventricular arrhythmias.
- Pheochromocytoma.
- Essential tremor.
- Prophylaxis for migraine headaches.
- Symptomatic treatment of hypertrophic subaortic stenosis.
- Mild-to-severe heart failure of ischemic or cardiomyopathic origin (carvedilol and metoprolol only).
- See Table 4–15 for specific FDA indications for each beta-blocker.

Mechanism

- Beta-blockers compete with adrenergic neurotransmitters (e.g., catecholamines) for binding at sympathetic receptor sites, which results in a decreased heart rate, cardiac output, and both systolic and diastolic blood pressure.

FORMS

- See Table 4-15.

USUAL ADULT DOSING

- JNC 7 recommended usual adult dose for the treatment of hypertension (see Table 4-15 for dosing recommendations for other indications).
- **Atenolol:** 25–100 mg once daily.
- **Bisoprolol:** 2.5–10 mg once daily.
- **Metoprolol:** 50–100 mg per day in 1–2 divided doses or metoprolol XL 50–100 mg once daily.
- **Nadolol:** 40–120 mg once daily.
- **Propranolol:** 40–160 mg in 2 divided doses or propranolol LA 60–180 mg once daily.
- **Timolol:** 20–40 mg in 2 divided doses.
- **Carvedilol:** 12.5–50 mg in 2 divided doses.
- **Labetalol:** 200–800 mg in 2 divided doses.

MEDICATIONS

DOSING IN SPECIAL POPULATIONS
Renal

- **Atenolol, bisoprolol, nadalol, and timolol** (especially with concurrent hepatic impairment): need dose adjustment with renal failure.

Hepatic

- **Metoprolol, propranolol, timolol, labetolol, and carvedilol:** need dose adjustment with hepatic insufficiency. Carvedilol should be avoided in severe hepatic impairment.

Pregnancy

- Atenolol is FDA Category D. All other beta-blockers are FDA Category C, but many experts recommend avoiding in second and third trimester of pregnancy.

Breastfeeding

- Human and/or animal data suggest that all beta-blockers are excreted into breast milk. Atenolol should be avoided in breastfeeding patients. Bisoprolol and carvedilol should be used only if the benefit outweighs the risk. The American Academy of Pediatrics considers metoprolol, nadolol, propranolol, timolol, and labetolol to be compatible with breastfeeding.

ADVERSE DRUG REACTIONS
Common

- Bronchospasm in patients with asthma and COPD
- Fatigue

Occasional

- Sinus bradycardia (AV block).
- Hypotension.
- Hyperglycemia.
- GI (e.g., diarrhea, nausea, vomiting).
- CNS side effects (e.g., dizziness, vertigo, fatigue).
- Exacerbation of peripheral vascular disease (avoid beta-blockers in patients with severe peripheral vascular disease).
- Slightly increased serum triglyceride and decrease HDL (may occur less commonly with carvedilol and labetalol).
- Depression, dreams, hallucinations (more common in elderly patients).

Rare

- CHF (especially in patients with preexisting left ventricular dysfunction)
- Agranulocytosis and thrombocytopenia
- Rash

DRUG INTERACTIONS

- The addition of other antihypertensive agents (e.g., ACE inhibitors, ARBs, calcium channel blockers, clonidine) may result in additive antihypertensive effect.
- **Insulin, sufonylureas:** beta-blockers can (1) blunt the tachycardic response to hypoglycemia; (2) exaggerate the hypertensive response to hypoglycemia due to unopposed alpha-adrenergic stimulation.
- Since beta-2 receptor blockade can decrease insulin secretion and worsen insulin sensitivity, nonselective beta-blockers (e.g., propranolol, nadolol, timolol) may decrease the efficacy of sulfonylureas such as glyburide and glipizide.
- **CYP2D6 inhibitors** (e.g., ritonavir, amiodarone, quinidine, propafenone, nicardipine, citalopram, fluoxetine) may increase serum concentrations of metoprolol, timolol, and propranolol. Use low-dose metoprolol, timolol, and propanalol with slow tritration.

PHARMACOKINETICS
TABLE 4-15. SPECIFIC FDA INDICATIONS, FORMS, AND PHARMACOKINETICS OF BETA-BLOCKERS

Cardioselective Beta-Blocker	FDA Indications	Usual Adult Dose for "Other" Indications	Dose Adjustment with Renal or Hepatic Insufficiency	Absorption, Metabolism, Excretion, T$\frac{1}{2}$	Brand Name/ Formulation/ Cost
Atenolol	Treatment of HTN alone or in conjunction with others; management of angina pectoris; secondary prevention of post-MI	**Post-MI:** Give after IV dose, with 100 mg/ day or 50 mg BID for 6–9 days after MI.	**CrCl 15–35 ml/min:** 50 mg/day max **CrCl <15 ml/ min:** 50 mg every other day max **HD:** dose after dialysis, or 25–50 mg additional dose.	**Absorption:** incomplete. **Metabolism:** limited hepatic. **Excretion:** 50% feces, 40% urine. **T$\frac{1}{2}$:** 6–9 hrs in normal renal function. Prolonged with renal impairment. 15–35 hrs in ESRD.	Tenormin. Generic available Generic: 25 mg (90 tabs): $14.99 Generic: 100 mg (90 tabs): $19.99
Bisoprolol	Treatment of HTN, alone or in combination with other agents		**CrCl, 40 ml/ min:** 2.5 mg/ day initially. Increase cautiously. Not dialyzable.	**Absorption:** rapid and almost complete. **Metabolism:** Extensively-hepatic, 20% first-pass effect. **Excretion:** 50%. **T$\frac{1}{2}$:** 9–12 hrs in normal renal function. 27–36 hrs in Clcr < 40 ml/min. 8–22 hrs in hepatic cirrhosis.	Zebeta. Generic available Generic: 5 mg (30 tabs);$35.99 Generic: 10 mg (30 tabs): $35.15

(Continued)

TABLE 4-15. SPECIFIC FDA INDICATIONS, FORMS, AND PHARMACOKINETICS OF BETA-BLOCKERS *(CONT.)*

Cardioselective Beta-Blocker	FDA Indications	Usual Adult Dose for "Other" Indications	Dose Adjustment with Renal or Hepatic Insufficiency	Absorption, Metabolism, Excretion, $T_{\frac{1}{2}}$	Brand Name/ Formulation/ Cost
Metoprolol	Treatment of angina pectoris, HTN, or hemodynamically stable acute MI. Extended release: as above, in addition to reduction of mortality and hospitalization in patients with heart failure (HYHA Class II and III) already receiving ACE inhibitor, digoxin, and/or diuretics	**Angina:** Oral: Immediate release: Initial: 50 mg twice daily; usual dosage range: 50–200 mg twice daily; maximum: 400 mg/day; increase dose at weekly intervals to desired effect. Extended release: Initial: 100 mg/ day (maximum: 400 mg/day). **Heart failure:** Oral: Extended release: Initial: 25 mg once daily (reduce to 12.5 mg once daily in NYHA class II class higher than class II); may double	May need to dose-adjust in hepatic insufficiency.	**Absorption:** rapid and complete. **Metabolism:** extensively hepatic via CYP2D6, 50% first-pass effect. **Excretion:** urine (<5% to 10%). $T_{\frac{1}{2}}$: 3–8 hrs, dependant on rate of CYP2D6 metabolism.	Toprol-XL, Lopressor. Generic available. **Immediate release:** Generic metoprolol tartrate: 25 mg (30 tabs) $12.99 Generic metoprolol tartrate: 50 mg (60 tabs): $12.99 Generic metoprolol succinate: 100 mg (60 tabs) $15.99 **Extended release:** Generic metoprolol succinate: 25 mg (30 tabs): $34.99 Generic metoprolol succinate: 50 mg (30 tabs): $33.88 Generic metoprolol succinate: 100 mg

| Metoprolol (CONT.) | dosage every 2 weeks as tolerated (maximum: 200 mg/day). **Myocardial infarction:** Acute: IV: 5 mg every 2 minutes for 3 doses in early treatment of myocardial infarction; thereafter, give 50 mg orally every 6 hours beginning 15 minutes after last IV dose and continue for 48 hours; then administer a maintenance-dose of 100 mg twice daily | (30 tabs): $41.99 Generic metoprolol succinate: 200 mg (90 tabs): $204.58 |

(Continued)

TABLE 4-15. SPECIFIC FDA INDICATIONS, FORMS, AND PHARMACOKINETICS OF BETA-BLOCKERS (CONT.)

Cardioselective Beta-Blocker	FDA Indications	Usual Adult Dose for "Other" Indications	Dose Adjustment with Renal or Hepatic Insufficiency	Absorption, Metabolism, Excretion, $T\frac{1}{2}$	Brand Name/ Formulation/ Cost
Nadolol	Treatment of HTN and angina pectoris; prophylaxis for migraine headaches	**Angina:** Oral: Initial: 40–80 mg/day, increase dosage gradually by 40–80 mg increments at 3- to 7-day intervals until optimum clinical response is obtained with profound slowing of heart rate. Doses up to 160–240 mg/ day.	**CrCl 31–40 ml/ min:** Give dose every 24–36 hrs, or give 50% of usual dose. **CrCl 10–30 ml/min:** Give ever 24–48 hrs, or give 50% of usual dose. **CrCl <10 ml/ min:** Give every 40–60 hrs, or give 25% of usual dose. **HD:** 20%–50% dialyzable. Administer dose postdialysis, or give 40 mg supplemental dose. Hepatic-impaired patients do not need adjustments.	**Absorption:** 30%–40%. **Metabolism:** not metabolized. **Excretion:** urine. **T$\frac{1}{2}$:** 10–24 hrs in normal renal function. 45 hrs in ESRD.	Corgard. Generic available. Generic 20 mg (30 tabs): $13.99 Generic 40 mg (30 tabs): $15.99 Generic 80 mg (30 tabs): $19.99 Generic 160 mg (30 tabs): $33.59

| Propranolol | Management of HTN; angina pectoris; pheo-chromocytoma; essential tremor; supraventricular arrhythmias (such as atrial fibrillation and flutter, AV nodal reentrant tachycardias), ventricular tachycardias (catecholamine-induced arrhythmias, digoxin toxicity); prevention of MI; migraine headache prophylaxis; symptomatic treatment of hypertrophic | **Hypertrophic subaortic stenosis:** Oral: 20–40 mg 3–4 times/day Inderal LA: 80–160 mg once daily. **Migraine headache prophylaxis:** Oral: Initial: 80 mg/day divided every 6–8 hours; increase by 20–40 mg/dose every 3–4 weeks to a maximum of 160–240 mg/day given in divided doses every 6–8 hours. **Pheochromo-cytoma:** Oral: 30–60 mg/day in divided doses. | Drug is not dia-lyzable, no need for additional dose postdi-alysis. In chronic liver disease patients, there is noticeable decreased heart rate on normal dose; give low initial dose, and monitor heart rate regularly. | **Absorption:** rapid and complete. **Metabolism:** he-patic via CYP2D6 and CYP1A2 to active and inactive compounds. Extensive first-pass effect. **Excretion:** urine. $T_{\frac{1}{2}}$: immediate release: 3–6 hrs. Extended release: 8–10 hrs. | Inderal. Ge-neric available. **Immediate release:** Generic 10 mg (100 tabs): $12.99 Generic 20 mg (100 tabs): $13.99 Generic 40 mg (30 tabs): $12.99 Generic 60 mg (60 tabs): $55.99 Generic 80 mg (90 tabs): $15.99 **Extended release:** Generic 60 mg (100 caps): $115.97 Generic 80 mg (100 caps): $134.99 Generic 120 mg (30 caps): $59.99 Generic 160 mg (100 caps): $219.99 |

(Continued)

TABLE 4-15. SPECIFIC FDA INDICATIONS, FORMS, AND PHARMACOKINETICS OF BETA-BLOCKERS *(CONT.)*

Cardioselective Beta-Blocker	FDA Indications	Usual Adult Dose for "Other" Indications	Dose Adjustment with Renal or Hepatic Insufficiency	Absorption, Metabolism, Excretion, $T_{\frac{1}{2}}$	Brand Name/ Formulation/ Cost
	subaortic stenosis (hypertrophic obstructive cardiomyopathy)	**Post-MI mortality reduction:** Oral: 180–240 mg/dayn 3–4 divided doses. **Stable angina:** Oral: 80–320 mg/day in doses divided 2–4 times/day Inderal LA: Initial: 80 mg once daily; maximum dose: 320 mg once daily **Tachyarrhythmias:** Oral: 10–30 mg/dose every 6–8 hours IV: 1–3 mg/dose slow IVP; repeat every			

Propranolol (CONT.)		2–5 minutes, up to a total of 5 mg; titrate initial dose to desired response.		
Timolol	**Oral:** Treatment of HTN and angina; to reduce mortality following MI; prophylaxis of migraine	**Prevention of MI:** Oral: 10 mg twice daily initiated within 1–4 weeks after infarction. **Migraine prophylaxis:** Oral: Initial: 10 mg twice daily, increase to maximum of 30 mg/day.	**CrCl <10 ml/min:** adjust dose based on clinical response, and monitor blood pressure; significant hypotensive responses have occurred in dialysis patients after receiving 20 mg by mouth daily maintenance dose. Dose reduction (up to 50%) may be needed in patients with hepatic impairment.	**Absorption:** rapid and complete. **Metabolism:** extensively hepatic; extensive first-pass effect. **Excretion:** urine. **T½:** 2–2.7 hrs. Longer in those with renal impairment.	Generic available Generic 5 mg (60 tabs): $22.99 Generic 10 mg (60 tabs): $25.99 Generic 20 mg (60 tabs): $41.99

(Continued)

TABLE 4-15. SPECIFIC FDA INDICATIONS, FORMS, AND PHARMACOKINETICS OF BETA-BLOCKERS *(CONT.)*

Mixed Alpha- and Beta-Blocker	FDA Indications	Usual Adult Dose for "Other" Indications	Dose Adjustment with Renal or Hepatic Insufficiency	Absorption, Metabolism, Excretion, $T_{\frac{1}{2}}$	Brand Name/ Formulation/ Cost
Labetalol	Treatment of mild-to-severe HTN	**HTN:** Initial: 100 mg twice daily, may increase as needed every 2–3 days. Usual dose range (JNC 7): 200–800 mg/day in 2 divided doses.	Not removed by dialysis; no need for additional dose post-dialysis. Dosage reduction may be necessary in hepatically impaired patients.	**Absorption:** complete. **Metabolism:** hepatic via glucoronide conjugation. Extensive first-pass effect. **Excretion:** urine. $T_{\frac{1}{2}}$: 6–8 hrs.	Trandate Generic available. Generic 100 mg (60 tabs): $20.99 Generic 200 mg (60 tabs): $28.99 Generic 300 mg (60 tabs): $38.99
Carvedilol	Mild-to-severe heart failure of ischemic or cardiomyopathic origin (usually in addition to standard therapy); left ventricular dysfunction following MI (clinically stable with	**Heart failure:** Oral: Immediate release: 3.125 mg twice daily for 2 weeks; if this dose is tolerated, may increase to 6.25 mg twice daily. Double the dose every 2 weeks to	No need to adjust dose in renal impairment. Use is contraindicated in patients with severe hepatic impairment.	**Absorption:** rapid and extensive. **Metabolism:** Extensively hepatic, via CYP2C9, CYP2D6, CYP3A4, and CYP2C19; 3 active metabolites; first-pass effect; plasma levels in with cirrhotic liver disease are 4–7 times higher, respectively.	Coreg immediate-release formulation has generic availability. Extended release is still brand name only. **Immediate release:** Generic 3.125 mg (30 tabs): $25.99 Generic 6.25 mg (30 tabs): $14.99

Carvedilol (*CONT.*)	LVEF <40%); management of HTN	the highest dose tolerated by patient. Maximum recommended dose: Mild-to-moderate heart failure: <85 kg: 25 mg twice daily >85 kg: 50 mg twice daily Severe heart failure: 25 mg twice daily.	**Excretion:** primarily feces. **T½:** 7–10 hrs.	Generic 12.5 mg (30 tabs): $14.99 Generic 25 mg (30 tabs): $16.00 **Extended release:** 10 mg (30 caps): $135.28, 20 mg (30 caps): $135.28, 40 mg (30 caps): $135.28, 80 mg (30 caps): $135.28

Courtesy of Paul Pham, PharmD, Johns Hopkins University School of Medicine.

MEDICATIONS

- **CYP2C9 inhibitors** (e.g., etravirine, fluconazole, ketoconazole, gemfibrozil, nicardipine) may increase serum concentrations of carvedilol. Use low-dose carvedilol with slow titration.
- **CYP3A4 inhibitors** (e.g., protease inhibitors, azole antifungal, macrolides) may increase bisoprolol serum concentrations. Use low-dose bisoprolol with slow titration.
- **Rifampin** may decrease serum concentrations of metoprolol, timolol, propranolol, carvedilol, and bisoprolol. May need to increase beta-blocker dose.
- Any agents that decreases AV nodal conduction (e.g., digoxin; disopyramide; class IC antiarrhythmics such as flecainide, propafenone) may result in additive AV nodal conduction with beta-blocker coadministration.

EXPERT OPINION

- Beta-blockers can mask symptoms of hypoglycemia (e.g., tremor, tachycardia, palpitations). Diaphoretic response to hypoglycemia is generally not masked.
- Incidence of hypoglycemia similar between captopril and atenolol (UKPDS 39), suggesting no adverse effect of beta-blockers on undetected hypoglycemia.
- Cardioselective beta-blockers (e.g., atenolol, metoprolol) bind more selectively at B1 than B2 receptors. At lower doses, cardioselective beta-blockers may be preferred in patients with diabetes and peripheral vascular disease.
- Selective beta-blockers (e.g., atenolol, metoprolol) may also have less adverse effect on glycemic control.
- Although beta-blockers may have a mildly negative effect on glycemic control, this can be easily overcome with antidiabetic therapy, and reduction of cardiovascular disease and mortality benefit post-MI have been demonstrated in people with diabetes treated with beta-blockers.
- Beta-blockers vary in their pharmacokinetic and pharmacodynamic effects, but their antihypertensive effects are comparable.
- Beta-blockers with intrinsic sympathomimetic effects (e.g., acebutolol, pindolol, and penbutolol) are generally not recommended since they do not reduce cardiovascular events as well as other beta-blockers.
- Beta-blockers may be preferred for use in patients with history of recent myocardial infarction.
- Beta-blockers may increase the risk of diabetes development by up to 28% after 6 years (Gress, Dahlof).

REFERENCES

Dahlöf B, Devereux RB, Kjeldsen SE, et al. Cardiovascular morbidity and mortality in the Losartan Intervention For Endpoint reduction in hypertension study (LIFE): a randomised trial against atenolol. *Lancet,* 2002; Vol. 359: pp. 995–1003.

> **Comments:** 9193 patients with hypertension and LVH were randomized to receive losartan-based or atenolol-based antihypertensive regimen for at least 4 years. Blood pressure reduction was comparable between the two groups with SBP and DBP decrease of ~30 and 17 mmHg, respectively. However, higher proportion of losartan versus atenolol-treated pts had fatal or nonfatal stroke (0·75, p = 0·001). Losartan was associated with less cardiovascular morbidity and death compared to atenolol. New-onset diabetes was less frequent with losartan.

Gress TW, Nieto FJ, Shahar E, et al. Hypertension and antihypertensive therapy as risk factors for type 2 diabetes mellitus. Atherosclerosis Risk in Communities Study. *NEJM,* 2000; Vol. 342: pp. 905–12.

> **Comments:** In an observational study, development of diabetes in patients treated with a beta-blocker was increased by 28% at six years.

Freemantle N, Cleland J, Young P, et al. Beta blockade after myocardial infarction: systematic review and meta regression analysis. *BMJ*, 1999; Vol. 318: pp. 1730–7.

  Comments: In this meta-analysis, beta-blockers with intrinsic sympathomimetic activity (ISA) had a reduction in cardioprotective benefit. The authors recommend against the use of beta-blocker with ISA properties (e.g., acebutolol, penbutolol, pindolol).

UK Prospective Diabetes Study Group (UKPDS) 39. Efficacy of atenolol and captopril in reducing risk of macrovascular and microvascular complications in type 2 diabetes: UKPDS 39. *BMJ*, 1998; Vol. 317: pp. 713–20.

  Comments: 1148 hypertensive patients with type 2 DM were randomized to receive captopril or atenolol to tightly control BP to a goal of <150/<85 mmHg. Captopril and atenolol were equally effective in reducing blood pressure to a mean of 144/83 mmHg and 143/81 mmHg, respectively. In addition, captopril and atenolol were equally effective in reducing the risk of macrovascular outcomes, retinopathy, and clinical grade albuminuria ≥300 mg/L. More significant weight gain was observed in the atenolol-treated patients (3.4 kg vs 1.6 kg). Although undetected hypoglycemia is a concern in beta-blocker–treated patients, the incidence was not different between captopril and atenolol.

CALCIUM CHANNEL BLOCKERS

Brian Pinto, PharmD, MBA

INDICATIONS

FDA

- Hypertension.
- See Table 4-16 for calcium channel blocker-specific indications.

NON-FDA APPROVED USES

- Diabetic nephropathy (diltiazem)

MECHANISM

- Though chemically dissimilar, all of the calcium channel blockers inhibit the influx of extracellular calcium across the myocardial and vascular smooth muscle cell membranes.
- Classes include dihydropyridine (amlodipine, felodipine, nifedipine) and non-dihydropyridine (verapamil, diltiazem).

FORMS

- See Table 4-16

USUAL ADULT DOSING

- **Amlodipine:** initial dose 5 mg daily; maximum dose 10 mg daily.
- **Nifedipine (extended-release):** initial 30 or 60 mg once daily; maximum: 90–120 mg/day.
- **Diltiazem extended-release (once daily):** initial 180–240 mg once daily; dose adjustment may be made after 14 days; maximum: 480 mg/day.
- **Verapamil (immediate-release):** 80–320 mg/day divided in two daily doses.
- **Verapamil (extended-release):** 120–480 mg/day in 1–2 divided doses.

DOSING IN SPECIAL POPULATIONS

Renal

- Verapamil clearance may be reduced in patients with advanced renal failure.
- Diltiazem is not removed by dialysis; no supplemental dose needed.

Hepatic

- Verapamil dosage should be decreased to 30% of the normal dose.
- Amlodipine should be initiated at 2.5 mg oral daily for hypertension.

MEDICATIONS

- Nifedipine clearance is reduced in patients with cirrhosis, which may result in increased drug exposure.
- Diltiazem half-life is increased in patients with cirrhosis.

Pregnancy
- Amlodipine, nifedipine, felodipine, verapamil, and diltiazem are Class C.

Breastfeeding
- Diltiazem and nifedipine are known to be excreted in breast milk.

ADVERSE DRUG REACTIONS

Common
- Edema (amlodipine, nifedipine, felodipine)
- Bradycardia (verapamil, diltiazem)
- Constipation (verapamil)

DRUG INTERACTIONS
- **Potent CYP3A4 inhibitors** have the potential to significantly reduce the metabolism of dihydropyridine calcium channel blockers leading to increased or prolonged effects of these agents.
- **Grapefruit juice** and nifedipine should be avoided in combination.. Studies demonstrate significant increases in plasma concentrations.

PHARMACOKINETICS

TABLE 4-16. SPECIFIC FDA INDICATIONS, FORMS, AND PHARMACOKINETICS OF CALCIUM CHANNEL BLOCKERS

Dihydro-pyridine	FDA Indications	Pharmacoki-netics	Pregnancy Risk Category/ Breast-feeding Risk	Cost and Formulation
Amlodipine	Treatment of HTN; treatment of chronic stable angina	**A:** ~ 65% oral **M:** extensive oxidative metabolism **E:** 60% renal, 25% fecal $T\frac{1}{2} =$ 30- 50 hours	Category C. Excretion in breast milk unknown	Generic available 2.5 mg (30 tab): $5.69, 5 mg (30 tab): $7.67, 10 mg (30 tab): $8
Nifedipine (extended-release)	Treatment of HTN	**A:** 65–90% **M:** Hepatic via CYP3A4 **E:** urine 60–80% $T\frac{1}{2} = 7$ hrs	Category C. Enters breastmilk (AAP considers compatible)	Generic extended-release 30 mg (30 tab): $38, 60 mg (30 tab): $60, 90 mg (30 tab): $68

Dihydro-pyridine	FDA Indications	Pharmacokinetics	Pregnancy Risk Category/ Breast-feeding Risk	Cost and Formulation
Felodipine	Treatment of HTN	**A:** 100% **M:** CYP3A4 substrate, extensive first-pass **E:** urine 70% as metabolites $T\frac{1}{2}$ = 10–16 hours	Category C. Enters breast milk/ not recommended	Generic available 2.5 mg (30 tab): $43, 5 mg (30 tab): $50, 10 mg (30 tab): $ 57.72

Non-dihydro-pyridine	FDA Indications	Pharmacokinetics	Pregnancy Risk Category/ Breast-feeding Risk	Cost and Formulation
Verapamil	Treatment of HTN, angina pectoris, supraventricular tachyarrhythmia	**A:** 90% **M:** extensive first-pass via multiple CYP isoenzymes **E:** urine 70% as metabolites $T\frac{1}{2}$: 5–12 hours, 14–16 hours (severe hepatic impairment)	Category C. Enters breastmilk. WHO Rating: compatible AAP Rating: usually compatible	Generic available Verapamil, 24 hr capsule 100 mg (100): $149.98, 120 mg (30): $27.31, 180 mg (30): $26.99, 200 mg (30): $72.91, 240 mg (30): $27.43, 300 mg (30): $104.09, 360 mg (30): $62.99
Diltiazem	Treatment of HTN, chronic stable angina, or angina from coronary spasm	**A:** ~95% **M:** extensive first-pass metabolism **E:** urine 35% $T\frac{1}{2}$: 5–10 hours	Category C. Enters breastmilk. AAP Rating: compatible	Generic capsule available120 mg (30): $23.99, 180 mg (30): $27.99, 240 mg (30): $43.99, 300 mg (30): $75.99

A = absorption; M = metabolism; E = excretion; AAP = American Academy of Pediatrics
Courtesy of Paul Pham, PharmD, Johns Hopkins University School of Medicine.

MEDICATIONS

EXPERT OPINION

- While dihydropyridine calcium channel blockers (e.g., nifedipine and amlodipine) may worsen proteinuria, in contrast, nondihydropyridine calcium channel blockers (e.g., diltiazem and verapamil) may reduce overt proteinuria in diabetic nephropathy (Bakris; Smith; Remuzzi).
- Non-dihydropyridine calcium channel blockers are considered second-line therapy for diabetic nephropathy and may be best used in combination with ACE inhibitors (Ruggenenti).
- Immediate-release nifedipine and nisoldipine should not be used for acute blood pressure reduction due to increased risk of adverse events (e.g., death, stroke, acute myocardial infarction) (Estacio).
- Calcium channel blockers (e.g., verapamil, diltiazem) may be associated with hyperglycemia as an uncommon side effect; however, this does not usually preclude their use in diabetes given its benefit as a potent antihypertensive agent (Louters, Levine).

REFERENCES

Louters LL, Stehouwer N, Rekman J, et al. Verapamil inhibits the glucose transport activity of GLUT1. *J Med Toxicol*, 2010; 6: 100–5.

   Comments: Discusses the association of verapamil with hyperglycemia, and contribution in a dose-dependent manner of GLUT1 transport activity inhibition.

Levine M, Boyer EW, Pozner CN, et al. Assessment of hyperglycemia after calcium channel blocker overdoses involving diltiazem or verapamil. *Crit Care Med*, 2007; 35: 2071–5.

   Comments: Severity of calcium channel blocker (dilitazem, verapamil) overdose correlated directly with resulting serum glucose concentrations, with a median increase in blood glucose of 71%.

Ruggenenti P, Fassi A, Ilieve AP, et al. Preventing microalbuminuria in type 2 diabetes. *N Engl Med*. 2004; 351: 1941–51.

   Comments: In persons with type 2 diabetes and hypertension but with normoalbuminuria, the use of trandolapril plus verapamil and trandolapril alone were similarly associated with a lower incidence of microalbuminuria. The effect of verapamil alone was no different from placebo.

Remuzzi G, Schieppati A, Ruggenenti P. Clinical practice. Nephropathy in patients with type 2 diabetes. *N Engl J Med*, 2002; 346: 1145–51.

   Comments: Discusses treatment of diabetic nephropathy with various agents including calcium channel blockers.

Estacio RO, Jeffers BW, Hiatt WR, et al. The effect of nisoldipine as compared with enalapril on cardiovascular outcomes in patients with non-insulin-dependent diabetes and hypertension. *N Engl J Med*, 1998; 338: 645–52.

   Comments: In a population of patients who had diabetes and hypertension, calcium channel blockers (nisoldipine) were associated with a higher incidence of fatal and nonfatal myocardial infarction compared to enalapril.

Smith AC, Toto R, Bakris GL. Differential effects of calcium channel blockers on size selectivity of proteinuria in diabetic glomerulopathy. *Kidney Int*, 1998; 54: 889–96.

   Comments: This study found that use of diltiazem, but not nifedipine, led to sustained reductions in proteinuria in diabetic nephropathy, by improving glomerular size.

Bakris GL. Renal effects of calcium antagonists in diabetes mellitus. An overview of studies in animal models and in humans. *Am J Hypertens*, 1991; 4: 487S–93S.

   Comments: Reviews use of calcium channel blockers in diabetes.

DIURETICS

Lipika Samal, MD, MPH, and Paul A. Pham, PharmD

INDICATIONS

FDA

- Hypertension.
- Congestive heart failure.
- See Table 4-17 for diuretic-specific FDA indications.

Mechanism

- Diuretics are classified according to their mechanism: thiazide diuretics, loop diuretics, distal tubule or potassium-sparing diuretics, osmotic diuretics, and carbonic anhydrase inhibitors.
- **Thiazide diuretics** increase the excretion of sodium, chloride, and water by inhibiting both sodium ion transport across the renal tubular epithelium and active chloride reabsorption.
- **Loop diuretics** inhibit the reabsorption of sodium and chloride by interfering with the chloride-binding of the Na+/K+/2Cl-cotransport system.
- **Potassium-sparing diuretics** either inhibit the sodium-potassium ion exchange mechanism in the distal renal tubule independently of aldosterone (amiloride and triamterene) or only in the presence of aldosterone (spironolactone).
- **Osmotic diuretics** increase the osmotic pressure of the glomerular filtrate and inhibit reabsorption of water and solutes.
- **Carbonic anhydrase inhibitors** decrease hydrogen ion concentrations in the renal tubule lumen and increase excretion of bicarbonate, sodium, potassium, and water.

USUAL ADULT DOSING

- **Hydrochlorothiazide:** 12.5–50 mg/day.
- **Chlorothiazide:** 125–250 mg daily initially. Can titrate up to 500 mg daily.
- **Metolazone:** 2.5–10 mg once daily (max 20 mg once daily for edema). For HTN: 2.5–5 mg/dose once daily.
- **Spironolactone:** 25–200 mg/day in 1–2 divided doses (edema); HTN: 25–50 mg/day in 1–2 divided doses. Heart failure (NYHA Class III, IV): 12.5–25 mg/day (max 50 mg).
- **Triamterene:** 50–100 mg/day (max 300 mg/day).
- **Furosemide:** for edema/heart failure, initially 20–80 mg/dose (edema/heart failure); if response not adequate, may increase dose by 20–40 mg/dose every 6–8 hours (max 600 mg/day).
- **Bumetanide:** for edema/heart failure, initially 0.5–2 mg/dose (max dose 10 mg/day) 1–2 times/day.

FORMS

- See Table 4-17 for more information.

ADVERSE DRUG REACTIONS

Occasional

- Hypokalemia, hyponatremia, and hypochloremic alkalosis (thiazide and loop diuretics)
- Hyperkalemia (potassium-sparing diuretics)
- Photosensitivity
- Profound diuresis resulting in dehydration and prerenal acute tubular necrosis (more common with loop diuretics)

MEDICATIONS

PHARMACOKINETICS
TABLE 4-17. SPECIFIC FDA INDICATIONS, FORMS, AND PHARMACOKINETICS OF DIURETICS

Thiazide Diuretics	FDA Indications	Pharmacokinetics	Pregnancy Risk Category/Breast-feeding Risk	Cost and Formulation
Hydrochlorothiazide	Treatment of mild to moderate HTN; treatment of edema in heart failure and nephrotic syndrome	**A:** ~50–80% **M:** minimal metabolism **E:** Urine T½ = 5.6–14.8 hrs	Category B Enters breast milk/use caution	Generic available. 12.5 mg (30 cap): $36.71, 25mg (100 tab): $12.99, 50 mg (100 tab): $15.99
Chlorothiazide	Management of mild to moderate HTN; adjunct treatment for edema	**A:** poor **M:** saturable. Single dose 250 or 500 mg has similar systemic absorption **E:** urine. T½ = 1–2 hrs.	Category C, but most experts do not recommend. Enters breast milk; use caution	Generic tablets available. Oral suspension still brand. 250 mg (30 tab): $12.99, 500 mg (30 tab): $13.99
Metolazone	Management of mild-to-moderate hypertension; treatment of edema in heart failure and nephrotic syndrome, impaired renal function	**A:** 40–65% **M:** minimal metabolism **E:** urine. T½ = 20 hrs	Category B Enters breast milk; not recommended.	Generic available. 2.5 mg (30 tab): $42.99, 5 mg (30 tab): $37.37

Potassium-sparing Diuretics	FDA Indications	Pharmacokinetics	Pregnancy Risk Category/Breast-feeding Risk	Cost and Formulation
Spironolactone	Management of edema associated with excessive aldosterone excretion; hypertension; primary hyperaldosteronism; hypokalemia; cirrhosis of liver accompanied by edema or ascites; nephritic syndrome; severe heart failure (NYHA class III–IV) to increase survival and reduce hospitalization when added to standard therapy	**A:** 73% **M:** hepatic, multiple metabolites **E:** urine and feces **T½:** 1.3–2 hrs. Active metabolites **T½** = >10 hrs.	Category C (teratogenic in animal studies) Enters breast milk	Generic available 25 mg (30 tabs): $15.99, 50 mg (30 tabs): $21.99
Triamterene	Alone or in combination with other diuretics in treatment of edema and hypertension; decreases potassium excretion caused by kaliuretic diuretics	**A:** rapid **M:** rapid metabolism **E:** < 50% by urine, the rest by biliary/fecal **T½:** 1–2 hrs	Category C No data available in breastfeeding	No generic available. Brand: Dyrenium. 50 mg (30 caps): $44.09, 100 mg (30 caps): $67.24

(Continued)

TABLE 4–17. SPECIFIC FDA INDICATIONS, FORMS, AND PHARMACOKINETICS OF DIURETICS (CONT.)

Loop Diuretics	FDA Indications	Pharmacokinetics	Pregnancy Risk Category/Breast-feeding Risk	Cost and Formulation
Furosemide	Management of edema associated with heart failure and hepatic or renal disease; acute pulmonary edema; treatment of hypertension (alone or in combination with other antihypertensives)	**A:** erratic **M:** minimally hepatic **E:** urine, feces **T½:** 0.5–2 hrs	Category C. Enters breast-milk/use caution	Generic available, in both tablet and solution form. 10 mg/ml (60 ml): $17.99, 10 mg/ml (120 ml): $15.98, 20 mg (100 tabs): $13.99, 40 mg (100 tabs): $13.99, 80 mg (30 tabs): $12.99
Bumetanide	Management of edema secondary to heart failure or hepatic or renal disease including nephritic disease; may be used alone or in combination with antihypertensives for treatment of HTN; can be used in furosemide-allergic patients.	**A:** 85–95% absorbed **M:** partially hepatic **E:** urine **T½:** 1–1.5 hrs	Category C. (per manufacturer); D (per expert analysis)Excretion in breast milk unknown; use caution	Generic available 0.5 mg (90 tabs): $17.00, 1 mg (90 tabs): $28.97, 2 mg (30 tabs): $20.99, 2 mg (100 tabs) $82.39

PK = pharmacokinetics; A = absorption; M = metabolism; E = excretion.
Courtesy of Paul Pham, PharmD, Johns Hopkins University School of Medicine.

- Gynecomastia (spirinolactone)
- Loss of blood glucose control (thiazides)

Rare
- Sulfa cross-allergy
- Ototoxicity (loop diuretics, especially with aminoglycoside coadministration)
- Hyperuricemia (loop diuretics)

DRUG INTERACTIONS
- **Lithium:** all diuretics may increase lithium serum concentration. Coadminister with close monitoring for lithium toxicity and serum concentrations.
- **Thiazide and loop diuretics–amiodarone:** hypokalemia may reduce the effect of amiodarone, or cause it to become arrhythmogenic.
- **Thiazide and loop diuretics–dofetilide:** electrolyte imbalance can cause pro-arrhythmic events. Dofetilide clearance reduced by 16%.
- **Potassium-sparing diuretics (e.g., spironolactone, triamterene) interactions:** coadministration with eplerenone, angiotensin II receptor antagonists, ACE inhibitors, tacrolimus, trimethoprim, and cyclosporine can cause hyperkalemia. Use with close monitoring for hyperkalemia. Lithium clearance may be decreased with potassium-sparing diuretics.
- **Furosemide-bile acid sequestrants:** colestipol and cholestyramine decrease furosemide bioavailability by 80% and 95%, respectively. Avoid coadministration.
- **Furosemide-sucralfate:** sucralfate may significantly decrease furosemide serum concentrations.
- **Furosemide-risperidone:** several trials involving elderly patients with dementia-related psychosis observed an increased mortality with furosemide and risperidone coadministration.
- Agents that result in electrolyte wasting (e.g., amphotericin, foscarnet) may worsen hypokalemia with diuretics coadministration.

EXPERT OPINION
- Tight blood pressure control is advantageous regardless of agent used, with target generally considered to be <130/80.
- Diuretics modestly decrease HDL.
- Thiazide diuretics, particularly in the setting of hypokalemia, increase insulin resistance such that treatment of blood glucose may have to be intensified.
- A number of studies show that conventional dose thiazide diuretics decrease insulin sensitivity (Pollare).
- However, the benefits of thiazide diuretics on hypertension are considered to outweigh the relatively minor effect on blood glucose.
- However, studies comparing low-dose thiazide (bendrofluazide) to conventional dose show that low dose is as effective with less adverse metabolic effects (Harper).

REFERENCES
ACCORD Study Group, Cushman WC, Evans GW, et al. Effects of intensive blood-pressure control in type 2 diabetes mellitus. *NEJM*, 2010; Vol. 362: pp. 1575–85.

Comments: The ACCORD study randomly assigned people at high risk for CVD with diabetes to target more or less tight BP control. With average systolic BP <119, there was no added benefit over average systolic BP 133 mmHg.

MEDICATIONS

Barzilay JI, Davis BR, Cutler JA, et al. Fasting glucose levels and incident diabetes mellitus in older nondiabetic adults randomized to receive 3 different classes of antihypertensive treatment: a report from the Antihypertensive and Lipid-Lowering Treatment to Prevent Heart Attack Trial (ALLHAT). *Arch Intern Med,* 2006; Vol. 166: pp. 2191–201.

Comments: A post hoc analysis that suggested that chlorthalidone causes impaired glucose metabolism in people who do not have preexisting diabetes.

Kasiske BL, Ma JZ, Kalil RS, et al. Effects of antihypertensive therapy on serum lipids. *Ann Intern Med,* 1995; Vol. 122: pp. 133–41.

Comments: A meta-analysis that suggested that diuretics produce a small (0.08 mmol/L) deleterious effect on HDL cholesterol level in patients with diabetes.

Harper R, Ennis CN, Heaney AP, et al. A comparison of the effects of low and conventional-dose thiazide diuretic on insulin action in hypertensive patients with NIDDM. *Diabetologia,* 1995; Vol. 38: pp. 853–9.

Comments: A small trial reporting similar efficacy and decreased metabolic side effects using low-dose thiazide diuretic (bendrofluazide) as compared to a conventional dose.

Pollare T, Lithell H, Berne C A comparison of the effects of hydrochlorothiazide and captopril on glucose and lipid metabolism in patients with hypertension. *NEJM,* 1989; Vol. 321: pp. 868–73.

Comments: A small trial showing that hydrochlorothiazide decreases insulin sensitivity at conventional dose.

ACETYLCYSTEINE

Lipika Samal, MD, MPH, and Paul A. Pham, PharmD

INDICATIONS

FDA

- Adjuvant mucolytic therapy for patients with abnormal, viscid, or inspissated mucous secretions secondary to respiratory diseases such as emphysema, tuberculosis, and bronchitis, or for treatment of respiratory complications of cystic fibrosis and tracheostomy care.

Non-FDA Approved Uses

- Nephrotoxicity prophylaxis (focus of this section)
- Acetaminophen overdose

USUAL ADULT DOSING

- For nephrotoxicity prophylaxis in patients with chronic renal insufficiency (including persons with diabetes) before CT scan with nonionic, low-osmolality contrast agent: 600 mg PO twice daily, given the day prior to and the day of administration of the contrast agent (total of 4 doses).
- Prevention of contrast-associated nephropathy in patients (including persons with diabetes) undergoing angioplasty: 1200-mg IV bolus before angioplasty followed by 1200 mg PO twice daily for the 48 hours following angioplasty.

FORMS

Brand Name (mfr)	Preparation	Forms†	Cost*
Mucomyst (Bristol-Myers Squibb and various generic manufacturers)	acetylcysteine	oral/inhalation vial 30 ml 20% or 200 mg/ml 10% or 100 mg/ml	$12.00 $6.49
Acetadote (Cumberland Pharmaceutical)	acetylcysteine	IV vial 200 mg/ml (30 ml)	$181.25

*Prices represent cost per unit specified, are representative of "Average Wholesale Price" (AWP).
†Dosage is indicated in mg unless otherwise noted.

DOSING IN SPECIAL POPULATIONS

Renal

- Usual dose

Hepatic

- Although there was a 3-fold increase in acetylcysteine plasma concentrations in patients with hepatic cirrhosis, no acetylcysteine dose reduction is recommended.

MEDICATIONS

Pregnancy
- FDA pregnancy risk Category B. Does not cross the placenta and case report of pregnant patients receiving acetylcysteine to treat acetaminophen overdose has found acetylcysteine to be safe and effective.

Breastfeeding
- Avoid. It is not known if acetylcysteine is distributed into human milk.

ADVERSE DRUG REACTIONS

Common
- Strong odor of "rotten eggs" can cause dysgeusia in many patients. Dilute the solution prior to oral administration as recommended to help mask the odor.
- Gastrointestinal: diarrhea, nausea (2%–7%), vomiting (9%–12%).

Occasional
- Acute flushing and erythema of the skin during infusion. No intervention is needed.
- Respiratory: bronchospasm and respiratory distress (with inhaled acetylcysteine). Use inhaled acetylcysteine with caution in patient with history of bronchospasm and asthma.
- Anaphylactoid reaction (0.1%–19%): generally occurs in the first hour of IV acetylcysteine bolus. Consider diphenhydramine and slowing the infusion over 1 hour.

Rare
- Neurologic: status epilepticus (association unclear)
- Cardiovascular: abnormal ECG, decreased cardiac function (association unclear)
- Dermatologic: pruritus and urticaria

DRUG INTERACTIONS
- **Nitroglycerin:** pharmacologic effect of nitrates may be increased. Use with close monitoring.
- **Charcoal:** may decrease the serum concentrations of acetylcysteine.

PHARMACOKINETICS
- **Absorption:** 6% to 10% (oral)
- **Metabolism and excretion:** Hepatic metabolism and 30% renal excretion
- **Protein binding:** 83%
- **T$\frac{1}{2}$:** 5.6 hrs
- **Distribution:** Vd = 0.47 L/kg

EXPERT OPINION
- Also known as N-acetylcysteine or N-acetyl-L-cysteine (abbreviated as NAC).
- Patients with diabetic nephropathy are often subject to multiple diagnostic contrast studies (e.g., CT scan, cardiac catherization); in these patients, acetylcysteine should be considered to prevent contrast-associated nephropathy in addition to adequate hydration where possible, with careful monitoring of renal function afterwards.
- May be especially useful in patients who have problems with volume overload (i.e., comorbid congestive heart failure) and may not be good candidates for pre- and poststudy hydration to prevent contrast-induced nephropathy.
- Incidence of contrast-induced nephropathy significantly reduced in patients with chronic renal insufficiency given oral acetylcysteine compared to placebo (2% vs 21%; Tepel).
- Also, effective in prevention of contrast-induced nephropathy prior to angioplasty when given intravenously (8% vs 15%; Marenzi).

BASIS FOR RECOMMENDATIONS

Marenzi G, Assanelli E, Marana I, et al. N-acetylcysteine and contrast-induced nephropathy in primary angioplasty. *NEJM,* 2006; Vol. 354: pp. 2773–82.

Comments: In patients undergoing angioplasty (large contrast load) after acute myocardial infarction, lower incidence of nephrotoxicity (Scr increased >25% from baseline) was observed with high-dose (1200 mg twice daily) acetylcysteine group compared to standard-dose (600 mg twice daily) group (15% vs 8%, p <0.001).

Tepel M, van der Giet M, Schwarzfeld C, et al. Prevention of radiographic-contrast-agent-induced reductions in renal function by acetylcysteine. *NEJM,* 2000; Vol. 343: pp. 180–4.

Comments: In patients with chronic renal insufficiency, acetylcysteine (600 mg twice daily × 48 hrs) plus hydration were effective in preventing contrast-induced nephropathy compared to control (2% vs 21%, p = 0.01).

Neuropathy

TREATMENT OF NEUROPATHIC PAIN

Michael Polydefkis, MD, MHS, and Brian Pinto, PharmD, MBA

INDICATIONS

FDA

- **Pregabalin** for painful diabetic polyneuropathy (DPN).
- **Duloxetine** for painful DPN.

Non-FDA Approved Uses

- **Gabapentin** most commonly used non-FDA approved medication (Backonja).
- Non FDA-approved DPN pain medications include antidepressants, opiates or opiate-like agents, and anti epileptic medications.
- **Antidepressants** include tricyclic antidepressants (amitriptyline, nortriptyline) and selective serotonin and norepinephrine reuptake inhibitors (SNRIs: venlafaxine, duloxetine).
- **Antiepileptic** medications include gabapentin, valproate, lamotrigine, carbamazepine, phenytoin, and lacrosamide.
- **Opiate** or opiate-derivative agents include oxycodone, morphine sulfate, hydromorphone, fentanyl, and tramadol.
- Other agents include topical agents (lidocaine cream, lidoderm patches), neutriceuticals (Metanx, alpha-lipoic acid), and devices (spinal stimulators, transcutaneous electrical nerve stimulation).

MECHANISM

- **Pregabalin:** GABA analog with affinity for the alpha2-delta subunit of voltage-gated calcium channels.
- **Duloxetine:** selective serotonin and norepinephrine reuptake inhibitor.
- **Gabapentin:** unknown.

USUAL ADULT DOSING

- **Pregabalin:** start 50 mg three times a day, then titrate to 100 mg three times a day if tolerated after one week. Pregabalin ~6 times more potent than gabapentin (i.e., 1800 mg gabapentin = 300 mg pregabalin) with more rapid onset. Can be dosed twice a day.
- **Duloxetine:** start 30 mg for one week, then increase to 60 mg if needed. Doses >60 mg/day have relatively modest additional pain relief but associated with more side effects. Benefit as early as 1–2 weeks after initiating treatment but continues until 4–6 weeks before plateauing. Taken once daily in morning since bedtime doses can result in insomnia.
- **Gabapentin:** start 300 mg (one tablet) at bedtime, additional tablets added first at the morning dose, then in the afternoon with dose increased every 2–3 days. Stop titration if patients either experience pain relief or develop side effects such as sedation. Usual

effective dose 1800 mg/day given in three divided doses of 600 mg. Higher doses (up to 5 grams/day) rarely effective.

- **Tricyclic antidepressants:** amitriptyline is the prototype. Requires long titration schedules of 6–8 weeks before efficacy seen (Wernicke).
- **Antiepileptic agents:** similar pain relief as gabapentin or pregabalin but with more side effects (i.e., phenytoin [Sindrup]). Many older agents also require monitoring of serum levels with potential bone marrow toxicity and multiple drug interactions.

FORMS

Brand Name (mfr)	Generic	Forms†	Cost*
Lyrica (Pfizer)	Pregabalin	oral capsule 25, 50, 75, 100, 150, 200, 225, 300	$225 (90 tabs)
Cymbalta (Eli Lilly)	Duloxetine	oral capsule 20 oral capsule 30 oral capsule 60	$300 (60 tabs) $168 (30 tabs) $168 (30 tabs)
Neurontin (Pfizer, Various Generic)	Gabapentin	oral capsule 100 oral capsule 300 oral capsule 400 oral capsule 600 oral capsule 800 oral capsule 250/5 ml	$53 (100 tabs) $133 (100 tabs) $160 (100 tabs) $73 (90 tabs) $93 (90 tabs) $160 (470 ml)

*Prices represent cost per unit specified, are representative of "Average Wholesale Price" (AWP).
†Dosage is indicated in mg unless otherwise noted.

- **Opiate and opiate-like agents:** can be given alone or in combination with acetaminophen for synergistic effects, allowing for similar pain relief with lower doses of opiate-like agents.
- **Topical agents:** no systemic absorption and lower rates of side effects or drug interactions. Capsaicin applied to the painful area 2–4 times per day. Lidoderm patches applied to painful areas on a 12 hour on/off schedule.
- **Neutraceuticals:** supplements have not been systematically studied in controlled trials. Exception is alpha lipoic acid, which demonstrates benefit on neuropathy symptom severity, with trend toward improved symptoms at >600 mg daily using pharmaceutical-grade alpha lipoic acid (not available in US) (Ziegler).
- **Devices:** spinal cord stimulators not associated with systemic side effects although invasive and expensive. Additional studies needed (Tesfaye). Other approaches being investigated include near infrared light therapy. Not subject to FDA approval process with potential for inappropriate marketing.

MEDICATIONS

DOSING IN SPECIAL POPULATIONS
Renal
- Duloxetine not recommended for GFR <30 ml/min.
- See Tables 4–19 and 4–20 for gabapentin and pregabalin renal dosage adjustments.

Hepatic
- Duloxetine is hepatically metabolized; use with caution in liver disease.

Pregnancy
- All (gabapentin, pregabalin, duloxetine) Category C.

Breastfeeding
- All: infant risk cannot be ruled out (Thomson).

ADVERSE DRUG REACTIONS
General
- Duloxetine CONTRAINDICATED with concomitant use of MAO inhibitors, and black box warning for pediatric patients and increased risk of suicidal thinking. Duloxetine also contraindicated with uncontrolled narrow-angle glaucoma. Other warnings include hepatotoxicity, orthostatic hypotension, and abnormal bleeding.
- Pregabalin warnings include angioedema, hypersensitivity reactions, withdrawal seizures, suidical behavior, and peripheral edema.
- Gabapentin warnings include suicidal behavior, withdrawal seizures, and tumorigenic potential in preclinical studies with unclear clinical significance.

Common
- Pregabalin: edema, weight gain, constipation, increased appetite, sedation, dizziness.
- Gabapentin: edema, sedation, dizziness, fatigue, fever.
- Duloxetine: constipation, dizziness, headache, sedation, fatigue, nausea, dry mouth.

Rare
- Pregabalin: angioedema (especially with concomitant ACE inhibitor use) can be serious
- Gabapentin: Stevens-Johnson syndrome, suicidal thoughts, drug-induced coma

DRUG INTERACTIONS
- Gabapentin and pregabalin have no major drug interactions that require dosage adjustments.
- Duloxetine is contraindicated with MAO inhibitors (i.e., isocarboxazid, linezolid, moclobemide, phenelzine, procarbazine, rasagiline, selegiline, tranylcypromine)
- Inhibitors of CYP1A2 (i.e., cimetidine, quinolone antibotics) and CYP2D6 (i.e., fluoxetine) should be avoided.
- Pregabalin may increase risk of angioedema with concomitant use of ACE inhibitors.

PHARMACOKINETIC
TABLE 4-18. PHARMACOKINETICS

Drug	Absorption	Metabolism	Excretion	Half-Life
Pregabalin	>90%	Minimal hepatic metabolism	90% renal unchanged	6.3 hours
Duloxetine	Well absorbed	Via CYP1A2, 2D6 to inactive metabolites	~70% renal unchanged, 20% feces	12 hours
Gabapentin	50%–60%	No hepatic metabolism	Renal unchanged	5–7 hours
Courtesy of Paul Pham, PharmD, Johns Hopkins University School of Medicine.				

TABLE 4-19. PREGABALIN RENAL DOSAGE ADJUSTMENT

GFR (ml/min)	Total Daily Dose (mg)	Dosage Regimen
>60	150–600	two or three times a day
0–60	75–300	two or three times a day
15–30	50–150	once or twice daily
<15	25–75	once daily

Courtesy of Paul Pham, PharmD, Johns Hopkins University School of Medicine.

TABLE 4-20. GABAPENTIN RENAL DOSAGE ADJUSTMENT

GFR (ml/min)	Total Daily Dose (mg)	Dosage Regimen
>60	300–1200	three times a day
30–60	200–700	twice daily
15–30	200–700	once daily
<15	100–300	once daily

Courtesy of Paul Pham, PharmD, Johns Hopkins University School of Medicine.

EXPERT OPINION

- General principles: start with the lowest effective dose and titrate; higher doses generally associated with increasing side effects.
- Treatment focused on reducing pain levels (i.e., level of ~3 on a 0 to 10 visual analog scale [VAS]) to improve quality of life and functional limitations, rather than complete pain resolution, which is less realistic.
- In general, number needed-to-treat analyses suggest that neuropathic agents have similar degrees of efficacy, so side effect profiles, titration schedules, potential drug interactions, and cost often play a central role in choosing an agent.
- New guidelines released by the American Academy of Neurology in 2011 suggest that pregabalin is established as effective and should be offered for DPN; venlafaxine, duloxetine, amitriptyline, gabapentin, valproate, opioids (morphine sulfate, tramadol, and oxycodone controlled-release), and capsaicin are probably effective and should be considered for DPN (Bril).
- Gabapentin and pregabalin are not hepatically metabolized and are attractive in patients with liver disease.
- Pregabalin with concomitant use of thiazolidinediones increases risk of weight gain and edema.
- Duloxetine may be associated with small increases in fasting glucose and HbA1c.
- Combining agents from different classes results in synergistic effects (Gilron, 2005; Gilron, 2009) and lower doses of medications from the opiate, antidepressant, and antiepileptic classes.

MEDICATIONS

- Anti-inflammatory agents that are effective in treating inflammatory pain are generally not helpful for neuropathic pain.
- Selective serotonin reuptake inhibitors (SSRIs) are not as effective for painful DPN.

BASIS FOR RECOMMENDATIONS

Bril V, England H, Franklin GM, et al. Evidence-based guideline: Treatment of painful diabetic neuropathy: Report of the American Academy of Neurology, the American Association of Neuromuscular and Electrodiagnostic Medicine, and the American Academy of Physical Medicine and Rehabilitation. *Neurology*, 2011. Prepublished online before print April 11, 2011.

Comments: New consensus guidelines on effective treatments for DPN based on a systematic review of the literature between 1960–2008.

Wernicke JF, Pritchett YL, D'souza DN, et al. A randomized controlled trial of duloxetine in diabetic peripheral neuropathic pain. *Neurology*, 2006; Vol. 67: pp. 1411–20.

Comments: One of the registration trials for duloxetine.

Rosenstock J, Tuchman M, LaMoreaux L, et al. Pregabalin for the treatment of painful diabetic peripheral neuropathy: a double-blind, placebo-controlled trial. *Pain*, 2004; Vol. 110: pp. 628–38.

Comments: One of the FDA registration trials for pregabalin.

Backonja M, Beydoun A, Edwards KR, et al. Gabapentin for the symptomatic treatment of painful neuropathy in patients with diabetes mellitus: a randomized controlled trial. *JAMA*, 1998; Vol. 280: pp. 1831–6.

Comments: The first trial to demonstrate pain relief with gabapentin. Many subsequent trials adopted the same design.

OTHER REFERENCES

Gilron I, Bailey JM, Tu D, et al. Nortriptyline and gabapentin, alone and in combination for neuropathic pain: a double-blind, randomised controlled crossover trial. *Lancet*, 2009; Vol. 374: pp. 1252–61.

Comments: Similar to the Backonja et al. study but with gabapentin and a tricyclic agent.

Ziegler D, Ametov A, Barinov A, et al. Oral treatment with alpha-lipoic acid improves symptomatic diabetic polyneuropathy: the SYDNEY 2 trial. *Diabetes Care*, 2006; Vol. 29: pp. 2365–70.

Comments: A well-designed study of alpha lipoic acid.

Gilron I, Bailey JM, Tu D, et al. Morphine, gabapentin, or their combination for neuropathic pain. *N Engl J Med*, 2005; Vol. 352: pp. 1324–34.

Comments: Landmark publication showing that combination of morphine and gabapentin was better than either agent alone.

Sindrup SH, Jensen TS. Pharmacologic treatment of pain in polyneuropathy. *Neurology*, 2000; Vol. 55: pp. 915–20.

Comments: A nice comparison of different classes of agents.

Tesfaye S, Watt J, Benbow SJ, et al. Electrical spinal-cord stimulation for painful diabetic peripheral neuropathy. *Lancet*, 1997; Vol. 348: pp. 1698–701.

Comments: A nice early report of spinal cord stimulators in painful diabetic neuropathy.

Max MB, Lynch SA, Muir J, et al. Effects of desipramine, amitriptyline, and fluoxetine on pain in diabetic neuropathy. *N Engl J Med*, 1992; Vol. 326: pp. 1250–6.

Comments: A classic reference on tricyclic agents and neuropathic pain in diabetes.

Obesity

ORLISTAT

Reza Alavi, MD, MHS, MBA, and Paul A. Pham, PharmD

INDICATIONS
FDA
- Obesity management including weight loss and weight maintenance in patients with a body mass index (BMI) ≥ 30 kg/m^2 OR ≥ 27 kg/m^2 in the presence of other risk factors (e.g., hypertension, diabetes, dyslipidemia).

MECHANISM
- Orlistat blocks the absorption of dietary fat by inhibiting gastrointestinal lipase.

USUAL ADULT DOSING
- 120 mg (1 capsule) orally 3 times a day with each main fat-containing meal, taken during the meal or up to 1 hour after the meal.
- Doses above 120 mg 3 times a day have not been shown to provide additional benefit.

FORMS

Brand Name (mfr)	Preparation	Forms†	Cost*
Xenical (Roche Pharmaceuticals)	orlistat	oral capsule 120 mg	90 capsules: $284.33

*Prices represent cost per unit specified, are representative of "Average Wholesale Price" (AWP).
†Dosage is indicated in mg unless otherwise noted.

DOSING IN SPECIAL POPULATIONS
Renal
- Usual dose

Hepatic
- Usual dose likely

Pregnancy
- Category B

Breastfeeding
- No data. Generally not recommended.

ADVERSE DRUG REACTIONS
General
- Gastrointestinal side effects are most common, especially with diets high in fat (>30% total daily calories from fat).

Common
- Flatulence with discharge
- Fecal urgency and incontinence

MEDICATIONS

- Steatorrhea
- Oily spotting and oily evacuation
- Increased defecation

Occasional
- Abdominal pain
- Nausea/vomiting
- Dizziness
- Infectious diarrhea
- Rectal pain

Rare
- Hypersensitivity reaction: pruritus, rash (unspecified), urticaria, angioedema, bronchospasm, and anaphylactoid reactions
- Bullous rash or eruption
- Elevated hepatic enzymes
- Increased alkaline phosphatase

DRUG INTERACTIONS
- Due to orlistat's mechanism of action, the potential exists for the malabsorption of fat-soluble drugs and dietary supplements.
- **Vitamin A, D, E, and K, beta-carotene:** fat-soluble vitamin supplements (and analogues) should be administered at least 2 hrs before or after the administration of orlistat.
- **Warfarin:** INR may be increased secondary to lower absorption of vitamin K. Warfarin dose may need to be decreased.
- **Cyclosporine:** reduces the absorption of cyclosporine. Cyclosporine should be administered at least 2 hrs before or after orlistat.
- **Amiodarone and propafenone:** absorption may be decreased. Administer these drugs 2 hrs before or after orlistat.
- **Levothyroxine:** absorption may be significantly decreased. Administer levothyroxine 4 hrs before or after orlistat.
- **Pravastatin, digoxin, phenytoin, oral contraceptives, nifedipine, and glyburide:** pharmacokinetics were not affected by orlistat coadministration.

PHARMACOKINETICS
- **Absorption:** Less than 1%.
- **Metabolism and excretion:** Metabolized within the gastrointestinal wall; forms inactive metabolites. Excretion: feces (~97%, 83% as unchanged drug); urine (<2%)
- $T\frac{1}{2}$: 48 hr.

EXPERT OPINION
- Compared to placebo, orlistat produces a modest weight reduction of 3 kg over 4 years.
- Patients should be strongly encouraged to take a multivitamin supplement that contains fat-soluble vitamins (A, D, E, and K).
- May have beneficial effects on lipids.
- Not reported to have the same increased risk of cardiovascular disease as the obesity drug sibutramine, which is now unavailable in the US.
- Orlistat is contraindicated in patients with chronic malabsorption syndromes or cholestasis.

REFERENCES

Siebenhofer A, Horvath K, Jeitler K, et al. Long-term effects of weight-reducing drugs in hypertensive patients. *Cochrane Database Syst Rev*, 2009; (3): CD007654.

Comments: A meta-analysis of orlistat trials showed safe cardiovascular profile and an average reduction in systolic blood pressure of 2.5 mmHg.

Chou KM, Huang BY, Fanchiang JK, et al. Comparison of the effects of sibutramine and orlistat on obese, poorly controlled type 2 diabetic patients. *Chang Gung Med J*, 2008; Vol. 30: pp. 538–46.

Comments: This study found that sibutramine treatment produced greater reduction in weight than orlistat in obese, poorly controlled type 2 diabetic patients.

Rucker D, Padwal R, Li SK, et al. Long term pharmacotherapy for obesity and overweight: updated meta-analysis. *BMJ*, 2007; Vol. 335: pp. 1194–9.

Comments: A meta-analysis of 3 pharmacologic agents for weight loss.

PHENTERMINE

Reza Alavi, MD, MHS, MBA, and Paul A. Pham, PharmD

INDICATIONS

FDA

- Short-term (a few weeks) management of obesity (in adjunct to weight reduction program of exercise, behavioral modification, and caloric restriction) in patients with an initial BMI $\geq$30 kg/m^2, or BMI $\geq$27 kg/m^2 in the presence of other risk factors (e.g., hypertension, diabetes, hyperlipidemia).

MECHANISM

- Sympathomimetic amine with pharmacologic properties similar to the amphetamines.
- Mechanism of action in reducing appetite appears to be secondary to CNS effects, including stimulation of the hypothalamus to release norepinephrine.

USUAL ADULT DOSING

- Oral: 18.75–37.5 mg/day (phentermine hydrochloride) or 15–30 mg/day (phentermine resin).
- Administer before breakfast or 1–2 hours after breakfast.
- To decrease insomnia, phentermine should be administered 10–14 hours before bedtime.

FORMS

Brand Name (mfr)	Preparation	Forms†	Cost*
Adipex-P (Gate Pharmaceuticals and generic manufacturers)	phentermine	oral capsule 37.5 mg; oral tablet 37.5 mg	$1.52–$2.19; $1.52–$2.15
Ionamin (UCB Pharmaceuticals and generic manufacturers)	phentermine	oral capsule 15 mg, 30 mg	$1.25

*Prices represent cost per unit specified, are representative of "Average Wholesale Price" (AWP).
†Dosage is indicated in mg unless otherwise noted.

MEDICATIONS

DOSING IN SPECIAL POPULATIONS

Renal

- Use lower doses in patients with decreased renal function.

Hepatic

- Use with caution, consider lower doses with decreased hepatic function.

Pregnancy

- Category C

Breastfeeding

- Avoid due to potential for serious adverse reactions in nursing infant.

ADVERSE DRUG REACTIONS

General

- Compared to amphetamines, phentermine causes less euphoriant properties and causes less central nervous system or cardiovascular toxicity.

Common

- Palpitations, tachycardia, elevation of blood pressure
- **CNS:** overstimulation, restlessness, dizziness, insomnia, euphoria, dysphoria, tremor, headache

Occasional

- **Genitourinary/endocrine:** impotence; changes in libido
- **GI:** dry mouth; unpleasant taste; diarrhea; constipation
- **Dermatologic:** allergic urticaria

Rare

- BLACKBOX WARNING: Primary pulmonary hypertension (PPH) most commonly reported with concurrent use of phentermine with fenfluramine or dexfenfluramine, but rare reports of PPH have been reported in patients taking phentermine alone.
- BLACKBOX WARNING: serious regurgitant cardiac valvular disease affecting the mitral, aortic and/or tricuspid valves reported with concurrent use of phentermine with fenfluramine or dexfenfluramine, but rare reports of valvular heart disease have been reported with phentermine alone.
- Psychosis (associated with doses above the recommended range).

DRUG INTERACTIONS

- **Guanethidine, guanadrel, methyldopa, and reserpine:** may decrease hypotensive effect of these agents.
- **MAOIs (e.g., phenelzine), furazolidone:** may cause hypertensive crisis and intracranial hemorrhage. Phentermine should not be administered during or within 14 days following the use of MAOIs or drugs with MAO-inhibiting activity.
- **Selective serotonin reuptake inhibitors (e.g., fluoxetine):** sympathomimetic effects of phentermine and risk of serotonin syndrome may be increased. Avoid coadministration.
- **Tricyclic antidepressant:** pressor response to phentermine may be exaggerated. Avoid coadministration.
- **Phenothiazines:** efficacy of phentermine may be decreased. Avoid coadministration if possible.
- Any agents with sympathomimetic properties (e.g., amphetamine, dextroamphetamine, ephedra alkaloids, Ma huang) may result in additive sympathomimetic side effects (e.g., hypertensive crisis, cardiac arrhythmias, severe agitation). Avoid coadministration.

PHARMACOKINETICS

- **Absorption:** Well absorbed; resin absorbed slower.
- **Metabolism and excretion:** Metabolism is hepatic; not significantly biotransformed. Excretion is primarily renal (70%–80% excreted unchanged); excretion is increased by acidifying the urine.
- $T\frac{1}{2}$: 19–24 h.

EXPERT OPINION

- Contraindicated in patients with advanced arteriosclerosis, cardiovascular disease, moderate to severe hypertension, hyperthyroidism, and glaucoma.
- Drug dependence: Psychological and physical dependence may occur with continued use; this class of drugs has been extensively abused.
- Avoid in patients with history of drug abuse.
- Compared to amphetamine products, phentermine produces the same degree of weight loss, but causes less euphoriant properties and central nervous system or cardiovascular toxicity.
- Tolerance to the anorexiant effects of phentermine develops within a few weeks of therapy. Dose may be increased to a maximum of 37.5 mg/d, but phentermine should be discontinued if tolerance develops to the maximum recommended dose.
- Use with caution in patients with diabetes mellitus; antidiabetic agent requirements may be altered with anorexigens and concomitant dietary restrictions.
- Average weight loss at 6 months is 3.6 kg compared to placebo.
- Currently being studied as a combination drug with topiramate. When used at low doses, may have synergistic effects.

REFERENCES

Snow V, Barry P, Fitterman N, et al. Pharmacologic and surgical management of obesity in primary care: a clinical practice guideline from the American College of Physicians. *Ann Intern Med*, 2005; Vol. 142: pp. 525–31.
Comments: Guidelines on the management of obesity.

Li Z, Maglione M, Tu W, et al. Meta-analysis: pharmacologic treatment of obesity. *Ann Intern Med*, 2005; Vol. 142: pp. 532–46.
Comments: Excellent meta-analysis of obesity medications including phentermine.

McTigue KM, Harris R, Hemphill B, et al. Screening and interventions for obesity in adults: summary of the evidence for the U.S. Preventive Services Task Force. *Ann Intern Med*, 2003; Vol. 139: pp. 933–49.
Comments: Pharmacogic therapy appears safe in the short term; long-term safety has not been as strongly established.

Abenhaim L, Moride Y, Brenot F, et al. Appetite-suppressant drugs and the risk of primary pulmonary hypertension. International Primary Pulmonary Hypertension Study Group. *NEJM*, 1996; Vol. 335: pp. 609–16.
Comments: When phentermine is coadministered with fenfluramine for >3 months, there is a 23-fold increased risk of primary pulmonary hypertension.

MEDICATIONS

BETHANECHOL

Lipika Samal, MD, MPH, and Paul A. Pham, PharmD

INDICATIONS

FDA

- Treatment of acute postoperative and postpartum nonobstructive (functional) urinary retention, and neurogenic atony of the urinary bladder with retention

Non-FDA Approved Uses

- Ileus
- Gastric reflux

MECHANISM

- Parasympathomimetic effects mediated by a direct agonist action on muscarinic (cholinergic) receptors in the urinary tract causing increased bladder contraction.
- Also stimulates GI motility.

USUAL ADULT DOSING

- For atonic neurogenic bladder: initially 5–10 mg at increased at hourly intervals until maximum of 50 mg PO. Usual maintenance dose: 10–50 mg PO 3–4 times daily.

FORMS

Brand Name (mfr)	Preparation	Forms†	Cost*
Bethanechol Chloride (Abrika Pharmaceuticals and other generic manufacturers)	bethanechol chloride	oral tablet 5 mg	$0.71
		oral tablet 10 mg	$1.33
		oral tablet 25 mg	$1.78
		oral tablet 50 mg	$2.85

*Prices represent cost per unit specified, are representative of "Average Wholesale Price" (AWP).
†Dosage is indicated in mg unless otherwise noted.

DOSING IN SPECIAL POPULATIONS

Renal

- No dosage adjustment needed

Hepatic

- Specific guidelines not available

Pregnancy

- FDA pregnancy risk Category C

Breastfeeding

- Not known if bethanechol is excreted into breast milk

ADVERSE DRUG REACTIONS

General

- Cholinergic agonists can cause flushing and warmth of the skin, miosis, diaphoresis, lacrimation, hypersalivation, and bronchospasm.

Common
- GU: urinary urgency, increased urinary frequency
- GI: abdominal pain/cramps, diarrhea, flatulence, nausea/vomiting, and borborygmi (stomach growling, or rumbling)

Occasional
- Blurred vision (secondary to myosis)
- Headache
- Retrograde urine flow
- Orthostatic hypotension, or a sudden drop in blood pressure in hypertensive patients

Rare
- Seizures
- Hypothermia

DRUG INTERACTIONS
- **Antimuscarinic drugs:** maprotiline, mecamylamine, tricyclic antidepressants, phenothiazines, amoxapine, bupropion, clozapine, disopyramide, maprotiline, olanzapine, procainamide, and quinidine may significantly decrease the efficacy of bethanechol. Avoid coadministration if possible.
- **Antidiarrheal agents:** carbinoxamine, chlorpromazine, clemastine, diphenhydramine, mesoridazine, olanzapine, opiate agonists, parasympathomimetics, promazine, promethazine, quinidine, and sympathomimetics can also interfere with the action of bethanechol. Avoid coadministration if possible.

PHARMACOKINETICS
- **Absorption:** Poorly absorbed, with the onset of action in 30–90 mins.
- **T$\frac{1}{2}$:** Duration of action typically lasts 1 hour.

EXPERT OPINION
- Can be used for treatment of diabetic neurogenic bladder (Frimodt-Moller).
- An effective treatment of urinary retention, perhaps more so when combined with an alpha-blocker, but use of this old drug is limited by cholinergic side effects such as diarrhea and abdominal cramping (Yamanishi).
- Clinicians should rule out bladder or urinary tract obstruction before using bethanechol.
- Contraindicated in patients with bradycardia, hypotension, or CAD. Bethanechol should also be avoided in hyperthyroidism, seizure disorder, and parkinsonism since it may exacerbate these conditions.
- Avoid in patients with asthma or COPD because of potential airway obstruction.

REFERENCES

Taylor JA, Kuchel GA. Detrusor underactivity: clinical features and pathogenesis of an underdiagnosed geriatric condition. *J Am Geriatr Soc,* 2006; Vol. 54: pp. 1920–32.
  Comments: A good review of the clinical features of detrusor underactivity.

Yamanishi T, Yasuda K, Kamai T, et al. Combination of a cholinergic drug and an alpha-blocker is more effective than monotherapy for the treatment of voiding difficulty in patients with underactive detrusor. *Int J Urol,* 2004; Vol. 11: pp. 88–96.
  Comments: Total urinary symptom scores (International Prostate Symptom Score, IPSS) remained unchanged after the cholinergic therapy, but were significantly lower after the alpha-blocker treatment and the combination therapy (p = 0.0001). Combination therapy with a cholinergic drug and an alpha-blocker appears to be more useful than monotherapy for the treatment of underactive detrusor.

Frimodt-Møller C, Mortensen S. Treatment of diabetic cystopathy. *Ann Intern Med,* 1980; Vol. 92: pp. 327–8.
  Comments: Describes treatments for diabetic cystopathy including bethanechol.

MEDICATIONS

OXYBUTYNIN

Lipika Samal, MD, MPH, and Paul A. Pham, PharmD

INDICATIONS

FDA

- Uninhibited or reflex neurogenic bladder (i.e., urgency, frequency, urinary leakage, urge incontinence, dysuria)

MECHANISM

- Oxybutynin, a tertiary amine ester, exerts antimuscarinic (atropine-like) and antispasmodic (papaverine-like) actions, thereby inhibiting effect of acetylcholine on smooth muscle. In reflex neurogenic bladder, oxybutynin inhibits detrusor muscle hyperreflexia.

USUAL **A**DULT **D**OSING

- **Nonelderly adults:** immediate-release oxybutynin 5 mg PO 4 times per day; dosage may be adjusted weekly by 5-mg increments based on efficacy and tolerability.
- **Elderly:** extended-release oxybutynin 5 mg PO once daily is more appropriate for elderly patients based on the Beers criteria.
- Maximum dose 30 mg/day.
- Transdermal patch: 3.9 mg/day system applied twice weekly to dry, intact skin on the abdomen, hip, or buttock.
- Topical gel 10%: apply the content of one sachet to a dry, intact skin on the abdomen, upper arms/shoulders, or thighs.
- Patch and gel require patient to rotate sites.

FORMS

Brand Name (mfr)	Preparation	Forms†	Cost*
Ditropan (Major Pharmaceuticals Inc. and other generic manufacturers)	oxybutynin chloride	oral tablet 5 mg	$0.61
Ditropan XL (Ortho Womens Health & Urology: a Division of OMP and other generic manufacturers)	oxybutynin chloride extended release	oral extended-release tablet 5 mg	$3.30
		oral extended-release tablet 10 mg	$3.30
		oral extended-release tablet 15 mg	$3.40
Ditropan (Pharmaceutical Association Inc. and other generic manufacturers)	oxybutynin chloride	oral syrup 5 mg/5 ml	$66.32 (per 16 oz)
Oxytrol Transdermal System (Watson Pharmaceuticals)	oxybutynin chloride	transdermal patch 3.9 mg/24 hr	$19.53
Gelnique 10% gel (Watson Pharmaceuticals)	oxybutynin chloride	topical gel 10%	$4.78

*Prices represent cost per unit specified, are representative of "Average Wholesale Price" (AWP).

†Dosage is indicated in mg unless otherwise noted.

DOSING IN SPECIAL POPULATIONS

Renal

- Extended-release formulations of oxybutynin have not been evaluated in severe renal impairment and are not recommended.

Hepatic

- Lower dosages may be needed in hepatic disease because the drug is extensively metabolized in the liver.
- Extended-release formulations of oxybutynin have not been evaluated and are not recommended.

Pregnancy

- Although oxybutynin is classified as FDA pregnancy risk Category B, safe use during pregnancy has not been established.

Breastfeeding

- It is not known if oxybutynin is excreted in breast milk. Lactation suppression has been reported during post marketing use of immediate-release oxybutynin.

ADVERSE DRUG REACTIONS

General

- Side effects are related to the anticholinergic effects and the antimuscarinic effects on GI smooth muscle.

Common

- GI: constipation, gastroenteritis, nausea, xerostomia
- CNS: dizziness, headache, somnolence

Occasional

- Cardiac: palpitations, sinus tachycardia, fluid retention, peripheral edema
- Endocrine: hyperglycemia

Rare

- Severe allergic reactions, urticaria

DRUG INTERACTIONS

- Oxybutynin is metabolized primarily by the cytochrome P450 3A4 isoenzyme in the liver and gut wall.
- Potent inhibitors of CYP450 3A4 (e.g., HIV protease inhibitors, azole antifungals, macrolide antibiotics) should be avoided.
- Drugs that induce CYP450 3A4 (e.g., carbamazepine, phenytoin, phenobarbital, rifamycin antibiotics, nevirapine, efavirenz) may reduce the effects of oxybutynin.

PHARMACOKINETICS

- **Absorption:** 1.6%–10.9% for immediate release.
- **Metabolism and excretion:** Intestinal wall and extensive liver metabolism, very low renal excretion.
- **T$\frac{1}{2}$:** Immediate release: 2–3 hr; extended release 10 mg: 12–19 hr.

EXPERT OPINION

- Commonly used for outpatient treatment of diabetic overactive bladder; some evidence for reduction of daytime urinary frequency in the elderly.
- Caution with diabetic gastroparesis, due to GI smooth muscle effects. Do not use in patients with urinary retention and/or bladder outflow obstruction.

MEDICATIONS

- Close angle glaucoma and urinary retention are absolute contraindications.
- May be useful in the treatment of diabetic gustatory sweating and severe diarrhea associated with autonomic dysfunction in diabetes.

REFERENCES

Abrams P, Cardozo L, Chapple C, et al. Comparison of the efficacy, safety, and tolerability of propiverine and oxybutynin for the treatment of overactive bladder syndrome. *Int J Urol,* 2006; Vol. 13: pp. 692–8.

   Comments: Oxybutynin 15 mg was more effective than propiverine 20 mg in reducing symptomatic and asymptomatic involuntary detrusor contractions.

Blair DI, Sagel J, and Taylor I. Diabetic gustatory sweating. *South Med J,* 2002; Vol. 95: pp. 360–2.

   Comments: Oxybutinin can be considered for diabetic gustatory sweating.

Szonyi G, Collas DM, Ding YY, et al. Oxybutynin with bladder retraining for detrusor instability in elderly people: a randomized controlled trial. *Age Ageing,* 1995; Vol. 24: pp. 287–91.

   Comments: Oxybutynin is effective in controlling overactive bladder.

Chideckel EW. Oxybutynin for diabetic complications. *JAMA,* 1990; Vol. 264: p. 2994.

   Comments: The author reports successful treatment of diabetic gustatory sweating and severe diarrhea with oxybutynin.

SECTION 5
CLINICAL TESTS

Bone

BONE MINERAL DENSITY

Kendall F. Moseley, MD, and Todd T. Brown, MD, PhD

DESCRIPTION

- Bone mineral density (BMD) is a measure of mineral content for a given bone area or volume.
- Osteoporosis is a systemic skeletal disorder characterized by low bone mineral density and microarchitectural deterioration of bone tissue with consequent increase in bone fragility and susceptibility to fracture.
- Bone architecture consists of minerals (calcium, phosphorus), which form hydroxyapatite crystals, as well as type I collagen and other proteins.
- Type 1 diabetes mellitus (T1DM): BMD lower than age-matched healthy population; at higher risk for fracture compared to age-matched population (Schwartz).
- Type 2 diabetes mellitus (T2DM): BMD higher than age-matched healthy population; may be at higher risk for fracture despite higher BMD (Schwartz; Brandi).

ASSAYS

- Dual X-ray absorptiometry (DXA) considered the clinical gold standard for measuring BMD at the lumbar spine, total hip, femoral neck, and forearm.
- DXA quantifies bone mineral content (BMC) in grams and bone area (BA) in centimeters squared, with BMD equaling BMC/BA in grams per centimeters squared.
- Vertebral fracture assessment may also be done for high-risk patients.
- Quantitative computed tomography (CT) measures volumetric bone density rather than areal density (product of DXA) but is expensive and not used for regular clinical evaluation (Khoo).
- Calcaneal ultrasound, radiographic absorptiometry, and single energy X-ray absorptiometry have also been employed for BMD calculation (Nayak).
- New imaging technologies (MICRO CT and magnetic resonance imaging [MRI]) are in development to better assess bone microarchitecture and quality for clinical use.

INDICATIONS

- No specific guidelines for BMD measurement in type 1 or type 2 diabetes mellitus, necessitating use of guidelines established for the age- and sex-matched healthy population.
- The National Osteoporosis Foundation (NOF) recommends BMD screening for women >65 years old and men >70 years old regardless of fracture risk (Heinemann).
- DXA evaluation should be considered in younger postmenopausal women and men age 50–69 years who have additional fracture risk factors. Per NOF, diabetes mellitus is considered an additional fracture risk factor.
- Other clinical risk factors that may prompt BMD measurement include a low BMI, family history of hip fracture, tobacco or alcohol abuse, chronic inflammatory disease (rheumatoid arthritis, ulcerative colitis, etc.), long-term steroid or antiepileptic use, or hormonal dysregulation (prolonged vitamin D deficiency, hyperparathyroidism, hypogonadism, hyperthryoidism, Cushing's syndrome, etc.) (Kanis).

- DXA evaluation should be performed in all persons with a fragility fracture (fall from standing height or less resulting in fracture), regardless of age, and for persons treated with osteoporosis medications (bisphosphonates, teriparatide, SERMs, etc.) or those considered candidates for therapy.
- Thiazolidenedione use associated with low BMD and fracture.

DIFFERENTIAL DIAGNOSIS

- Bone mineral density defined on a spectrum of normal, osteopenia, and osteoporosis (see Interpretation section here).

INTERPRETATION

- DXA BMD reported as a T-score and Z-score at the lumbar spine, total hip, femoral neck, or forearm (may require separate request at some institutions).
- T-score calculated as the mean BMD of <30 year old reference population minus patient BMD, divided by the standard deviation (SD) of the young population (Heinemann).
- Z-score calculated as the mean BMD of peers (age and sex-matched) minus patient BMD, divided by the SD of referenced peers.
- Normal bone density is defined as a T-score above −1.0.
- Osteopenia defined as a T-score between −1 and −2.5.
- Osteoporosis defined as a T-score less ≤−2.5.
- Severe (or established) osteoporosis defined as a T-score ≤−2.5 in the presence of one or more fragility fractures.
- Changes in BMD evaluated with sequential DXA evaluation, with significant percent change at a specific body site defined by institution and machine standards (Baim).
- In premenopausal women and men <50 years, Z-score should be used, rather than T-score. Z-scores ≤−2.0 considered low BMD, but should not alone be the basis for treatment decisions.

LIMITATIONS OR CONFOUNDERS

- DXA, quantitative CT, and other noted imaging modalities describe bone quantity, not quality (also important in fracture risk).
- DXA accuracy and precision dependent on machine calibration, technologist skill, and appropriate interpretation of BMD data and imaging (Kanis).
- Proper patient positioning on the scanner table is required for accurate BMD, and is the most common error in densitometry testing.
- Those with scoliosis cannot be positioned correctly on the table, invalidating spine BMD measurements.
- Local structural and degenerative changes (osteophytes, compression fractures, aortic calcification, spondylosis, etc.) can falsely elevate BMD at local sites.
- Artifacts including surgical clips, metal jewelry, and radiopaque tablets will spuriously elevate BMD.
- Obese patients, such as those with T2DM, may not fit properly on the scanning table; half-body DXA scanner may be needed.
- Excessive lean mass and fat mass (obese individuals) at the skeletal region of interest may increase DXA-derived BMD inaccuracies (Bolotin).

EXPERT OPINION

- BMD can help predict fracture risk, but it cannot replace clinical judgment and risk factor assessment for people with diabetes who likely have reduced bone quality (i.e., impaired bone microarchitecture and mechanics) (Burghardt).
- Bone density testing 1–2 years following initial screening DXA indicated in people on medication for osteoporosis or those considered at high risk for fracture if medication might be indicated later.
- Fracture risk assessment tool (*http://www.shef.ac.uk/FRAX/*) put femoral neck BMD and patient risk factors for osteoporosis into a multivariate model, helping to predict 10-year major osteoporotic and hip fracture; T1DM considered a risk factor for bone loss in the FRAX model (Kanis).

BASIS FOR RECOMMENDATIONS

National Osteoporosis Foundation. *Clinician's Guide to Prevention and Treatment of Osteoporosis.* Washington, DC: National Osteoporosis Foundation; 2010. Available at: http://www.nof.org/sites/default/files/pdfs/NOF_ClinicianGuide2009_v7.pdf. Accessed 4/25/11.

  Comments: Consensus guidelines on the management of osteoporosis in postmenopausal women and men >50 years.

OTHER REFERENCES

Brandi ML Microarchitecture, the key to bone quality. *Rheumatology (Oxford),* 2009; Vol. 48 Suppl 4: pp. iv, 3–8.

  Comments: Bone as comprised of a macrostructure and microstructure, and the imaging techniques used for measuring each one.

Burghardt AJ, Issever AS, Schwartz AV, et al. High-resolution peripheral quantitative computed tomographic imaging of cortical and trabecular bone microarchitecture in patients with type 2 diabetes mellitus. *J Clin Endocrinol Metab,* 2010; Vol. 95: pp. 5045–55.

  Comments: Describes increased BMD but impaired bone strength in patients with type 2 diabetes.

Khoo BC, Brown K, Cann C, et al. Comparison of QCT-derived and DXA-derived areal bone mineral density and T scores. *Osteoporos Int,* 2009; Vol. 20: pp. 1539–45.

  Comments: Quantitative CT compared to gold standard DXA was found to accurately diagnose osteoporosis.

Baim S, Binkley N, Bilezikian JP, et al. Official positions of the International Society for Clinical Densitometry and executive summary of the 2007 ISCD Position Development Conference. *J Clin Densitom,* 2008; Vol. 11: pp. 75–91.

  Comments: Position paper highlighting current recommendations, standards, and guidelines in the clinical use of densitometry testing.

Schwartz AV, Sellmeyer DE. Diabetes, fracture, and bone fragility. *Curr Osteoporos Rep,* 2007; Vol. 5: pp. 105–11.

  Comments: Description of low BMD in T1DM and high BMD in T2DM with speculation as to why both groups are at higher risk for fracture.

Kanis JA, Oden A, Johnell O, et al. The use of clinical risk factors enhances the performance of BMD in the prediction of hip and osteoporotic fractures in men and women. *Osteoporos Int,* 2007; Vol. 18: pp. 1033–46.

  Comments: Meta-analysis serving as foundation of WHO risk factor assessment tool (FRAX).

Nayak S, Olkin I, Liu H, et al. Meta-analysis: accuracy of quantitative ultrasound for identifying patients with osteoporosis. *Ann Intern Med,* 2006; Vol. 144: pp. 832–41.

  Comments: Meta-analysis to evaluate the sensitivity and specificity of calcaneal ultrasound (US) in detecting osteoporosis compared to gold standard DXA.

Kanis JA, Borgstrom F, De Laet C, et al. Assessment of fracture risk. *Osteoporos Int,* 2005; Vol. 16: pp. 581–9.

  Comments: Discussion of additional risk factors for bone loss which, combined with BMD, aid in determining a patient's risk for fracture.

Bolotin HH, Sievänen H, Grashuis JL. Patient-specific DXA bone mineral density inaccuracies: quantitative effects of nonuniform extraosseous fat distributions. *J Bone Miner Res,* 2003; Vol. 18: pp. 1020–7.

Comments: Discussion of inaccuracies in BMD interpretation caused by fat mass and lean mass attenuation artifacts.

VITAMIN D

Kendall F. Moseley, MD, and Todd T. Brown, MD, PhD

DESCRIPTION

- Estimated that 1 billion people worldwide have vitamin D deficiency or insufficiency (Holick 2007).
- Studies ongoing to determine prevalence of hypovitaminosis D in type 1 diabetes (T1DM) and type 2 diabetes (T2DM); preliminary data suggest prevalence may be as high as 30% in T2DM (Targher).
- Vitamin D optimizes intestinal calcium and phosphorus absorption to maintain skeletal mineral content.
- Sources of vitamin D include sunlight exposure, dietary intake, and dietary supplements.
- Vitamin D derived from sunlight or dietary sources metabolized in the liver to form 25-hydroxyvitamin D (25(OH)D).
- 25-hydroxyvitamin D metabolized by 1-alpha-hydroxylase in kidneys to active form, 1,25-dihydroxyvitamin D (1,25(OH)D).
- Vitamin D deficiency in adults can lead to development of osteopenia, osteoporosis, and/or osteomalacia; muscle weakness; and increased risk of fractures and falls (Holick 2007).
- Vitamin D may have other roles in human health including modulation of immune function and reduction of inflammation.

ASSAYS

- Gold standard: high-performance liquid chromatography, but expensive and cumbersome (Holick 2009).
- Two assay types are in common use: immunoassay and liquid chromatography tandem mass spectroscopy (LC-MS). Immunoassays give a total 25(OH)D measurement, whereas LC-MS measures serum D2 and D3, the sum of which gives the total 25(OH)D concentration. Relative accuracy of these two methodologies is debated.
- Radioimmunoassays (RIA) used today in clinical practice measure both 1,25(OH)D2 and 1,25(OH)D3.
- Calcium and parathyroid hormone (PTH) tests may also be helpful if hypocalcemia suspected.

INDICATIONS

- No definite guidelines for screening for vitamin D deficiency or insufficiency in the otherwise healthy population or in diabetes.
- 25(OH)D levels determine a person's vitamin D stores and thus status (Holick 2009).
- Consider screening with 25(OH)D level in the elderly or those with limited sunlight exposure, excessive sunscreen use, minimal dairy intake, dark skin, obesity, or malnutrition.

- Consider checking 25(OH)D level in workup for secondary causes of osteoporosis, persons with known or suspected celiac disease (CD), or persons with other malabsorption conditions (ulcerative colitis, gastric bypass, etc.) (Taxel).
- Hypocalcemia on routine bloodwork or symptoms of tetany, paresthesias, or muscle cramps may be a reason to check vitamin D levels.
- Symptoms such as fatigue, muscle weakness, and bony pain may be nonspecific.

DIFFERENTIAL DIAGNOSIS

- Low 25(OH)D due to reduced synthesis: dark skin pigmentation, sunscreen use, older age, winter season, higher latitudes, liver disease (Holick 2007).
- Low 25(OH)D due to decreased absorption: celiac disease, cystic fibrosis, Whipple's disease, gastric bypass, obesity (vitamin D sequestered in fat).
- Low 25(OH)D due to decreased dietary intake.
- Low 25(OH)D due to increased catabolism: HIV therapy, antirejection medications, antiseizure medications, steroids.
- Elevated 1,25(OH)D and low 25(OH)D: primary hyperparathyroidism, granulomatous disease, lymphoma.

INTERPRETATION

- No definite consensus defining normal range of 25(OH)D or what defines vitamin D insufficiency versus deficiency (Holick 2009).
- PTH plateaus at 25(OH)D levels between 30 and 40 ng/ml, defining "normal" serum D levels as greater than 30 ng/ml.
- Vitamin D insufficiency: 20–30 ng/ml.
- Vitamin D deficiency: <20 ng/ml.
- Vitamin D intoxication: 25(OH)D levels >150 ng/ml in association with hypercalcemia, hypercalciuria, and hyperphosphatemia.

LIMITATIONS OR CONFOUNDERS

- Immunoassays and LC-MS assays are used most often, but discrepancies occur based on the assay used; efforts to standardize assays underway.
- 1,25(OH)D, though a biologically active form of vitamin D, is not a good measure of vitamin D status due to short half-life (4–6 hours).
- Persons with vitamin D deficiency may have transient elevations in 1,25(OH)D due to elevated PTH in secondary hyperparathyroidism.
- Although 25(OH)D level of >30 ng/ml may be considered "normal," each person has an individualized setpoint for normal vitamin D, often appreciated with a concurrently normal PTH (no evident secondary hyperparathyroidism).
- A person may be within 25(OH)D range considered insufficient or deficient and still have normal PTH (no evident secondary hyperparathyroidism).

EXPERT OPINION

- Serum 25(OH)D level is the best indicator of vitamin D status.
- Prevalence of celiac disease in children and adolescents with T1DM may be as high as 10% (8% in adults); practitioners may screen for celiac antibodies (anti-tissue transglutaminase, anti-endomysial, antigliadin) and malabsorption of vitamin D (25(OH)D levels) in people with T1DM (Larsson).
- Supplementation of vitamin D in pregnancy and early childhood may reduce risk of T1DM via reduction of islet autoantibodies; this is controversial (Hyppönen).

- Low serum 25(OH)D levels are associated with cardiovascular disease, obesity, beta-cell dysfunction, insulin resistance, impaired glucose tolerance, metabolic syndrome, and T2DM in observational studies, although causality unclear (Cheng; Chiu; Pittas; Chonchol).
- Both T1DM and T2DM are associated with increased risk of fracture; so vitamin D screening and appropriate supplementation is indicated in deficient and insufficient states to reduce fracture risk.
- Diagnosis of vitamin D insufficiency or deficiency requires treatment with higher doses of vitamin D (e.g., ergocalciferol 50,000 IU orally once weekly for 8 weeks; repeat if vitamin D levels remain <30 ng/ml).
- Adequate calcium intake is essential for vitamin D function and should also be optimized.
- A recent 2011 Institute of Medicine Report suggested that current evidence supports the benefits of vitamin D in skeletal health but is inconsistent for extraskeletal outcomes, including diabetes. The recommended daily allowance was 600 IU for ages 1–70 years and 800 IU for ages >70 years, corresponding to a vitamin D level >20 ng/ml.

REFERENCES

Ross AC, Manson JE, Abrams SA, et al. The 2011 Report on Dietary Reference Intakes for Calcium and Vitamin D from the Institute of Medicine: What Clinicians Need to Know. *J Clin Endocrinol Metab*; epub ahead of print November 29, 2010.

Comments: Summarizes the new IOM report on dietary requirements for calcium and vitamin D. Suggests that vitamin D level of >20 ng/ml is adequate and that levels >50 ng/ml may be associated with adverse effects.

Holick MF. Vitamin D status: measurement, interpretation, and clinical application. *Ann Epidemiol*, 2009; Vol. 19: pp. 73–8.

Comments: Overview of vitamin D synthesis, sources, assays, degrees of sufficiency, and treatment recommendations.

Cheng S, Massaro JM, Fox CS, et al. Adiposity, cardiometabolic risk, and vitamin D status: the Framingham Heart Study. *Diabetes*, 2010; Vol. 59: pp. 242–8.

Comments: 25(OH)D levels positively correlated with insulin sensitivity, negatively correlated with beta-cell function in T2DM.

Holick MF. The vitamin D deficiency pandemic and consequences for nonskeletal health: mechanisms of action. *Mol Aspects Med*, 2008; Vol. 29: pp. 361–8.

Comments: Role of vitamin D in multiple organ systems and nonskeletal consequences that deficiency might precipitate.

Chonchol M, Cigolini M, Targher G. Association between 25-hydroxyvitamin D deficiency and cardiovascular disease in type 2 diabetic patients with mild kidney dysfunction. *Nephrol Dial Transplant*, 2008; Vol. 23: pp. 269–74.

Comments: Inverse association between vitamin D levels and CVD prevalence in T2DM with mild renal dysfunction.

Larsson K, Carlsson A, Cederwall E, et al. Annual screening detects celiac disease in children with type 1 diabetes. *Pediatr Diabetes*, 2008; Vol. 9: pp. 354–9.

Comments: Because celiac disease with 10% prevalence in T1DM, recommended screening at time of diagnosis and yearly for minimum of 2 years.

Smyth DJ, Plagnol V, Walker NM, et al. Shared and distinct genetic variants in type 1 diabetes and celiac disease. *NEJM*, 2008; Vol. 359: pp. 2767–77.

Comments: T1DM and CD share common alleles (HLA-DR3, HLA-DQ2) and genetic variations, suggestive that the diseases have common pathogenesis.

Holick MF. Vitamin D deficiency. *NEJM,* 2007; Vol. 357: pp. 266–81.

Comments: Review article highlighting vitamin D metabolism, conditions associated with deficiency, and hypovitaminosis D as potentially causal in other disease states.

Pittas AG, Lau J, Hu FB, et al. The role of vitamin D and calcium in type 2 diabetes. A systematic review and meta-analysis. *J Clin Endocrinol Metab,* 2007; Vol. 92: pp. 2017–29.

Comments: Calcium and vitamin D as positive mediators of glycemic control, while deficient states associated with progression to metabolic syndrome and T2DM.

Levin A, Bakris GL, Molitch M, et al. Prevalence of abnormal serum vitamin D, PTH, calcium, and phosphorus in patients with chronic kidney disease: results of the study to evaluate early kidney disease. *Kidney Int,* 2007; Vol. 71: pp. 31–8.

Comments: Vitamin D and other mineral metabolism disrupted at varied levels of GFR.

Pittas AG, Dawson-Hughes B, Li T, et al. Vitamin D and calcium intake in relation to type 2 diabetes in women. *Diabetes Care,* 2006; Vol. 29: pp. 650–6.

Comments: Prospective Nurse's Health Study showing >1200 mg calcium and >800 IU vitamin D intake associated with 33% lower risk of developing T2DM.

Targher G, Bertolini L, Padovani R, et al. Serum 25-hydroxyvitamin D3 concentrations and carotid artery intima-media thickness among type 2 diabetic patients. *Clin Endocrinol (Oxf),* 2006; Vol. 65: pp. 593–7.

Comments: Hypovitaminosis D independently associated with increased carotid intima-media thickness in T2DM.

Chiu KC, Chu A, Go VL, et al. Hypovitaminosis D is associated with insulin resistance and beta cell dysfunction. *Am J Clin Nutr,* 2004; Vol. 79: pp. 820–5.

Comments: 25(OH)D levels inversely associated with visceral and subcutaneous adiposity, the fat mass that contributes to cardiovascular disease.

Hyppönen E, Läärä E, Reunanen A, et al. Intake of vitamin D and risk of type 1 diabetes: a birth-cohort study. *Lancet,* 2001; Vol. 358: pp. 1500–3.

Comments: Cohort study indicating that vitamin D supplementation following birth could reduce risk of T1DM development.

Taxel P, Kenny A. Differential diagnosis and secondary causes of osteoporosis. *Clin Cornerstone,* 2000; Vol. 2: pp. 11–21.

Comments: Vitamin D as a component of secondary osteoporosis workup.

Lampasona V, Bonfanti R, Bazzigaluppi E, et al. Antibodies to tissue transglutaminase C in type I diabetes. *Diabetologia,* 1999; Vol. 42: pp. 1195–8.

Comments: 10% prevalence of CD and 30% anti-tissue transglutaminase antibodies in T1DM; possible that the antibody may arise from pancreatic beta-cell destruction.

Endocrine

HYPOALDOSTERONISM

Amin Sabet, MD

DESCRIPTION

- State of aldosterone deficiency or resistance, often associated with hyperkalemia and mild non-anion gap metabolic acidosis.
- Associated with type 4 renal tubular acidosis (RTA) in patients with diabetic nephropathy.
- May also be seen in patients with diabetes and hypertension treated with ACE-inhibitors, ARBs, or potassium-sparing diuretics.
- In autoimmune conditions such as type 1 diabetes, may be associated with primary adrenal insufficiency.

ASSAYS

- Plasma renin activity (PRA) measured by radioimmunoassay (RIA) for angiotensin I after plasma incubation at 37°C.
- Serum aldosterone and cortisol measured by RIA or chemiluminescence immunoassay (CLIA).
- Serum and urine potassium and osmolality should be checked to calculate transtubular potassium gradient (TTKG).
- TTKG = (urine potassium X serum osmolality)/(serum potassium X urine osmolality).

INDICATIONS

- Persistent or recurrent hyperkalemia without other apparent causes such as acute renal failure or severe illness with marked intravascular volume depletion (e.g., severe congestive heart failure, dehydration), though these conditions often exacerbate hyperkalemia in diabetes.

DIFFERENTIAL DIAGNOSIS

- In general, 3 causes of hypoaldosteronism (hyporeninemic hypoaldosteronism, primary aldosterone deficiency, aldosterone resistance).
- **Hyporeninemic hypoaldosteronism:** causes include diabetic nephropathy, chronic interstitial nephritis, medication use (NSAID, ACE-I, ARB, cyclosporine), and HIV.
- **Primary aldosterone deficiency:** causes include primary adrenal insufficiency (Addison's disease), some forms of congenital adrenal hyperplasia (CAH, most commonly 21-hydroxylase deficiency), aldosterone synthase deficiency (rare), or heparin use.
- **Aldosterone resistance:** causes include K-sparing diuretics (spironolactone, eplerenone, amiloride, triamterene), trimethoprim, pentamidine, pseudohypoaldosteronism (rare).

INTERPRETATION

- In hyperkalemia, aldosterone action should increase potassium excretion causing TTKG >10.
- TTKG <6 with hyperkalemia suggests hypoaldosteronism (Choi). Further interpretation is then based on upright PRA, serum aldosterone, and serum cortisol.

- Low PRA, low aldosterone, and normal cortisol suggests hyporeninemic hypoaldosteronism.
- Low cortisol, low aldosterone, and high PRA suggest primary adrenal insufficiency or CAH.
- Low aldosterone, normal cortisol, and high PRA are consistent with aldosterone synthase deficiency (seen in infants with recurrent hypovolemia, failure to thrive).
- High PRA and high aldosterone are consistent with pseudohypoaldosteronism.

LIMITATIONS OR CONFOUNDERS

- TTKG is unreliable with urine sodium concentration <25 mEq/L, as sodium delivery to distal nephron may become rate limiting for potassium excretion.
- TTKG also unreliable with urine osmolality < plasma osmolality since ADH is needed for optimal potassium excretion.

EXPERT OPINION

- Hyporeninemic hypoaldosteronism is a common cause of hyperkalemia in diabetic patients age >50 years, with mild to moderate nephropathy and exacerbating medications (e.g., ACE-I) or acute illness (e.g., dehydration).
- Patients with hyperkalemia due to hypoaldosteronism often have renal insufficiency with associated volume expansion that may be exacerbated by mineralocorticoid therapy (fludrocortisone).
- Most patients with hyporeninemic hypoaldosteronism respond well to low potassium diet and, if necessary, a loop or thiazide diuretic to enhance potassium excretion.

REFERENCES

Nyirenda MJ, Tang JI, Padfield PL, et al. Hyperkalaemia. *BMJ*, 2009; Vol. 339: p. b4114.
    Comments: Clinical review of hyperkalemic disorders.

Choi MJ, Ziyadeh FN. The utility of the transtubular potassium gradient in the evaluation of hyperkalemia. *J Am Soc Nephrol*, 2008; Vol. 19: pp. 424–6.
    Comments: TTKG <6 indicates impaired aldosterone action as a cause of hyperkalemia.

White PC. Disorders of aldosterone biosynthesis and action. *NEJM*, 1994; Vol. 331: pp. 250–8.
    Comments: Review of disorders of mineralocorticoid deficiency and resistance including CAH, aldosterone synthase deficiency, and pseudohypoaldosteronism.

Ethier JH, Kamel KS, Magner PO, et al. The transtubular potassium concentration in patients with hypokalemia and hyperkalemia. *Am J Kidney Dis*, 1990; Vol. 15: pp. 309–15.
    Comments: Defined expected values for TTKG in hypokalemia and hyperkalemia.

West ML, Marsden PA, Richardson RM, et al. New clinical approach to evaluate disorders of potassium excretion. *Miner Electrolyte Metab*, 1986; Vol. 12: pp. 234–8.
    Comments: Described the use of TTKG in assessing renal mineralocorticoid action.

SEX HORMONES

Ana Emiliano, MD, and Rita Rastogi Kalyani, MD, MHS

DESCRIPTION

- Testosterone (T) and estradiol (E2) have important metabolic actions that are gender-specific (sex-dimorphic).
- Most T and E2 circulate bound to sex hormone-binding globulin (SHBG), a glycoprotein that regulates the amount of sex steroids available for biological action.

- Of total T, 54% weakly bound to albumin and other proteins, 44% bound to SHBG, 2% unbound (free T) (Dunn).
- In reproductive age women, one-third of T is directly secreted by the ovary, whereas two-thirds arises from the peripheral conversion of androstenedione to T.
- Androstenedione directly produced by the ovary but also from peripheral conversion of adrenal dehydroepiandrosterone sulfate (DHEA-S).
- Male hypogonadism (for example, with androgen deprivation therapy for prostate cancer) is linked to the metabolic syndrome, type 2 diabetes, and an increased risk for cardiovascular disease (Basari).
- Hyperandrogenism in women (for example, with polycystic ovarian syndrome [PCOS]) is linked to the metabolic syndrome, type 2 diabetes, and cardiovascular disease (Moran). High T in postmenopausal women is also linked to an increased risk of type 2 diabetes (Ding 2006; Kalyani).
- High endogenous E2 is associated with an increased risk for type 2 diabetes in males and postmenopausal women (Ding 2006; Kalyani).
- Low SHBG is a risk factor for type 2 diabetes in both males and females (Ding 2009).

ASSAYS

- **Total testosterone:** commonly measured using chemiluminescence immunoassay or radioimmunoassay; gold standard is liquid chromatography tandem mass spectrometry (LC-MS). LC-MS is especially helpful in cases of low T concentration, for example in females and prepubertal individuals, as the immunoassays perform poorly at low T concentrations (Wang).
- **Bioavailable testosterone:** represents biologically active T; includes both free T and albumin-bound T. Calculated based on the binding of T to SHBG and albumin. Also, measured directly by the ammonium sulfate precipitation method, which precipitates SHBG and SHBG-bound T.
- **Free testosterone:** gold standard is direct measurement by equilibrium dialysis. Can also be calculated based on total T and SHBG (Vermeulen).
- **Estradiol:** commonly measured using chemiluminescence immunoassay or radioimmunoassay, but gold standard also LC-MS (Kushnir).
- **SHBG:** chemiluminescence immunoassay, radioimmunoassay, ammonium sulfate precipitation method.
- **DHEA-S:** biologically inert steroid produced by the adrenals that becomes active after being converted to androstenedione and then T in the periphery. Measured with chemiluminescence immunoassay, radioimmunoassay, or LC-MS.
- **LH and FSH:** measured using chemiluminescence immunoassay or radioimmunoassay.

INDICATIONS

- **Male hypogonadism:** sexual dysfunction (including erectile dysfunction), muscle weakness, depression, cognitive difficulties, osteoporosis. Measure morning total (and free) T, on two different mornings. LH and FSH should be checked to differentiate primary versus secondary hypogonadism.
- **Female menstrual cycle disturbances:** irregular menses or amenorrhea, subfertility, and signs of hyperandrogenism (as in suspected PCOS). Measure total T, DHEA-S, LH, FSH, prolactin, E2, and thyroid function tests.
- **Moderate to severe hirsutism:** measure total T, free T, and DHEA-S.
- **Postmenopausal status:** measure FSH.

DIFFERENTIAL DIAGNOSIS

- SHBG increased in: aging, hyperthyroidism, estrogen use, chronic inflammatory states
- SHBG decreased in: obesity, hyperinsulinemia (i.e., type 2 diabetes), liver disease, androgen excess, hypothyroidism, glucocorticoid use, nephrotic syndrome
- T increased in: ovarian tumors, hyperthecosis, adrenocortical carcinoma, nonclassical congenital adrenal hyperplasia
- T decreased in: aging, androgen deprivation therapy, male type 2 diabetes (Dhindsa)
- E2 increased in: pregnancy, ovarian sex-cord stromal tumor
- E2 decreased in: menopause, amenorrhea
- LH and FSH increased in: primary hypogonadism, menopause
- LH and FSH decreased in: secondary hypogonadism
- DHEA-S increased in: PCOS, adrenocortical carcinoma

INTERPRETATION

- High T or DHEA-S, low FSH/LH: androgen producing tumor
- High T and DHEA-S, elevated LH/FSH ratio: consistent with PCOS but not necessarily a requirement for the diagnosis
- Low T, high FSH/LH: primary male hypogonadism, which can be in seen in the setting of type 2 diabetes
- Low T, low FSH/LH: secondary male hypogonadism, more commonly seen in type 2 diabetes
- Low E2, high FSH/LH: primary female hypogonadism, menopause
- Low E2, low FSH/LH: secondary female hypogonadism
- High E2, low FSH/LH: pregnancy, ovarian sex-cord stromal tumor

LIMITATIONS OR CONFOUNDERS

- T levels should be obtained at about 8 AM, since there is diurnal variation and the highest levels occurring in the morning.
- In women of childbearing age, E2 is lowest in the early follicular phase and highest in the midcycle.

EXPERT OPINION

- Total T (by immunoassay or LC-MS) is an adequate test to evaluate male hypogonadism in individuals with type 2 diabetes who are not overweight.
- In the setting of overweight/obesity, check free and total T and SHBG levels when considering male hypogonadism. Free T to be checked by equilibrium dialysis or by the Vermeulen method.
- Although male hypogonadism is common in type 2 diabetes, T replacement is not generally recommended unless symptoms are present and treatment needs to be individualized.
- Measurement of sex hormones for the assessment of diabetes risk is subject of ongoing research.

REFERENCES

Moran LJ, Misso ML, Wild RA, et al. Impaired glucose tolerance, type 2 diabetes and metabolic syndrome in polycystic ovary syndrome: a systematic review and meta-analysis. *Hum Reprod Update,* 2010; Vol. 16 Supp. 4: pp. 347–63.
   Comments: A systematic review and meta-analysis of the literature on prevalence and incidence of impaired glucose tolerance, type 2 diabetes, or metabolic syndrome in women with and without PCOS, concluding that women with PCOS have a higher prevalence of impaired glucose tolerance, type 2 diabetes and metabolic syndrome.

Kalyani RR, Franco M, Dobs AS, et al. The association of endogenous sex hormones, adiposity, and insulin resistance with incident diabetes in postmenopausal women. *J Clin Endocrinol Metab,* 2009; Vol. 94: pp. 4127–35.

Comments: Prospective study of 1612 postmenopausal women aged 45–84, not taking hormone replacement therapy, which showed that women with higher quartiles of bioavailable T and E2 and lower quartiles of SHBG had a greater risk for developing type 2 diabetes.

Ding EL, Song Y, Manson JE, et al. Sex hormone-binding globulin and risk of type 2 diabetes in women and men. *NEJM,* 2009; Vol. 361: pp. 1152–63.

Comments: A nested case-control study of postmenopausal women in the Women's Health Study not on hormone therapy showed that a low circulating SHBG is associated with a higher risk of type 2 diabetes in men and women.

Kushnir MM, Rockwood AL, Bergquist J, et al. High-sensitivity tandem mass spectrometry assay for serum estrone and estradiol. *Am J Clin Pathol,* 2008; Vol. 129: pp. 530–9.

Comments: This study describes the use of a high-sensitivity liquid chromatography-tandem mass spectrometry assay for measurement of E2, showing its superiority over radioimmunoassay and chemiluminescent immunoassay.

Basaria S, Muller DC, Carducci MA, et al. Hyperglycemia and insulin resistance in men with prostate carcinoma who receive androgen-deprivation therapy. *Cancer,* 2006; Vol. 106: pp. 581–8.

Comments: Cross-sectional study of 18 men with prostate cancer who had received androgen deprivation therapy (ADT), 17 age-matched controls with prostate cancer who had not received ADT, and 18 age-matched healthy controls, showed that men in the ADT group had higher fasting blood glucose, insulin level, and leptin level, and a higher HOMA-IR.

Ding EL, Song Y, Malik VS, et al. Sex differences of endogenous sex hormones and risk of type 2 diabetes: a systematic review and meta-analysis. *JAMA,* 2006; Vol. 295: pp. 1288–99.

Comments: Systematic review and meta-analysis of 43 prospective and cross-sectional studies, including 6974 women and 6427 men, found that high T levels are associated with an increased risk for type 2 diabetes in females but a lower risk in males; and an inverse correlation between SHBG level and type 2 diabetes risk in males but stronger in females.

Wang C, Catlin DH, Demers LM, et al. Measurement of total serum testosterone in adult men: comparison of current laboratory methods versus liquid chromatography-tandem mass spectrometry. *J Clin Endocrinol Metab,* 2004; Vol. 89: pp. 534–43.

Comments: The comparison of automated immunoassay instruments, manual immunoassay methods, and liquid chromatography-tandem mass spectrometry (LC-MS) showed that LC-MS had a much greater accuracy and precision, especially in the detection of low levels of T.

Dhindsa S, Prabhakar S, Sethi M, et al. Frequent occurrence of hypogonadotropic hypogonadism in type 2 diabetes. *J Clin Endocrinol Metab,* 2004; Vol. 89: pp. 5462–8.

Comments: Cross-sectional study that evaluated total T, free T, SHBG, LH, and FSH of 103 male patients with type 2 diabetes, showing that 33% of patients were hypogonadal.

Vermeulen A, Verdonck L, Kaufman JM. A critical evaluation of simple methods for the estimation of free testosterone in serum. *J Clin Endocrinol Metab,* 1999; Vol. 84: pp. 3666–72.

Comments: Study showing that calculation of free T based on total testosterone and SHBG as determined by immnunoassay is a reliable index of bioavailable T and comparable to free T measured by equilibrium dialysis.

Dunn JF, Nisula BC, Rodbard D. Transport of steroid hormones: binding of 21 endogenous steroids to both testosterone-binding globulin and corticosteroid-binding globulin in human plasma. *J Clin Endocrinol Metab,* 1981; Vol. 53: pp. 58–68.

Comments: Study describing the plasma distribution of steroid hormones into fractions bound to sex-hormone binding globulin, albumin-bound and unbound under equilibrium conditions using a solid phase method.

Gastrointestinal

LIVER FUNCTION

Mariana Lazo, MD, ScM, PhD, and Jeanne M. Clark, MD, MPH

DESCRIPTION

- Multiple serum chemistries assayed to assess hepatic function and/or injury.
- Tests indicative of (1) *liver inflammation:* ALT (alanine aminotransferase) and AST (aspartate aminotransferase); (2) *cholestasis or biliary obstruction:* bilirubin (total includes both direct and indirect bilirubin), ALP (alkaline phosphatase), and GGT (gamma-glutamyltransferase); and (3) *synthetic function:* albumin and PT (prothrombin time).
- Abnormal liver function due to nonalcoholic fatty liver disease (NAFLD) is common in diabetes (see p. 259).

ASSAYS

- Serum ALT, AST, ALP and bilirubin (total and direct) are measured indirectly by using a spectrophotometer.
- PT, reported as the international normalized ratio (INR), measured from citrated whole blood: 1 full blue top, mixed gently. The vacutainer must be filled to the tube's drawing capacity to achieve the proper blood to anticoagulant ratio.

INDICATIONS

- **Symptoms suggestive of liver disease:** jaundice, dark urine, light-colored bowel movements, loss of appetite, fatigue, vomiting of blood, bloody or black bowel movements, swelling or pain in the abdomen, unusual weight changes.
- **Signs suggestive of liver disease:** hepatomegaly, ascites.
- **Medications:** Exposure to medications associated with liver damage (e.g., HMG Co-A reductase inhibitors, thiazolidinediones).
- Contact with people that have viral hepatitis.
- Excessive alcohol consumption. **Comorbidities:** those additionally associated with liver disease among persons with diabetes include extreme obesity, hypertriglyceridemia, alcohol use.
- To monitor response to treatment or track course of disease in patients with liver disease.

DIFFERENTIAL DIAGNOSIS

- **Increased AST:** primary liver disease, acute myocardial infarction, muscle trauma and diseases, pancreatitis, intestinal surgery, burns, renal infarction, pulmonary embolism.
- **Increased ALT:** primary liver disease, biliary obstruction, pancreatitis. ALT >AST viral hepatitis; AST >ALT alcoholic liver disease.
- ALT >AST viral hepatitis; AST >ALT alcoholic liver disease.
- **Increased ALP:** biliary obstruction, primary liver disease (changes parallel GGT), infiltrative liver disease, bone diseases, hyperparathyroidism, hyperthyroidism.
- **Increased GGT:** biliary obstruction, primary liver disease (changes parallel ALP), alcohol consumption, pancreatitis.

- **Increased bilirubin:** biliary obstruction, primary liver disease, hemolytic anemias, hypothyroidism.
- Medications may cause increases in one or more liver chemistry tests because of direct hepatotoxicity or cholestasis (See American Gastroenterological Association [AGA] Technical Review for full list of medications.)

INTERPRETATION

- ALT and AST are abundant liver enzymes. AST is also present in heart muscle.
- ALP is present in nearly all tissues, primarily bone and liver.
- GGT is abundant in liver, kidney, pancreas, and intestine.
- ALT and AST normal ranges vary depending on lab, in general: <40 U/L.
- **Mild ALT and AST elevations** (ALT and AST less than 5 times the upper limit of normal [ULN]) should be rechecked before extensive workup is undertaken. Possible causes: chronic hepatitis C or B, acute viral hepatitis, NAFLD, hemachromatosis, autoimmune hepatitis, medications, alcohol-related liver injury, Wilson's disease.
- **Moderately elevated ALT and AST** (ALT and AST 5–15 times the ULN) should be investigated without waiting to confirm the persistence of abnormal ALT; possible causes: entire spectrum of liver diseases that may cause either mild or severe elevations.
- **Severe ALT and AST elevations** (ALT and AST >15 times the ULN) suggest severe acute liver cell injury: acute viral hepatitis, ischemic hepatitis or other vascular disorder, toxin-mediated hepatitis, acute autoimmune hepatitis.
- Bilirubin is a heme degradation product excreted in the bile; it requires conjugation in the liver before its secretion.
- **Increased GGT:** alcohol consumption.
- **Increased ALP and GGT:** bile duct obstruction, primary biliary cirrhosis, primary sclerosing cholangitis, benign recurrent cholestasis, infiltrative disease of the liver (sarcoidosis, lymphoma, metastasic disease).
- **Isolated elevated ALP (extrahepatic disease):** bone disease, pregnancy, chronic renal failure, lymphoma, congestive heart failure.
- **Hyperbilirubinemia:** investigate if caused by direct (conjugated) or indirect (unconjugated) fraction of bilirubin. Prehepatic causes (increased production, decreased liver uptake) lead to increase of indirect. Intrahepatic or posthepatic causes (decreased hepatic excretion) lead to increase of direct. Increased production: hemolysis. Decreased liver uptake: Gilbert's syndrome, found in 5% population, benign. Decreased hepatic excretion: bile duct obstruction, primary biliar cirrhosis, primary sclerosing cholangitis, benign recurrent cholestasis, hepatitis, cirrhosis, medications, sepsis, total parenteral nutrition, Dubin-Johnson syndrome, medications. (See AGA Technical Review for full list of medications.)
- **Abnormal PT** (expressed in seconds or as INR) and albumin levels: indicate severe hepatic synthetic dysfunction and indicates progression to cirrhosis or impending hepatic failure.
- Other commonly used tests to assess potential causes of hepatic diseases include: viral markers (IgM hepatitis A virus, HBsAg, total anti-HBc, IgM anti-HBc, anti-hepatitis C antibody), immunologic markers (ANA, SMA, anti-LKM-1, AMA), genetic diseases (hereditary hemochromatosis: transferrin saturation, ferritin, hepatic iron index;

Wilson's disease: serum ceruloplasmin, urinary copper; alpha-1-antitrypsin deficiency: serum electrophoresis), hepatocellular carcinoma marker (AFP: alpha-fetoprotein), and imaging studies (ultrasound, CT, MRI).

LIMITATIONS OR CONFOUNDERS

- Poor correlation between ALT and AST levels and hepatic fibrosis. Patients with cirrhosis may have normal or only mildly elevated ALT.
- For ALT, AST, ALP and bilirubin samples, hemolysis can cause significant increases. Samples need to be stable at 0° to 4°C over 1–3 days.
- ALT and AST: increase with strenuous exercise and muscle injury. Meals have no effect.
- ALT is increased with higher BMI.
- ALP levels increase with food intake, pregnancy, and smoking.
- Bilirubin levels increase with fasting. Light exposure decreases bilirubin.

EXPERT OPINION

- Among people with type 2 diabetes (T2DM), liver disease is one of the leading causes of death.
- In addition, patients with T2DM have a higher incidence and prevalence not only of NAFLD, but of hepatitis C and hepatocellular carcinoma compared to the general population.
- Liver tests are not always specific for the liver because there are extrahepatic sources.
- Normal levels of liver chemistry tests (including ALT) do not exclude the presence of liver disease.

BASIS FOR RECOMMENDATIONS

Green RM, Flamm S. AGA technical review on the evaluation of liver chemistry tests. *Gastroenterology,* 2002; Vol. 123: pp. 1367–84. Available online from the American Gastroenterological Association at *http://www. gastro.org*.

Comments: Formal recommendations on how to interpret liver function tests and comprehensive list of medications that may cause liver toxicity or injury.

OTHER REFERENCES

Dufour DR, Lott JA, Nolte FS, et al. Diagnosis and monitoring of hepatic injury. I. Performance characteristics of laboratory tests. *Clin Chem,* 2000; Vol. 46: pp. 2027–49.

Comments: Very detailed review of the characteristics of all liver tests, reference values, individual factors influencing their levels. An approved guideline not only by the National Academy of Clinical Biochemistry but also by the American Association for the Study of Liver Diseases.

Dufour DR, Lott JA, Nolte FS, et al. Diagnosis and monitoring of hepatic injury. II. Recommendations for use of laboratory tests in screening, diagnosis, and monitoring. *Clin Chem,* 2000; Vol. 46: pp. 2050–68.

Comments: Detailed review of the different patterns of liver injuries and their laboratory findings. An approved guideline by the National Academy of Clinical Biochemistry.

Glucose Monitoring

CONTINUOUS GLUCOSE MONITORING SYSTEMS

Ari Eckman, MD, and Christopher D. Saudek, MD

DESCRIPTION

- A continuous glucose monitoring (CGM) system consists of sensor, transmitter, and receiver providing real-time readings, graphs, trends, glucose levels, and projected glucose alarms directly to patient.
- Calibrated by self-monitored blood glucose, used to indicate immediate interstitial glucose as well as patterns of high and low glucose throughout the day.
- Real-time monitoring of interstitial fluid glucose, with continuous display of glucose level for up to 5–7 days before changing sensor.
- Displays results on an external palm-held device or on an insulin pump.
- Glucose reported every 5–10 minutes, with capability of every minute for some CGMs.

ASSAYS

- Small, flexible glucose oxidase sensor inserted under skin in abdomen or arm measuring interstitial glucose concentrations; water-resistant transmitter sits on skin, sends glucose readings wirelessly to receiver, downloads values to personal computer, and generates glycemic profiles.
- Portion of membrane polymer remains in skin after sensor removed. Long-term effects of this not yet determined, although no health effects initially reported in clinical studies.
- Devices currently available: Abbott Free Style Navigator Continuous Glucose Monitor, DexCom SEVEN Plus, Medtronic Guardian Real-Time Continuous Glucose Monitoring System, and MiniMed Paradigm and Revel Real-Time Systems.

INDICATIONS

- Specific indications are yet to be established, but may be indicated for patients with unstable diabetes for purposes of improving diabetes management.
- May be useful for patients with type 1 diabetes who use intensive insulin therapy, with or without insulin pump, to help recognize fluctuations in glycemia and their causes.
- May be used to evaluate glucose control in specific clinical situations such as gestational diabetes or intensive care units.
- Useful in patients with hypoglycemia unawareness, repeated severe hypoglycemic episodes, or undetected hypoglycemia.
- JDRF (Juvenile Diabetes Research Foundation) study found that children and adolescents used it less regularly, and with limited use there was no benefit.

INTERPRETATION

- JDRF study suggested more frequent CGM use associated with greater reduction in HbA1c after 6 months (Tamborlane).
- Adults (>25 years old) with diabetes associated with greater CGM use compared to children and adolescents.
- With regular use, more time within target glucose range 71–180 mg/dl.

- Patients using CGM may spend less time in hypoglycemic and hyperglycemic range, and may have less nocturnal hypoglycemia (Garg).
- Valuable in guiding therapy adjustments: changing mealtime bolus dosage, adjusting basal insulin rate, changing insulin-to-carbohydrate ratio, etc.
- Used to diagnose and prevent postprandial hypoglycemia.

LIMITATIONS OR CONFOUNDERS

- Results are not as accurate as with SMBG. Mean error about 15%.
- Physiological lag between capillary blood glucose data and interstitial fluid sensor data can be as much as 4–10 minutes, depending on rate of glucose change (Boyne).
- Not approved as replacement for SMBG; abnormally high or low reading should prompt SMBG before acting upon CGM result.
- Can have inflammation, slight bleeding, or, rarely, infection at glucose sensor insertion site.
- If sensor dislodges, new sensor must be inserted; sensors needs to be changed every 3–7 days, depending on CGM brand.
- Receiver must be within 5–10 feet of sensor for wireless range.
- No data collected during warm-up period (can be between 2 and 10 hours depending on CGM device) required before 1st calibration each time new sensor inserted.
- Calibrations only permitted when blood glucose levels not changing rapidly, so calibrate after overnight fasting or at least 2–3 h postprandially.
- Not a good choice for people who are technically challenged, and not adapted for visually impaired.
- Expensive; confirm insurance coverage prior to initiating CGM.

EXPERT OPINION

- CGM may enhance management of diabetes in highly motivated people, who are technically capable to incorporate it into personal daily diabetes management.
- Most commonly used in patients on insulin therapy with difficult to control blood glucose (both highs and lows).
- Provides complete picture of glycemic control by increasing number of glucose values available to make appropriate changes to insulin therapy, food intake, and activity in patients with diabetes.
- CGM useful for detecting unrecognized hypoglycemia in type 1 and type 2 diabetes.
- Projected glucose alarms may prevent severe, potentially dangerous hypoglycemic events.
- Useful in self-education of motivated patients, showing them what self-care events (insulin doses, diet, exercise) cause highs and lows.
- Valuable in controlling daily fluctuations in blood glucose, which may not be reflected in HbA1c levels.

REFERENCES

Juvenile Diabetes Research Foundation Continuous Glucose Monitoring Study Group. Factors predictive of use and of benefit from continuous glucose monitoring in type 1 diabetes. *Diabetes Care,* 2009; Vol. 32 Suppl 11: pp. 1947–53.

Comments: Factors associated with greater CGM use was age >25 years and more frequent self-reported prestudy blood glucose meter measurements per day. More frequent CGM use associated with greater reduction in HbA1c after 6 months, in all age groups.

Juvenile Diabetes Research Foundation Continuous Glucose Monitoring Study Group. Sustained benefit of continuous glucose monitoring on HbA1c, glucose profiles, and hypoglycemia in adults with type 1 diabetes. *Diabetes Care,* 2009; Vol. 32 Suppl 11: pp. 2047–9.

Comments: Evaluated long-term effects of CGM in intensively treated adults with type 1 diabetes. CGM use and benefit sustained for 12 months in this population.

Juvenile Diabetes Research Foundation Continuous Glucose Monitoring Study Group. The effect of continuous glucose monitoring in well-controlled type 1 diabetes. *Diabetes Care,* 2009; Vol. 32: pp. 1378–83.

Comments: Study examined CGM benefits for patients with type 1 diabetes who have already achieved HbA1c levels <7.0 %. Most outcomes, including those combining A1c and hypoglycemia, better with CGM group.

Juvenile Diabetes Research Foundation Continuous Glucose Monitoring Study Group, Tamborlane WV, Beck RW, et al. Continuous glucose monitoring and intensive treatment of type 1 diabetes. *NEJM,* 2008; Vol. 359: pp. 1464–76.

Comments: Landmark study evaluating the value of CGM in management of type 1 diabetes mellitus. Results suggested CGM can be associated with lower HbA1c levels in adults with T1DM.

Garg S, Zisser H, Schwartz S, et al. Improvement in glycemic excursions with a transcutaneous, real-time continuous glucose sensor: a randomized controlled trial. *Diabetes Care,* 2006; Vol. 29: pp. 44–50.

Comments: Study revealed patients using CGM spent less time in hypoglycemic and hyperglycemic range, more time at target glucose range, and had less nocturnal hypoglycemia; no difference in A1C levels.

Klonoff DC. Continuous glucose monitoring: roadmap for 21st century diabetes therapy. *Diabetes Care,* 2005; Vol. 28: pp. 1231–9.

Comments: Real-time recognition of both the absolute magnitude of glycemia and trend patterns provides enormous, useful information to patient.

Tanenberg R, Bode B, Lane W, et al. Use of the Continuous Glucose Monitoring System to guide therapy in patients with insulin-treated diabetes: a randomized controlled trial. *Mayo Clin Proc,* 2004; Vol. 79: pp. 1521–6.

Comments: Study revealed fewer hypoglycemic events per day (1.4 + 1.1 vs 1.7 + 1.2; p = .30) as well as a shorter duration of the event (49.4 + 40.8 minutes per event vs 81.0 + 61.1 minutes per event; p = .009) in a group of patients using the CGM as compared to a control group using SMBG.

Chico A, Vidal-Ríos P, Subirà M, et al. The continuous glucose monitoring system is useful for detecting unrecognized hypoglycemias in patients with type 1 and type 2 diabetes but is not better than frequent capillary glucose measurements for improving metabolic control. *Diabetes Care,* 2003; Vol. 26: pp. 1153–7.

Comments: CGM useful for detecting unrecognized hypoglycemias in type 1 and type 2 diabetic subjects, but not better than standard capillary glucose measurements for improving metabolic control of type 1 diabetic subjects.

Boyne MS, Silver DM, Kaplan J, et al. Timing of changes in interstitial and venous blood glucose measured with a continuous subcutaneous glucose sensor. *Diabetes,* 2003; Vol. 52: pp. 2790–4.

Comments: Physiological lag between capillary blood glucose data and interstitial fluid sensor data can be as much as 4–10 minutes, depending on rate of glucose change.

FRUCTOSAMINE, 1-5 AG

Vanessa Walker Harris, MD, and Rita Rastogi Kalyani, MD, MHS

DESCRIPTION

- **Fructosamine** is the common name for 1-amino-1-deoxy-fructose.
- Fructosamine is a ketoamine formed from the joining of fructose to protein molecules (mostly albumin) through glycation (Armbruster).

- As the half-life of albumin is 14–21 days, fructosamine reflects the average blood sugar concentration over the prior 2–3 weeks (Armbruster; Goldstein; Austin; Baker, 1985; Baker, 1984).
- **1,5-anhydroglucitol (1,5-AG),** the 1-deoxy form of glucose, is a metabolically inert polyol composed of six-carbon chain monosaccharides derived mainly from food and well absorbed by the intestine.
- 1,5-AG competes with glucose for reabsorption into the kidneys. When glucose levels rise (>180 mg/dl), even transiently, urinary loss of 1,5-AG occurs, and circulating levels of 1,5-AG fall.
- 1,5-AG levels more tightly associated with rapid glucose fluctuations, responding within 24 hours (Buse).
- 1,5-AG has been measured and used clinically in Japan for over a decade to monitor short-term glycemic control.

ASSAYS

- **Fructosamine:** first-generation assays suffered from lack of specificity, lack of standardization among laboratories, susceptibility to interference by hyperlipidemia, and difficulty in calibrating the assay.
- However, second-generation fructosamine assays are rapid, inexpensive, highly specific, and free from interference by urates and triglycerides (Austin).
- The fructosamine assay commonly used today is the nitroblue tetrazolium colorimetric procedure, which separates glycated from nonglycated species based on differences in chemical reactivity.
- Multiple studies indicate that there is generally good correlation between serum fructosamine and HbA1c values (correlation coefficient, r = 0.76). Like HbA1c, fructosamine is a marker of mean blood glucose (Gebhart; Negoro).
- Whether fructosamine measurements should be corrected for either total protein or albumin concentrations is debatable; currently, no formal correction method is recommended (Goldstein).
- Fructosamine test results performed on automated instruments are available for same-day clinic visits (Austin; Goldstein).
- **1,5-AG:** GlycoMark is the automated, commercially available assay for 1,5-AG in the US (Dungan).
- The GlycoMark assay involves two enzymatic steps: the first step uses glucokinase to convert glucose to glucose-6-phophate in order to avoid its interference with the second enzymatic step; in the second step, 1,5-AG is oxidized with pyranose oxidase, and the resulting hydrogen peroxide is detected colorimetrically (Dungan).
- The assays for fructosamine and 1,5-AG can be performed using serum or plasma samples.

INDICATIONS

- No definite guideline for using fructosamine or 1,5-AG as an adjunct or alternative to other tests of glycemia, such as HbA1c, fasting serum glucose, or self-monitored blood glucose measures (Goldstein).
- Consider fructosamine in patients with patient visits less than 1 month apart. Because the half-life of albumin and other serum proteins is shorter than that of hemogloblin, concentrations of fructosamine will change more rapidly than HbA1c. Fructosamine can serve as an index of intermediate-term glycemic control (Armbruster).

- Consider fructosamine in patients with hemoglobinopathies (i.e., thalassemias or hemoglobin variants) that may falsely elevate or lower HbA1c (Saudek).
- Consider fructosamine in patients with comorbidities that may affect erythrocyte life span and falsely elevate or lower HbA1c (i.e., kidney disease, liver disease, hemolytic anemia, HIV, iron-deficiency anemia, aplastic anemia) (Saudek).
- Fructosamine may be useful in pregnancy to detect short-term changes in glucose.
- Fructosamine and 1,5-AG correlate better with post-load glucose levels compared to fasting values (Herdzik; Dungan), and may be helpful in patients for whom postprandial hyperglycemia is suspected.
- 1,5-AG may be most useful when day-to-day glucose changes are being monitored (Yamanouchi) or as an adjunct to self-monitoring of blood glucose to confirm stable glycemic control (Buse).
- 1,5-AG probably superior to HbA1c and fructosamine in detecting near-normoglycemia and glycemic excursions

DIFFERENTIAL DIAGNOSIS

- **High fructosamine:** hyperglycemia over the preceding 2–3 weeks, supported by self-monitored blood glucose measures and/or fasting or random blood glucose measures.
- **Low fructosamine:** hypoalbuminemia and/or hypoproteinemia from liver failure, protein-losing enteropathy, or nephrotic syndrome (Armbruster; Austin).
- **Low 1,5-AG:** hyperglycemia within the preceding 24 hours.
- 1,5-AG not significantly affected by hypoglycemia and better differentiates patients with extensive glycemic excursions who have similar HbA1c values.

INTERPRETATION

- Fructosamine levels depends upon patient's age and sex.
- In general, fructosamine levels <265 umol/L are normal and >350 umol/L (approximately equivalent to HbA1c 7.5–8%) considered poor glycemic control.
- The trend of fructosamine levels over time may have greater importance than the absolute value.
- Normal 1,5 AG concentration: women 6.8–29.3 mcg/ml, men 10.7–32.0 mcg/ml (Dungan).
- Fructosamine also associated with presence of microvascular conditions in diabetes (Selvin).

LIMITATIONS OR CONFOUNDERS

- Remains unclear whether serum fructosamine values should be corrected for protein and/or albumin concentration.
- The within subject variation for serum fructosamine is higher than that for HbA1c, which means that fructosamine levels must change much more before a significant difference can be determined (Howey).
- Studies on the clinical usefulness of home fructosamine testing have yielded conflicting results. One study found that mean glycemia over a prior 2-week period was better predicted by HbA1c. Additionally, when used as an adjunct to home blood glucose monitoring, weekly fructosamine did not improve HbA1c levels (Saudek; Goldstein).
- High fructosamine can be due to high levels of glycated immunoglobulins, specifically IgA.
- Similar to HbA1c, fructosamine and 1,5 AG interpretation may be limited in renal disease (Chen).
- 1,5-AG of limited clinical utility in gestational diabetes (Buse).

- Chinese herbal supplement Polygalae radix is a crude form of 1,5-AG and may artifactually increase levels.

EXPERT OPINION

- Several studies recommend cautious interpretation of serum fructosamine values unless they are performed frequently.
- Patients can improve their fructosamine levels by increasing compliance during the week or two prior to their clinic visit (Goldstein).
- The clinical usefulness of intermediate-term measures of glycemia, such as serum fructosamine, remains debatable and may be best applied to specific subsets of diabetic patients, such as those with hemoglobinopathies or abnormal erythrocyte life spans for whom HbA1c may be less reliable.
- Fructosamine may be particularly suitable, at least in an adjunctive role to other measures of glycemia, for monitoring outpatients with diabetes.
- The low cost and convenience of the fructosamine assay may make it a useful alternative to HbA1c in developing countries (Austin).
- 1,5-AG may be useful as an adjunct to self-monitoring of blood glucose and reflects day-to-day changes in glucose levels.

REFERENCES

Selvin E, Francis LM, Ballantyne CM, et al. Nontraditional markers of glycemia: associations with microvascular conditions. *Diabetes Care*, 2011; Vol. 34: pp. 960–7.
  Comments: This study examined the association of fructosamine, glycated albumin, and 1,5-AG versus standard glycemic markers with risk of microvascular conditions associated with diabetes. Fructosamine and glycated albumin were as or more strongly associated with microvascular conditions as HbA1c.

Chen HS, Wu TE, Lin HD, et al. Hemoglobin A(1c) and fructosamine for assessing glycemic control in diabetic patients with CKD stages 3 and 4. *Am J Kidney Dis*, 2010; Vol. 55: pp. 867–74.
  Comments: This study suggests that estimated average glucose calculated from HbA1c and fructosamine underestimates mean blood glucose in patients with CKD stages 3–4.

Dungan KM. 1,5-anhydroglucitol (GlycoMark) as a marker of short-term glycemic control and glycemic excursions. *Expert Rev Mol Diagn*, 2008; Vol. 8: pp. 9–19.
  Comments: Comprehensive review of 1,5-AG as a marker of short-term glycemia.

Saudek CD, Derr RL, Kalyani RR. Assessing glycemia in diabetes using self-monitoring blood glucose and hemoglobin A1c. *JAMA*, 2006; Vol. 295: pp. 1688–97.
  Comments: Literature review assessing the evidence underlying the use of self-monitored blood glucose and hemoglobin A1c.

Dungan KM, Buse JB, Largay J, et al. 1,5-anhydroglucitol and postprandial hyperglycemia as measured by continuous glucose monitoring system in moderately controlled patients with diabetes. *Diabetes Care*, 2006; Vol. 29: pp. 1214–9.
  Comments: Describes utility of 1,5-AG in assessing postprandial hyperglycemia in patients with diabetes.

Goldstein DE, Little RR, Lorenz RA, et al. Tests of glycemia in diabetes. *Diabetes Care*, 2004; Vol. 27: pp. 1761–73.
  Comments: Technical review of the tests most widely used in monitoring blood glucose control by the National Academy of Clinical Biochemistry and published as a position statement by the American Diabetes Association.

Buse JB, Freeman JL, Edelman SV, et al. Serum 1,5-anhydroglucitol (GlycoMark): a short-term glycemic marker. *Diabetes Technol Ther*, 2003; Vol. 5: pp. 355–63.
  Comments: Describes clinical utility of 1,5-AG.

Herdzik E, Safranow K, Ciechanowski K. Diagnostic value of fasting capillary glucose, fructosamine and glycosylated haemoglobin in detecting diabetes and other glucose tolerance abnormalities compared to oral glucose tolerance test. *Acta Diabetol*, 2002; Vol. 39: pp. 15–22.
Comments: This study found that fructosamine correlated better with 2h-post-load glucose than fasting glucose values.

Austin GE, Wheaton R, Nanes MS, et al. Usefulness of fructosamine for monitoring outpatients with diabetes. *Am J Med Sci*, 1999; Vol. 318: pp. 316–23.
Comments: Prospective case-control study evaluating impact of same-day serum fructosamine levels on clinical decision making.

Yamanouchi T, Akanuma Y. Serum 1,5-anhydroglucitol (1,5 AG): new clinical marker for glycemic control. *Diabetes Res Clin Pract*, 1994; Vol. 24 Suppl: pp. S261–8.
Comments: Good review of 1,5-AG.

Gebhart SS, Wheaton RN, Mullins RE, et al. A comparison of home glucose monitoring with determinations of hemoglobin A1c, total glycated hemoglobin, fructosamine, and random serum glucose in diabetic patients. *Arch Intern Med*, 1991; Vol. 151: pp. 1133–7.
Comments: Study comparing four objective measures of glycemic control with home glucose monitoring in diabetic patients.

Howey JE, Bennet WM, Browning MC, et al. Clinical utility of assays of glycosylated haemoglobin and serum fructosamine compared: use of data on biological variation. *Diabet Med*, 1989; Vol. 6: pp. 793–6.
Comments: Describes the relative variation of HbA1c and fructosamine with changes in glycemia.

Negoro H, Morley JE, Rosenthal MJ. Utility of serum fructosamine as a measure of glycemia in young and old diabetic and non-diabetic subjects. *Am J Med*, 1988; Vol. 85: pp. 360–4.
Comments: Comparison of fructosamine levels with other measures of glycemia in young and old diabetic and nondiabetic subjects.

Armbruster DA. Fructosamine: structure, analysis, and clinical usefulness. *Clin Chem*, 1987; Vol. 33: pp. 2153–63.
Comments: Details the mechanisms, usefulness, and limitations of available fructosamine assays.

Baker JR, Metcalf PA, Holdaway IM, et al. Serum fructosamine concentration as measure of blood glucose control in type I (insulin-dependent) diabetes mellitus. *BMJ (Clin Res Ed)*, 1985; Vol. 290: pp. 352–5.
Comments: Evaluation of fructosamine as a measure of glycemia in type 1 diabetics.

Baker JR, Johnson RN, Scott DJ. Serum fructosamine concentrations in patients with type II (non-insulin-dependent) diabetes mellitus during changes in management. *BMJ (Clin Res Ed)*, 1984; Vol. 288: pp. 1484–6.
Comments: Prospective study evaluating usefulness of fructosamine in monitoring metabolic control in noninsulin-dependent diabetics during changes in management.

HEMOGLOBIN A1C

Christopher D. Saudek, MD

Description

- Hemoglobin A1c (HbA1c) is a stable adduct of glucose on the beta-chain of hemoglobin (N-[1-deoxyfructosyl]hemoglobin).
- Formed by a largely irreversible reaction, posttranslationally and nonenzymatically, when hemoglobin circulating in a red blood cell is exposed to ambient glucose.
- Alternate terms: A1c (preferred for use in communication with patients), glycated hemoglobin (the most accurate term), and glycosylated hemoglobin.

- Expressed most often as the percent of hemoglobin that is glycated (alternatively, as mmol glycated hemoglobin per mole total hemoglobin).
- The single best test to monitor overall blood glucose control in diabetes (Saudek, 2006).
- Reflects the average blood glucose over about 3 months previously, although somewhat disproportionately weighted to recent blood glucose levels (Tahara).
- A strong indicator of risk for long-term diabetic complications, especially retinopathy, neuropathy, and nephropathy (DCCT).
- Also an indicator of cardiovascular disease (CVD) risk, although glucose control may be less strong of a risk factor for CVD than lipids, blood pressure, and smoking (Selvin).
- Recently, HbA1c >6.5% is recommended as a criterion for diagnosing diabetes (International Expert Committee; American Diabetes Association; Saudek, 2008).

ASSAYS

- Many specific methods, divided into those that are based on charge (cation-exchange high pressure liquid chromatography [HPLC], electrophoresis, isoelectric focusing), structure (boronate-affinity chromatography, immunoassays) or chemical analysis (mass spectroscopy). Most commonly used methods in US are HPLC and immunoassay.
- Hospital or commercial laboratory assays should be standardized through the National Glycohemoglobin Standardization Program (NGSP), a rigorous quality control program.
- Point-of-care (POC) equipment available for clinics and offices, requires careful standardization and quality control; often used for diabetes screening programs (Lenters-Westra).
- Generally, good correlation between point-of-care and laboratory A1c testing. However, 18% of patients with an HbA1c ≥7% by laboratory analysis were not similarly identified by the POC test (Schwartz).
- Kits for home use not recommended due to lack of quality control.

INDICATIONS

- Recommended for monitoring blood glucose control in all people with diabetes.
- Recommended every 3–6 months, more often if treatment is changing rapidly.
- Can be used for screening and diagnosis of people at high risk for diabetes (International Expert Committee).

INTERPRETATION

- Directly correlated with average blood glucose over about 3 months' time
- Normal (non-diabetic) range is ~4%–6%; recent criteria suggest A1c 5.7–6.4% is category of high risk for diabetes (International Expert Committee).
- Recommended A1c target for most people with diabetes is <6.5%–7%, individualized according to the clinical situation.
- Over 8% generally considered poor blood glucose control; over 10% is very poor.
- Table 5-1 describes relationship between A1c and average blood glucose.
- Most accurate, recent equation to convert A1c to estimated average glucose (eAG): eAG (mg/dl) = $28.7 \times$ A1c − 46.7; eAG (mmol/l) = $1.59 \times$ A1c − 2.59.
- Be aware of confounders and effect modifiers (see Limitations or Confounders section, expanded in NGSP website).
- Not meaningfully affected by glycemic variability after accounting for mean blood glucose levels (Derr).

MORE

TABLE 5-1. RELATIONSHIP BETWEEN A1c AND ESTIMATED AVERAGE BLOOD GLUCOSE*

HbA1c (%)	eAG (estimated Average Glucose)	
	(mmol/L)	(mg/dl)
5	5.4 (4.2–6.7)	97 (76–120)
6	7.0 (5.5–8.5)	126 (100–152)
7	8.6 (6.8–10.3)	154 (123–185)
8	10.2 (8.1–12.1)	183 (147–217)
9	11.8 (9.4–13.9)	212 (170–249)
10	13.4 (10.7–15.7)	240 (193–282)
11	14.9 (12.0–17.5)	269 (217–314)
12	16.5 (13.3–19.3)	298 (240–347)

*Data in parentheses are 95% CIs.
Source: Nathan DM, Kuenen J, Borg R, et al. Translating the A1C assay into estimated average glucose values. *Diabetes Care*, 2008; Vol. 31(8:) pp. 1473–8. Epub 2008 Jun 7. Reproduced with permission of The American Diabetes Association.

LIMITATIONS OR CONFOUNDERS

- Anything that lowers red blood cell survival time (such as hemolytic anemia) lowers A1c independent of blood glucose.
- Conversely, anything that increases the average age of red cells (such as aplastic anemia) increases A1c independent of blood glucose.
- Hemoglobinopathies interfere with valid A1c in some assays.
- For complete list of confounders and effect modifiers according to the method of assay, search NGSP website (*http://www.ngsp.org/interf.asp*).

EXPERT OPINION

- Even in the case of hemoglobinopathies, measurements from most commonly used A1c assays are a valid reflection of glycemia, assuming red cell survival is normal.
- Laboratory quality control is essential.
- A1c is the test we use most often to indicate when treatment of blood glucose should be intensified.
- Not the preferred test for evaluating glycemic control in pregnancy, since A1c reflects control too slowly. In pregnancy, improvement of glucose control should be more quickly accomplished than possible based on A1c.
- Use of A1c in diagnosing diabetes is still new and controversial. Question about whether criteria should be adjusted according to racial/ethnic group.

CLINICAL TESTS

- ADA statement in 2007 proposed worldwide use of International Federation of Clinical Chemistry (IFCC) new mass-spectroscopy-based reference method to standardize A1c assay; also recommended laboratory reporting value as conventional %, but also as mmol/mol, and as estimated average glucose.
- Despite 2007 ADA statement, most clinicians continue reporting HbA1c as %.

BASIS FOR RECOMMENDATIONS

American Diabetes Association. Standards of medical care in diabetes—2011. *Diabetes Care*, 2011; Vol. 34 Suppl 1: pp. S11–61.

Comments: Most recent summary of the standards of medical care in diabetes from the American Diabetes Association including recommendations for annual measurement of renal function.

International Expert Committee. International Expert Committee report on the role of the A1C assay in the diagnosis of diabetes. *Diabetes Care*, 2009; Vol. 32: pp. 1327–34.

Comments: An expert committee report recommending the use of hemoglobin A1c be the preferred method of diagnosing diabetes.

OTHER REFERENCES

National Glycohemoglobin Standardization Program. HbA1c methods and Hemoglobin Variants (HbS, HbC, HbE and HbD traits). *http://www.ngsp.org/prog/index3.html*, Updated 2/2010, accessed 3/16/2011.

Comments: National Glycohemoglobin Standardization Program website, providing comprehensive list of factors that interfere with HbA1c by measurement method.

Lenters-Westra E, Slingerland RJ. Six of eight hemoglobin A1c point-of-care instruments do not meet the general accepted analytical performance criteria. *Clin Chem*, 2010; Vol. 56: pp. 44–52.

Comments: A careful comparison of 8 different point-of-care devices used to measure HbA1c. Valuable information in choosing POC equipment.

Schwartz KL, Monsur J, Hammad A, et al. Comparison of point of care and laboratory HbA1c analysis: a MetroNet study. *J Am Board Fam Med*, 2009; Vol. 22: pp. 461–3.

Comments: In five clinical practices which performed paired point-of-care and laboratory A1c tests on 99 samples, correlation was good (coefficient = 0.88) but 18% of individuals with A1c >7% using laboratory assays missed by point-of-care testing.

Nathan DM, Kuenen J, Borg R, et al. Translating the A1C assay into estimated average glucose values. *Diabetes Care*, 2008; Vol. 31: pp. 1473–8.

Comments: A discussion of the various options for reporting results of HbA1c.

Saudek CD, Herman WH, Sacks DB, et al. A new look at screening and diagnosing diabetes mellitus. *J Clin Endocrinol Metab*, 2008; Vol. 93: pp. 2447–53.

Comments: Results of a consensus panel, reviewing the rationale for use of hemoglobin A1c in screening and diagnosing diabetes.

American Diabetes Association, European Association for the Study of Diabetes, International Federation of Clinical Chemistry and Laboratory Medicine, and the International Diabetes Federation. Consensus Committee statement on the worldwide standardization of the hemoglobin A1C measurement. *Diabetes Care*, 2007; Vol. 30: pp. 2399–400.

Comments: Consensus statement on use of IFCC reference method to standardize A1c assay.

Saudek CD, Derr RL, Kalyani RR. Assessing glycemia in diabetes using self-monitoring blood glucose and hemoglobin A1c. *JAMA*, 2006; Vol. 295: pp. 1688–97.

Comments: A review of the use of hemoglobin A1c and self-monitoring in clinical diabetes care.

Sacks DB, ADA/EASD/IDF Working Group of the HbA1c Assay Global harmonization of hemoglobin A1c. *Clin Chem*, 2005; Vol. 51: pp. 681–3.

Comments: Discusses the issue of hemoglobin A1c being reported in various ways: using conventional DCCT-validated units (% of total hemoglobin), as Average Blood Glucose, or as mmol/mol hemoglobin.

Selvin E, Marinopoulos S, Berkenblit G, et al. Meta-analysis: glycosylated hemoglobin and cardiovascular disease in diabetes mellitus. *Ann Intern Med,* 2004; Vol. 141: pp. 421–31.

Comments: A meta-analysis describing the statistically significant association between hemoglobin A1c and macrovascular (cardiovascular) disease.

Derr R, Garrett E, Stacy GA, et al. Is HbA(1c) affected by glycemic instability? *Diabetes Care,* 2003; Vol. 26: pp. 2728–33.

Comments: A demonstration that hemoglobin A1c reflects average, not variability, of blood glucose.

UK Prospective Diabetes Study (UKPDS) Group. Intensive blood-glucose control with sulphonylureas or insulin compared with conventional treatment and risk of complications in patients with type 2 diabetes (UKPDS 33). *Lancet,* 1998; Vol. 352: pp. 837–53.

Comments: The UKPDS description of the relationship between intensive glycemic control and complication risk in type 2 diabetes. One of many UKPDS publications.

The Diabetes Control and Complications Trial Research Group. Hypoglycemia in the Diabetes Control and Complications Trial. *Diabetes,* 1997; Vol. 46: pp. 271–86.

Comments: The DCCT description of adverse effect of intensive blood glucose control: the increase in hypoglycemic events as hemoglobin A1c is lowered.

Tahara Y, Shima K. Kinetics of HbA1c, glycated albumin, and fructosamine and analysis of their weight functions against preceding plasma glucose level. *Diabetes Care,* 1995; Vol. 18: pp. 440–7.

Comments: A study of the kinetics of hemoglobin glycation, indicating that about 50% of the value of HbA1c is determined by the previous 30 days' glycemia.

The Diabetes Control and Complications Trial Research Group (DCCT). The effect of intensive treatment of diabetes on the development and progression of long-term complications in insulin-dependent diabetes mellitus. *NEJM,* 1993; Vol. 329: pp. 977–86.

Comments: The main DCCT article describing the relationship of intensive glycemic control, as assessed by hemoglobin A1c, to microvascular complications (retinopathy, nephropathy, and neuropathy) in type 1 diabetes. One of many DCCT publications.

Koenig RJ, Peterson CM, Jones RL, et al. Correlation of glucose regulation and hemoglobin A1c in diabetes mellitus. *NEJM,* 1976; Vol. 295: pp. 417–20.

Comments: An early description of the relationship between hemoglobin A1c and blood glucose.

SELF-MONITORING OF BLOOD GLUCOSE

Christopher D. Saudek, MD

DESCRIPTION

- With self-monitoring of blood glucose (SMBG), the patient measures his or her own blood glucose level using a drop of blood applied to a reagent stick.
- A meter displays the blood glucose level at the moment it is tested.
- Wide variety of different meters and strips, each with strengths and weaknesses.
- Usually, a small drop of blood is taken from a finger prick, although some meters can use blood from alternate sites such as forearm.
- Results are usually stored in meter by date, time, and result, and can be downloaded with simple software packages; some meters display their results on an external insulin pump ("smart pumps").

ASSAYS

- Either glucose oxidase or glucose dehydrogenase enzymes are impregnated on test strips, with measurement of hydrogen peroxide or electron production.
- Accuracy highly technique-dependent, ideally ±10%, but generally about ±10%–15% accurate compared to laboratory values.
- Most meters calibrated to display result as plasma glucose, although testing whole blood.
- SMBG is not as accurate as laboratory plasma glucose but far more useful since it is done repeatedly at home.
- Strips must also be shipped and stored properly, and some meters require entry of a code on the vial.

INDICATIONS

- Uniformly agreed that people with type 1 diabetes should self-monitor regularly and frequently (i.e., several times daily).
- Evidence of benefit of regular SMBG in all insulin-requiring diabetes, either type 1 (T1DM) or 2 (T2DM) diabetes (Soumerai).
- Controversy over cost effectiveness of using SMBG in non-insulin-requiring type 2 diabetes, likely most effective if continued over longer times (Tunis).
- In non-insulin-requiring type 2 diabetes, a meta-analysis found modest (−0.16%) improvement in A1c (St. John).

INTERPRETATION

- Healthcare professional must evaluate results and provide feedback to the patient.
- Patients must understand the meaning of results, and how to *respond* to high or low results.
- Interpretation greatly facilitated by downloading results with convenient, graphic displays.
- SMBG can confirm whether symptoms are caused by high or low blood glucose or whether a change in treatment is effective.
- Controversial whether or when routine premeal or postmeal SMBG is most useful.

LIMITATIONS OR CONFOUNDERS

- User error is the most common cause of serious inaccuracy (Bergenstal).
- Strips may be defective upon purchase or become defective if improperly stored in extreme temperature or humidity.
- Less accurate at low (<50 mg/dl) or high (>300 mg/dl) glucose levels, but accuracy even at extremes is adequate.
- Accuracy also requires that hands be dry and clean of any contact with sugar, and that the drop of blood be of adequate volume.
- Many meters require calibration and/or inputting a code for vial of strips into meter.
- Unusually, interference can occur. Glucose oxidase strips may have interference from high-dose acetaminophen, salicylates, ascorbic acid, or low oxygen. Glucose dehydrogenase strips may be affected by maltose or galactose sometimes used on inpatient settings or peritoneal dialysis.

EXPERT OPINION

- Regular use of SMBG helps diabetes self-care *only if results are translated into changes in treatment.*

- SMBG empowers patients to take part in their own self-care, to know when their glucose level is high or low.
- We encourage people with type 1 diabetes to monitor at least 2–4 times daily.
- With type 2 diabetes, we recommend SMBG depending on instability of glucose levels and treatment changes.
- Particularly recommend SMBG in T2DM if A1c is unexpectedly high, or there is a change in treatment.
- We usually recommend premeal and bedtime testing, except for suspected isolated postmeal hyperglycemia.
- Profiling various times of day rather than only one time can be helpful.
- Strongly recommend reviewing downloads of glucometer data, which easily display summary statistics (e.g., average and standard deviation of glucose; number of tests performed per day; patterns over day, week, or month; frequency and timing of serious highs or lows).
- If SMBG readings do not correlate with A1c, consider confounders, more frequent testing (including postmeal or nocturnal testing) or continuous glucose monitoring.

REFERENCES

St John A, Davis WA, Price CP, et al. The value of self-monitoring of blood glucose: a review of recent evidence. *J Diabetes Complications,* 2010; Vol. 24: pp. 129–141.
  Comments: Meta-analysis and review of SMBG in type 2 diabetes, finding SMBG-related decrease in hemoglobin A1c.

Neeser K, Weber C. Cost impact of self-measurement of blood glucose on complications of type 2 diabetes: the Spanish perspective. *Diabetes Technol Ther,* 2009; Vol. 11: pp. 509–16.
  Comments: A Spanish study showing cost savings in the use of SMBG.

Murata GH, Duckworth WC, Shah JH, et al. Blood glucose monitoring is associated with better glycemic control in type 2 diabetes: a database study. *J Gen Intern Med,* 2009; Vol. 24: pp. 48–52.
  Comments: Increasing use of SMBG along with intensification of treatment was associated with better glycemic control.

Towfigh A, Romanova M, Weinreb JE, et al. Self-monitoring of blood glucose levels in patients with type 2 diabetes mellitus not taking insulin: a meta-analysis. *Am J Manag Care,* 2008; Vol. 14: pp. 468–75.
  Comments: A recent meta-analysis of SMBG in non-insulin-requiring type 2 diabetes; found small benefit but such studies are hard to interpret because people with more unstable or worse glycemic control tend to monitor more often.

Simon J, Gray A, Clarke P, et al. Cost effectiveness of self monitoring of blood glucose in patients with non-insulin treated type 2 diabetes: economic evaluation of data from the DiGEM trial. *BMJ,* 2008; Vol. 336: pp. 1177–80.
  Comments: A health economics group evaluated cost benefit of SMBG in non-insulin-treated type 2 diabetes, found no benefit.

Kristensen GB, Monsen G, Skeie S, et al. Standardized evaluation of nine instruments for self-monitoring of blood glucose. *Diabetes Technol Ther,* 2008; Vol. 10: pp. 467–77.
  Comments: Evaluation of 9 meters, showing improvement in recent years but still the need for using an evaluation protocol.

SMBG International Working Group. Self-monitoring of blood glucose in type 2 diabetes: an inter-country comparison. *Diabetes Res Clin Pract,* 2008; Vol. 82: pp. e15–8.
  Comments: A multinational study, finding unexpectedly high use of SMBG in non-insulin-treated diabetes.

Tunis SL, Minshall ME. Self-monitoring of blood glucose in type 2 diabetes: cost-effectiveness in the United States. *Am J Manag Care,* 2008; Vol. 14: pp. 131–40.
Comments: Positive cost effectiveness of SMBG, especially over a longer (10-year) time frame.

Farmer A, Wade A, Goyder E, et al. Impact of self monitoring of blood glucose in the management of patients with non-insulin treated diabetes: open parallel group randomised trial. *BMJ,* 2007; Vol. 335: p. 132.
Comments: Randomized trial, no improvement with SMBG in non-insulin-treated type 2 diabetes.

Saudek CD, Derr RL, Kalyani RR. Assessing glycemia in diabetes using self-monitoring blood glucose and hemoglobin A1c. *JAMA,* 2006; Vol. 295: pp. 1688–97.
Comments: Review of the use of SMBG and hemoglobin A1c.

Diabetes Research in Children Network (Direcnet) Study Group, Buckingham BA, Kollman C, et al. Evaluation of factors affecting CGMS calibration. *Diabetes Technol Ther,* 2006; Vol. 8: pp. 318–25.
Comments: A detailed study of calibration approaches.

Moreland EC, Volkening LK, Lawlor MT, et al. Use of a blood glucose monitoring manual to enhance monitoring adherence in adults with diabetes: a randomized controlled trial. *Arch Intern Med,* 2006; Vol. 166: pp. 689–95.
Comments: Joslin Diabetes Center randomized clinical trial of SMBG in type 1 diabetes, discusses use of their manual.

Davidson MB, Castellanos M, Kain D, et al. The effect of self monitoring of blood glucose concentrations on glycated hemoglobin levels in diabetic patients not taking insulin: a blinded, randomized trial. *Am J Med,* 2005; Vol. 118: pp. 422–5.
Comments: Randomized trial of SMBG in a large inner-city diabetes center, found no benefit to its use.

Soumerai SB, Mah C, Zhang F, et al. Effects of health maintenance organization coverage of self-monitoring devices on diabetes self-care and glycemic control. *Arch Intern Med,* 2004; Vol. 164: pp. 645–52.
Comments: Evaluation of policy that provided SMBG equipment and instruction for insulin-treated diabetes. Use of SMBG reduced HbA1c by 0.63%.

Bellazzi R, Arcelloni M, Bensa G, et al. Design, methods, and evaluation directions of a multi-access service for the management of diabetes mellitus patients. *Diabetes Technol Ther,* 2003; Vol. 5: pp. 621–9.
Comments: A multicenter trial of alternate site testing.

Bergenstal R, Pearson J, Cembrowski GS, et al. Identifying variables associated with inaccurate self-monitoring of blood glucose: proposed guidelines to improve accuracy. *Diabetes Educ,* 2002; Vol. 26: pp. 981–9.
Comments: Demonstrated that various errors in user technique are common and correctable by good education.

Hematology

ANEMIA

Nisa M. Maruthur, MD, MHS

DESCRIPTION
- Hemoglobin <13 g/dl in men, <12.0 g/dl in women (World Health Organization).
- Anemia is most commonly caused by chronic kidney disease in diabetes.

ASSAYS
- Complete blood count with differential (includes mean corpuscular volume): electrical impedance
- Reticulocyte count: flow cytometry
- Peripheral blood smear: light microscopy
- Other laboratory tests: basic metabolic panel to assess glomerular filtration rate

INDICATIONS
- Symptoms of anemia: fatigue, weakness, dizziness, shortness of breath, chest pain, coldness of the extremities.
- Presence of diabetic nephropathy.
- Bleeding, most commonly menstrual and gastrointestinal (hematemesis, hematochezia, or melena).
- Restrictive diets (e.g., vegetarian diets).
- A lower than expected level of hemoglobin A1c (based on plasma glucose levels) could indicate the presence of a hemolytic anemia.
- Iron deficiency anemia has been associated with increased hemoglobin A1c but does not significantly affect HbA1c levels in diabetes (Ford).

DIFFERENTIAL DIAGNOSIS
- Chronic kidney disease
- Nutritional deficiency (e.g., vitamin B12 and folate)
- Inflammation ("anemia of chronic disease") including from acute infection, cancer, and autoimmune disease
- Iron deficiency from bleeding (e.g., gastrointestinal) or malabsorption (e.g., celiac disease)
- Bone marrow disorder
- Acquired hemolytic anemias (e.g., drug-induced)
- Hemoglobinopathies (e.g., thalassemia, sickle cell disease)
- Other: thyroid disease, liver disease, HIV

INTERPRETATION
- **Microcytic:** low mean corpuscular volume with elevated red cell distribution width indicates iron deficiency. Low mean corpuscular volume with normal red cell distribution width indicates thalassemia.
- **Macrocytic:** elevated mean corpuscular volume suggests vitamin B12 deficiency, folate deficiency, hypothyroidism, alcohol abuse, or liver disease.

- **Normocytic:** normal mean corpuscular volume suggests chronic kidney disease, anemia of inflammation, sickle cell disease, or bone marrow disease.
- Iron studies, reticulocyte count, and peripheral blood smear can help to evaluate for iron deficiency, anemia of inflammation, and bone marrow disease.
- See Table 5-2 for overview of anemia by severity.

MORE

TABLE 5-2. SEVERITY OF ANEMIA

Severity	Hb Range (g/dl)	Symptoms	Medical Attention
Mild	9.5–13.0	Often no signs or symptoms	Commonly remains untreated
Moderate	8.0–9.5	May present with symptoms	Requires management to prevent complications from developing
Severe	<8.0	Symptoms usually present	May be life threatening and requires prompt management

Source: Elsevier Oncology. *The Elsevier Guide to Oncology Drugs & Regimens.* New York: Elsevier Health; 2006. Reprinted with permission of Elsevier.

LIMITATIONS OR CONFOUNDERS
- Dehydration can mask anemia.
- Recent transfusion can confuse interpretation of red blood cell indices and peripheral blood smear.
- Iron deficiency anemia may be associated with higher HbA1c.
- Higher hemoglobin concentrations are positively associated with HbA1c (Ford).

EXPERT OPINION
- Hemolytic anemias (i.e., shortened red blood cell life span) may be associated with falsely low hemoglobin A1c levels.
- Vitamin B12 deficiency should be considered in patients with megaloblastic anemia on long-term metformin therapy.
- Check complete blood count periodically (at least yearly or with decreases in kidney function) if glomerular filtration rate <60 ml/min per 1.73 m².
- There is a paucity of data to determine optimal transfusion levels in anemia.
- Symptomatic anemia and active bleeding should be treated with transfusion.
- In general, erythropoeitin treatment should only be used for chronic kidney disease-associated anemia (hemoglobin level to be maintained 11–12 g/dl).

REFERENCES

American Diabetes Association. Standards of medical care in diabetes—2011. *Diabetes Care,* 2011; Vol. 34 Suppl 1: pp. S11–61.

   Comments: American Diabetes Association report on general standards of diabetes care, which suggests the potential for HbA1c to be misleading in the presence of anemia or chronic kidney disease.

Ford ES, Cowie CC, Li C, et al. Iron-deficiency anemia, non-iron-deficiency anemia and HbA1c among adults in the US. *J Diabetes*, 2011; Vol. 3: pp. 67–73.

Comments: This cross-sectional national study found higher mean adjusted HbA1c in persons with iron deficiency versus those without (5.56% vs. 5.46%; p=0.095). Higher hemoglobin concentration was also associated with higher HbA1c.

Thomas DR. Anemia in diabetic patients. *Clin Geriatr Med*, 2008; Vol. 24: pp. 529–40, vii.

Comments: Review of approach to anemia in diabetes patients emphasizing importance of diabetic nephropathy in development of anemia.

Saudek CD, Derr RL, Kalyani RR. Assessing glycemia in diabetes using self-monitoring blood glucose and hemoglobin A1c. *JAMA*, 2006; Vol. 295: pp. 1688–97.

Comments: A review of methods, use, and interpretation of HbA1c and self-monitoring of blood glucose.

Weiss G, Goodnough LT. Anemia of chronic disease. *NEJM*, 2005; Vol. 352: pp. 1011–23.

Comments: Review of pathophysiology, laboratory testing, and management of anemia of inflammation.

Panzer S, Kronik G, Lechner K, et al. Glycosylated hemoglobins (GHb): an index of red cell survival. *Blood*, 1982; Vol. 59: pp. 1348–50.

Comments: Study showing that glycosylated hemoglobins are lower in patients with hemolytic anemia compared with those with nonhemolytic anemia or in normal controls.

World Health Organization. *http://whqlibdoc.who.int/publications/2008/9789241596657_eng.pdf*. Accessed March 5, 2010.

Comments: Report of worldwide anemia based on WHO Global Database on anemia.

National Kidney Foundation. *http://www.kidney.org/professionals/KDOQI/guidelines_anemia/cpr21.htm*. Accessed March 5, 2010.

Comments: National Kidney Foundation Disease Outcomes Quality Initiative (NKF KDOQI) practice guideline on anemia related to chronic kidney disease.

CLINICAL TESTS

AUTOANTIBODIES IN TYPE 1 DIABETES

Shivam Champaneri, MD, and Christopher D. Saudek, MD

DESCRIPTION

- Four autoantibodies are markers of beta-cell autoimmunity in type 1 diabetes: islet cell antibodies (ICA) against cytoplasmic proteins in the beta cell, glutamic acid decarboxylase (GAD65), insulin autoantibodies (IAA), and islet antigen-2 antibodies (IA-2A) to protein tyrosine phosphatase (Taplin).
- Autoantibodies against GAD65 are found in 80% of patients with type 1 diabetes at clinical presentation (Isermann).
- Presence of ICA and IA-2A at diagnosis for type 1 diabetes range from 69%–90% and 54%–75%, respectively (Winter).
- IAA prevalence correlates inversely with age at onset of diabetes; it is usually the first marker in young children at risk for diabetes (Franke) and found in approximately 70% of young children at time of diagnosis (Bingley).

ASSAYS

- Radioimmunoassay (RIA) has superior diagnostic sensitivity and specificity compared to enzyme-linked immunosorbent assay (ELISA) (Greenbaum).
- In the Diabetes Autoantibody Standardization Program 2000 workshop, the ELISA for the insulin autoantibody (IAA) assay ranged in sensitivity of 4%–42%; the standardization of the insulin antibody assay continues to be more challenging than for GAD or IA-2A antibodies (Greenbaum).

INDICATIONS

- When the classification of type of diabetes is unclear, for instance when considering latent autoimmune diabetes of the adult (LADA) in an individual with surprisingly rapid development of insulin dependence (e.g., <2 years in an adult), or in a person who does not fit the type 2 diabetes phenotype (Falorni).
- Assessing risk for developing type 1 diabetes in patients with gestational diabetes; patients who have autoantibodies at delivery either have type 1 diabetes or are at high risk for developing it (Füchtenbusch).
- Screening for possible incipient type 1 diabetes in high-risk people such as first-degree relatives of people with type 1 diabetes.
- Surveillance of autoantibodies in pancreas or islet-cell transplant patients, as presence is predictive of graft survival rates (Shapiro).

DIFFERENTIAL DIAGNOSIS

- Positivity of one or more autoantibodies in the presence of diabetes is pathognomonic of type 1 diabetes.
- People who screen positive for one or more autoantibodies but do not yet have diabetes, however, will *not* necessarily develop diabetes. Risk is proportional to number and titer of antibodies (Achenbach).

INTERPRETATION

- Antibodies may be present several years before a patient develops hyperglycemia, indicating that the autoimmune process is in progress.
- First-phase insulin response is impaired in patients with multiple positive antibodies and high titers of insulin antibodies, suggesting early beta-cell failure (Achenbach, Keskinen).
- In the diabetes prevention trial (DPT1), 882 first-degree relatives of type 1 diabetes had GAD, IAA, and insulin antibodies measured. With 11-year follow-up, 5-year risk of developing diabetes was 68% with 2 or more antibodies, and 100% if all 3 antibodies were present (Verge).
- In DPT1, 91% of individuals with GAD antibody positivity were also positive for other antibodies (Verge).
- GAD antibodies have a sensitivity of 84% and are of higher sensitivity for adult onset type 1 diabetes; unlike insulin antibodies, GAD antibodies remain at a high titer even if the patient no longer produces c-peptide (Yu).
- IAA have 49%–92% sensitivity for type 1 diabetes (Yu).

LIMITATIONS OR CONFOUNDERS

- People can have transient autoantibodies disappear months or years later without the development of diabetes as found in the DIPP (Finnish Type I Diabetes Prediction and Prevention; Kimpimäki) and DAISY (Diabetes Autoimmunity Study in the Young; Barker) cohorts.
- Since insulin-treated patients develop insulin antibodies with treatment, analysis of IAA is not useful in insulin-treated people (Falorni).
- Antibodies may be transferred transplacentally to infants of type 1 diabetic mothers so caution must be used for interpretation (Ziegler).
- A small proportion of patients with type 2 diabetes may also have positive GAD antibodies or IA-2A (Umpaichitra).

EXPERT OPINION

- Given that positive autoantibodies define type 1 diabetes, we screen for them when it is unclear whether a given patient has type 1 or type 2.
- Positivity of most autoantibodies declines over the years with type 1 diabetes, so measuring them years after the onset of disease is not as useful.

REFERENCES

Bingley PJ. Clinical applications of diabetes antibody testing. *J Clin Endocrinol Metab,* 2010; Vol. 95: pp. 25–33.
  Comments: This 2009 review provides a summary of literature review and consensus statements on diabetes antibody testing.

Taplin CE, Barker JM. Autoantibodies in type 1 diabetes. *Autoimmunity,* 2008; Vol. 41: pp. 11–8.
  Comments: This 2008 review provides a basic overview of the described antibodies associated with type 1 diabetes and their role as a predictive marker for overt diabetes.

Yu L, Eisenbarth GS. Humoral autoimmunity. In Eisenbarth GS (Ed.) *Type 1 diabetes: molecular, cellular, and clinical immunology.* Denver: Barbara Davis Center for Childhood Diabetes; 2007.
  Comments: This review examines the immunologic basis underlying type 1 diabetes.

Isermann B, Ritzel R, Zorn M, et al. Autoantibodies in diabetes mellitus: current utility and perspectives. *Exp Clin Endocrinol Diabetes,* 2007; Vol. 115: pp. 483–90.
  Comments: This review focuses on knowledge about antibody assays for diabetes associated autoimmunity, their clinical value, and their role in diagnosing and predicting autoimmune-associated diabetes mellitus.

Shapiro AM, Ricordi C, Hering BJ, et al. International trial of the Edmonton protocol for islet transplantation. *NEJM,* 2006; Vol. 355: pp. 1318–30.

    Comments: This international, multicenter trial looked at 36 type 1 diabetes patients who underwent islet cell transplantation and reported cases of long-term restoration of endogenous insulin production.

Falorni A, Brozzetti A. Diabetes-related antibodies in adult diabetic patients. *Best Pract Res Clin Endocrinol Metab,* 2005; Vol. 19: pp. 119–33.

    Comments: This 2005 review provides an overview of different markers of autoimmunity in type 1 diabetes and their role in the clinical setting.

Pihoker C, Gilliam LK, Hampe CS, et al. Autoantibodies in diabetes. *Diabetes,* 2005; Vol. 54 Suppl 2: pp. S52–61.

    Comments: This 2005 article is a review of the different autoantibodies seen in diabetes and pathogenesis and clinical significance of autoimmunity in type 1 diabetes.

Franke B, Galloway TS, Wilkin TJ. Developments in the prediction of type 1 diabetes mellitus, with special reference to insulin autoantibodies. *Diabetes Metab Res Rev,* 2005; Vol. 21: pp. 395–415.

    Comments: This 2005 review provides an overview of antibodies in type 1 diabetes and assays for its detection.

Achenbach P, Warncke K, Reiter J, et al. Stratification of type 1 diabetes risk on the basis of islet autoantibody characteristics. *Diabetes,* 2004; Vol. 53: pp. 384–92.

    Comments: The study found a strong association between risk of developing type 1 diabetes and high titer, with the highest risks associated with high-titer IA-2A and IAA, IgG2, IgG3, and/or IgG4 subclass of IA-2A and IAA, and antibodies to the IA-2-related molecule IA-2beta.

Barker JM, Goehrig SH, Barriga K, et al. Clinical characteristics of children diagnosed with type 1 diabetes through intensive screening and follow-up. *Diabetes Care,* 2004; Vol. 27: pp. 1399–404.

    Comments: This study assessed whether earlier diagnosis of diabetes in prospectively followed autoantibody-positive children lowered onset morbidity and improved the clinical course after diagnosis, and the authors found that such patients did have a milder clinical course in the first year after diagnosis.

Barker JM, Barriga KJ, Yu L, et al. Prediction of autoantibody positivity and progression to type 1 diabetes: Diabetes Autoimmunity Study in the Young (DAISY). *J Clin Endocrinol Metab,* 2004; Vol. 89: pp. 3896–902.

    Comments: This prospective study reveals that determination of islet autoantibodies in 1972 children found a large number of individuals being either false or transiently positive.

Umpaichitra V, Banerji MA, Castells S. Autoantibodies in children with type 2 diabetes mellitus. *J Pediatr Endocrinol Metab,* 2002; Vol. 15: Suppl 1: pp. 525–30.

    Comments: In 37 children and adolescents with type 2 diabetes who had positive meal-stimulated C-peptide levels, 10.8% also had positive GAD and/or IA2 antibodies.

Keskinen P, Korhonen S, Kupila A, et al. First-phase insulin response in young healthy children at genetic and immunological risk for Type I diabetes. *Diabetologia,* 2002; Vol. 45: pp. 1639–48.

    Comments: This study noted a decreased first-phase insulin response as potentially an early phenomenon in the course of prediabetes in young children, implying a rapid autoimmune destruction or loss of function of beta cells as well as possible metabolic compensation mechanisms.

Winter WE, Harris N, Schatz D. Type 1 diabetes islet autoantibody markers. *Diabetes Technol Ther,* 2002; Vol. 4: pp. 817–39.

    Comments: This 2002 article provides a basic overview of antibodies seen in type 1 diabetes and their diagnostic role in the clinical setting.

Kimpimäki T, Kupila A, Hämäläinen AM, et al. The first signs of beta-cell autoimmunity appear in infancy in genetically susceptible children from the general population: the Finnish Type 1 Diabetes Prediction and Prevention Study. *J Clin Endocrinol Metab,* 2001; Vol. 86: pp. 4782–8.

    Comments: In this population-based prospective cohort study, monitoring for the appearance of diabetes-associated autoantibodies and development of type 1 diabetes from birth was performed. The authors noted children with a strong human-leukocyte-antigen-DQ-defined genetic risk of type 1 diabetes show signs of beta-cell autoimmunity proportionally more often than those with a moderate genetic risk with generally IAA emerging as the first detectable antibody more commonly than any other antibody.

Ziegler AG, Hummel M, Schenker M, et al. Autoantibody appearance and risk for development of childhood diabetes in offspring of parents with type 1 diabetes: the 2-year analysis of the German BABYDIAB Study. *Diabetes,* 1999; Vol. 48: pp. 460–8.

Comments: This prospective trial of 1353 offspring of parents with type 1 diabetes looked at the development of autoantibodies. They noted a cumulative risk for disease of 1.8% by 5 years of age and a 50% risk for offspring with more than one autoantibody in their 2-year sample.

Füchtenbusch M, Ferber K, Standl E, et al. Prediction of type 1 diabetes postpartum in patients with gestational diabetes mellitus by combined islet cell autoantibody screening: a prospective multicenter study. *Diabetes,* 1997; Vol. 46: pp. 1459–67.

Comments: This prospective multicenter study of 437 gestational diabetes patients assessed the predictive value of autoantibody markers for the development of type 1 diabetes. The authors noted the risk for type 1 diabetes 2 years postpartum increased with the number of antibodies present at delivery from 17% (6%–28%) for one antibody, to 61% (30%–91%) for two antibodies, and to 84% (55%–100%) for 3 antibodies.

Verge CF, Gianani R, Kawasaki E, et al. Prediction of type I diabetes in first-degree relatives using a combination of insulin, GAD, and ICA512bdc/IA-2 autoantibodies. *Diabetes,* 1996; Vol. 45: pp. 926–33.

Comments: This study looked at 882 first-degree relatives of patients with type 1 diabetes, 50 of whom later developed diabetes with a median follow-up of 2.0 years. The authors concluded that the presence of 2 or more autoantibodies (out of IAAs, GAAs, and ICA512bdcAAs) is highly predictive of the development of type 1 diabetes among relatives.

Greenbaum CJ, Palmer JP, Kuglin B, et al. Insulin autoantibodies measured by radioimmunoassay methodology are more related to insulin-dependent diabetes mellitus than those measured by enzyme-linked immunosorbent assay: results of the Fourth International Workshop on the Standardization of Insulin Autoantibody Measurement. *J Clin Endocrinol Metab,* 1992; Vol. 74: pp. 1040–4.

Comments: This report compares the measurement of insulin autoantibodies (IAA) using RIA and ELISA assays, with the finding of labs that used RIA had a much higher percentage of sera to be IAA positive among both newly diagnosed patients and healthy individuals who later developed diabetes than laboratories using ELISA.

INSULIN ANTIBODIES

Shivam Champaneri, MD, and Christopher D. Saudek, MD

DESCRIPTION

- Antibodies to exogenously delivered insulin are common with insulin treatment but are not often clinically significant.
- IgG antibodies are most common while IgE antibodies are the cause of insulin allergy (Fineberg).
- At high titers, IgG antibodies may limit insulin action, which could delay or diminish insulin action.
- Rarely, antibodies can be agonists to the insulin receptor and cause hypoglycemia (usually postprandial hypoglycemia) (Koyama).
- The development of antibodies depends on the purity, molecular structure, and storage conditions of the insulin administered as well as patient factors such as age, HLA type, and delivery route (Fineberg).

- Most common when patients are exposed to beef or pork insulin, rather than only to human or analog insulins (Heinzerling).
- React equally to analog insulin and unmodified human insulins.
- Insulin autoantibodies, in people not previously treated with insulin, are an indication of developing Type 1 diabetes.

ASSAYS

- Radioligand binding (RLB) assays are the most common assay used for measurement of insulin antibodies (Fineberg).
- Standard immunoprecipitation and agglutination analytic methods cannot measure insulin antibodies since insulin antibody immune complexes do not precipitate (Fineberg).
- Higher sensitivity is required for evaluating insulin autoantibodies, which are in much lower concentration than antibodies to exogenous insulin (Greenbaum)

INDICATIONS

- Severe insulin resistance, unresponsive to high-dose insulin treatment.
- Evaluation of possible insulin allergy: IgE antibodies are seen in rapid type 1 allergy, whereas IgG are seen in delayed type III hypersensitivity reaction (Heinzerling).
- Evaluation of possible factitious hypoglycemia: surreptitious insulin administration in individuals without diabetes may be diagnosed by detecting insulin antibodies.
- Diagnosing autoimmune hypoglycemia: a rare condition but one to be distinguished from insulinoma (Koyama).

DIFFERENTIAL DIAGNOSIS

- The presence of insulin antibodies does not prove that they are causing insulin resistance or hypoglycemia.
- More soluble insulins, such as regular insulin, are less allergenic than intermediate- or long-acting insulins (Chance).
- Circulating IgE antibodies to insulin may cause dermal and systemic allergic reactions to animal-source insulin (Fineberg).
- Allergies to protamine and zinc (which help slow absorption of long-acting insulins) need to be distinguished from allergy to insulin (Feinglos).
- Autoimmune hypoglycemia can be due to endogenous antibodies to insulin or the insulin receptor (Koyama).

INTERPRETATION

- Most studies show no relationship between the presence of insulin antibodies and complications such as nephropathy, retinopathy, and neuropathy (Fineberg).
- Rarely, antibodies bind differently to different insulins from different species; clinical improvement may result from switching insulin sources (Grammer).
- No relationship between insulin dose and development of antibodies has been shown in clinical trials.
- Antibodies are only a cause of insulin resistance when found in unusually high titer (Fineberg).
- For severely insulin-resistant patients, positive antibody testing can lead to consideration of the following treatments: switching insulin formulations, glucocorticoid therapy, or rarely plasmaphoresis (Kahn; Koyama).
- Insulin allergy can be treated with antihistamines to control symptoms, switching insulin preparations, or immunotherapy in the form of desensitization (Heinzerling).

- Autoimmune hypoglycemia can be treated with tapering doses of corticosteroids to suppress endogenous insulin antibodies (Redmon).

LIMITATIONS OR CONFOUNDERS

- No standardization of the insulin antibody assay is available for proper quantification (Fineberg).
- Diagnosis of insulin allergy is not established by presence of IgE alone as it can be found in patients with no apparent allergy (Fineberg).
- Little evidence to show a causal relationship between presence of insulin antibodies and hypoglycemia in patients on insulin.
- Can also be seen in patients with viral disorders, other autoimmune disorders, paraneoplastic syndromes, or with a high likelihood of type 1 diabetes development (Fineberg).

EXPERT OPINION

- As indicated, IgG insulin antibodies are rarely pathogenic, so attributing insulin resistance to antibodies is valid only when very high titer and only having ruled out more common causes.

REFERENCES

Radermecker RP, Renard E, Scheen AJ. Circulating insulin antibodies: influence of continuous subcutaneous or intra-peritoneal insulin infusion, and impact on glucose control. *Diabetes Metab Res Rev*; 2009; Vol. 25 Suppl 6: pp. 491–501.
   Comments: This 2009 reference discusses the significance of different modalities of insulin administration toward development of insulin antibodies and its potential implications toward management.

Heinzerling L, Raile K, Rochlitz H, et al. Insulin allergy: clinical manifestations and management strategies. *Allergy* 2008; Vol. 63: pp. 148–55.
   Comments: This review provides an overview of insulin allergy, including presentation, diagnosis, and immunotherapy.

Fineberg SE, Kawabata TT, Finco-Kent D, et al. Immunological responses to exogenous insulin. *Endocr Rev*; 2007; Vol. 28: pp. 625–52.
   Comments: This reference provides an overview of the immunologic factors in the development of insulin antibodies and reviews its relationship toward diabetes complications.

Koyama R, Nakanishi K, Kato M, et al. Hypoglycemia and hyperglycemia due to insulin antibodies against therapeutic human insulin: treatment with double filtration plasmapheresis and prednisolone. *Am J Med Sci*, 2005; Vol. 329: pp. 259–64.
   Comments: This article discusses the role of plasmapheresis and subsequent use of steroid therapy to lower insulin antibodies to achieve better glycemic control by insulin.

Redmon JB, Nuttall FQ. Autoimmune hypoglycemia. *Endocrinol Metab Clin North Am*, 1999; Vol. 28: pp. 603–18, vii.
   Comments: This excellent review describes the clinical significance, pathogenesis, evaluation, and management of autoimmune hypoglycemia.

Salardi S, Cacciari E, Steri L, et al. An 8-year follow-up of anti-insulin antibodies in diabetic children: relation to insulin autoantibodies, HLA type, beta-cell function, clinical course and type of insulin therapy. *Acta Paediatr*, 1995; Vol. 84: pp. 639–45.
   Comments: This trial studied 105 children and adolescents with insulin-dependent diabetes and noted an inverse relationship between insulin autoantibodies and age at diagnosis; they compared levels of antibodies to A1c values, insulin requirement, HLA, and presence of early complications and concluded that antibodies did not have significant effects on the clinical course of the disease.

Greenbaum CJ, Palmer JP, Kuglin B, et al. Insulin autoantibodies measured by radioimmunoassay methodology are more related to insulin-dependent diabetes mellitus than those measured by enzyme-linked immunosorbent assay: results of the fourth International Workshop on the Standardization of Insulin Autoantibody Measurement. *J Clin Endocrinol Metab*, 1992; Vol. 74: pp. 1040–4.

Comments: This summarizes the findings of the fourth International Workshop on the Standardization of Insulin Autoantibody Measurement with the finding that the data suggest that insulin autoantibodies measured by radioimmunoassay are more disease related than those measured by enzyme-linked immunosorbent assay.

Sutton M, Klaff LJ, Asplin CM, et al. Insulin autoantibodies at diagnosis of insulin-dependent diabetes: effect on the antibody response to insulin treatment. *Metabolism*, 1988; Vol. 37: pp. 1005–7.

Comments: This study assessed whether insulin antibody response over the first year of treatment with insulin was different in individuals with or without insulin autoantibodies. They noted that patients with insulin autoantibodies at diagnosis develop higher insulin antibody measurements when subsequently treated with exogenous insulin.

Grammer LC, Roberts M, Patterson R. IgE and IgG antibody against human (recombinant DNA) insulin in patients with systemic insulin allergy. *J Lab Clin Med*, 1985; Vol. 105: pp. 108–13.

Comments: This paper notes the presence of IgE and IgG antibodies to human insulin as well as bovine and porcine insulin in patients found to have systemic insulin allergy.

Kahn CR, Rosenthal AS. Immunologic reactions to insulin: insulin allergy, insulin resistance, and the autoimmune insulin syndrome. *Diabetes Care*, 1980; Vol. 2: pp. 283–95.

Comments: This is a review from 1980 (one of the original papers) that provides a summary of insulin allergy and insulin resistance and what was known about the mechanisms at that time.

Feinglos MN, Jegasothy BV. "Insulin" allergy due to zinc. *Lancet*, 1979; Vol. 1: pp. 122–4.

Comments: This 1979 paper describes the phenomenon of allergy to zinc in commercially prepared insulins.

Chance RE, Root MA, Galloway JA. The immunogenicity of insulin preparations. *Acta Endocrinol Suppl* (Copenhagen), 1976; Vol. 205: pp. 185–98.

Comments: This review assessed antibody formation from differently prepared insulins (porcine and bovine) with the finding that more purely prepared insulins had less immunogenecity.

Schlichtkrull J, Brange J, Christiansen AH, et al. Clinical aspects of insulin—antigenicity. *Diabetes*, 1972; Vol. 21: pp. 649–56.

Comments: This is one of the original papers that describes the antigenicity of insulin.

Lipids

LIPIDS

Simeon Margolis, MD, PhD

DESCRIPTION
- Standard lipid profile includes total cholesterol, triglycerides (TG), HDL cholesterol (HDL-C), and LDL cholesterol (LDL-C).
- Apolipoproteins and lipoprotein lipase activity can also be measured.
- Chylomicrons carry fat absorbed from the intestine.
- High LDL-C ("bad cholesterol") is the strongest lipid risk factor for cardiovascular disease.
- Low HDL-C ("good cholesterol") is also a strong risk factor for cardiovascular disease.
- High TG are also associated with cardiovascular disease although less strongly than high LDL-C or low HDL-C.
- Severe hypertriglyceridemia is a cause of pancreatitis.

ASSAYS
- The most important assay is a fasting lipid profile performed by a standard chemical assay, usually with autoanalyzer, which measures total cholesterol, TG, and HDL-C (LDL is usually calculated).
- Immunoassays can measure apoproteins A, B, C-II, C-III, and E as well as the 3 major isoforms of apo E.
- Chylomicrons can be detected by finding a white layer of fat at the top of serum refrigerated overnight.

INDICATIONS
- Obtain fasting lipid profile at the time of diagnosis of type 2 diabetes and at least annually during the course of treatment.
- Consider obtaining an apo B if LDL-C is still above target of 70 mg/d or the patient develops cardiovascular disease (CVD), to determine if more aggressive statin treatment or addition of niacin is needed because of persistently high levels of small, dense, atherogenic LDL particles (Pischon; Contois).

DIFFERENTIAL DIAGNOSIS
- The Fredrickson classification may be useful to distinguish different phenotypes of hyperlipoproteinemia, though the classification system itself is no longer commonly used. Major phenotypes are described here.
- **Hyperchylomicronemia:** characterized by very high fasting triglycerides (often >1000 mg/dl), which can be seen as a large band of chylomicrons in overnight refrigerated serum. The familial disorder is due to deficient lipoprotein lipase activity or apo CII, the activator of lipoprotein lipase. Can be distinguished by measuring apo CII. Severe insulin deficiency can produce hyperchylomicronemia.
- **Hypercholesterolemia (HCH):** LDL-C is elevated. TG may be normal or high. LDL receptor deficiency is the major cause of familial hypercholesterolemia. Primary HCH can also result from other genetic defects. Other disorders and dietary excesses can also cause HCH.

- **Familial combined hyperlipoproteinemia:** elevated LDL-C and triglycerides and increased apo B (Veerkamp).
- **Dysbetalipoproteinemia:** suspected by nearly equal elevations of cholesterol and TG. Confirmed by finding apo E2:E2 isoform pattern (Kane).
- **Familial hypertriglyceridemia:** elevated VLDL-containing TG with normal or modest elevations in LDL-C.
- **Mixed hypertriglyceridemia:** elevated VLDL-containing TG and chylomicron-containing TG. In serum refrigerated overnight, a layer of chylomicrons appears on top of underlying turbid serum.
- **Familial combined hyperlipidemia** can be diagnosed by finding high levels of cholesterol, TG, and/or apo B in family members. Lipid abnormalities differ in members of the same family (Veerkamp). Acquired combined hyperlipidemia common in diabetes.
- It is important to identify patients with familial hypercholesterolemia, dysbetalipoproteinemia, and familial combined hyperlipidemia because of their especially high risk of CVD. Screening family members is indicated.
- The most common lipid disorder in type 2 diabetes is an elevation of both cholesterol and TG with low HDL (mixed hyperlipidemia).

INTERPRETATION

- LDL-C is not usually measured directly, but is estimated from the lipid profile by the following Friedewald equation (if triglycerides are below 400 mg/dl): LDL-C = total cholesterol − triglycerides/5 − HDL-C.
- Non-HDL cholesterol is used when treating hypertriglyceridemia. It is calculated as follows: Non-HDL cholesterol = total cholesterol − HDL-C.
- Target for LDL-C in type 2 diabetes is <100 mg/dl, and in cases considered high risk, <70 mg/dl. Target for non-HDL cholesterol in type 2 diabetes is either <100 mg/dl or <130 mg/dl.
- Hypertriglyceridemia is almost always associated with low HDL-C and an increased number of more atherogenic small dense LDL.
- Presence of chylomicrons may indicate a nonfasting sample.
- Risk of acute pancreatitis when triglycerides exceed 1000 mg/dl.

LIMITATIONS OR CONFOUNDERS

- LDL-C cannot be calculated accurately with the Friedewald equation when triglycerides exceed 400 mg/dl or in patients with dysbetalipoproteinemia; tests are available to directly measure LDL-C in these circumstances.
- When TG are very high, serum amylase and lipase usually cannot be used to make the diagnosis of acute pancreatitis.
- Worsening of glycemic control can lead to hyperchylomicronemia and the risk of acute pancreatitis.
- Triglycerides and HDL cholesterol can improve considerably with better glycemic control.
- LDL varies less with exercise or glycemic control.
- Lipid profile should be fasting since triglycerides can vary depending on recent food intake.
- Total and LDL cholesterol varies little between fed and fasted state unless TG are high.
- HDL does not significantly depend on fasting status.

EXPERT OPINION

- Though fasting lipid profiles are preferred (particularly for triglyceride levels), levels of total, HDL, and LDL cholesterol are likely not significantly affected by fasting status.
- High LDL cholesterol is commonly considered the strongest lipid risk factor for CVD.
- However, non-HDL cholesterol, total cholesterol, and especially apo B, may be better predictors of cardiovascular risk; changes in apo B provide an additional estimate of the effectiveness of lipid-lowering therapy (Pischon; Contois).
- Apo B can determine the number of LDL particles and the presence of more atherogenic, small dense LDL.
- Other than apo B, special tests like lipoliprotein lipase activity and apoprotein measurements are largely of research interest and are rarely if ever needed for patient care (Mora).
- Before initiating lipid-lowering therapy, baseline tests in patients with lipid abnormalities should include TSH and liver enzymes but not necessarily CK; however, CK must be obtained with complaints of either muscle pain or weakness.
- Recent studies indicate that nonfasting triglycerides may be better predictors of cardiovascular risk than fasting triglycerides, but upper limits of normal values have not yet been established for nonfasting triglycerides (Bansal; Nordestgaard).

REFERENCES

Mora S. Advanced lipoprotein testing and subfractionation are not (yet) ready for routine clinical use. *Circulation*, 2009; Vol. 119: pp. 2396–404.

> **Comments:** It is not necessary to measure apoproteins or particle size and number to determine risk of cardiovascular disease or to follow treatment outcomes in most patients with type 2 diabetes.

Mora S, Otvos JD, Rifai N, et al. Lipoprotein particle profiles by nuclear magnetic resonance compared with standard lipids and apolipoproteins in predicting incident cardiovascular disease in women. *Circulation*, 2009; Vol. 119: pp. 931–9.

> **Comments:** At least in healthy women, lipoprotein profiles evaluated by nuclear magnetic resonance (NMR) were comparable but not superior to measurements of standard lipids or apolipoproteins.

Contois JH, McConnell JP, Sethi AA, et al. Apolipoprotein B and cardiovascular disease risk: position statement from the AACC Lipoproteins and Vascular Diseases Division Working Group on Best Practices. *Clin Chem*, 2009; Vol. 55: pp. 407–19.

> **Comments:** This paper from clinical chemists recommends the use of apo B rather than LDL-C to assess cardiovascular disease risk.

Martin SS, Qasim AN, Mehta NN, et al. Apolipoprotein B but not LDL cholesterol is associated with coronary artery calcification in type 2 diabetic whites. *Diabetes*, 2009; Vol. 58: pp. 1887–92.

> **Comments:** Plasma apo B, but not LDL cholesterol, levels were associated with coronary artery calcification scores in type 2 diabetic whites.

El Harchaoui K, van der Steeg WA, Stroes ES, et al. Value of low-density lipoprotein particle number and size as predictors of coronary artery disease in apparently healthy men and women: the EPIC-Norfolk Prospective Population Study. *J Am Coll Cardiol*, 2007; Vol. 49: pp. 547–53.

> **Comments:** The additional value of LDL particle number was comparable to non-HDL-C, and it was abolished after adjusting for triglycerides and HDL-C.

Ingelsson E, Schaefer EJ, Contois JH, et al. Clinical utility of different lipid measures for prediction of coronary heart disease in men and women. *JAMA*, 2007; Vol. 298: pp. 776–85.

Comments: During a 15-year follow-up of subjects from the Framingham study, results did not support measurement of apo B or apo A-I to predict risk of coronary heart disease in clinical practice when total cholesterol and HDL-C measurements are available.

Nordestgaard BG, Benn M, Schnohr P, et al. Nonfasting triglycerides and risk of myocardial infarction, ischemic heart disease, and death in men and women. *JAMA,* 2007; Vol. 298: pp. 299–308.
Comments: Nonfasting triglycerides were as good or better than fasting triglycerides for predicting risk of coronary heart disease events and death.

Bansal S, Buring JE, Rifai N, et al. Fasting compared with nonfasting triglycerides and risk of cardiovascular events in women. *JAMA,* 2007; Vol. 298: pp. 309–16.
Comments: Nonfasting triglycerides were more effective than fasting triglycerides in predicting cardiovascular events in women.

Pischon T, Girman CJ, Sacks FM, et al. Non-high-density lipoprotein cholesterol and apolipoprotein B in the prediction of coronary heart disease in men. *Circulation,* 2005; Vol. 112: pp. 3375–83.
Comments: In this study of men, the plasma concentration of atherogenic lipoprotein particles (measured by apo B) was more predictive for the development of CHD than LDL-C or the cholesterol carried by atherogenic particles, measured by non-HDL-C.

Veerkamp MJ, de Graaf J, Hendriks JC, et al. Nomogram to diagnose familial combined hyperlipidemia on the basis of results of a 5-year follow-up study. *Circulation,* 2004; Vol. 109: pp. 2980–5.
Comments: Familial combined hyperlipidemia is associated with a very high risk of cardiovascular complications. Identification of the disorder can be made from detailed family information, but it is also possible to identify the disorder in an individual patient by measuring total cholesterol, triglcerides, and apo B.

Huang ES, Meigs JB, Singer DE. The effect of interventions to prevent cardiovascular disease in patients with type 2 diabetes mellitus. *Am J Med,* 2001; Vol. 111: pp. 633–42.
Comments: Improvement in cholesterol levels reduce the risk of cardiovascular disease in patients with type 2 diabetes.

Kane JP, Havel RJ. Disorders of the biogenesis and secretion of lipoproteins containing the B apoproteins. In Scriver CR, Beaudet AL, Sly WS, Valle DS, (Eds.), *The Metabolic and Molecular Bases of Inherited Disease,* 8th edition. New York: McGraw-Hill; 2001: pp. 2717–62.
Comments: Description of normal and abnormal production and metabolism of B-containing lipoproteins— VLDL and LDL—along with criteria for diagnosis of dysbetaliproteinemia.

Renal

RENAL FUNCTION

Donna I. Myers, MD

DESCRIPTION

- **Serum creatinine:** useful and convenient measure to monitor renal status. Serum creatinine in the normal range may not reflect normal glomerular filtration rate (GFR). Age, gender, and muscle mass need to be considered.
- The reciprocal serum creatinine curve is useful but cumbersome, plotting change in creatinine over time. Sudden acceleration of the slope of deterioration suggests a potentially reversible component such as volume depletion resulting in acute on chronic kidney injury. Similarly, a successful intervention such as blood pressure or glycemic control may flatten the curve over time.
- **GFR:** simplest measure of renal function; 24-hour urine collection not required. Elevated GFR indicates hyperfiltration, an early predictor of subsequent diabetic renal disease. GFR then declines as renal disease progresses. The four variable MDRD equation calculates GFR based on serum creatinine, age, race, and gender. The six-variable expanded MDRD equation also includes blood urea nitrogen (BUN) and serum albumin. The Cockcroft-Gault equation calculates GFR based on serum creatinine, weight, gender, and age. It is of limited value in patients with obesity in whom weight may not reflect muscle mass, but useful in lean patients.
- **BUN:** varies inversely with GFR, but can be affected by factors other than GFR (see Limitations or Confounders section on p. 595).
- **Microalbuminuria:** earliest evidence of diabetic nephropathy, especially in type 1 diabetes, and should be monitored routinely in diabetes.
- The spot urine albumin:creatinine ratio to assess microalbuminuria preferred for monitoring the impact of therapeutic interventions such as renin-angiotensin blockade on proteinuria. 24-hour urine protein collections rarely required.
- **Microscopic urinalysis:** a bland sediment may be seen with either prerenal or postrenal failure. *Glomerulonephritis:* documented proteinuria and hematuria with dysmorphic red blood cells (RBCs), RBC casts, granular casts, and lipiduria. *Nephrosis:* proteinuria and lipiduria with a bland sediment. *Infection:* dipstick positive leukocyte esterase and nitrites and confirmed by the microscopic finding of pyuria, hematuria, and bacteriuria with or without white blood cell (WBC) casts and a positive urine culture. *Acute interstital nephritis:* WBCs and WBC casts without infection; finding eosinophiluria confirms suspicion of an allergic reaction. *Acute tubular necrosis:* muddy brown granular casts.
- **Radiographic examinations:** include renal and bladder ultrasound to detect anatomic changes; functional nuclear medicine scans for split renal function, GFR and obstruction; and CT angiography, renal MRA, or Doppler flow studies for renal artery stenosis (see Limitations or Confounders section on p. 595).

Assays

- **Serum creatinine and BUN:** serum creatinine measured by the alkaline picrate method, a colorimetric assay. Values more reproducible at the lower end of the scale.
- **GFR** (ml/min/1.73m^2): most laboratories will report an estimated GFR on the basis of the measured serum creatinine, gender, race, and age (MDRD).
- **Urine albumin and creatinine** (to assess microalbuminuria): see Albuminuria, p. 597.

Indications

- Preventive annual screening for microalbuminuria starting at diagnosis in type 2 diabetes and beginning 5 years after diagnosis in type 1 diabetes (ADA Standards of Medical Care).
- Measure serum creatinine at least annually in all adults with diabetes, regardless of the degree of urine albumin excretion, to stage chronic kidney disease (CKD) using GFR (ADA Standards of Medical Care).
- Signs or symptoms of renal failure including frothy urine, edema, uncontrolled hypertension, congestive heart failure, uremia.
- Presence of electrolyte abnormalities often associated with chronic renal insufficiency (e.g., hyperkalemia, hyponatremia, hypocalcemia, hyperphosphatemia, metabolic acidosis) or anemia.
- Medications with potential nephrotoxic effects (i.e., metformin) or predominantly renal clearance (i.e., insulin, sulfonylureas).

Differential Diagnosis

- **Elevated creatinine:** prerenal, renal, or postrenal failure; drug reaction (see below)
- **Elevated BUN:** prerenal, renal, or postrenal failure; nonrenal factors (see below)
- **Reduced GFR:** prerenal, renal, or postrenal failure; 24-hr urine collection error
- **Elevated urinary albumin:** micro- or macroalbuminuria from intrinsic glomerular disease; renal vein thrombosis; congestive heart failure; febrile states; benign postural proteinuria

Interpretation

- Chronic kidney disease is classified by GFR and urinary albumin: Stage 1: proteinuria, GFR $\geq$90 ml/min; Stage 2: proteinuria, GFR = 60–89 ml/min; Stage 3: GFR = 30–59 ml/min; Stage 4: GFR = 15–29 ml/min; Stage 5: GFR <15 ml/min.
- A doubling of the serum creatinine results in halving of the GFR. A serum creatinine of 0.6 mg/dl at baseline and 1.2 mg/dl at follow-up may reflect advanced kidney disease although the creatinine level remains in the "normal" laboratory range.
- The curve of creatinine and GFR is nonlinear. At the lower end a small rise in creatinine reflects a large change in GFR; at the upper end a small change in creatinine is of less significance. Plotting the reciprocal creatinine obviates these difficulties. An awareness of the fact that every doubling of creatinine indicates a 50% reduction in GFR is helpful; a rise in serum creatinine from 0.6 to 1.2 mg/dl is similar in magnitude to a rise from 4.0 to 8.0 mg/dl change.
- The reciprocal creatinine over time plot may predict when the patient reaches stage 5 CKD but the actual initiation of maintenance dialysis depends on the patient's comorbidities and symptoms.
- Spot urine albumin:creatinine ratio of 30–300 mg/g creatinine indicates microalbuminuria; >300 mg/g creatinine indicates macroalbuminuria.

LIMITATIONS OR CONFOUNDERS

- The MDRD formula for GFR was developed in a population of chronic kidney disease patients and is not useful when the GFR is >60 ml/min (uniformly reported as ">60 ml/min" rather than a specific number).
- The alkaline picrate assay for serum creatinine may be affected by creatinine chromogens such as acetoacetate in diabetic ketoacidosis, spuriously elevating the serum creatinine by up to 2.0 mg/dl.
- The serum creatinine may fluctuate as a function of prerenal factors such as volume status, cardiac performance, and serum oncotic pressure. Increasing muscle mass from exercise or decreasing muscle mass from wasting or amputation may affect the serum creatinine irrespective of a change in GFR.
- Enhanced creatinine production may occur with a large meat meal or with enhanced muscle breakdown (rhabdomyolysis) with release of creatine.
- Wasting disorders with severe malnutrition (cirrhosis, cancer, bulimia, low protein intake) may present with low serum creatinine (poor muscle mass) and low BUN even in the setting of acute kidney failure such as the hepatorenal syndrome.
- Drugs that block proximal tubular secretion of creatinine, resulting in a spurious elevation of the serum creatinine without a fall in GFR, include trimethoprim and cimetidine.
- The blood urea nitrogen may be elevated during dehydration (prerenal azotemia), with increased protein in the diet (certain fad diets) or gut (GI bleeding), during increased catabolism from sepsis or steroids. Prerenal azotemia is characterized by a BUN:creatinine ratio ≥20:1.
- Urine microalbumin should be verified on two separate collections and is affected by exercise and hypermetabolic states including fever and congestive heart failure.
- CT contrast should be avoided once the serum creatinine is elevated above 1.8 mg/dl, especially in patients with diabetes and proteinuria or heart disease. If contrast needed, consider using N-acetylcysteine and IV hydration beforehand.
- Gadolinium to enhance MRI examination of renal arteries is contraindicated with GFR <60 ml/min because of the associated risk of nephrogenic systemic fibrosis.
- Doppler evaluation of renal blood flow is limited by body habitus (obesity) and technician expertise.

EXPERT OPINION

- Earliest clinical evidence of diabetic nephropathy is microalbuminuria (30–300 mg/day), typically 10 years after disease. Without tight glycemic control and renin angiotensin system blockade by ACE-I or ARB therapy, can evolve into macroalbuminuria (>300 mg/day) within several years, followed by a fall in GFR, hypertension, and progressive renal failure within 3–5 years.
- Only 25% of diabetic patients develop classic diabetic nephropathy (diabetic glomerulosclerosis or Kimmelstiel-Wilson disease). After 20 years, unlikely to occur. Long-term survivors of diabetes may go on to develop arteriosclerotic renal disease (nephrosclerosis), typically nonproteinuric and often very slowly progressive.
- Renovascular disease (RAS) commonly present with diabetic nephropathy, and should be suspected in persons with history of peripheral vascular disease with or without vascular bruits, asymmetric kidneys, a sudden rise in the serum creatinine after initiating ACE-I or ARB therapy, or flash pulmonary edema (bilateral RAS).

- Serum electrolyte abnormalities directly associated with renal function include hyponatremia, hyperkalemia, and metabolic acidosis and may reflect CKD. Hyperkalemia in a diabetic patient with early CKD raises suspicion of hyporenin-hypoaldosteronism (type IV RTA) (see Hypoaldosteronism, p. 557).
- Day-to-day minor fluctuations in serum creatinine reflect volume changes and hydration status.
- Physicians should avoid overzealous use of diuretics, particularly in conjunction with RAAS blockade.
- The fractional excretion of sodium (FENa) or urea (FEurea) may be helpful in distinguishing acute kidney injury from volume depletion, but not important in the evaluation of stable renal function.
- Dipstick evaluation of the urine does not provide information on renal function but provides indirect evidence of infection (positive leukocyte esterase and nitrites), nephritis, and nephrosis.
- At each clinical visit the patient should be assessed for orthostatic hypotension.
- Renal consult should be considered for CKD Stage 3.

BASIS FOR RECOMMENDATIONS

Levey AS, Schoolwerth AC, Burrows NR, et al. Comprehensive public health strategies for preventing the development, progression, and complications of CKD: report of an expert panel convened by the Centers for Disease Control and Prevention. *Am J Kidney Dis*, 2009; Vol. 53: pp. 522–35.

   Comments: Physician awareness of the patient's GFR is recommended for timely referral and appropriate management of CKD.

High WA, Ayers RA, Chandler J, et al. Gadolinium is detectable within the tissue of patients with nephrogenic systemic fibrosis. *J Am Acad Dermatol*, 2007; Vol. 56: pp. 21–6.

   Comments: The toxicity of gadolinium in patients with kidney disease was suspected when gadolinium was detected in tissue of a number of patients with nephrogenic systemic fibrosis (NSF). This association has been confirmed and new guidelines established for the use of this agent.

Schwab SJ, Christensen RL, Dougherty K, et al. Quantitation of proteinuria by the use of protein-to-creatinine ratios in single urine samples. *Arch Intern Med*, 1987; Vol. 147: pp. 943–4.

   Comments: This article describes the utility of single voided urine samples to measure protein-to-creatinine ratios, an observation that obviated the need, in most instances, of a 24-hr urine collection.

OTHER REFERENCES

American Diabetes Association. Standards of medical care in diabetes—2011. *Diabetes Care*, 2011; Vol. 34 Suppl 1: pp. S11–61.

   Comments: Most recent summary of the standards of medical care in diabetes from the American Diabetes Association including recommendations for annual measurement of renal function.

Kanbay M, Kasapoglu B, Perazella MA. Acute tubular necrosis and pre-renal acute kidney injury: utility of urine microscopy in their evaluation—a systematic review. *Int Urol Nephrol*, 2010; Vol. 42 Suppl 2: pp. 425–33.

   Comments: Urine microscopy is useful for the diagnosis of acute kidney injury.

Tanemoto M. Treatment for hyperkalemia in hyporeninemic hypoaldosteronism. *Kidney Int*, 2009; Vol. 75: p. 1113; author reply 1113–4.

   Comments: Type IV RTA, which is prevalent in diabetic patients, may limit the ability to treat proteinuria with renin-angiotensin blocking agents such as ACE-I and ARB therapy.

Diskin CJ, Stokes TJ, Dansby LM, et al. The comparative benefits of the fractional excretion of urea and sodium in various azotemic oliguric states. *Nephron Clin Pract*, 2009; Vol. 114: pp. c145–c150.

   Comments: This compares the utility of FENa versus FEurea in oliguric azotemia.

Miller WG. Reporting estimated GFR: a laboratory perspective. *Am J Kidney Dis*, 2008; Vol. 52: pp. 645–8.

   Comments: Setting up estimated GFR from a laboratory's perspective.

Levey AS, Bosch JP, Lewis JB, et al. A more accurate method to estimate glomerular filtration rate from serum creatinine: a new prediction equation. Modification of Diet in Renal Disease Study Group. *Ann Intern Med*, 1999; Vol. 130: pp. 461–70.

   Comments: Historical derivation of the MDRD equation following analysis of the Modification of Diet in Renal Disease Study.

Geyer SJ. Urinalysis and urinary sediment in patients with renal disease. *Clin Lab Med*, 1993; Vol. 13: pp. 13–20.

   Comments: Patterns on microscopic examination also help distinguish chronic injury based on findings of red cells, white cells, tubular cells, and various casts.

Webb JA. Ultrasonography in the diagnosis of renal obstruction. *BMJ*, 1990; Vol. 301 pp. 944–6.

   Comments: Ultrasonography is a valuable tool in diagnosing renal disease as it has no risk. (Author's comment: CT scan without intravenous contrast is more costly, exposes the patient to radiation, and in general is not necessary in the workup of medical renal disease.)

ALBUMINURIA

Donna I. Myers, MD

DESCRIPTION

- **Microalbuminuria** is defined as an albumin:creatinine ratio (ACR) between 30–300 mg/g.
- **Macroalbuminuria** is defined as an ACR >300 mg/g.
- Confirmation is required on 2 out of 3 samples over 3–6 months from initial detection in the absence of a urinary tract infection.

ASSAYS

- Immunochemistry method offers highly sensitive and specific measure of urinary albumin either from a 24-hour collection or a randomly voided ("spot") sample.
- Immunoassays for urine albumin utilize an antibody to human albumin. The antibody-albumin complexes are measured if albumin is present.
- Four methods to measure antibody to human albumin complexes: (1) turbidimetric analyzer (simple to perform but greater up-front expense); (2) radioimmunoassay (RIA); (3) ELISA assay (more labor intensive); and (4) radioimmunodiffusion.
- Immunoturbidimetric analysis (ITA) is available for commercial use. One example, "The Albumin Tina-Quant" (Roche) has, as its primary linearity, urine albumin levels from 3–400 mg/L with an extended linearity to 4400 mg/L. Values >4400 mg/L may be estimated by using dilutions up to 20-fold.
- Point-of-care testing utilizing table top immunoturbidimetric reactions such as the DCA2000 (Bayer analyzer) and the HemoCue Albumin 201 system has a rapid turnaround of results (7 minutes).
- Spectrophotometric assays measuring a colored end product are used for 24-hour urine total protein (vs albumin) collections.
- On routine urinalysis, protein is detected by a reagent stick with tetrabromophenol. Albumin combines with the blue divalent anionic form of the indicator changing color from yellow to green to blue. A colorimetric analyzer (reflectance spectroscopy) is used; it has a sensitivity of 10 mg/dl with a specificity of 97%. A correction pad compensates for the natural color of urine.

- A technician-dependent spot urine protein by dipstick is a useful tool in a clinic practice.
- Sulfosalicylic acid 3% turbidity test offers a semi-quantitative estimate of total urinary protein, measuring albumin, globulins and Bence Jones proteins. It is most useful in making a preliminary diagnosis of nephrotic range proteinuria, dramatically demonstrated by thick white clumps in the test tube.
- High-performance liquid chromatography (HPLC) accurately measures urine albumin but is time consuming and limited to research studies.

INDICATIONS

- Guidelines recommend annual screening for chronic kidney disease starting from the diagnosis of type 2 diabetes (T2DM) and starting 5 years after the diagnosis of type 1 diabetes (T1DM).
- Screening for kidney disease should consist of a serum creatinine with estimation of glomerular filtration rate (GFR) and a spot urinary albumin:creatinine ratio (ACR).
- A 24-hour urine collection for protein is seldom needed.
- In patients with diabetes and hypertension, both low levels (microalbuminuria) and high levels (macroalbuminuria in nephrotic range) of urinary protein are a risk predictor of heart failure, in addition to nephropathy.
- In patients with diabetes or a history of cardiovascular disease, microalbuminuria increases the risk of developing heart failure almost 2-fold.
- High macroalbuminuria ($\geq$3 g/g creatinine) in T2DM is associated with a 3-fold higher risk of heart failure versus those with lower levels of macroalbuminuria ($<$1.5 g/g).
- In the general population, microalbuminuria increases the chance of developing hypertension, diabetes, and cardiovascular disease. It should be part of a comprehensive cardiovascular risk profile for healthy individuals.
- Point-of-care testing provides immediate results during consultation, offers an added risk assessment for cardiovascular disease, and allows physicians to motivate patients to make appropriate lifestyle changes at the time of the clinic visit.

LIMITATIONS OR CONFOUNDERS

- High levels of conjugated bilirubin ($>$66 mg/dl), hemolysis ($>$300 mg/dl), and hyperlipidemia interfere with the Albumin Tina-Quant assay, with results flagged or not reported in presence of these interfering substances.
- Interference with the Tina-Quant assay also from very high levels of urinary acetone, ascorbic acid, calcium, creatinine, glucose, hemoglobin, and urea and uric acid.
- Patients with uric acid kidney stones may be hyperuricosuric ($>$800 mg/day in males), interfering with the assay with up to 10% inaccuracy on the Tina-Quant assay.
- Do point of care testing for microalbuminuria only when negative for leukocytes, nitrites, and blood.
- Measurements of urinary protein by assays sensitive only to albumin excludes measurement of other tubular proteins such as Bence Jones protein, missing the diagnosis of multiple myeloma.
- The colorimetric dipstick analysis for protein is semi-quantitative; has greater sensitivity to albumin than to Bence Jones proteins and globulins; requires a fresh specimen (refrigerated $<$4 hrs); and may give a false positive in the presence of alkaline urine (pH $>$8), hemoglobin, and contrast medium.

- Another limitation to the dipstick analysis is interobserver variability.
- Collection of a 24-hour urine is cumbersome and not generally used, requiring strict adherence to instructions, adequate hydration, and voiding that is both timely and complete. Useful in measuring urine creatinine as this is stable for a given patient unless body mass changes.

EXPERT OPINION

- The measurement of urinary albumin is critical to identification of early diabetic nephropathy. Microalbuminuria is relatively specific in type 1 diabetes, although not nearly as specific to diabetic nephropathy in type 2 diabetes.
- A spot urine albumin:creatinine ratio is recommended for detecting albuminuria.
- Both micro- and macroalbuminuria are associated with a higher risk of cardiovascular disease in normal and at-risk populations.
- The reason for the link between albuminuria and cardiovascular disease is unclear, but may be due to impaired systemic endothelial function.
- Albuminuria is an important therapeutic target for renal and cardiovascular protection.

BASIS FOR RECOMMENDATIONS

National Kidney Foundation-Kidney Disease Outcomes Quality Initiative (NFK-KDOQI). NFK-KDOQI Clinical Practice Guidelines and Clinical Practice Recommendations for Diabetes and Chronic Kidney Disease. *Am J Kidney Dis*, 2007; Vol. 49: pp. S12–154.

> **Comments:** Comprehensive practice guidelines for diabetes and chronic kidney disease by the National Kidney Foundation-Kidney Disease Outcomes Quality Initiative (NFK-KDOQI).

Arnlöv J, Evans JC, Meigs JB, et al. Low-grade albuminuria and incidence of cardiovascular disease events in nonhypertensive and nondiabetic individuals: the Framingham Heart Study. *Circulation*, 2005; Vol. 112: pp. 969–75.

> **Comments:** Urinary albumin:creatinine ratios below normal (<30 mg/g) predicted the development of de novo cardiovascular disease in a population healthy at baseline.

OTHER REFERENCES

Guy M, Borzomato JK, Newall RG, et al. Protein and albumin-to-creatinine ratios in random urines accurately predict 24 h protein and albumin loss in patients with kidney disease. *Ann Clin Biochem*, 2009; Vol. 46: pp. 468–76.

> **Comments:** Evidence that a random spot urinary albumin to creatinine ratio is adequate to detect proteinuria.

Dobre D, Nimade S, de Zeeuw D. Albuminuria in heart failure: what do we really know? *Curr Opin Cardiol*, 2009; Vol. 24: pp. 148–54.

> **Comments:** A comprehensive review article of the association of albuminuria with cardiovascular disease citing many important references.

Sarafidis PA, Riehle J, Bogojevic Z, et al. A comparative evaluation of various methods for microalbuminuria screening. *Am J Nephrol*, 2008; Vol. 28: pp. 324–9.

> **Comments:** HemoCue system was compared to a central laboratory system for measuring urine albumin and found to be comparable.

Lambers Heerspink HJ, Witte EC, Bakker SJ, et al. Screening and monitoring for albuminuria: the performance of the HemoCue point-of-care system. *Kidney Int*, 2008; Vol. 74: pp. 377–83.

> **Comments:** The HemoCue system using a first voided urine of the day accurately measures urinary albumin. It does not provide a urinary albumin:creatinine determination.

Contois JH, Hartigan C, Rao LV, et al. Analytical validation of an HPLC assay for urinary albumin. *Clin Chim Acta*, 2006; Vol. 367: pp. 150–5.

> **Comments:** The immunoturbidimetric assay (ITA) was compared to the high-performance liquid chromatography (HPLC) assay. HPLC has the advantage of measuring immunoreactive urinary albumin species and may provide earlier detection of microalbuminuria in diabetic subjects.

de Zeeuw D, Remuzzi G, Parving HH, et al. Albuminuria, a therapeutic target for cardiovascular protection in type 2 diabetic patients with nephropathy. *Circulation,* 2004; Vol. 110: pp. 921–7.

Comments: In the RENAAL Study (Reduction in End Points in NIDDM with Losartan) albuminuria was the strongest predictor of cardiovascular outcome.

Arnold JM, Yusuf S, Young J, et al. Prevention of Heart Failure in Patients in the Heart Outcomes Prevention Evaluation (HOPE) Study. *Circulation,* 2003; Vol. 107: pp. 1284–90.

Comments: In this trial to prevent heart failure in 9297 patients, microalbuminuria has a risk ratio of 1.82.

Collins AC, Vincent J, Newall RG, et al. An aid to the early detection and management of diabetic nephropathy: assessment of a new point of care microalbuminuria system in the diabetic clinic. *Diabet Med,* 2001; Vol. 18: pp. 928–32.

Comments: This study describes a point of care microalbuminuria detection system (DCA2000) in a clinic setting with rapid and reliable results.

HYPOALDOSTERONISM

See Hypoaldosteronism on p. 557.

Index